Instructor's Resource Manual
for

Medical–Surgical Nursing Care

Second Edition

Karen M. Burke
Priscilla LeMone
Elaine L. Mohn-Brown

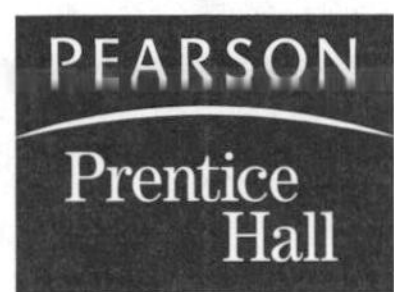

Upper Saddle River, New Jersey 07458

Notice: Care has been taken to confirm the accuracy of the information presented in this book. The authors, editors, and the publisher, however, cannot accept any responsibility for errors or omissions or for consequences from application of the information in this book and make no warranty, express or implied, with respect to its contents.

The authors and the publisher have exerted every effort to ensure that drug selections and dosages set forth in this text are in accord with current recommendations and practice at time of publication. However, in view of ongoing research, changes to government regulation, and the constant flow of information relating to drug therapy and drug reactions, the reader is urged to check precautions. This is particularly important when the recommended agent is a new and/or infrequently employed drug.

The authors and publisher disclaim all responsibility for any liability, loss, injury, or damage incurred as a consequence, directly or indirectly, of the use and application of any of the contents of this volume.

All photography/illustrations not credited on page, under or adjacent to the piece, were photographed/rendered on assignment and are the property of Pearson Education/Prentice Hall Health.

Cover and unit opening photographs copyright Nick Zungoli, The Exposures Gallery.

This work is protected by United States copyright laws and is provided solely for the use of instructors in teaching their courses and assessing student learning. Dissemination or sale of any part of this work (including on the World Wide Web) will destroy the integrity of the work and is not permitted. The work and materials from it should never be made available to students except by instructors using the accompanying text in their classes. All recipients of this work are expected to abide by these restrictions and to honor the intended pedagogical purposes and the needs of other instructors who rely on these materials. Anywhere.

All Rights Reserved.

Copyright © 2007, 2003 by Pearson Education, Inc., Upper Saddle River, New Jersey 07458. Pearson Prentice Hall. All rights reserved. Printed in the United States of America. This publication is protected by Copyright and permission should be obtained from the publisher prior to any prohibited reproduction, storage in a retrieval system, or transmission in any form or by any means, electronic, mechanical, photocopying, recording, or likewise. For information regarding permission(s), write to: Rights and Permissions Department.

Pearson Prentice Hall™ is a trademark of Pearson Education, Inc.
Pearson® is a registered trademark of Pearson plc
Prentice Hall® is a registered trademark of Pearson Education, Inc.

Pearson Education Ltd.
Pearson Education Singapore, Pte. Ltd.
Pearson Education Canada, Ltd.
Pearson Education—Japan
Pearson Education Australia PTY, Limited
Pearson Education North Asia Ltd.
Pearson Educación de Mexico, S.A. de C.V.
Pearson Education Malaysia, Pte. Ltd.
Pearson Education, Upper Saddle River, New Jersey

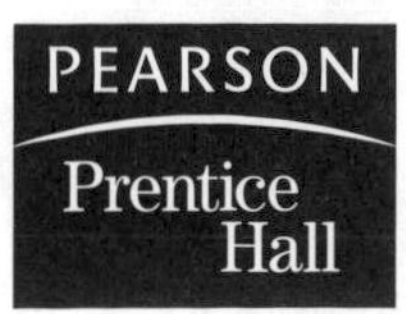

10 9 8 7 6 5 4 3 2 1
ISBN 0-13-237110-3

Contributors

Instructor's Resource Manual Chapters

Cheryl DeGraw, RN, MSN, CRNP
Faculty/Course Coordinator
Florence-Darlington Technical College
Florence, SC

JoAnne Carrick, RN, MSN
Instructor
Penn State University
Sharon, PA

Diane M. Bligh, RN, MS, CNS
Associate Professor, Nursing
Front Range Community College
Westminster, CO

Linda F. Roy, RN, MSN, CRNP
Assistant Professor of Nursing
Montgomery County Community College
Blue Bell, PA

NCLEX® Test Bank

Maragert M. Gingrich, RN, MSN
Professor
Harrisburg Area Community, College
Harrisburg, PA

Dawna Martich, RN, MSN
Manager, Training
American Healthways
Pittsburgh, PA

CONTENTS

PREFACE

The nature of nursing embodies the ever-changing rewards and challenges for today's practical and vocational nursing students. Streamlined yet thorough content provides easy access to need-to-know information and the essential skills needed to deliver safe and effective medical–surgical nursing care. This accompanying **Instructor's Resource Manual** is designed to support your teaching in this stepped-up environment, and to reduce your preparation time for class. It will help you focus your energy on teaching students what they need to know and do as practical nurses, and is intended to assist you provide an optimal learning experience for your students and their many learning needs.

Each chapter in the Instructor's Resource Manual is thoroughly integrated with the corresponding chapter in the textbook ***Medical Surgical Nursing Care, 2/E*** by Burke, Lemone, and Mohn-Brown. Chapters are organized by objectives, and the teaching unit flows from these objectives. You will find the following features to support the objectives:

- The Concepts for Lecture in this manual may be used in their entirety for class presentation or they may be merged with the classroom activities for a mixture of teaching styles that will meet the needs of students with various learning styles.
- The Lecture Outlines can be found on your Instructor's Resource CD-ROM in PowerPoint
- Suggestions for Classroom and Clinical Experiences attempt to go beyond the traditional activities that have been the mainstay of nursing education for many years.
- The Resource Library identifies for you—the instructor—all the specific media resources and activities available for that chapter on the Student CD-ROM, Companion Website and Instructor's Resource CD-ROM. Chapter by chapter, the Resource Library helps you decide what resources from the CD-ROM, Companion Website, and Instructor's Resource CD-ROM to use to enhance your course and your students' ability to apply concepts from the book into practice.

To organize your course further please see the sections at the beginning of this manual that provides you with an overall guide to the media resources and activities available from the Student CD-ROM, Companion Website, and Instructor's Resource CD-ROM. Also, included in this beginning section of this manual is a guide on "Teaching Medical Surgical Nursing Care to Students who Speak English as a Nonnative Language." This tool is intended to guide you in reaching across cultural barriers to train nurses.

Finally, the following additional resources are also available to accompany this textbook. For more information or sample copies, please contact your Prentice Hall Sales Representative:

- **Student Workbook ISBN 0-13-188461-1**—This workbook incorporates strategies for students to focus their study and increase comprehension of concepts of medical surgical nursing care. It contains a variety of activities, MediaLinks referring students to the Student CD-ROM and Companion Website, and more.
- **Student CD-ROM**—This CD-ROM is packaged with the textbook. It provides an interactive study program that allows students to practice answering NCLEX-PN style questions with rationales for right and wrong answers. It also contains an audio glossary, animations and video tutorials, and a link to the Companion Website (an Internet connection is required).
- **Companion Website www.prenhall.com/burke**—This on-line Study Guide is designed to help students apply the concepts presented in the book. Each chapter specific module features Objectives, NCLEX-PN Review Questions with rationales, Chapter Outlines for lecture notes, Case Studies, Critical Thinking WebLinks, Audio Glossary, and more. Faculty adopting this textbook have access to the online ***Syllabus Manager*** feature of the Companion Website, www.prenhall.com/burke. Syllabus Manager offers a whole host of features that facilitate the students' use of the Companion Website, and allows faculty to post syllabi and course information online for their students. For more information or a demonstration of Syllabus Manager, please contact a Prentice Hall Sales Representative.
- **Instructor's Resource CD-ROM ISBN 0-13-226999-6**—This cross-platform CD-ROM provides text slides and illustrations in PowerPoint for use in classroom lectures. It also contains an electronic test bank, answers to the textbook critical thinking exercises, and animations and video clips from the Student CD-ROM. This supplement is available to faculty free upon adoption of the textbook.

It is our hope that the information provided in this manual will decrease the time it takes you to prepare for class and will optimize the learning experience for your students.

Guidelines for Incorporating Prentice Hall's Nursing Media Resources into Your Course

Media resources for ***Medical Surgical Nursing Care, 2/E*** by Burke et al. are available for both the instructor and the student. These resources enhance your teaching, as well as help your students visualize and comprehend difficult concepts. Furthermore, the media resources and activities enable your students to apply concepts from the textbook to real nursing scenarios, hone critical thinking skills, and reinforce basic knowledge gained from textbook reading assignments.

The table below identifies where these media resources are available among the free supplements accompanying this textbook. Resources located on the textbook's Companion Website are available to both the instructor and student at *www.prenhall.com/burke*.

Resource	Companion Website	Instructor's Resource CD-ROM	Student CD-ROM
Objectives	√	Electronic Instructor's Manual	√
Audio Glossary	√		√
Chapter Outline	√		√
Practice NCLEX-PN Review Questions	√		√
Animations and/or Video Clips		√	√
Toolbox	√		
Case Studies	√		
Study Tips	√		
Challenge Your Knowledge	√		
Matching	√		
Faculty Office	√		
Web Links	√		
Syllabus Manager™	√ (See Guide for using this resource within this Instructor's Resource Manual.)		
Customizable and Printable Instructor's Resource Manual		√	
PowerPoint Images from the textbook		√	
PowerPoint text slides—Discussion Points		√	
NCLEX-style Test Items		√	
Additional Resources		√	

Suggestions for Incorporating These Media Resources and Activities into Your Course

1. Students who have difficulty identifying the main idea when reading the full chapter may use the chapter summary on the website to highlight major concepts.
2. Students who are visual learners can use the animations and/or video clips to reinforce their understanding of difficult concepts. Instructors may use the animations and/or video clips to enhance lecture presentations.
3. Students may use practice NCLEX-PN style review questions to prepare for course tests and to improve test-taking skills. Students may be expected to use these independently on the Companion website and submit their answers to receive an instant score. Instructors may assign these quizzes and exercises as homework, and ask students to route their answers to the instructor using the Email Results function on the Companion Website. Or, these practice questions may be used as a discussion for the end of the classroom lecture or discussion in small groups.
4. Students may be assigned case studies to analyze as a group and present results to the class in a post conference activity. They may respond to case study questions to prepare for clinical learning experiences as an independent study activity. Or, Instructors may assign these activities as homework and ask students to route their essay-style answers to the instructor using the Email Results Function on the Companion Website.
5. Students may use the MediaLinks as additional resources in support of written assignments or for enhancement of course requirements.
6. Instructors may use PowerPoint images and PowerPoint text slides, i.e., the Discussion Points, to enhance classroom presentations and discussions.

How to Use Prentice Hall's Syllabus Manager™ and Companion Website

Syllabus Manager™ provides an easy, step-by-step process to create and revise syllabi, with direct links to Companion Websites and other online content. It can be used by a non-technical person to build and maintain one or more syllabi on the web. Students may "turn on" an instructor's syllabus from within any Companion Website. Your complete syllabus is hosted on Prentice Hall servers, allowing convenient updates from any computer by only you and your students. Changes you make to your syllabus are immediately available to your students at their next login.

All features and content on the Companion Website were developed in accordance with the chapter and textbook objectives. Thus, all the exercises meet the goals of the objectives, making the Companion Website a pedagogically sound study and teaching tool. The features on the Companion Website for ***Medical Surgical Nursing Care 2/E,*** include the following modules for each chapter:

- Objectives
- Chapter Outline
- Audio Glossary
- NCLEX-PN Multiple Choice Questions
- Case Study
- Challenge Your Knowledge
- Matching
- Study Tip
- Web Links
- Faculty Office
- Toolbox

To access Syllabus Manager™, go to the home page for this textbook at **www.prenhall.com/burke**. On the top navigation bar, click on **Syllabus**. New users can click on **Instructor Help** for assistance on the syllabus creation process.

To create your own secure course syllabus online, click on **New Account**. After entering your Personal Information, School Information, and Log in Information, click **Continue**. From here, you begin the easy four-step process to creating your syllabus.

Step 1 Course Details

This step allows you to create the basic information for your syllabus: Course Name (including start date and end date), Course Description (including policies and objectives), Class Time and Location, Course Pre-requisites, and Grading Policy. Some of the fields have drop-down capability. You can even cut and paste your current syllabus into these fields or link the school's URL to your current syllabus. *Scroll to the bottom of the screen, and click on Next or on drop-down menu select STEP 2: Assignment Schedule.*

Step 2 Assignment Schedule

On this screen you are choosing dates for the assignments, and making notations about the assignments. It contains the course calendar in a pane on the left side of the page. Notice the days when your class meets are highlighted in blue. When you create assignments their due dates appear in orange on the calendar. To create an assignment, click on the day of the assignment in the calendar. Next, you will give the assignment a name. Under notes/instructions, you may choose to mention clinical days, guest speakers, activities, or simply describe a set of assignments due that day. Then, you can add a component to the assignment, either from the textbook's Companion Website or a custom assignment from your current syllabus online by adding a link.

To add an activity from the textbook's Companion Website, begin by clicking on **Add CW Resource**. A window opens and displays your Companion Website title and parts. Click through the Companion Website to locate the element you want to include as an assignment resource and the click **Select** to add the component. When the student views your syllabus, they will click on the date of the assignment, and immediately be linked to the exercises you selected on the textbook Companion Website. You may add any combination of components. When you finish creating the assignment click the **Save** button. You may copy this assignment or add additional assignments for other days before clicking on **Next to** continue creating your syllabus. *Click on Next or on drop-down menu select STEP 3: Password for Students.*

Step 3 Password for Students

You may want to protect this syllabus by entering a password. This password should be given out to only those that should have access to this syllabus. If you choose not to enter any password, your syllabus will be viewable by anyone. On this screen you can designate a secure password so only your students can access this syllabus. You can change the password as often as you like. *Click on Next or on drop-down menu select STEP 4: Finish.*

Step 4 Finish

Here you designate whether your syllabus is finished and able to be viewed by students, or still under construction and available only to you. *Click on **Log Off** to log out of Syllabus Manager™ and return to your Companion Website.*

Your students will now be able to access your course syllabus by searching your name, your email address, or your school name under Student Login. To view or update any of your existing syllabi, begin by logging in under Instructor Login. For additional demonstrations of Syllabus Manager™, or for help in creating your syllabus, please contact your Prentice Hall Sales Representative.

Teaching Medical Surgical Nursing Care to Students Who Speak English as a Nonnative Language

We are fortunate to have so many multi-national and multi-lingual nursing students in the United States in the 21st century. As our classrooms become more diverse, there are additional challenges to communication, but we in the nursing education community are ready. Our goal is to educate competent and caring nurses to serve the health needs of our diverse communities.

We know that ENNL students experience higher attrition rates than their native English-speaking counterparts. This is a complex problem. However, there are teaching strategies that have helped many students be successful.

The first step toward developing success strategies is understanding language proficiency. Language proficiency has four interdependent components. Each component is pertinent to nursing education. *Reading* is the first aspect of language. Any nursing student will tell you that there are volumes to read in nursing education. Even native speakers of English find the reading load heavy. People tend to read more slowly in their nonnative language. They also tend to recall less. Nonnative speakers often spend inordinate amounts of time on reading assignments. These students also tend to take longer to process exam questions.

Listening is the second component of language. Learning from lectures can be challenging. Some students are more proficient at reading English than at listening to it. It is not uncommon for ENNL students to understand medical terminology, but to become confused by social references, slang, or idiomatic expressions used in class. The spoken language of the teacher may be different in accent or even vocabulary from that experienced by immigrant students in their language education. ENNL students may not even hear certain sounds that are not present in their native languages. Amoxicillin and Ampicillin may sound the same. Asian languages do not have gender-specific personal pronouns (he, she, him, her, etc.). Asian students may become confused when the teacher is describing a case study involving people of different genders.

Speaking is the third component of language proficiency. People who speak with an accent are often self-conscious about it. They may hesitate to voice their questions or to engage in discussion. Vicious cycles of self-defeating behavior can occur in which a student hesitates to speak, resulting in decreased speaking skills, which results in more hesitation to speak. Students may develop sufficient anxiety about speaking that their academic outcomes are affected. Students tend to form study groups with others who have common first languages. Opportunities to practice English are therefore reduced, and communication errors are perpetuated. When the teacher divides students into small groups for projects, ENNL students often do not participate as much as others. If these students are anxious about speaking, they may withdraw from classroom participation. ENNL students may feel rejected by other students in a small group situation when their input is not sought or understood.

The fourth aspect of language is *writing*. Spelling and syntax errors are common when writing a nonnative language. Teachers often respond to student writing assignments with feedback that is too vague to provide a basis for correction or improvement by ENNL students. When it comes to writing lecture notes, these students are at risk of missing important details because they may not pick up the teacher's cues about what is important. They might miss information when they spend extra time translating a word or concept to understand it, or they might just take more time to write what is being said.

Another major issue faced by ENNL nursing students is the culture of the learning environment. International students were often educated in settings where students took a passive role in the classroom. They may have learned that faculty are to be respected, not questioned. Memorization of facts may have been emphasized. It may be a shock to them when the nursing faculty expect assertive students who ask questions and think critically. These expectations cannot be achieved unless students understand them.

Finally, the European-American culture, which forms the context for nursing practice, creates challenges. Because they are immersed in Euro-American culture and the culture of nursing, faculty may not see the potential sources of misunderstanding. For example, if a teacher writes a test question about what foods are allowed on a soft diet, a student who understands therapeutic diets may miss the question if s/he does not recognize the names of the food choices. Nursing issues with especially high culture connection are: food, behavior, law, ethics, parenting, games, or choosing the right thing to say. These topics are well represented in psychiatric nursing, which makes it a difficult subject for ENNL students.

Minimizing Culture Bias on Nursing Exams

Our goal is not really to eliminate culture from nursing or from nursing education. Nursing exists in a culture-dependent context. Our goal is to practice transcultural nursing and to teach nursing without undue culture bias.

Sometimes our nursing exam questions will relate to culture-based expectations for nursing action. The way to make these questions fair is to teach transcultural nursing and to clarify the cultural expectations of a nursing student in the Euro-American-dominated health care system.

Students must learn the cultural aspects of the profession before they can practice appropriately within it. Like other cultures, the professional culture of nursing has its own language (medical terminology and nursing diagnosis, of course). We have our own accepted way of dress, our own implements, skills, taboos, celebrations, and behavior. The values accepted by our culture are delineated in the ANA Code of Ethics, and are passed down to our young during nursing education.

It is usually clear to nursing educators that students are not initially aware of all the aspects of the professional culture, and that these must be taught. The social context of nursing seems more obvious to educators, and is often overlooked in nursing education. Some aspects of the social context of nursing were mentioned above (food, games, social activities, relationships, behavior, what to say in certain situations). Students must also learn these social behaviors and attitudes if they are to function fully in nursing. If they do not already know about American hospital foods, what to say when someone dies, how to communicate with an authority figure, or what game to play with a 5-year-old child, they must learn these things in nursing school.

Try for yourself the following test. It was written without teaching you the cultural expectations first.

CULTURE BIASED TEST

1. Following radiation therapy, an African American client has been told to avoid using her usual hair care product due to its petroleum content. Which product should the nurse recommend that she use instead?
   A. Royal Crown hair treatment
   B. Dax Wave and Curl
   C. Long Aid Curl Activator Gel
   D. Wave Pomade

2. A Jewish client is hospitalized for Pregnancy Induced Hypertension during Yom Kippur. How should the nurse help this client meet her religious needs based on the tradition of this holy day?
   A. Order meals without meat-milk combinations
   B. Ask a family member to bring a serving of *Marror* for the client
   C. Encourage her to fast from sunrise to sunset
   D. Remind her that she is exempt from fasting

3. Based on the Puerto Rican concept of *compadrazco*, who is considered part of the immediate family and responsible for care of children?
   A. Parents, grandparents, aunts, uncles, cousins, and godparents
   B. Mother and father, older siblings
   C. Mother, father, any blood relative
   D. Parents and chosen friends (*compadres*) who are given the honor of childcare responsibility

4. A 60-year-old Vietnamese immigrant client on a general diet is awake at 11 P.M. on a summer night. What is the best choice of food for the nurse to offer to this client?
   A. warm milk
   B. hot tea
   C. ice cream
   D. iced tea

5. Which of the following positions is contraindicated for a client recovering from a total hip replacement?
   A. Side-lying using an abductor pillow
   B. Standing
   C. Walking to the restroom using a walker
   D. Sitting in a low recliner

When you took this test, did it seem unfair? It was intended to test nursing behaviors that were based on culture-specific situations. Your immigrant and ENNL students are likely to face questions like these on every exam.

Item #1 is about hair care products for black hair. Option C is the only one that does not contain petroleum products. Students could know this, if they were given the information before the exam. Otherwise the item is culture-biased.

Item #2 is about the Jewish holiday Yom Kippur. To celebrate this holiday, it is customary to fast from sunrise to sunset, but people who are sick, such as the client in the question, are exempted from fasting. This is only unfair if students did not have access to the information.

Item #3 expects you to know about *compadrazco*, in which parents, grandparents, aunts, uncles, cousins, and godparents are all considered immediate family. This can be an important point if you are responsible for visiting policies in a pediatrics unit.

Item #4 tests knowledge about the preferred drink for an immigrant Vietnamese client. Many people in Asia feel comforted by hot drinks and find cold drinks to be unsettling.

Item #5 does not seem so biased. If you understand total hip precautions, it is a pretty simple question, unless you have never heard of a "low recliner". An ENNL student who missed this question, said, "I saw the chairs in clinical called 'geri chairs' and I know that the client cannot bend more than 90 degrees, but 'low recliner' was confusing to me. I imagined someone lying down (reclining) and I think this would not dislocate the prosthesis."

The best way to avoid culture bias on exams is to know what you are testing. It is acceptable to test about hip precautions, but not really fair to test about the names of furniture. The same is true of foods. Test about therapeutic diets, but not about the recipes (an African immigrant student advised us to say "egg-based food" instead of custard).

Behavior in social and professional situations is especially culture-bound. Behavior-based questions are common on nursing exams. Make behavior expectations explicit. Especially when a student is expected to act in a way that would be inappropriate in his or her social culture, these are very difficult questions. For example, we expect nurses to act assertively with physicians and clients. It is inappropriate for many Asian students to question their elders. When a client is their elder, these students will choose the option that preserves respect for the client over one that provides teaching. We must make our expectations very clear.

Finally, talk with your ENNL and immigrant students after your exams. They can provide a wealth of information about what confused them or what was ambiguous. Discuss your findings with your colleagues and improve your exams. Ultimately your exams will be clearer and more valid.

Success Strategies

The following strategies were developed originally to help ENNL students. An interesting revelation is that they also help native English speakers who have learning styles that are not conducive to learning by lecture, or who read slowly, or have learning disabilities or other academic challenges.

Strategies for Promoting ENNL Student Success

1. You cannot decrease the reading assignment because some students read slowly, but you can help students prioritize the most important areas.
2. Allow adequate time for testing. The NCLEX is not a 1-minute-per-question test anymore. Usually 1.5 hours is adequate for a 50 item multiple-choice exam.
3. Allow students to tape lectures if they want to. You might have lectures audio-taped and put in the library for student access.
4. Speak clearly. Mumbling and rapid anxious speech are difficult to understand. If you have a problem with clarity, provide handouts containing the critical points. Provide the handouts anyway. You want to teach and test nursing knowledge, not note-taking skills.
5. Avoid slang and idiomatic expressions. This is harder than heck to do, but you can do it with practice. When you do use slang, explain it. This is especially important on exams. When in doubt about whether a word is confusing, think about what the dictionary definition would be, if there are two meanings, use another word.
6. Allow the use of translation dictionaries on exams. You can say that students must tell you what they are looking up, so they cannot find medical terminology that is part of the test.
7. Be aware of cultural issues when you are writing exams. Of course you will test on culture-specific issues, but be sure you are testing what you want to test (the student's knowledge of diets, not of recipes).
8. Feel free to use medical terminology, after all this is nursing school. However, when you use an important new term, write it on the board so students can spell it correctly in their notes.
9. In clinical, make the implied explicit. It seems obvious that safety is the priority, but if a student thinks the priority is respecting her elders, when a client with a new hip replacement demands to get out of bed there could be a disaster.
10. Hire a student who takes clear and accurate lecture notes to post his/her notes for use by ENNL and other students. The students will still attend class and take their own notes, but will have this resource to fill in the details that they miss.
11. SOA (spell out abbreviations).
12. Many international students learned to speak English in the British style. If something would be confusing to a British person, they will find it confusing.
13. Provide opportunities for students to discuss what they are learning with other students and faculty. A faculty member might hold a weekly discussion group where students bring questions. It can be interesting to find a student having no trouble tracing the path of a red cell from the heart to the portal vein, but having difficulty understanding what cream of wheat is ("I thought it was a stalk of grain in a bowl with cream poured on it").
14. Make it clear that questions are encouraged. When a student is not asking, and you think they may not understand, ask the student after class if s/he has questions. Make it easier for students to approach you by being approachable. Learn their names, and learn to pronounce them correctly. Hearing you try to pronounce their name might be humorous for them, and it will validate how difficult it is to speak other languages.
15. Take another look at basing grades on class participation. You may be putting inordinate demands on the ENNL students. Of course nurses must learn to work with others, but the nurse who talks most is not necessarily the best.
16. Be a role model for communication skills. You might even say in class when you talk about communication that if you respect a person who is trying to communicate with you, you will persist until you understand the message. Say, "Please repeat that," or "I think you said to put a chicken on my head, is that correct?" or "You want me to do what with the textbook?" It may be considered socially rude to ask people to repeat themselves repeatedly. Make it clear that this is not a social situation. In the professional role, we are responsible for effective communication. We cannot get away with smiling and nodding our heads.
17. In clinical, if a student has an accent that is difficult for the staff to understand, discuss clarification techniques (#16 above) to the student and staff member. Make it explicit that it is acceptable for the student to ask questions and for the staff to ask for clarification.
18. If your college has a writing center where students can receive feedback on grammar and style before submitting papers, have students use it. If you are not so fortunate, view papers as a rough draft instead of a final product. Give specific feedback about what to correct and allow students to resubmit.
19. Make any services available to ENNL students available to all students (such as group discussions and notes). These services may meet the learning needs of many students while preventing the attitude that "they are different and they get something I don't."
20. Faculty attitudes are the most important determinant of a successful program to promote the success of ENNL nursing students. Talk with other faculty about the controversial issues. Create an organized program with a consistent approach among the faculty. The rewards will be well worth the work.

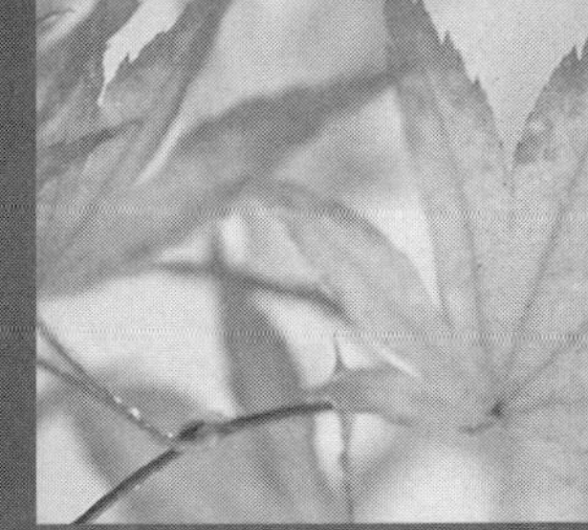

CHAPTER 1
THE MEDICAL–SURGICAL NURSE

RESOURCE LIBRARY

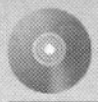 **CD-ROM**

Video: LPN and LVN
Video: Assessment vs. Diagnosis

IMAGE LIBRARY

Figure 1-1 In the role of caregiver, the nurse provides comprehensive, individualized care to the adult client.
Figure 1-2 The nurse's role as teacher is an essential component of care. As part of the discharge planning process, this nurse is providing teaching for self-care at home.
Figure 1-3 Steps of the nursing process. Notice that the steps are interrelated and interdependent. For example, evaluation of the client might reveal the need for further assessment, additional nursing diagnoses, and/or a revision of the plan of care.

LEARNING OUTCOME 1

Describe the licensed practical/vocational nurse's role as caregiver, manager of care, advocate, and teacher.

CONCEPTS FOR LECTURE

1. Medical–surgical nurses promote health and provide care during illness or injury to adult clients.
2. The roles of the medical–surgical nurse include caregiver, manager of care, client advocate, and teacher.
3. The nurse provides interventions to meet the physical, psychosocial, spiritual, environmental, and cultural needs of clients and families.

POWERPOINT LECTURE SLIDES

1 Nurses assume roles to promote and maintain health, to prevent illness, and to help clients cope with disability or death in any setting

2 Roles of the Medical–Surgical Nurse
- Caregiver
  - Assess, plan, implement client care.
- Manager of care
  - Direct, delegate, coordinate, evaluate quality of care
- Client advocate
  - Speaks for, mediates, and protects rights of the client
- Teacher
  - Assess learning needs and teach to meet those needs

3 Box 1-1 Culturally Sensitive Nursing

SUGGESTIONS FOR CLASSROOM ACTIVITIES

1. Initiate a discussion on the role of the medical–surgical nurse using the following scenarios:
   Scenario A: As a caregiver, how would the nurse help a 72-year-old male admitted with left-sided paralysis due to a cerebral vascular accident?
   Scenario B: As a client advocate, how would the nurse participate in the care of a 34-year-old mother admitted with severe blood loss, who is refusing blood transfusion due to religious reasons?

SUGGESTIONS FOR CLINICAL ACTIVITIES

Have students identify the roles of the medical–surgical nurse in the clinical setting and discuss the roles in postconference.

Suggestions for Classroom Activities *continued*

2. As a teacher, how can the nurse help promote health and prevent the onset of complications for a 43-year-old woman newly diagnosed with type 2 diabetes?
3. As a leader, what directions can the nurse give to a certified nursing assistant who is having problems with timely completion of personal care tasks?

Learning Outcome 2

Discuss the steps of the nursing process: assessment, diagnosis, planning, implementation, and evaluation.

Concepts for Lecture

1. The nursing process is a model of care that differentiates nursing practices from the practices of other health care providers.
2. The five interdependent and cyclic steps of the nursing process are assessment, diagnosis, planning, implementation, and evaluation.
3. Licensed practical/vocational nurses use all steps of the nursing process except making a nursing diagnosis.
4. The nursing process serves as a base for improving clinical practice and evaluating quality of care.

PowerPoint Lecture Slides

1 Nursing Process
- Model of care
- Series of activities nurses perform as they provide care to clients
- Legitimized by the American Nurses Association Standards of Practice and by state nurse practice acts

2, 3 Steps of the Nursing Process
- Assessment
- Diagnosis (by registered nurses only)
- Planning
- Implementation
- Evaluation

4 Benefits of Nursing Process
- Provides common reference system and terminology
- Provides framework for evaluating quality of care
- Provides structure for planned, individualized interventions
- Involves the client and increases client satisfaction
- Ensures continuity of care through a written care plan
- Leads to better resource utilization and improved documentation

Suggestions for Classroom Activities

Discuss the benefits of the nursing process to the practice of nursing, the clients, and health care facilities.

Suggestions for Clinical Activities

Have students record their clinical activities in a diary for 1 to 3 days. Then categorize each activity according to the steps in the nursing process. In postconference have the students discuss the method and rationale used to categorize each activity. Have students discuss their thoughts and feelings about their competency in using the nursing process.

Learning Outcome 3

Define critical thinking and explain how it contributes to nursing care.

Concept for Lecture

1. Critical thinking is self-directed thinking that is focused on what to believe or do in a specific situation. It

PowerPoint Lecture Slides

1 Critical Thinking
- Self-directed thinking

© 2007 Pearson Education, Inc.

CONCEPTS FOR LECTURE *continued*

involves both attitudes and skills. Critical thinking and the nursing process are essential in nursing practice.

POWERPOINT LECTURE SLIDES *continued*

- Uses knowledge to consider a client care situation
- Uses judgments and decisions about what to do in that situation

SUGGESTIONS FOR CLASSROOM ACTIVITIES

Discuss the role of the licensed practical nurse in each step of the nursing process, and the attributes of a critical thinker.

SUGGESTIONS FOR CLINICAL ACTIVITIES

Have students review the use of the nursing process in the area of clinical rotation, and document the findings.

LEARNING OUTCOME 4

Explain how critical thinking and the nursing process are used to determine priorities of nursing care activities to promote, maintain, or restore health.

CONCEPTS FOR LECTURE

1. Critical thinking involves the cognitive (knowledge) skills, attitude, and mental habits of the nurse.
2. Critical thinking skills are the mental abilities that are used.

POWERPOINT LECTURE SLIDES

1 Attitudes and Mental Habits of Critical Thinking
- Being able to think independently
- Having intellectual courage
- Having intellectual empathy
- Having an intellectual sense of justice and being intellectually humble
- Being disciplined
- Being creative and confident in self

2 Major Critical Thinking Skills
- Ability to use divergent thinking
- Ability to use reasoning
- Use of clarifying
- Use of reflection

SUGGESTIONS FOR CLASSROOM ACTIVITIES

Discuss the importance of critical thinking in establishing nursing diagnoses as defined by the North American Nursing Diagnosis Association.

LEARNING OUTCOME 5

Describe the importance of codes for nursing and nursing standards in medical-surgical nursing care.

CONCEPTS FOR LECTURE

1. Nursing codes of ethics (principles of conduct) and standards guide nursing practice and protect the public.
2. The American Nurses Association (ANA) Code for Nurses states principles of ethical concern. It guides the behavior of nurses and defines nursing for the general public.
3. The National Association for Practical Nurse Education and Service developed the code of ethics for licensed practical/vocational nurses.

POWERPOINT LECTURE SLIDES

1 Ethics
- Principles of conduct
- Moral duty, values, obligations, distinction between right and wrong

1a Nursing Code of Ethics
- Framework of reference for "professionally valued and ideal nursing behaviors"

2 ANA Code for Nurses
- Nurse's primary commitment is to the patient
- Nurse promotes, advocates for, and strives to protect the health, safety, and rights of the patient
- Nurse owes the same duties to self as to others

3 Box 1-2 The Licensed Practical/Vocational Nurse Code of Ethics

Suggestions for Classroom Activities

If the school has an honor code, ask five students to review the code of honor and lead a discussion on the pros and cons of having an honor code.

Learning Outcome 6

Discuss examples of legal and ethical dilemmas in client care.

Concepts for Lecture

1. The National Association for Practical Nurse Education and Service (NAPNES) set a foundation for providing safe and competent nursing practice, guided by a commitment to ethical/legal principles.
2. The American Nurses Association sets standards of clinical nursing practice for care and professional practice, including quality of care, education, ethics, collaboration, use of resources.
3. Nurses often face dilemmas—a choice between two unpleasant alternatives—in clinical practice. Some dilemmas arise in the areas of client rights, issues of death and dying, and caring for clients with AIDS.

PowerPoint Lecture Slides

1 Box 1-3 NAPNES Standards for Nursing Practice of LPN/LVNs

2 Standards for Care of Clinical Nursing Practice
- Set by ANA
- Criterion used by a profession and the general public to measure quality of practice
- Nurse who provides care has responsibility or obligation to account for own behaviors within the role

3 Legal and Ethical Dilemmas in Nursing
- Client rights
  - Advance directive, living will, power of attorney
- Issues of dying and death
- Caring for the client with AIDS
  - Moral obligation to provide care unless risk exceeds responsibility

Suggestions for Classroom Activities

Divide the class into groups of five to six students. Using the nursing codes of ethics and the standards for nursing practice, assign each group to discuss the following situations: (1) A young man was involved in a motor vehicle accident and is now in a brain-damaged state, and the health care facility is asking the family to donate his organs. (2) How can the nurse working in a clinic for chemical and substance abuse assist the client in maintaining dignity and uniqueness? (3) How does the nurse who has had a personal experience involving a drunken driver objectively care for an alcoholic who has been involved in a motor vehicle accident where the victim died? (4) When caring for a client with AIDS, what code of ethical behavior is mandated by the American Nurses Association?

Suggestions for Clinical Activities

Discuss legal and ethical dilemmas based on nursing care assignments in the clinical setting.

© 2007 Pearson Education, Inc.

CHAPTER 2
THE ADULT CLIENT IN HEALTH AND ILLNESS

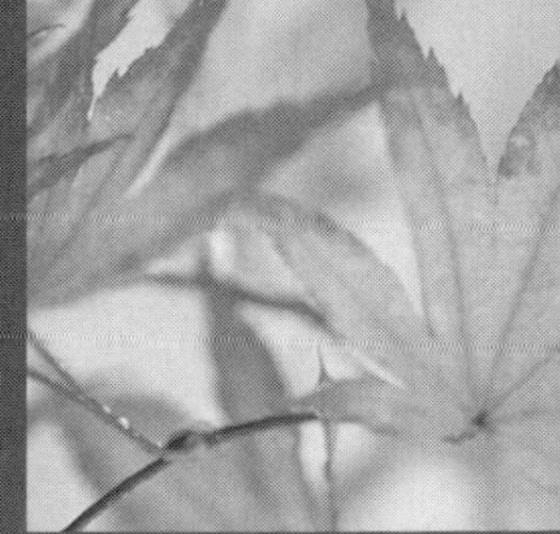

RESOURCE LIBRARY

CD-ROM

Video: Defining Family
Video: Health Promotion & Health Maintenance

IMAGE LIBRARY

Figure 2-1 The health-illness continuum.

LEARNING OUTCOME 1

Compare and contrast the physical status, risks for alterations in health, and health behaviors of the young adult and the middle adult.

CONCEPTS FOR LECTURE

1. Growth and development are continuous processes throughout life. The adult years are commonly divided into three stages: the young adult, ages 18 to 40; the middle adult, ages 40 to 65; and the older adult, over 65.
2. With aging, specific changes occur in intellectual, psychosocial, and spiritual development and in physical structures and functions.
3. Havighurst identified developmental tasks of the young and middle adult.

POWERPOINT LECTURE SLIDES

1 Growth and Development of the Adult
- Three stages
  - Young adult—ages 18 to 40
  - Middle adult—ages 40 to 65
  - Older adult—ages over 65

2 Changes with Aging
- Intellectual
- Psychosocial
- Spiritual development
- Physical changes and functions

2a Box 2-1 Healthy Behaviors in the Young Adult

2b Table 2-1 Physical Status and Changes in the Young Adult Years

2c Box 2-2 Healthy Behaviors in the Middle Adult

2d Table 2-2 Physical Changes in the Middle Adult Years

3 Developmental Tasks of Young Adults
- Select and learn to live with mate
- Have and raise children
- Have a job
- Manage a home
- Take on civic responsibility

3a Developmental Tasks of Middle Adults
- Establish and maintain economic standard of living
- Help adolescent children become responsible adults
- Develop leisure activities
- Accept and adjust to physical changes
- Adjust to aging parents

Suggestions for Classroom Activities

1. Initiate a discussion on the developmental stages of the adult client.
2. Partner students in groups of two. Have the students assess each other at their developmental stage, including the risks for alterations in health and health behaviors. Then, using the nursing process, set up a teaching plan to correct a health deficit or decrease the risk for a health alteration.
3. Divide the class into three large groups. The groups should discuss the developmental stage for the young adult and middle adult. Each group should describe the nursing role in promoting health and decreasing the risks for health alterations in each stage.

Suggestions for Clinical Activities

Assign students to care for clients in the adult developmental stages. Have each student compare the health–illness continuum, risks for health alterations, and health behaviors for that age group with the actual developmental stage of the client. In postconference, have the students share their findings and identify any of the psychosocial, economical, and physical factors that have been incorporated into the nursing care plan.

Learning Outcome 2

Describe the functions and developmental stages and tasks of the family.

Concepts for Lecture

1. The nurse includes the family as an integral component of care in all health care settings.
2. The nurse must consider both the needs of the client at a specific developmental stage and the needs of the client within a family with specific developmental tasks.

PowerPoint Lecture Slides

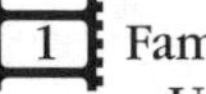

Family
- Unit of people related by marriage, birth, or adoption
- Two or more people who are emotionally involved with each other and live close to each other
- Family structure
  - Roles and relationships
- Family function
  - Interactions that provide support, guidance, and stability

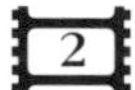

Developmental Stages and Tasks of the Couple
- Adjust to living together
- Establish a mutually satisfying relationship
- Relate to kin
- Decide whether to have children or not

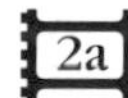

Developmental Stage and Tasks of the Family with Infants and Preschoolers
- Support the needs and economic costs of more than two members
- Develop an attachment between parents and children
- Cope with lack of energy and privacy
- Carry out activities that promote growth and development of the children

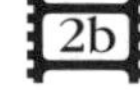

Developmental Stage and Tasks of the Family with School-Age Children
- Adjust to expanded world of children in school
- Encourage educational achievement
- Promote joint decision making between children and parents

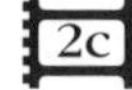

Developmental Stage and Tasks of the Family with Adolescents and Young Adults
- Provide supportive home base
- Maintain open communications

© 2007 Pearson Education, Inc.

PowerPoint Lecture Slides *continued*

- Balance freedom with responsibility
- Encourage adult children to become independent

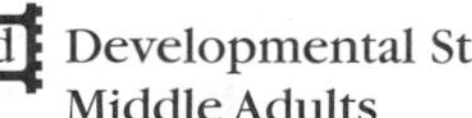

2d Developmental Stage and Tasks of Family with Middle Adults
- Maintain ties with older and younger generations
- Plan for retirement
- Reestablish the couple's relationship
- Acquire role of grandparents

2e Developmental Stage and Tasks of Family with Older Adults
- Adjust to retirement and aging
- Cope with loss if spouse dies
- Adjust to living alone or close to family home

Suggestions for Classroom Activities

Have each student do a paper defining his or her type of family, the family development stage, and how its functions and tasks differ from the family stages present in the chapter. How do the family and its members deal with concerns about its health and illness?

Suggestions for Clinical Activities

Assign student to provide nursing care to adults of different developmental stages. Discuss the differences in their tasks and changes of aging.

Learning Outcome 3

Define health, the health–illness continuum, and the concept of high-level wellness.

Concepts for Lecture

1. Health is "a state of complete physical, mental, and social well-being, and not merely the absence of disease or infirmity."
2. The health–illness continuum is a dynamic process with high-level wellness at one extreme of the continuum and death at the opposite extreme.
3. High-level wellness is a way of functioning to reach one's maximum potential at a particular point in time.

PowerPoint Lecture Slides

1 Health
- "State of complete physical, mental, social well-being, and not merely the absence of disease or infirmity."

2 Health–Illness Continuum
- Dynamic process with high-level wellness at one extreme of the continuum and death at the opposite end

3 High-Level Wellness
- Way of functioning to reach one's maximum potential at a particular point in time
- Wellness is influenced by:
    - Self-concept
    - Environment
    - Culture
    - Spiritual values

Suggestions for Classroom Activities

Discuss the wellness-illness continuum. How does its definition differ from the definition of health by the World Health Organization? In what ways does it differ from Dunn's description of wellness?

Suggestions for Clinical Activities

Interview clients to determine their concept of health and wellness.

© 2007 Pearson Education, Inc.

LEARNING OUTCOME 4

Explain factors affecting health status, health promotion, and health maintenance.

CONCEPTS FOR LECTURE

1. Many different factors affect a person's health or level of wellness.
2. Teaching health promotion and maintenance provides learning for clients to maintain wellness, identify risk factors, and be informed of how to decrease risk factors.

POWERPOINT LECTURE SLIDES

1 Major Factors Affecting Health Status
- Genetic makeup
- Cognitive abilities and educational level
- Race, ethnicity, and cultural background
- Age, gender, and developmental level
- Lifestyle and environment
- Socioeconomic background
- Geographic area

2 Practices to Promote Health and Wellness
- Eating three balanced meals/day
- Eating moderately to maintain a healthy weight
- Exercising 30 to 60 minutes/day
- Sleeping 7 to 8 hours/day
- Limiting alcohol consumption
- Eliminating smoking
- Keeping sun exposure to minimum

SUGGESTIONS FOR CLASSROOM ACTIVITIES

Initiate the discussion on factors affecting health status, promotion, and maintenance by having the students compare their present health status and the ways in which they promote personal and family health.

SUGGESTIONS FOR CLINICAL ACTIVITIES

Have students help with teaching health promotion and maintenance at a health fair.

LEARNING OUTCOME 5

Compare and contrast disease and illness.

CONCEPTS FOR LECTURE

1. *Disease* is a medical term describing disruptions in structure and function of the body or mind. Diseases have mechanical causes, biologic causes, or normative causes.
2. Illness is a response a person has to a disease. Illness integrates pathophysiologic alterations; psychologic effects of those alterations; effects on roles, relationships, and values; and cultural and spiritual beliefs.

POWERPOINT LECTURE SLIDES

1 Disease
- Medical term describing disruptions in structure and function of the body or mind
- Diseases have:
  - Mechanical causes—trauma
  - Biologic causes—body function
  - Normative causes—mind-body interaction
- Manifestations are signs and symptoms exhibited by disruption

2 Illness
- Response a person has to a disease
- Illness integrates:
  - Pathophysiologic alterations
  - Psychologic effects of alterations
  - Effects on roles, relationships, and values
  - Cultural and spiritual beliefs

© 2007 Pearson Education, Inc.

Suggestions for Classroom Activities

Divide the class into small groups of four. Have the students develop the following scenarios and role-play the nurse–client interaction.
Scenario A: A 22-year-old male seen in the hematology clinic with sickle cell disease
Scenario B: A 45-year-old recently divorced female who had a hysterectomy
Scenario C: A 55-year-old postmenopausal female with a high cholesterol level
Scenario D: A 75-year-old with chronic obstructive lung disorder

Learning Outcome 6

Describe the sequence of acute illness behaviors.

Concepts for Lecture

1. Acute illness occurs rapidly, lasts a relatively short period of time, and is self-limiting usually with a full recovery and return to normal preillness functioning.
2. Suchman describes five stages of acute illness behaviors.

PowerPoint Lecture Slides

1 Acute Illness
- Occurs rapidly
- Lasts a relatively short period of time
- Is self-limiting
- Usually with full recovery

2 Suchman's Stages of Acute Illness
- First stage—experiences manifestations of illness
- Second stage—assumes sick role
- Third stage—seeks medical care
- Fourth stage—assumes dependent role
- Final stage—recovery and rehabilitation

Suggestions for Classroom Activities

Define and discuss acute illness and chronic illness. Describe the steps of the sick role in acute illness.

Suggestions for Clinical Activities

Assign students to observe clients in a physician's office. Have them identify the stages of an acute illness that the clients exhibit.

Learning Outcome 7

Discuss chronic illness, including characteristics, needs of clients who are chronically ill, and the effects of chronic illness on the family.

Concepts for Lecture

1. The National Commission on Chronic Illness defines a chronic illness as any impairment or deviation from normal functioning that has one or more characteristic. Chronic illness is characterized by impaired function of more than one body system.
2. The intensity of a chronic illness and its related symptoms ranges from mild to severe, and the illness is usually characterized by periods of remission and exacerbation.
3. Responses to chronic illness are interrelated and result in individualized illness behaviors and needs.
4. Nursing interventions for the person with a chronic illness focus on education to promote independent functioning, reduce health care costs, and improve well-being and quality of life.
5. Chronic illness in a family member is a major stressor that may cause changes in family structure and function, as well as changes in performing family developmental tasks.

PowerPoint Lecture Slides

1 Chronic Illness
- Any impairment or deviation from normal functioning that has one or more characteristic of chronic illness
- Impaired function in more than one body system.
  - Sensory perception
  - Self-care abilities
  - Mobility
  - Cognition
  - Social skills

1a Characteristics of Chronic Illness
- Permanent
- Leaves permanent disability
- Caused by nonreversible pathologic alterations
- Requires special teaching of the client for rehabilitation
- Requires long period of care

© 2007 Pearson Education, Inc.

PowerPoint Lecture Slides *continued*

2 Attributes of Chronic Illness
- Impaired function in more than one body system
- Mild to severe symptoms
- Periods of remission and exacerbation

3 Needs of a Person with Chronic Illness
- Live as normally as possible
- Learn to adapt activities of daily living and self-care activities
- Grieve over loss of physical abilities, income, status, roles, and dignity
- Learn to live with chronic pain
- Follow a medical treatment plan
- Maintain a positive self-concept and sense of hope
- Maintain a feeling of being in control
- Confront the inevitability of death at an earlier age

4 Nursing Interventions with Chronic Illness
- Educate to promote independent functioning
- Reduce health care costs
- Improve well-being and quality of life

5 Effects of Chronic Illness on Family
- Changes in family structure and function
- Changes in performing family developmental tasks
- Family response affects client's response to and perception of illness
- Changes in personal, social, and economic resources
- Response to nature and course of the disease
- Demands of illness as perceived by family members

Suggestions for Clinical Activities

Assign students to care for clients in a rehabilitation facility. They should compare the care of a client with a chronic illness to a client with an acute illness in an acute health care facility.

 © 2007 Pearson Education, Inc.

Chapter 3
The Older Adult Client in Health and Illness

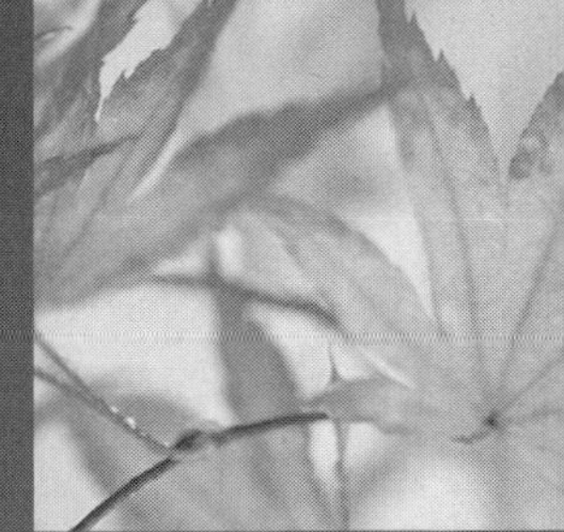

Resource Library

IMAGE LIBRARY

Figure 3-1 Number of people age 65 and over, by age group, for selected years 1900–2000 and projected 2010–2050. (Source: Federal Interagency Forum on Aging-Related Statistics. [2004]. Older Americans 2004: Key Indicators of Well-Being.)
Figure 3-2 The older population is increasing more rapidly than any other age group, making gerontologic nursing a major part of medical-surgical nursing.
Figure 3-3 Many older adults find creative outlets during retirement.
Figure 3-4 A regular program of exercise is important for maintenance of joint mobility and muscle tone and can promote socialization.

Learning Outcome 1

Describe what is meant by the term *old,* including who is considered an older adult.

Concepts for Lecture

1. Aging may be defined in many ways, including age in years as well as by personal definition. Older adulthood may be divided into three periods: *young-old* (ages 65 to 74), *middle-old* (ages 75 to 84), and *old-old* (ages 85 and older).
2. The rapid increase in older adults in the United States is the result of the baby boom and an increased growth of minority populations.

PowerPoint Lecture Slides

1 Three Divisions of Older Adulthood
- Young-old—ages 65 to74
- Middle-old—ages 75 to 84
- Old-old—ages 85 and older

1a Table 3-1 Age and Socioeconomic Characteristics of Older Adults

2 Reasons for Increase in Older Population
- Due to "baby boom" in post-World War II period
- Growth in migration from other countries

Learning Outcome 2

Discuss selected theories of aging, including those involving genetics, immunity, free radicals, and apoptosis.

Concepts for Lecture

1. The theories of why people age include genetics, immune factors, free radicals, and cell death (apoptosis). Scientists also study the factors that influence having a long and healthy life, which include genetic inheritance, physical environment, physical activity, and diet.

PowerPoint Lecture Slides

1 Biologic Aging Theories
- Genetic theories
- Immunity theories
- Free-radical theory
- Apoptosis theory

2 Longevity and Senescence Theories
- Genetic factors
- Physical environment
- Physical activity throughout life
- Consumption of alcohol
- Sexual activity
- Dietary factors
- Social environment

Suggestions for Classroom Activities

Discuss healthy behaviors that lead to people living longer.

Suggestions for Clinical Activities

Interview clients in a nursing home and compare their beliefs about living longer.

Learning Outcome 3

Define ageism, incorporating common myths of older adults.

Concepts for Lecture

1. Ageism is a form of prejudice in which older adults are stereotyped by characteristics found in only a small number of their age group. Most older adults are satisfied with their lives, have adequate income, live in their own homes, are close to family and friends, and take part in community activities.
2. Myths and stereotypes may lead health care workers to have negative perceptions of older adults.

PowerPoint Lecture Slides

1 Ageism
- Form of prejudice in which older adults are stereotyped by characteristics found only in a small number of their age group

2 Table 3-2 Common Myths about Older Adults

Learning Outcome 4

Compare and contrast cognitive, psychosocial, moral, and spiritual development of the older adult to that of the young and middle adult.

Concepts for Lecture

1. Older adults continue to have developmental tasks. Cognition does not normally change with age. As people age it is important to review their lives through reminiscence in order to achieve ego integrity. Most older adults are at the moral development stage of conventional level, and find strength in spirituality and transcendence.
2. Havinghurst developed tasks for old age and later maturity.
3. Health care workers need to respect the moral and spiritual development of the older adult.

PowerPoint Lecture Slides

1 Developmental Aspects of Aging
- Cognitive development
- Psychosocial development
- Ego integrity versus despair and disgust (Erikson)

2 Havighurst's Tasks of Old Age
- Maintain social contacts and relationships
- Adjust to decreasing physical strength and health
- Adjust to retirement and reduced income
- Adjust to death of a spouse
- Establish an affiliation with one's age group
- Adjust and adapt social roles in a flexible way
- Establish satisfactory physical living arrangement

3 Moral and Spiritual Development
- Kohlberg's stages of moral development
  - Conventional level—follow societal rules and meet expectations of others
- Spirituality
  - Integrate faith and truth to see reality of their own
  - Acceptance without regretting past mistakes or fear of future

Suggestions for Classroom Activities

1. Initiate a discussion on the developmental stages of the older adult client.
2. Divide the class into three large groups. The groups should discuss the developmental stage for the young adult, middle adult, and older adult. Each group should describe the nursing role in promoting health and decreasing the risks for health alterations in each stage.

Suggestions for Clinical Activities

Assign students to care for older adults. Have them compare and contrast cognitive, psychosocial, moral, and spiritual development of the older adult to that of the young and middle adult.

© 2007 Pearson Education, Inc.

Learning Outcome 5

Explain age-related physical and psychosocial changes common to older adults.

Concepts for Lecture

1. Aging does bring physical changes as well as the strong probability of psychosocial changes involving widowhood, retirement, and living arrangements.

PowerPoint Lecture Slides

1 Table 3-3 Age-Related Physical Changes in the Older Adult

2 Age-Related Psychosocial Changes
- Illness or death of a spouse
- Decreased or limited income
- Retirement
- Isolation from friends and family
- Relocation to a long-term health care facility
- Role loss or reversal

Suggestions for Classroom Activities

Identify psychosocial changes related to the older adult. Discuss ways to assist the older adult with these changes.

Suggestions for Clinical Activities

Perform physical assessments on the older adult. Identify changes related to the aging process.

Learning Outcome 6

Describe common threats to the health of the older adult, including chronic illness, accidental injuries, medication management, and dementia and confusion.

Concepts for Lecture

1. The older adult is at risk for alterations in health from chronic illnesses, accidental injuries, medication, management, and dementia.

PowerPoint Lecture Slides

1 Threats to the Health of the Older Adult
- Chronic illness
  - Arthritis
  - Hypertension
  - Hearing and vision impairments
  - Cardiovascular disease
  - Cataracts
  - Sinusitis
  - Orthopedic disorders
  - Diabetes
  - Alzheimer's disease

1a Threats to the Health of the Older Adult
- Accidental injuries
  - Falls
  - Fires
  - Motor vehicle crashes

1b Threats to the Health of the Older Adult
- Medication management
  - Increased use of over-the-counter medications
  - Adverse reactions that have more serious consequences
  - Decreased metabolism
  - Nutritional problems
  - Visual deficits
  - Memory changes
  - Cost
  - Noncompliance

© 2007 Pearson Education, Inc.

POWERPOINT LECTURE SLIDES *continued*

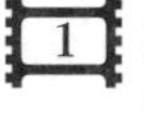

1c Threats to the Health of the Older Adult
- Confusion and dementia
  - Alzheimer's disease
  - Circulatory or metabolic problems
  - Electrolyte imbalances
  - Effects of medications
  - Nutritional deficiencies
  - Too many changes or losses at one time
  - Different environment
  - Sundowning syndrome

SUGGESTIONS FOR CLASSROOM ACTIVITIES

Discuss interventions to decrease and/or manage health threats to the older adult.

SUGGESTIONS FOR CLINICAL ACTIVITIES

Assign students to care for older adults in the clinical setting. Have them discuss their client's health threats and what interventions they took to manage them.

LEARNING OUTCOME 7

Incorporate actions to promote health and quality of life into nursing care of the older adult.

CONCEPTS FOR LECTURE

1. Nursing care to promote health in older adults includes teaching healthy behaviors and encouraging healthy lifestyles, preventive medication (including screening examinations and immunizations), injury prevention, and self-management of illness.

POWERPOINT LECTURE SLIDES

1 Nursing Interventions to Promote Health and Quality of Life
- Adapt teaching methods to the older adult
- Promote healthy lifestyle
- Screen for early detection of diseases
- Administer immunizations
- Teach injury prevention
- Teach self-management techniques

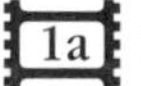

1a Box 3-2 Healthy Behaviors in the Older Adult

1b Table 3-4 Nursing Care to Promote Health in Older Adults

SUGGESTIONS FOR CLASSROOM ACTIVITIES

Discuss ways to promote healthy behaviors in the older adult client, especially screening for diseases and the necessity of immunizations.

SUGGESTIONS FOR CLINICAL ACTIVITIES

1. Have students develop charts or posters with large print to teach healthy behaviors to a group of older adults.
2. Administer immunizations at a health clinic or long-term care facility.

© 2007 Pearson Education, Inc.

Chapter 4
Settings of Care

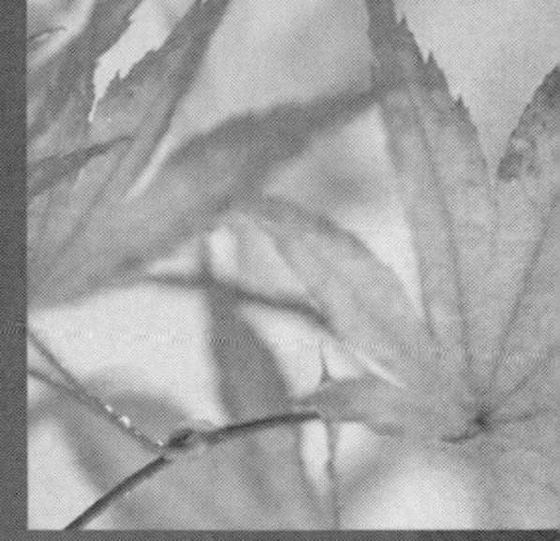

Resource Library

IMAGE LIBRARY

Figure 4-1 The home health nurse often provides client education. This nurse is teaching the client and family member how to apply dressings.

Figure 4-2 The rehabilitation team discusses the client's plan of care.

Learning Outcome 1

Define community-based nursing care.

Concepts for Lecture

1. Community-based nursing care focuses on individual and family health care needs, with nurses providing care in a variety of community settings, including community centers and clinics, day care programs, churches, long-term facilities, and homes.

PowerPoint Lecture Slides

1 Community-Based Nursing Care
- Provides culturally competent individual and family health care needs
- Provides direct services to individuals to manage acute or chronic health problems
- Promotes self-care
- Provides care in many different settings

Suggestions for Classroom Activities

1. Discuss the history of health care service and the changes in provider services that moved health care from hospital to community-based care.
2. Discuss the meaning of community-based care and contrast it with community health nursing.

Learning Outcome 2

Identify types of community-based health care services.

Concepts for Lecture

1. Long-term care facilities provide health care and activities of daily living for people who are mentally or physically unable to care for themselves.
2. Community centers and clinics, day care programs, parish nursing, and Meals-on-Wheels provide a wide range of services and often meet the health needs of clients who are unable to get care elsewhere.
3. Licensed practical/vocational nurses are often employed in community centers and clinics to carry out basic assessments, to assist the physician or advanced practice nurse with examinations, and to teach the client how to provide any needed self-care activities.

PowerPoint Lecture Slides

1,2 Box 4-1 Community-Based Nursing Care Settings

3 Community Services Provided by Licensed Practical/Vocational Nurses
- Basic assessments
- Assist physicians or advanced practice nurses with examinations
- Teach client to provide self-care activities
- Supervision during the day at day care centers

Suggestions for Classroom Activities

1. Discuss the different types of home health care agencies related to the care provided, whether it is private or not-for-profit, and the funding.
2. Discuss types of clients utilizing home health care agencies.
3. Have each student write a description of her or his community using the elements described in the chapter. Have the student evaluate the services in the community and document the needs of the community using the nursing process.

Suggestions for Clinical Activities

Arrange for students to spend a day in a community-based health care setting and assist with care and teaching of the clients.

Learning Outcome 3

Discuss the components of home health and the roles of the home health nurse.

Concepts for Lecture

1. Home health agencies are organizations that provide skilled nursing and other therapeutic services in the client's home. Nurses make the initial visit and collect data to develop a plan of care. The plan of care is implemented and evaluated within the special characteristics of the home as a nursing care setting.
2. Nurses who practice home health do so within a system where clients, referrals, and reimbursement sources interact.
3. The roles of the home health nurse are similar to those of nurses in any setting: provider of care, educator, and advocate.

PowerPoint Lecture Slides

1 Home Health Agencies
- Official or public agencies
- Voluntary or private not-for-profit agencies
- Private, proprietary agencies
- Institution-based agencies
- 20,000 providers deliver home health care services to 7.6 million people

2 Components of Home Health Care
- Care of clients in the home
  - Observe family dynamics
  - Identify caregiver burden
- Referrals for home care
  - Discuss funding
- Reimbursement sources for home care
  - Medicare, Medicaid, insurance, public funding, self-pay

3 Roles of the Home Health Nurse
- Provider of care
- Teacher
- Advocate

Suggestions for Classroom Activities

Compare and contrast the role of the medical-surgical nurse with the role of the home health nurse as a caregiver, educator, coordinator of care, and advocate.

Learning Outcome 4

Understand nursing care guidelines and special considerations for home health care.

Concepts for Lecture

1. Home health nurses are responsible for adhering to the same codes and standards that guide all other nurses. The American Nurses Association has established Standards for Home Health Nursing Practice and Standards of Community Health Nursing as basic for the practice of nursing in the home. Nurses are required by law to review the National Association for

PowerPoint Lecture Slides

1 Guidelines for Home Health Care Nurses
- ANA Standards for Home Health Nursing Practice
- ANA Standards of Community Health Nursing
- National Association for Home Care Bill of Rights

2 Legal Issues in Home Health
- Privacy and confidentiality

© 2007 Pearson Education, Inc.

Concepts for Lecture *continued*

Home Care Bill of Rights with clients on the initial visit.

2. Nurses can avoid lawsuits by familiarizing themselves with standards of practice, providing care that is consistent with standards and with their agency's policies, and documenting all care fully and accurately.
3. Safety and infection control in the home are priority concerns for the home health nurse.

PowerPoint Lecture Slides *continued*

- Client access to health information
- Freedom from unreasonable restraint
- Witnessing of documents
- Informed consent
- Negligence or malpractice

Concerns for the Home Health Nurse

- Safety
  - Assessment of, documentation of, and teaching of safety measures
- Infection Control
  - Effective hand washing
  - Use of gloves
  - Disposal of wastes and soiled dressings
  - Handling of linens
  - Practice Standard Precautions

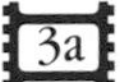

Table 4-1 Suggestions for Effective Home Health Care

Suggestions for Classroom Activities

1. Discuss legal and ethical issues of providing nursing care in the home setting.
2. Review standards of care for home health nursing.
3. Have the students volunteer to role-play a home health nurse and a client in the following home care settings:

   Scenario A: A 78-year-old male with a history of congestive heart failure has been discharged from the hospital after stabilization. He lives alone, is visually impaired, and is having problems seeing how to take his daily medications and prepare his meals.

   Scenario B: A 54-year-old male with terminal cancer is refusing further treatment for cancer, and is requesting to die at home.

   Scenario C: A 43-year-old female with type 2 diabetes is having home health visits for the treatment of a nonhealing cellulitis of the right lower leg. Treatment includes IV antibiotic therapy every 12 hours. The client verbalizes that she is having a problem adjusting to being a diabetic.

   Scenario D: A 25-year-old male severely injured in a motor vehicle accident, with multiple fractures of the lower extremities, is discharged from a rehabilitation hospital. His concerns are his physical and social limitations.

Suggestions for Clinical Activities

1. Assign students to care for clients in need of home care after discharge. Assign students to assess client home care needs and prepare a nursing care plan.
2. In the postconference setting, have students discuss their thoughts and feelings about receiving home care for an acute illness or follow-up care for a chronic illness.
3. Have students role-play the initial home visit performed by the home health nurse. Encourage students to make specific suggestions about what to do on the initial visit.

Learning Outcome 5

Apply the nursing process to care of the client in the home.

Concepts for Lecture

1. The nursing process is the same for home care as for any other setting. Differences lie is assessing how the home's unique environment affects the need or problem and in using outcome criteria and mutual participation to plan goals and interventions.

PowerPoint Lecture Slides

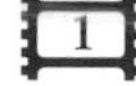

Nursing Process in Home Health

- Assessing
  - Conduct careful and complete data collection initially and on an ongoing basis
- Diagnosing
  - Identify actual or potential problems—LPN/LVNs contribute to this process

POWERPOINT LECTURE SLIDES *continued*

- Planning
  - Set priorities, establish goals, decide on interventions
- Implementing
  - Carry out interventions
- Evaluating
  - Compare plan of care with goals and review client's progress

SUGGESTIONS FOR CLASSROOM ACTIVITIES

Review the steps of the nursing process and the responsibilities of the licensed practical/vocational nurse in developing it.

SUGGESTIONS FOR CLINICAL ACTIVITIES

Develop a plan of care based on the nursing process for a client in a home health setting.

LEARNING OUTCOME 6

Describe the philosophy of and nursing care to facilitate rehabilitation.

CONCEPTS FOR LECTURE

1. Rehabilitation is the process of learning to live to one's maximum potential with a chronic impairment and the resulting functional disability.
2. Rehabilitation nursing care is often provided in community-based settings.The goal of rehabilitation nurses is to assist clients to again become a part of their family and community.

POWERPOINT LECTURE SLIDES

1 Rehabilitation Philosophy

- Process of learning to live to one's maximum potential
- Each person has a unique set of strengths and abilities
- Applies to both acute and chronic illnesses

1a Definitions used in Rehabilitation

- Impairment
  - Disturbance in structure or function resulting from physiologic or psychologic abnormalities
- Disability
  - Degree of observable and measurable impairment
- Handicap
  - Total adjustment to disability that limits functioning at a normal level.

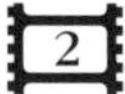
2 Rehabilitation Nursing Care Interventions

- Preventing infection
- Maintaining correct body alignment, position, and range of motion
- Preventing skin breakdown
- Providing adequate nutrition and fluids
- Providing care as necessary and appropriate, with the goal of achieving a level of independence realistic for the client
- Making referrals to community agencies

SUGGESTIONS FOR CLASSROOM ACTIVITIES

Discuss types of clients who need rehabilitative nursing care.

SUGGESTIONS FOR CLINICAL ACTIVITIES

Assign students to observe or provide care for clients in a rehabilitative care setting. In postconference, discuss the roles of the rehabilitative care nurse.

© 2007 Pearson Education, Inc.

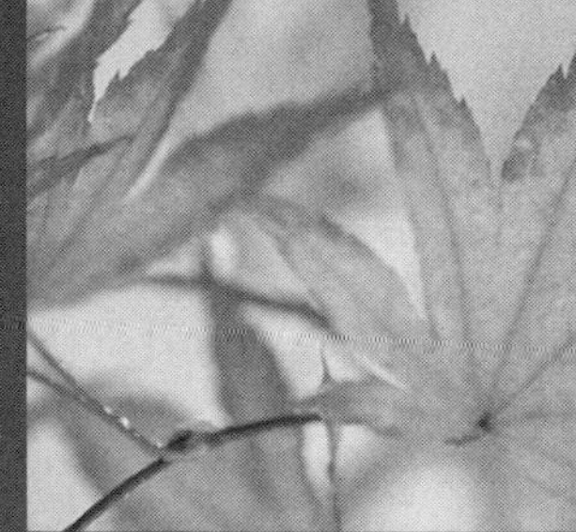

Chapter 5
Guidelines for Client Assessment

Resource Library

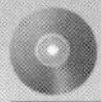
CD-ROM

Video: Taking Patient Histories
Video: Prepping the Exam Room

IMAGE LIBRARY

Figure 5-1 The position of the hand for light palpation.
Figure 5-2 Indirect percussion. Use the finger of one hand to tap the finger of the other.
Figure 5-3 Assessing edema. (**A**) Palpating for edema over the tibia. (**B**) Four-point scale for grading edema.
Figure 5-4 Size of pupil in millimeters.
Figure 5-5 Types of eye charts: the preschool children's chart (left), Snellen's standard chart (center), and the Snellen E chart for clients who are unable to read (right).
Figure 5-6 Lymph nodes of the head and neck.
Figure 5-7 Location of the apical impulse.
Figure 5-8 Possible pattern for palpation of the breast.
Figure 5-9 The four quadrants of the abdomen, with anatomic location of organs within each quadrant.
Figure 5-10 Body sites at which peripheral pulses are most easily palpated.

Learning Outcome 1

Discuss the purposes of a client assessment.

Concepts for Lecture

1. Assessment is the collection of data that provides information about the client's individualized health care needs. Assessment is mandated by nursing standards, nurse practice acts, accrediting bodies, and institutional bodies.
2. Nurses collect this data through the health assessment, comprised of a health history and a physical examination.

PowerPoint Lecture Slides

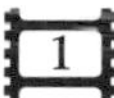
Assessment
- Collection of data that provides information about client's individualized health care needs
- First step of nursing process
- Mandated by nursing standards, nurse practice acts, accrediting bodies, institutional policies

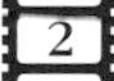
Purposes of Client Assessment
- Collect objective data (signs)
- Collect subjective data (symptoms)
- Collect information about client's family, community, culture, ethnicity, religion
- Identify past and present client behaviors that support health or increase risk of illness
- Identify data that suggest risk for or actual health problems

Suggestions for Classroom Activities

1. Initiate a discussion on the importance of performing the assessment according to the standards of the Joint Commission on Accreditation of Healthcare Organizations (JCAHO).
2. Discuss the difference between objective and subjective data. Have the students describe the sources for collection of data and give examples of subjective and objective data.

Learning Outcome 2

Describe the types of client assessment.

Concepts for Lecture

1. Types of assessments vary depending on the setting, the situation, and the needs of the client.

PowerPoint Lecture Slides

1 Types of Client Assessment
- Comprehensive assessment
  - Health history
  - Physical status
- Partial assessment
  - Ongoing assessment on a regular basis
- Focused assessment
  - Assessment of a specific client problem
  - Emergency assessment

Suggestions for Classroom Activities

Have students discuss when a certain type of assessment is appropriate to perform.

Suggestions for Clinical Activities

Have students practice the steps in performing an emergency assessment.

Learning Outcome 3

Compare sources and accuracy of assessment data.

Concepts for Lecture

1. The primary source of data is the client. Secondary sources include the client's family or friends, client records, and other health care professionals.
2. Assessment data must be accurate and factual.

PowerPoint Lecture Slides

1 Sources of Assessment Data
- Primary
  - Client
- Secondary
  - Client's family or friends
  - Client records
  - Health care professionals

2 Guidelines for Collection of Assessment Data
- Compare subjective and objective data
- Consider factors that may interfere with accurate measurements
- Clarify statements made by the client
- Double-check data that are very high or low
- Do not jump to conclusions

Suggestions for Classroom Activities

Have students discuss the methods of obtaining accurate and factual data.

Suggestions for Clinical Activities

Have student review client's record to obtain information needed to develop a plan of care.

Learning Outcome 4

Describe components of the health history.

Concepts for Lecture

1. The health history, collected through an interview of the client, provides subjective and objective data.
2. Principles of therapeutic communication help the nurse collect accurate data.

PowerPoint Lecture Slides

1 Table 5-1 Information Included in a Health History

2 Principles of Therapeutic Communication
- Use words client can understand
- Listen carefully
- Sit in a relaxed position and maintain eye contact

© 2007 Pearson Education, Inc.

PowerPoint Lecture Slides *continued*

- Use open-ended questions
- Be sensitive to cultural differences
- Use a translator if client speaks other than yours language

3 Barriers to Therapeutic Communication

- Offering advice
- Acting disgusted or defensive
- Disagreeing
- Offering false assurance
- Jumping to conclusions

Suggestions for Classroom Activities

1. Initiate a discussion on the importance of cultural and social differences when obtaining a health history or performing a physical assessment.
2. Partner students in groups of two or three. Have students role-play methods of collecting data for a health history. Have students use methods of therapeutic communication such as closed-ended and open-ended questions to collect data.

Suggestions for Clinical Activities

1. In the clinical setting, review a health assessment form with the students.
2. Have students interview clients using therapeutic communication techniques.

Learning Outcome 5

Demonstrate the methods of physical examination.

Concepts for Lecture

1. The four methods of physical examination are inspection, palpation, percussion, and auscultation. The skills of physical examination take practice.

PowerPoint Lecture Slides

1 Four Basic Methods of Physical Examination

- Inspection
- Palpation
- Percussion
- Auscultation

1a Guidelines for Inspection

- Provide comfortable room temperature
- Use good lighting
- Look before touching
- Completely expose body part being inspected
- Compare symmetrical parts
- Inspect for color, size, symmetry, patterns, location, consistency of tissue, movement, behavior, odors, sounds

1b Guidelines for Palpation

- Make sure hands are clean and warm, fingernails short
- Follow Standard Precautions
- Use pads of fingers to palpate pulses, texture, size, shape, crepitus
- Table 5-2 Characteristics Assessed by Palpation

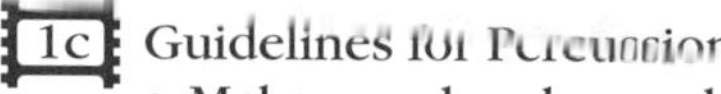

1c Guidelines for Percussion

- Make sure hands are clean and warm, fingernails short
- Follow Standard Precautions
- Direct percussion:
    - Use one or more fingertips to tap over area being percussed

© 2007 Pearson Education, Inc.

PowerPoint Lecture Slides *continued*

- Indirect percussion:
  - Place middle finger of nondominant hand over area to be percussed
  - Use pad of middle finger of dominant hand to strike area between knuckle and fingernail of hand over body part
  - Deliver two quick taps by flexing wrist and listen to the tone

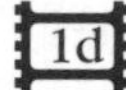

Guidelines for Auscultation
- Make sure hands are clean and warm, fingernails short
- Follow Standard Precautions
- Make environment as quiet as possible
- Auscultate over bare skin
- Press diaphragm of stethoscope firmly on body part being assessed
- Hold bell of stethoscope lightly on body part being assessed to listen to low-pitched sounds

Suggestions for Classroom Activities

Initiate a discussion on the methods of physical assessment. Have the students identify the methods of assessment to use in the following scenarios:

Scenario A: A 49-year-old male is admitted with a productive cough and shortness of breath.

Scenario B: A 30-year-old male is admitted with complaint of severe abdominal pain with nausea and vomiting.

Scenario C: A 68-year-old female is diagnosed with a fractured femur and has a cast applied to the right lower extremity.

Scenario D: A 78-year-old female admitted with an acute onset of congestive heart failure has a complaint of shortness of breath and edema of the lower extremities.

Suggestions for Clinical Activities

Pair up students in the clinical laboratory and have them practice methods of physical assessment on each other.

Learning Outcome 6

Prepare a client for a physical examination.

Concepts for Lecture

1. Prepare the client for a physical assessment to decrease anxiety and feelings of embarrassment.

PowerPoint Lecture Slides

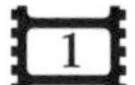

Preparation for a Physical Assessment
- Ensure comfortable room temperature, quiet and private area, adequate lighting
- Ensure equipment is clean and in good working order
- Wash hands before and after assessment
- Wear gloves and follow Standard Precautions
- Place client in comfortable position
- Adjust length of time to physical condition and age of client
- Assist client in removing clothes and putting on gown
- Have client empty bladder
- Place drape over client so only body part being assessed is exposed

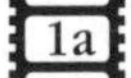

Box 5-1 Age-Related Assessment Findings in the Older Adult

© 2007 Pearson Education, Inc.

Learning Outcome 7

Describe the body systems and characteristics assessed in a physical examination.

Concepts for Lecture

1. A comprehensive physical examination is conducted in a head-to-toe sequence or system-by-system. If a focused or emergency assessment is being conducted, the nurse assesses only the specific client problem.

PowerPoint Lecture Slides

1 Table 5-3 Guidelines for a Physical Examination

1a General Survey
- Client's overall appearance and behavior
- Facial expressions, mood and speech patterns
- Hygiene, grooming, odors
- Posture, physical deformities, ability to move and walk
- Manifestations of illness
- Vital signs
- Height and weight

1b Integumentary System—Skin, Hair, Nails
- Assess skin for color, warmth, smooth, dry intact, lesions, turgor
- Assess nails for shape, color, consistency
- Assess hair for color, texture, distribution

1c Head and Neck
- Assess skull for shape, proportion, symmetry
- Assess face for color, symmetry, distribution of hair, functioning of muscles and nerves
- Assess eyes for alignment with eyebrows, eyelashes curl outward, eyelids cover eye, lacrimal gland is nontender, conjunctiva is pink, visual acuity
- Assess pupils for black and round, reaction to light, accommodation, convergence, Box 5-2 Assessing the Pupils

1d Head and Neck
- Assess ears for location, symmetry, lesions, redness, drainage, hearing
- Palpate ears for tenderness, swelling
- Assess nose for patency; mucous membranes for swelling, bleeding, or discharge; deviated septum
- Palpate sinuses for tenderness or pain
- Assess mouth for color, smooth, moist, odor, teeth in good repair
- Palpate lymph nodes for size, location, consistency, tenderness

1e Thorax
- Assess chest and back for color, size, shape, breathing movements, symmetry
- Assess lungs for respiratory rate, depth, rhythm, oxygen use, cough, sputum for color, amount, consistency
- Auscultate lungs for breath sounds
- Auscultate heart for heart sounds
- Assess heart for rate, rhythm, normal sounds (S_1, S_2)
- Assess breasts for size, symmetry, color, skin condition, nipple condition, discharge, tenderness or pain, abnormal consistency, presence of mass
- Assess lymph nodes for pain, size, consistency

© 2007 Pearson Education, Inc.

PowerPoint Lecture Slides *continued*

1f Abdomen

- Assess abdomen for slight rounding, umbilicus midline, skin condition, masses, distention
- Auscultate bowel sounds
- Palpate urinary bladder for distention

1g Extremities

- Assess extremities for color, temperature, lesions, condition of hair and nails, peripheral circulation, muscle strength
- Assess peripheral circulation for rate, rhythm, strength, capillary refill
- Assess musculoskeletal system for posture; ability to move, walk, and carry out activities of daily living; range of motion; muscle strength

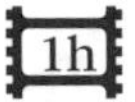

Mental Status

- Assess mental status for level of awareness (orientation), degree of wakefulness, ability to be aroused (level of consciousness)

Suggestions for Classroom Activities

Divide students into groups of three to four. Assign each group to perform an assessment on a body system and document its findings.

Suggestions for Clinical Activities

Assign students to perform a beginning-of-shift physical assessment on the assigned client and document findings using the principles of factual and accurate documentation found in the chapter.

Learning Outcome 8

Document a health assessment.

Concepts for Lecture

1. Documenting assessments factually and accurately provides the base for evaluation of health care outcomes, provides evidence to support health care cost reimbursement, and is legal evidence of the health status of the client at that point in time.

PowerPoint Lecture Slides

1 Principles of Documenting a Physical Assessment

- Document as soon as possible
- Document legibly or make computer entries accurately
- Organize data in a logical way
- Avoid inferences and judgments
- Record findings rather than methods of assessment
- Write concisely, using approved abbreviations and grammar
- Do not use the word "normal" for normal findings
- Charting by exception is documenting only abnormal findings

Suggestions for Classroom Activities

1. Review examples of documentation to discuss how to document accurately and factually.
2. Have students attend a documentation class at the health care facilities at which they will be doing clinical rotations.

Suggestions for Clinical Activities

Have students practice documenting factually and accurately before documenting in a client's medical record.

© 2007 Pearson Education, Inc.

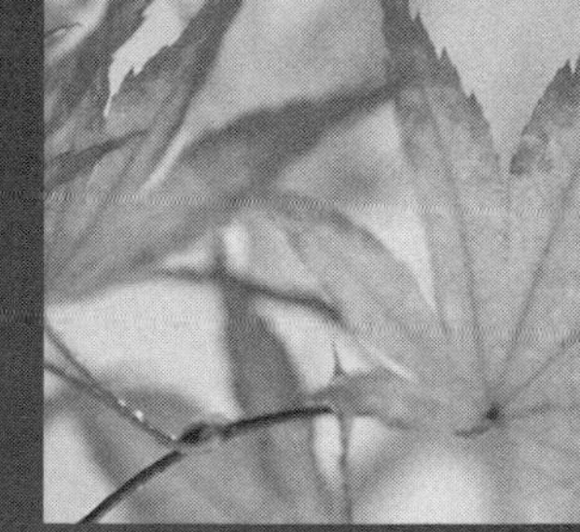

CHAPTER 6
ESSENTIAL NURSING PHARMACOLOGY

RESOURCE LIBRARY

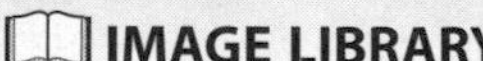

CD-ROM

Drug Metabolization
Agonist

IMAGE LIBRARY

Figure 6-1 The four processes of drug movement (pharmacokinetics): absorption, distribution, metabolism, and excretion.
Figure 6-2 First-pass effect.
Figure 6-3 Receptor site action: Drug A fits into the receptor site like a key into a lock to initiate a drug reaction. Drug B does not fit into this receptor site; therefore, no drug action occurs at this site.
Figure 6-4 Potency and efficacy. (**A**) Drug A has a higher potency than drug B. (**B**) Drug B has a higher efficacy than drug B.

LEARNING OUTCOME 1

Identify laws that govern the prescription, storage, and administration of drugs.

CONCEPTS FOR LECTURE

1. Pharmacology is the study of drugs and their uses in the body. Drugs are substances that alter body function to prevent or treat disease, aid in diagnosis, and restore or maintain function.
2. Drugs are made from natural resources, produced synthetically in the laboratory, or developed through genetic engineering.
3. Drugs have four names: chemical, generic, trade, and official.
4. Nurses must be familiar with both generic and trade names and with laws that regulate these drugs in order to prevent potential errors.
5. Nurses require reliable and up-to-date drug information to give medications safely and accurately.

POWERPOINT LECTURE SLIDES

1 Pharmacology
- Study of drugs and their uses in the body
- Drugs are used to
  - Prevent disease
  - Aid in diagnosis
  - Treat disease
  - Restore or maintain body system function

2 Drug Sources
- Natural sources
  - Plants, animal tissue, minerals
- Synthetics
- Genetic engineering
  - Uses recombinant DNA

3 Drug Names
- Chemical name
  - Describes chemical compounds and molecular structure of the drug
- Nonproprietary or generic name
  - Name approved by the United States Adopted Names Council
  - First letter in name is a lowercase letter
- Trade or brand name
  - Identifies drug sold by manufacturer
  - Symbols or trade mark after drug signify that name is registered
  - First letter in name is capitalized

PowerPoint Lecture Slides *continued*

- Official name
  - Official name is listed in the United States Pharmacopeia National Formulary

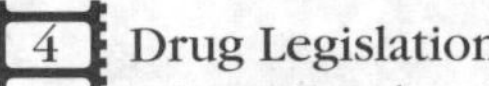

4 Drug Legislation
- Pure Food and Drug Act in 1906
  - Restricted manufacture and sale of drugs
- Food, Drug, and Cosmetic Act in 1938
  - Regulations regarding labeling and packaging of drugs
  - Required drug companies to perform toxicity tests on lab animals
  - Food and Drug Administration (FDA) enforces this legislation
- Controlled Substances Act of 1970
  - Identifies and regulates manufacture and sale of narcotics and dangerous drugs
  - Table 6-1 Schedule for Controlled Substances

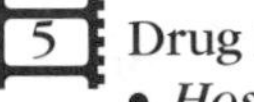

5 Drug Resources
- *Hospital Formulary*
- *Facts and Comparisons*
- *Physician's Desk Reference* (PDR)
- Drug package inserts
- Internet sites
  - www.fda.gov
  - http://rxmed.com

Suggestions for Classroom Activities

1. Develop a matching quiz to match generic names to trade names to help students identify drug names.
2. Compare and contrast drugs in each of the controlled substance schedules.

Suggestions for Clinical Activities

Have students look up assigned client's drugs in the *Hospital Formulary* or the *Physician's Drug Reference* while in the clinical setting.

Learning Outcome 2

Describe the processes of pharmacokinetics: absorption, distribution, metabolism, and excretion.

Concepts for Lecture

1. Pharmacokinetics is the study of how drugs are processed by the body.
2. The processes of absorption, distribution, metabolism, and excretion make up the pharmacokinetic action of a drug.
3. Older adults have physiologic changes, which affect pharmacokinetic processes.

PowerPoint Lecture Slides

1 Pharmacokinetics
- Study of how drugs are processed by the body
- Describes steps that occur from the time a drug is administered until it is eliminated

2 Absorption
- Time a drug enters the body until it enters the body fluids
- Absorption rate identifies how soon drug exerts its action
- Table 6-2 Drug Absorption Routes

2a Distribution
- Distribution of drug to various organs and tissues
- Factors affecting distribution
  - Blood flow
  - Plasma protein binding
  - Blood–brain barrier

© 2007 Pearson Education, Inc.

POWERPOINT LECTURE SLIDES *continued*

2b Metabolism (Biotransformation)
- Process by which body changes a drug from original chemical structure to a form that can be eliminated or excreted
- Most metabolism takes place in the liver
- Microsomal enzymes break down the drug and detoxify potentially harmful substances to the body
- Liver diseases inhibit enzyme action, resulting in excess drug accumulation in the body
- Oral drugs are subject to first-pass effect

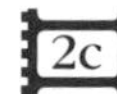
Excretion
- Process of elimination either unchanged or as metabolites
- Pathways of excretion are kidneys, lungs, feces
- Kidney damage
  - Impairs excretion
  - Leads to drug accumulation
  - Increases potential for severe drug reactions

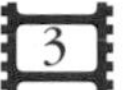
Box 6-1 Pharmacokinetic Changes in Older Adults

SUGGESTIONS FOR CLASSROOM ACTIVITIES

1. Discuss disease processes and physiologic changes of aging that may affect the processes of pharmacokinetics.
2. Discuss how to administer medications to bypass the blood-brain barrier.
3. Compare and contrast injection sites for speed of absorption.

LEARNING OUTCOME 3

Identify how pharmacodynamics affect drug action.

CONCEPTS FOR LECTURE

1. Pharmacodynamics is the study of how drugs produce their effects in the body to result in a pharmacologic response.
2. The effectiveness of a drug depends on its action and dose.
3. The response to any drug depends on the amount of drug given.
4. The nurse needs to understand that drug response varies in each client even when same dose and dosage regimen are followed.
5. Drug interactions are the effects that occur when actions of one drug are affected by another drug, food, or herbal therapy.
6. Adverse drug reactions (ADR) range from expected side effects to toxic effects. The most common toxic effects include liver and kidney damage.

POWERPOINT LECTURE SLIDES

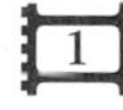
Pharmacodynamics
- Study of how drugs produce their effects in the body to result in a pharmacologic response
- Drug action begins after a drug attaches itself to a receptor site
  - Agonist
  - Antagonist
  - Agonist-antagonist
- Drugs have a local or systemic effect

2 Drug Effectiveness Factors
- Onset of action
- Peak action
- Duration of action
- Half-life
- Serum level
  - Loading dose
  - Maintenance dose

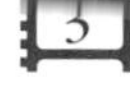
Drug Response Factors
- Potency
- Efficacy
- Ceiling effect

Variables in Drug Response
- Age
- Body weight

© 2007 Pearson Education, Inc.

PowerPoint Lecture Slides *continued*

- Genetics
- Ethnicity
- Disease conditions
- Emotional state

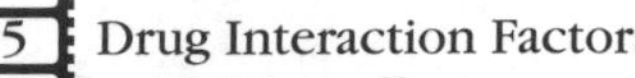

5 Drug Interaction Factors
- Additive effect
- Synergism
- Potentiation
- Nicotine (smoking)
- Drug incompatibility
- Foods
- Over-the-counter drugs
- Herbal therapy

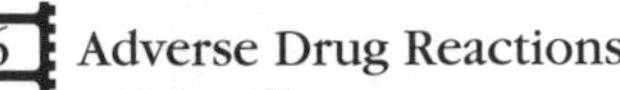

6 Adverse Drug Reactions
- Side effects
- Drug allergy
  - Anaphylaxis
- Idiosyncratic effects
- Toxic effects
- Teratogenic effect
- Carcinogenic effect

Suggestions for Classroom Activities

1. Discuss effective nursing interventions to help manage the adverse effects of medications.
2. Research foods or drugs that should be avoided with medication administration.
3. Assign students to present a case study on a client, including the factors of drug effectiveness, variables in drug response, and possible adverse reactions of the drugs the client is taking.

Suggestions for Clinical Activities

1. In postconference, discuss drugs in which the therapeutic effects vary when administered to different clients with different disease processes.
2. Have students look up medications on a drug incompatibility chart to determine which drugs are incompatible.
3. Interview a client with a hypersensitivity to a medication and explore the signs and symptoms the client exhibited.

Learning Outcome 4

Explain the six rights of medication administration and the importance of each right.

Concepts for Lecture

1. Safe medication administration means implementing the "Six Rights" in order to prevent a medication error.
2. Preventing medication errors requires everyone to make a commitment to client safety.

PowerPoint Lecture Slides

1 Six Rights of Medication Administration
- Right drug
- Right client
- Right time
- Right route
- Right dose
- Right documentation

2 Medication Errors
- Any preventable event that may cause or lead to inappropriate medication use or patient harm while medication is in control of the health care professional, patient, or consumer.

3 Most Common Types of Medication Errors
- Wrong dose
- Wrong drug
- Wrong route

© 2007 Pearson Education, Inc.

Suggestions for Classroom Activities

1. Compare and contrast medication administration routes and techniques.
2. Discuss the steps to take when a medication error occurs.

Suggestions for Clinical Activities

Administer medications in the clinical setting, using the "Six Rights" of medication administration.

Learning Outcome 5

Apply the nursing process to administering medications.

Concepts for Lecture

1. The nursing process is a systematic process for providing care to clients. When correctly applied to drug therapy, it can reduce the potential for errors.

PowerPoint Lecture Slides

[1] Nursing Process
- Systematic process for providing care to clients
- Reduces potential for drug errors
- Promotes sound decision making for safe drug administration

[1a] Assessment
- Collecting data on client's medication history
- Nonjudgmental interview about medication use
- Factors affecting compliance
- Box 6-3 Medication History
- Physical examination to determine problems that could affect ability to take medications
- Review pertinent laboratory test values

[1b] Diagnosis and Plan
- Identify client's actual or potential health problems
- Review drug's purpose, recommended dose, potential side effects, therapeutic effects
- Consider drug–food and drug–drug interactions

[1c] Implementation
- Interventions used to administer drug therapy
- Drug orders
  - Routine
  - Standing
  - Stat
  - prn
- Clarify unclear orders

[1d] Evaluation
- Monitor for manifestations that indicate that the medication is effective
- Determine side effects or any drug interactions
- Evaluate success in teaching medication administration
- Document administration, response of drug, and teaching completed

Suggestions for Classroom Activities

1. Have students develop patient teaching sheets on the most common drugs administered.
2. Discuss which assessments are necessary prior to administration of medications.

Suggestions for Clinical Activities

1. Develop a care plan for a client receiving medication, including the outcome criteria for evaluating the effectiveness of the medications.
2. Prepare drug cards to use in the clinical setting.

© 2007 Pearson Education, Inc.

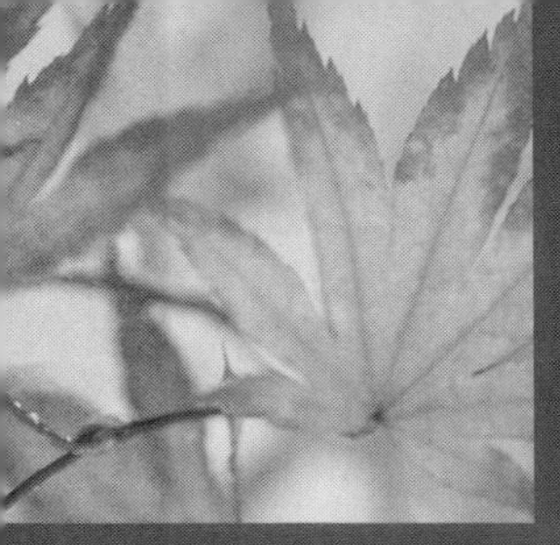

CHAPTER 7
CARING FOR CLIENTS WITH ALTERED FLUID, ELECTROLYTE, OR ACID–BASE BALANCE

RESOURCE LIBRARY

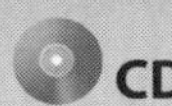 **CD-ROM**

Fluids
Furosemide

IMAGE LIBRARY

Figure 7-1 A comparison of the major fluid compartments of the body.
Figure 7-2 The principal electrolytes (in milliequivalents) of (**A**) extracellular fluid and (**B**) intracellular fluid.
Figure 7-3 Osmosis. Water moves across a selectively permeable membrane from an area of low solute concentration to an area of high solute concentration.
Figure 7-4 The effect of changes in the concentration of solutions on red blood cells. (**A**) Cells neither gain nor lose water, size, or shape in isotonic solutions. (**B**) Cells lose water and shrink in hypertonic solutions. (**C**) Cells absorb water, swell, and burst in hypotonic solutions.
Figure 7-5 In diffusion, molecules move across a semipermeable membrane from an area of higher solute concentration to an area of lower concentration.
Figure 7-6 The sodium–potassium pump. Active transport moves sodium and potassium ions across cell membranes against their concentration gradients.
Figure 7-7 Factors stimulating water intake through the thirst mechanism.
Figure 7-8 The renin–angiotensin–aldosterone system.
Figure 7-9 The effect of antidiuretic hormone (ADH) release.
Figure 7-10 A standard IV administration set.
Figure 7-11 An over-the-needle IV catheter.
Figure 7-12 Commonly used venipuncture sites of the (**A**) arm and (**B**) hand. Figure A also shows the site used for a peripherally inserted central catheter (PICC).
Figure 7-13 A central venous catheter inserted via the right subclavian vein.
Figure 7-14 Low serum calcium levels stimulate parathyroid hormone release, increasing serum calcium levels by triggering its release from bone, absorption in the intestine, and reabsorption in the kidneys.
Figure 7-15 (**A**) Positive Chvostek's sign and (**B**) positive Trousseau's sign.
Figure 7-16 As long as the ratio of bicarbonate to carbonic acid is 20:1, the pH remains within the normal range of 7.35 to 7.45.
Figure 7-17 Metabolic acid–base imbalances. (**A**) Metabolic acidosis. (**B**) Metabolic alkalosis.
Figure 7-18 Respiratory acid–base imbalances. (**A**) Respiratory acidosis. (**B**) Respiratory alkalosis.

LEARNING OUTCOME 1

Identify the functions and regulatory mechanisms that maintain water, electrolyte, and acid-base balance in the body.

CONCEPTS FOR LECTURE

1. The volume and composition of body fluid is normally maintained by a balance of fluid and electrolyte intake; elimination of water, electrolytes, and acids by the kidneys; and hormonal influences. Change in any of these factors can lead to a fluid, electrolyte, or acid–base imbalance that affects health.
2. Fluid, electrolyte, and acid–base imbalances can affect all body systems, especially the cardiovascular system, the central nervous system, and the transmission of nerve impulses.

POWERPOINT LECTURE SLIDES

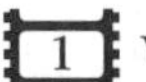

Water
- Primary component of body fluids
- Transports nutrients and oxygen to cells and waste products from cells
- Provides medium for metabolic reactions within cells
- Insulates and helps regulate and maintain body temperature
- Provides for body structure and acts as shock absorber
- Is a lubricant
- To maintain fluid balance, intake should equal output ~2500 mL/day

POWERPOINT LECTURE SLIDES *continued*

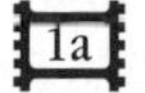
Electrolytes

- Substances that dissociate in solution to form ions
- Cations are positively charged; anions are negatively charged
- Help regulate water and acid-base balance
- Contribute to enzyme reactions
- Are essential to neuromuscular activity
- Table 7-1 Normal Laboratory Values for Electrolytes, Osmolality, and Urine specific Gravity

Body Fluid Distribution

- Intracellular fluid (ICF)
  - Fluid within cells—40% total body weight
  - Contains electrolytes, glucose, oxygen
- Extracellular fluid (ECF)
  - Interstitial fluid—15% total body weight
  - Intravascular fluid—5% total body weight
  - Transcellular fluid—<1% total body weight
  - Transports oxygen, electrolytes, and nutrients to cells
  - Transports waste products away from cells

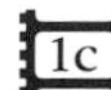
Body Fluid Movement

- Osmosis
  - Osmolality—concentration of solutes
  - Osmotic pressure—power of a solution
  - Tonicity—effect of osmotic pressure of a solution on cell within a solution
- Diffusion
- Filtration
- Active transport

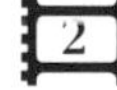
Body Fluid Regulation

- Thirst
  - Regulator of water intake
- Kidneys
  - Regulator of fluid volume and electrolyte balance
- Renin-angiotensin-aldosterone system
  - Maintains intravascular fluid balance and blood pressure
- Antidiuretic hormone (ADH)
  - Regulates water excretion from the kidneys
  - Diabetes insipidus—antidiuretic hormone is not produced
  - Syndrome of inappropriate ADH secretion—excess antidiuretic hormone is produced
- Atrial natriuretic factor (ANF)
  - Hormone released by cells in atria of heart in response to fluid overload
  - Inhibits renin secretion and blocks secretion and effects of aldosterone
  - Promotes sodium and water loss and causes blood vessels to dilate

© 2007 Pearson Education, Inc.

Suggestions for Classroom Activities

Divide the class into small groups. Assign each group to present one hormone associated with regulating the body fluids: renin-angiotensin-aldosterone system, the antidiuretic hormone, or the atrial natriuretic factor. Present the regulatory mechanisms and the disorders associated with each hormone.

Learning Outcome 2

Compare and contrast the causes and effects of fluid volume, electrolyte, and acid-base imbalances.

Concepts for Lecture

1. Fluid volume deficits may be due to excessive fluid losses, insufficient fluid intake, or both.
2. Fluid volume excess usually results from sodium and water retention.
3. Fluid and sodium imbalances commonly are related; both affect serum osmolality.
4. Potassium imbalances are due to excess or deficit in potassium intake, resulting in cardiac dysrhythmias.
5. Three hormones interact to regulate serum calcium levels: parathyroid hormone, calcitriol, and calcitonin.
6. Magnesium is critical to intracellular metabolism and extracellular functioning of neuromuscular transmission. The kidneys control extracellular magnesium.
7. Phosphorus is found in all body tissue, most combined with calcium in bones and teeth. It is the primary anion in intracellular fluid with very small amount in extracellular fluid. An inverse relationship exists between phosphorus and calcium levels.

PowerPoint Lecture Slides

1 Fluid Volume Deficit
- Due to excessive fluid losses, insufficient fluid intake, or both, resulting in hypovolemia
- Table 7-2 Fluid Imbalances
- Box 7-1 Fluid Volume Deficit in Older Adults
- Characterized by decrease in extracellular fluids, loss of water and electrolytes, interstitial fluid shifts into vascular space to maintain blood volume
- Third spacing
  - Shift of fluid from vascular space into soft tissue

2 Fluid Volume Excess
- Due to sodium and water retention, resulting in hypervolemia and interstitial edema
- Table 7-2 Fluid Imbalances
- Characterized by excess sodium that leads to water retention

3 Sodium Imbalances
- Most plentiful electrolyte in extracellular fluid
- Serum sodium range—135 to 145 mEq/L
- Regulates extracellular volume and distribution, contributes to neuromuscular activity and acid-base balance, affects osmolality of extracellular fluid
- Kidneys work with the renin-angiotensin-aldosterone system and atrial natriuretic factor to retain or excrete sodium

4 Potassium Imbalances
- Serum potassium range—3.5 to 5 mEq/L
- Regulates the transmission of nerve impulses and the normal contractility of smooth, skeletal, and cardiac muscle; can result in fatal dysrhythmias

5 Calcium Imbalances
- One of most abundant ions in body, mostly in bones and teeth with small amount in extracellular fluid
- Serum calcium range—8.5 to 10 mg/dL
- Three hormones interact to regulate serum calcium levels:
  - Parathyroid hormone—mobilizes calcium from bones, increases calcium absorption in intestines, and promotes calcium reabsorption by the kidneys
  - Calcitriol—assists parathyroid hormone processes

© 2007 Pearson Education, Inc.

PowerPoint Lecture Slides *continued*

  - Calcitonin—inhibits movement of calcium out of bone, reduces intestinal absorption of calcium, and promotes urinary calcium excretion

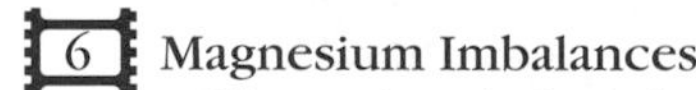

6 Magnesium Imbalances

- Magnesium is found mostly in bones with some in the intracellular and extracellular fluid
- Serum magnesium range—1.3 to 2.1 mEq/L or 1.6 to 2.6 mg/dL
- Extracellular magnesium affects neuromuscular irritability and contractility. The kidneys control conservation or excretion of magnesium

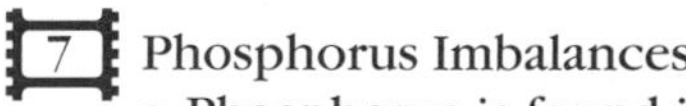

7 Phosphorus Imbalances

- Phosphorus is found in all body tissues and is the primary anion in intracellular fluid with very small amount in extracellular fluid
- Serum phosphorus range—2.5 to 4.5 mg/dL
- Phosphorus is important for energy (ATP) production, metabolism, and red blood cell function. Phosphate, ionized form of phosphorus, is responsible for its effects
- An inverse relationship exists between phosphorus and calcium. When one increases, the other decreases

Suggestions for Classroom Activities

1. Discuss the body's fluid composition, emphasizing the importance of water in the body, the process of fluid movement within the fluid compartments, and the function of electrolytes in body fluids. Assign the students to study the normal daily intake of water and the normal ranges of the electrolytes, and be prepared to discuss them in class.
2. Discuss the key terms used in transporting fluids across cell membranes and capillary walls

Suggestions for Clinical Activities

Compare and contrast the assessment data for fluid deficit and fluid excess and for electrolyte imbalances for assigned clients in the health care setting. What are the similarities in the assessment findings?

Learning Outcome 3

Identify tests used to diagnose and monitor treatment of fluid, electrolyte, and acid-base disorders.

Concepts for Lecture

1. Diagnostic studies, laboratory tests, and invasive monitoring help determine and monitor fluid status, electrolyte status, and acid-base disorders.

PowerPoint Lecture Slides

1 Laboratory Tests for Fluid Balance, Sodium, and Potassium Disorders

- Serum electrolytes
- Serum osmolality
- Hematocrit and hemoglobin
- Urine specific gravity and osmolality
- Liver and kidney function tests for fluid volume excess
- 24-hour urine specimen to evaluate sodium excretion
- Arterial blood gases
- Serum glucose

POWERPOINT LECTURE SLIDES *continued*

1a Laboratory Tests for Calcium, Phosphorus, and Magnesium Disorders
- Total serum calcium
- Serum magnesium
- Serum phosphate
- Serum parathyroid hormone

1b Diagnostic Studies and Invasive Monitoring
- Central venous pressure (CVP)
  - Box 7-2 Measuring Central Venous Pressure with a Manometer
- Electrocardiogram

1c Laboratory/Diagnostic Studies for Acid–Base Imbalances
- Arterial blood gas studies
  - Table 7-12 Normal Arterial Blood Gas Values
- Serum electrolytes
- Serum creatinine and BUN
- Electrocardiogram

SUGGESTIONS FOR CLASSROOM ACTIVITIES

1. Discuss the use of arterial blood gas findings to identify the types of acid–base imbalances present in a client.
2. Review the procedures for performing the laboratory and diagnostic studies. What preparation needs to be done prior to conducting the studies? What needs to be done after completing the procedure? What teaching needs to be done with the client?

SUGGESTIONS FOR CLINICAL ACTIVITIES

Assign students to hospital clients who are recovering in a post intensive care unit. Review with students the laboratory and diagnostic studies and arterial blood gas results of clients. When clients were experiencing significant imbalances, what was the clinical picture? What treatments were ordered? What was the client's response?

LEARNING OUTCOME 4

Recognize normal and abnormal values of electrolytes in the blood.

CONCEPTS FOR LECTURE

1. Hyponatremia and hypernatremia lead to neurologic manifestations. Excessively low or high sodium levels are considered critical and require immediate attention.
2. Both hypokalemia and hyperkalemia affect cardiac conduction and function. Carefully monitor cardiac rhythm and status in clients with very low or very high potassium levels.
3. Calcium imbalances primarily affect neuromuscular transmission: Too little calcium causes increased neuromuscular irritability; too much calcium depresses neuromuscular transmission. Magnesium imbalances have a similar effect.
4. Magnesium imbalances affect neuromuscular transmission, the central nervous system, cardiovascular system, and metabolism of potassium and calcium.
5. Phosphorus imbalances

POWERPOINT LECTURE SLIDES

1 Hyponatremia
- Loss of sodium or water gain that dilutes extracellular fluid
- Serum sodium < 135 mEq/L
- Affects functioning of voluntary and involuntary muscles; brain cells swell, leading to neurologic manifestations and possible brain damage
- Table 7-5 Sodium Imbalances

1a Hypernatremia
- Gain of sodium in excess of water or loss of water in excess of sodium
- Serum sodium > 145 mEq/L
- Dehydration of brain cells leads to neurologic manifestations and dry, sticky mucous membranes
- Table 7-5 Sodium Imbalances

2 Hypokalemia
- Excess potassium loss or insufficient intake
- Serum potassium level < 3.5 mEq/L

© 2007 Pearson Education, Inc.

PowerPoint Lecture Slides *continued*

- Loss through the kidneys, gastrointestinal tract, or shift into the intracellular space from alkalosis, rapid tissue repair, or high insulin levels affects transmission of nerve impulses and the normal contractility of smooth, skeletal, and cardiac muscle, resulting in cardiac dysrhythmias
- Table 7-6 Potassium Imbalances

3 Hyperkalemia

- Abnormally high serum potassium
- Serum potassium > 5 mEq/L
- Inadequate potassium excretion, excessive potassium intake, or shift of potassium from intracellular to extracellular fluid can alter neuromuscular function, resulting in decreased cardiac contractility, weakness of skeletal muscles and gastrointestinal symptoms
- Table 7-6 Potassium Imbalances

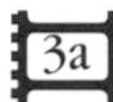

Hypocalcemia

- Low calcium levels due to having parathyroid glands removed, being an older adult or alcoholic, taking drugs that interfere with calcium absorption or promote calcium excretion
- Serum calcium < 8.5 mg/dL
- Insufficient ionized calcium in the extracellular fluid causes neuromuscular excitability or tetany. Critically low levels can cause respiratory or cardiac arrest or convulsions
- Table 7-8 Calcium Imbalances

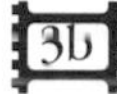

Hypercalcemia

- High calcium levels due to increased calcium release (resorption) from bones, increased calcium intake, and decreased renal excretion of calcium
- Serum calcium > 10.0 mg/dL
- Increased resorption of calcium from bones may result from hyperparathyroidism and excess hormone secretion, prolonged immobilization, malignancies (lung, breast, multiple myeloma), impaired renal excretion of calcium, resulting in sedative effect on neuromuscular transmission to skeletal, smooth, and cardiac muscles. Behavior is disturbed with excess calcium in cerebrospinal fluid. Kidney stones occur from excess calcium in urine. Critically high levels cause heart block and cardiac arrest
- Table 7-8 Calcium Imbalances

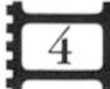

Hypomagnesemia

- Total body deficit of magnesium. Body stores may be depleted when serum magnesium levels are normal
- Serum magnesium < 1.3 mEq/L or 1.6 mg/dL
- Insufficient magnesium increases neuromuscular excitability, affects electrical conduction of the heart and the central nervous system, and affects potassium and calcium metabolism. Common in chronic alcoholism
- Table 7-10 Magnesium Imbalances

© 2007 Pearson Education, Inc.

PowerPoint Lecture Slides *continued*

4 Hypermagnesemia
- Excess amounts of magnesium caused by renal insufficiency or failure, excessive intake of magnesium-containing antacids or laxatives, and magnesium treatments in complications of pregnancy
- Serum magnesium > 2.1 mEq/L or 2.6 mg/dL
- Elevated levels interfere with neuromuscular transmission and depress the central nervous system; affects cardiovascular and respiratory functioning
- Table 7-10 Magnesium Imbalances

5 Hypophosphatemia
- Deficit in phosphate or shift of phosphate out of extracellular fluid into cells due to decreased absorption of phosphate from gastrointestinal tract or increased excretion by the kidneys
- Serum phosphate < 2.5 mg/dL
- Deficit of phosphate results in depletion of cellular energy resources for vital processes in the cell and tissue hypoxia due to decreased ability of red blood cells to transport oxygen. Alcoholism can cause severe hypophosphatemia
- Table 7-11 Phosphorus Imbalances

5a Hyperphosphatemia
- Excess phosphorus due to acute or chronic renal failure and impaired renal excretion, increased phosphate intake or absorption
- Serum phosphate > 4.5 mg/dL
- Phosphate is released into extracellular fluid when cells are damaged or destroyed, resulting in excess serum levels
- Table 7-11 Phosphorus Imbalances

Suggestions for Classroom Activities

Divide the class into four groups. Assign each group to present the functions of each major electrolyte. Include the manifestations of each excess or deficit, and the corrections for the excess or deficit. Have the groups formulate a nursing care plan for each imbalance.

Suggestions for Clinical Activities

Review with students which of their clients are receiving diuretic therapy. What are the classifications of diuretics? How do diuretics affect the electrolyte results? Do the clients follow any diet modifications or take supplements? What teaching should be given to the individual clients?

Learning Outcome 5

Use arterial blood gas results to identify the type of acid-base imbalance present in a client.

Concepts for Lecture

1. Acid-base imbalances may be caused by either metabolic or respiratory problems.
2. Buffers, lungs, and kidneys work together to maintain acid-base balance in the body. Buffers respond to changes almost immediately; the lungs respond within minutes; the kidneys, however, require hours to days to restore normal acid-base balance.

PowerPoint Lecture Slides

1 Acid-Base Regulation
- Acids are produced by metabolic processes in the body
- Volatile acids can be eliminated as gas, i.e., carbonic acid dissociates into carbon dioxide and water

© 2007 Pearson Education, Inc.

CONCEPTS FOR LECTURE *continued*

3. The lungs compensate for metabolic acid-base imbalances by excreting or retaining carbon dioxide. Increasing or decreasing the rate and depth of respirations accomplishes this.
4. The kidneys compensate for respiratory acid-base imbalances by producing and retaining or excreting bicarbonate, and by retaining or excreting hydrogen ions.
5. There are two major categories of acid-base imbalances: acidosis and alkalosis.

POWERPOINT LECTURE SLIDES *continued*

- Nonvolatile acids must be metabolized or excreted from the body in fluid, i.e., lactic acid, hydrochloric acid

2 Buffer System
- Buffers prevent changes in pH by attaching to or releasing hydrogen ions
- Major buffer systems are:
  - Bicarbonate-carbonic acid buffer system
  - Phosphate buffer system
  - Protein buffers
- Hemoglobin acts as a buffer in red blood cells

2a Buffer System
- Normal serum bicarbonate level: 24 mEq/L
- Normal carbonic acid serum level: 1.2 mEq/L
- Bicarbonate-to-carbonic acid ratio of 20:1 maintains a pH of 7.35 to 7.45

3 Respiratory System
- Regulates carbonic acid by eliminating or retaining carbon dioxide
- Increase in carbon dioxide or hydrogen ions stimulates respiratory center in brain to increase rate and depth of respirations
  - Eliminates carbon dioxide, carbonic acid levels fall, and pH becomes normal
- Alkalosis depresses the respiratory center, causing rate and depth of respirations to decrease; carbon dioxide is retained
  - Retained carbon dioxide combines with water; carbonic acid levels and pH return to normal

4 Renal System
- Regulate bicarbonate levels in extracellular fluid to excrete or retain hydrogen ions
- Excessive hydrogen ions cause pH to fall; kidneys excrete hydrogen ions and retain bicarbonate
- Excessive bicarbonate levels cause the kidneys to retain hydrogen ions and excrete bicarbonate to restore acid-base balance

5 Two Major Categories of Acid-Base Imbalances
- Acidosis
  - Hydrogen ion concentration increases above normal
  - pH falls below 7.35
- Alkalosis
  - Hydrogen ion concentration decreases below normal
  - pH rises above 7.45

5a Acidosis
- Metabolic acidosis
  - Bicarbonate is decreased
  - pH < 7.35, bicarbonate < 22 mEq/L, $Pa_{CO_2} < 35$ mm Hg
- Respiratory acidosis
  - Carbon dioxide is retained, increasing carbonic acid

© 2007 Pearson Education, Inc.

PowerPoint Lecture Slides *continued*

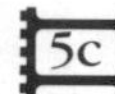 Alkalosis

- Metabolic alkalosis
  - Excessive bicarbonate
- Respiratory alkalosis
  - Carbon dioxide decreases, carbonic acid decreases

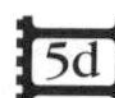 Acid-Base Disorders

- Primary or simple disorders
  - One cause respiratory or metabolic
  - Compensated by amount of change in pH
    - Kidneys alter bicarbonate and hydrogen
    - Lungs change rate and depth of respirations
- Mixed disorders
  - Metabolic and respiratory imbalances are present

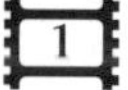 Acid-Base Disorders

- Box 7-13 Nursing Care Checklist: Interpreting Arterial Blood Gas

Suggestions for Classroom Activities

Divide the class into four groups. Have the groups present the causes and manifestations of primary acid-base imbalances. Include the normal lab values, the abnormal lab values, and compensatory mechanisms for each imbalance.

Suggestions for Clinical Activities

Arrange for students to observe arterial blood gases being drawn. Review the client's record for arterial blood gas results. Assist the students to determine the type of acid-base imbalance. Have the students identify causative factors in the client's case that led to the acid-base imbalance.

Learning Outcome 6

Provide appropriate nursing care and teaching for clients with fluid, electrolyte, or acid-base disorders.

Concepts for Lecture

1. Careful monitoring of respiratory and cardiovascular status, mental status, neuromuscular function, and laboratory values is an important nursing responsibility for all clients with fluid, electrolyte, or acid-base imbalances.

PowerPoint Lecture Slides

1 Fluid Volume Deficit

- Replace fluid and electrolytes enterally or intravenously
- Box 7-3 Nursing Care Checklist: Intravenous Infusion
- Table 7-3 Commonly Administered Intravenous Fluids
- Box 7-4 Assessing for Fluid Volume Deficit
- Priority of care is restoring blood and fluid volume
- Teach ways to prevent fluid volume deficit: recommended fluid intake, avoid overexposure to heat and exercise, and monitor weight
- Box 7-5 Assessing for Fluid Volume Imbalance

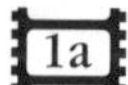 Fluid Volume Excess

- Sodium-restricted diet
  - Box 7-6 Foods High in Sodium
- Restricted fluid intake
  - Box 7-7 Nursing Care Checklist: Fluid Restriction Guidelines

© 2007 Pearson Education, Inc.

POWERPOINT LECTURE SLIDES *continued*

- Medications
  - Table 7-4 Nursing Implications for Pharmacology: Fluid Volume Excess
- Box 7-8 Assessing for Fluid Volume Excess
- Priorities of care are to decrease excess fluid volume and hypervolemia
- Teach fluid and sodium restrictions and medication administration
  - Box 7-9 Teaching Clients about a Low-Sodium Diet

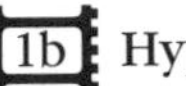

Hyponatremia

- Intake of foods high in sodium
  - Box 7-6 Foods High in Sodium
- Restrict oral fluids
- Administer sodium-containing intravenous fluids
- Medications
  - Administer loop diuretic and sodium replacement to remove excess water
- Priority of care is to increase sodium intake or decrease excess water
- Teach importance of drinking liquids containing sodium and other electrolytes when perspiring heavily, in hot environment, or experiencing prolonged watery diarrhea

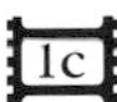

Hypernatremia

- Correct water deficit
- Medications
  - Administer diuretics to increase sodium excretion
- Prescribe low-sodium diet
- Priorities of care are to decrease sodium intake and increase water intake
- Teach low-sodium diet and sufficient water intake

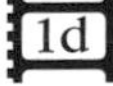

Hypokalemia

- Potassium replacement orally or intravenously
  - Table 7-7 Nursing Implications for Pharmacology: Hypokalemia
- Increased intake of foods high in potassium
  - Box 7-10 Foods High in Potassium
- Priorities of care are early identification and monitoring of cardiac status
- Teach high-potassium diet, administering potassium supplements, and regular follow-up assessment

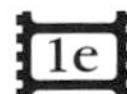

Hyperkalemia

- Medications
  - Administer loop diuretics, sodium polystyrene sulfonate (Kayexalate)
  - Administer intravenous insulin, glucose, sodium bicarbonate, and calcium gluconate
- Administer hemodialysis or peritoneal dialysis
- Priorities of care are early detection and monitoring of cardiac status
- Teach administration of medications, low-potassium diet, obtaining regular laboratory tests, and follow-up care

POWERPOINT LECTURE SLIDES *continued*

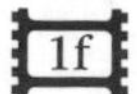 Hypocalcemia

- Medications
  - Administer oral calcium replacements and vitamin D
  - Administer intravenous calcium chloride, calcium gluconate, or calcium gluceptate via slow IV push or infusion
  - Table 7-9 Nursing Implications for Pharmacology: Hypocalcemia
- Increase dietary intake of calcium
- Priority of care is to replace deficient calcium to prevent dysrhythmias and seizures.
- Teach dietary intake of calcium foods and vitamin D, administration of medications, and follow-up care

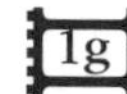 Hypercalcemia

- Medications
  - Administer intravenous normal saline solution
  - Administer diuretics
  - Administer biphosphonates, calcitonin, intravenous plicamycin, glucocorticoids
- Decrease dietary intake of calcium
  - Box 7-11 Foods High in Calcium
- Priorities of care are to monitor mental status, monitor respiratory and cardiac status, protect against injury due to falls from muscular weakness and fatigue, and decrease incidence of kidney stones
- Teach administration of medications, decreased dietary intake of calcium, increased dietary intake of fiber, and encourage weight-bearing activities

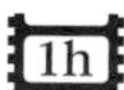 Hypomagnesemia

- Medications
  - Administer oral magnesium supplements, such as antacids
  - Administer magnesium via IV or deep intramuscular injection
- Increase dietary intake of foods high in magnesium
  - Box 7-12 Foods High in Magnesium
- Priorities of care are to monitor deep tendon reflexes and serum magnesium levels
- Teach administration of magnesium supplements, dietary intake of magnesium foods, and referrals for alcohol problems

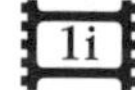 Hypermagnesemia

- Medications
  - Withhold all medications and solutions containing magnesium
  - Administer IV calcium to counteract cardiac effects
- Perform hemodialysis or peritoneal dialysis if renal failure
- Mechanical ventilation to support respirations

© 2007 Pearson Education, Inc.

POWERPOINT LECTURE SLIDES *continued*

- Priorities of care are to monitor cardiac and respiratory status, changes in neuromuscular excitability, and gastrointestinal function
- Teach to avoid magnesium-containing medications and to decrease dietary intake of magnesium foods

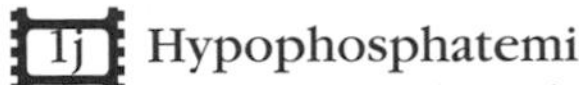

1j Hypophosphatemia

- Increase phosphorus in the diet, especially milk and milk products
- Medications
  - Administer oral phosphorus supplements
  - Administer intravenous phosphate solutions
- Priorities of care are to monitor for signs of phosphate imbalance and serum phosphate levels, and protect from infection
- Teach administration of medications, dietary intake of phosphorus, effects of phosphorus-binding antacids, referrals for alcohol use

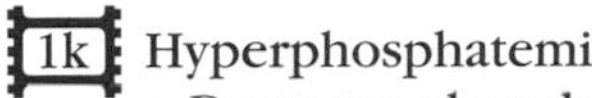

1k Hyperphosphatemia

- Decrease phosphorus in the diet
- Medications
  - Administer aluminum hydroxide (Amphogel)
  - Administer intravenous normal saline
  - Administer glucose and insulin to drive phosphate into cells
- Perform dialysis
- Priorities of care are to monitor and report signs of phosphate imbalance and monitor phosphate levels
- Teach to recognize signs of imbalance, avoid phosphate-containing laxatives and enemas, avoid dietary intake of phosphorus, and to take medications as ordered

1l Metabolic Acidosis

- Table 7-13 Causes and Manifestations of Primary Acid–Base Imbalances
- Insufficient oxygen leads to lactic acidosis
- Affects the central nervous system, gastrointestinal tract, cardiovascular function, Kussmaul's respirations
- Priorities of care are to treat the underlying cause and monitor cardiac and neurologic functioning
- Medications
  - Administer bicarbonate, lactate, acetate, or citrate solutions
- Teach proper diabetes mellitus care to prevent ketoacidosis, obtain treatment for alcoholism with proper diet and medications, manage renal failure with diet and dialysis, prevent or treat diarrhea

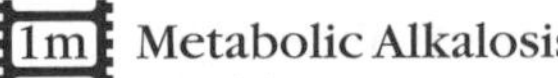

1m Metabolic Alkalosis

- Table 7-13 Causes and Manifestations of Primary Acid–Base Imbalances
- Loss of acid or excess bicarbonate in the body

© 2007 Pearson Education, Inc.

PowerPoint Lecture Slides *continued*

- Respiratory system attempts to return pH to normal by slowing respiratory rate
- Priorities of care are to treat underlying cause, restore normal fluid volume, and monitor respirations
- Medications
  - Administer potassium chloride and sodium chloride solutions
  - Administer dilute hydrochloric acid or ammonium chloride for critically high pH
- Teach how to prevent and manage acute gastroenteritis or vomiting, the advantages of a potassium-rich diet or potassium supplements, and to avoid use of antacids.

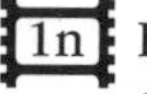

Respiratory Acidosis

- Table 7-13 Causes and Manifestations of Primary Acid–Base Imbalances
- Excess of dissolved carbon dioxide or carbonic acid
- Alveolar hypoventilation leads to carbon dioxide retention
- Bicarbonate is high because the kidneys compensate by retaining bicarbonate
- Priorities of care are to administer oxygen, clear the airways, support ventilation, and provide adequate hydration
- Medications
  - Administer bronchodilator medications
  - Administer antibiotics
  - Administer medications to reverse narcotic and anesthetic effects
- Teach to avoid respiratory infections, to immunize against pneumococcal pneumonia and influenza, and to obtain treatment for narcotic or drug abuse

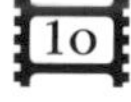

Respiratory Alkalosis

- Table 7-13 Causes and Manifestations of Primary Acid–Base Imbalances
- Hyperventilation leads to carbon dioxide deficit; low carbon dioxide levels cause cerebral blood vessels to constrict and cause a decrease in calcium ionization
- Priorities of care are to breathe slowly into a paper bag or rebreather mask to prevent excess loss of carbon dioxide
- Medications
  - Administer a sedative or antianxiety medication
- Teach to decrease anxiety, to seek counseling, and to identify hyperventilation and how to treat it

Suggestions for Classroom Experience

Use the nursing process case studies in the textbook to show the appropriate nursing care and teaching for clients with fluid, electrolyte, or acid–base disorders.

Suggestions for Clinical Experience

1. Assign the students to care for clients with acid–base imbalances. Have them report the clinical manifestations that the client exhibited, compare them with the textbook, and report observations.

© 2007 Pearson Education, Inc.

2. Assign the students to clients receiving intravenous therapy. Have them calculate the rate of infusion, and discuss the potential complications for a client with intravenous therapy.
3. Assign the students to care for clients who are receiving enteral feedings. Calculate the total calories and intake and output. Are daily/weekly weight measures being performed? How does weight relate to the intake and output? Do clients exhibit behavior consistent with fluid deficit or overload?

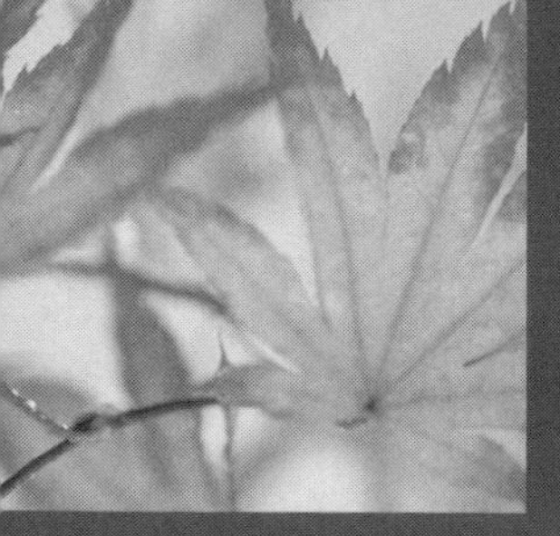

Chapter 8
Caring for Clients in Pain

Resource Library

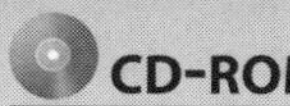

CD-ROM

Naproxen
Morphine

IMAGE LIBRARY

Figure 8-1 Pain conduction. (**A**) **Transduction:** Cutaneous nociceptors send impulses to spinal cord. (**B**) **Transmission:** Impulses synapse in the substantia gelatinosa. (**C**) **Perception:** Pain impulses processed in the thalamus and cerebral cortex. (**D**) **Modulation:** Along efferent fibers from cerebral cortex to substantia gelatinosa, pain may be inhibited or modulated.

Figure 8-2 (**A**) Substance-P transmits pain impulse across synapse between presynaptic neuron and postsynaptic neuron. (**B**) During modulation, endorphins are released from inhibitory neuron, which prevents the release of substance-P, and pain impulse is inhibited.

Figure 8-3 Diagram of gate-control theory. When small-diameter C fibers are stimulated, the gate is open and pain is transmitted. When large-diameter A-delta fibers are stimulated, the gate is closed and pain transmission is stopped.

Figure 8-4 Referred pain begins in one site but is felt in another area. For example, pain from an inflamed gallbladder may be felt in the shoulder, or angina from ischemia of the heart muscle may be felt in the left arm or jaw.

Figure 8-5 Transdermal patch. To apply the patch, clip any hair from the upper body, clean the site with clear water, and dry it. Apply immediately after opening the package by placing it in the palm and pressing firmly onto the prepared site for 30 seconds. Be sure that contact is complete around the edges. A patch lasts for 72 hours, and the next patch is applied on a different site.

Figure 8-6 PCA unit allows the client to self-manage severe pain. It can be mounted on an intravenous pole.

Figure 8-7 Surgical procedures are used to treat severe pain that does not respond to other types of management. They include cordotomy, neurectomy, sympathectomy, and rhizotomy.

Figure 8-8 TENS unit. Electrodes that deliver low-voltage electrical stimuli are placed directly on the client over painful areas.

Figure 8-9 The McGill Pain Questionnaire.

Figure 8-10 Examples of commonly used pain scales. Other examples include pictures of faces (from happy and relaxed to sad and frowning), or colors from bright red (terrible pain) to light blue (no pain).

Figure 8-11 A flow sheet for nursing documentation of pain management.

Figure 8-12 The WHO three-step analgesic ladder.

Learning Outcome 1

Define pain.

Concepts for Lecture

1. Pain affects an individual both physically and emotionally.
2. Pain management can be inadequate in all types of health care settings.
3. The American Pain Society designated pain assessment as the fifth vital sign. Standards for pain management have been developed to focus on client's right to appropriate pain management and intervention.

PowerPoint Lecture Slides

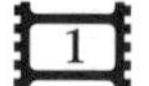

Pain

- "Whatever the person experiencing it says it is, and existing whenever the person says it does."
- All pain should be considered real
- A subjective response to physical and psychologic stressors
- Affected by biologic, psychologic, cognitive, social, cultural, and spiritual factors
- Most common reason for seeking health care

PowerPoint Lecture Slides *continued*

2 Factors Affecting Pain Perception and Management
- Lack of understanding about pain management
- Fear of addiction
- Positive or negative bias by nurse
- Subjective response may impair judgment

3 Pain as Fifth Vital Sign
- Pain should be routinely assessed (American Pain Society)
- Standards for pain management developed by
  - Agency for Health Care Policy and Research
  - Joint Commission for the Accreditation of Healthcare Organizations

Suggestions for Classroom Activities

1. Initiate a discussion on the causes of pain, and the rationale for pain as a fifth vital sign.
2. Discuss the organizations that set guidelines for pain management.

Suggestions for Clinical Activities

Students should check the standards of pain management that are being followed in the health care facilities they are using for clinical rotations.

Learning Outcome 2

Describe the steps of pain conduction: transduction, transmission, perception, and modulation.

Concepts for Lecture

1. Pain impulses are initiated by direct tissue damage and by release of internal chemicals.
2. Pain is transmitted through the four steps of transduction, transmission, perception, and modulation.
3. The gate-control theory of pain states that pain impulses traveling from the skin to the spinal cord can be stopped at the spinal cord or allowed to be transmitted to the brain by opening or closing the gate by stimulation of nerve fibers.

PowerPoint Lecture Slides

1 Physiology of Pain
- Table 8-1 Pain Stimuli
- Tissue damage causes inflammation
- Inflammation causes release of bradykinin and prostaglandin, which activate nociceptors
- Nociceptors are nerve endings that are activated by painful stimuli

2 Pain Conduction
- Transduction
  - Change of noxious stimulus into electrical action potential stimulus
  - Sends impulses transmitted by afferent A-delta fibers and small C nerve fibers throughout central nervous system
- Transmission
  - Sending impulses from afferent neurons to spinal cord
  - Substance-P sends impulse across synapse to travel to brain

2a Pain Conduction
- Perception
  - Processing of pain impulse in thalamus and cerebral cortex
  - Pain threshold—point at which pain is recognized
  - Pain tolerance—amount and duration of pain person can stand before seeking relief
- Modulation
  - Body attempts to decrease perception of pain
  - Endorphins bind with opiate receptors and inhibit release of substance-P

PowerPoint Lecture Slides *continued*

3 Gate-Control Theory
- Pain impulse travels from skin to spinal cord
- Stimulation of large and small nerve fibers can open or block the pain transmission to the brain

Suggestions for Classroom Activities

1. Initiate a discussion on the different methods of pain conduction.
2. Assign students to groups of four. Have each group present a theory of pain, and role-play the therapeutic measures for the theory.
3. Initiate a discussion on the types of pain pathways. Divide the class into groups of four, and assign each group to present a pathway.

Learning Outcome 3

Identify the characteristics of acute and chronic pain.

Concepts for Lecture

1. Acute pain is usually a short-term event, whereas chronic pain is prolonged.
2. Neuropathic pain is pain caused by damage to the central nervous system or peripheral nerves or following surgical or traumatic amputation of a limb.
3. Psychogenic pain results from emotional rather than physical causes.

PowerPoint Lecture Slides

1 Acute Pain
- Temporary, lasts less than 6 months
- Sudden onset
- Localized
- Has an identified cause
- Caused by tissue injury
- Has physical responses

1a Chronic Pain
- Prolonged, lasts more than 6 months
- May not have identifiable cause
- Unresponsive to conventional medical treatment
- Has psychologic responses
- Nonmalignant pain or malignant pain

1b Table 8-2 Comparison of Acute and Chronic Pain

2 Neuropathic Pain
- Caused by damage to central nervous system or peripheral nerves
- Burning or tingling sensation
- Allodynia
  - Pain that results from stimulus usually not causing pain
- Phantom pain
  - Surgical or traumatic removal of a limb
  - Itching, tingling, pressure, or burning, stabbing sensations

3 Psychogenic Pain
- Emotional rather than physical causes

Suggestions for Classroom Activities

Ask the students to relate their personal experiences with acute and chronic pain. Ask them to describe their pain threshold and pain tolerance levels. Are these levels different as a child? What cultural factors influence the coping skills for pain?

Suggestions for Clinical Activities

Interview a client with pain. Determine the signs and symptoms the client is exhibiting. Classify the type of pain as to whether acute or chronic.

© 2007 Pearson Education, Inc.

Learning Outcome 4

Differentiate characteristics of the four types of acute pain.

Concepts for Lecture

1. Acute pain is classified into four different types: cutaneous, deep somatic, visceral, and referred pain.

PowerPoint Lecture Slides

1 Types of Acute Pain
- Cutaneous pain
  - Injury to skin or superficial tissue
  - Sharp, burning, cutting, well localized
- Deep somatic pain
  - Injury to deep body structures
  - Dull, diffuse
- Visceral pain
  - Injury to body organs
  - Deep, dull, poorly localized
- Referred pain
  - Starts at one site but is perceived in another site

Suggestions for Classroom Activities

Discuss causes and signs and symptoms of the various types of pain.

Suggestions for Clinical Activities

Assign students in the clinical area to clients with each type of pain. Have student perform a pain assessment and present their findings in postconference.

Learning Outcome 5

Identify factors that may affect a client's response to pain.

Concepts for Lecture

1. A person's response to pain is shaped by age, sociocultural factors, emotional state, past experiences with pain, meaning of pain, and person's knowledge base.
2. Pain management includes medications such as nonopioids, opioids, and adjuvant analgesics, and nonpharmacologic therapies including relaxation, distraction, massage, and TENS.
3. Nonopioids are used to manage mild to moderate pain; opioids are given for moderate to severe pain; and adjuvant analgesics are used in chronic pain.
4. Route of administration affects the onset and duration of pain relief.

PowerPoint Lecture Slides

1 Factors Affecting Client Response to Pain
- Age
- Sociocultural factors
- Emotional status
- Past perception with pain
- Meaning of pain
- Knowledge deficit

2 Medications Used in Pain Management
- Analgesics
  - Opioids
  - Nonopioids
- Adjuvant Analgesics
  - Anticonvulsants, antidepressants, systemic anesthetics, corticosteroids, psychostimulants

3 Table 8-4 Equianalgesic Dosage Chart

4 Routes of Medication Administration
- Oral
- Rectal
- Transdermal
- Intramuscular
- Intravenous
- Subcutaneous
- Intraspinal
  - Box 8-1 Nursing Care of the Client Receiving Intraspinal Anesthesia
- Nerve block

© 2007 Pearson Education, Inc.

Suggestions for Classroom Activities

Divide the students into groups of four. Assign each group a method of pain relief, such as pharmacology and surgery.

Suggestions for Clinical Activities

Have the students evaluate pain management of assigned clients, and present the findings in postconference. Ask the students to assess what factors are affecting the client's response to his or her pain. Discuss effectiveness of different routes of pain medication administration.

Learning Outcome 6

Describe pain rating scales and their use in assessing pain.

Concepts for Lecture

1. The first step in relieving the client's pain is to conduct an accurate, unbiased, and thorough assessment of the client's pain.
2. Pain intensity is assessed by using a pain rating scale.

PowerPoint Lecture Slides

1 Box 8-2 Assessing for Pain

2 Pain Rating Scales
- Numerical scales from 1 to 10
- Word descriptor scale
- Color scales
- Wong-Baker Faces Pain Rating Scale

Suggestions for Classroom Activities

1. Discuss each step in assessing clients for pain.
2. Explain how to use various forms of pain-rating scales.

Suggestions for Clinical Activities

Have the students utilize pain-rating scales in the clinical setting. Discuss which pain-rating scale is appropriate to use based on age, developmental level, and culture.

Learning Outcome 7

Explain the nurse's role in administering medications to reduce or relieve pain.

Concepts for Lecture

1. The nurse assumes an important role in assessing the client's pain and working collaboratively with the physician to implement appropriate pain-reducing methods.
2. Clients receiving opioids must be monitored for side effects of sedation, respiratory, nausea, and constipation.

PowerPoint Lecture Slides

1 Responses to Pain
- Physiologic
  - Sympathetic nervous system responses
- Behavioral
  - May result from cultural factors, coping skills, fear, denial
  - May use relaxation or distraction

1a Box 8-4 Pain Management Guidelines for the Older Adult

2 Table 8-3—Nursing Implications of Pharmacology: Acetaminophen, NSAIDS, Opioids

Suggestions for Classroom Activities

1. Using Box 8-4, initiate a discussion on the guidelines and rationales for managing pain in the elderly.
2. Discuss the responsibilities of the nurse in pain management.
3. Discuss the Critical Thinking Care Map, and have the students answer the questions associated with the map.

Suggestions for Clinical Activities

In postconference, discuss pain management used with assigned clients in the clinical setting. Compare signs and symptoms of pain exhibited by the clients. Evaluate whether pain management was effective or not.

© 2007 Pearson Education, Inc.

Learning Outcome 8

Describe nonpharmacologic interventions clients may use in reducing or relieving pain.

Concepts for Lecture

1. Surgery for pain relief is performed only after all other methods have failed. The client needs to understand the implications of having surgery for pain relief.
2. To accomplish pain control, the client may use nonpharmacologic pain-relief strategies.

PowerPoint Lecture Slides

1 Pain Relief Surgeries
- Cordotomy
- Neurectomy
- Sympathectomy
- Rhizotomy

2 Alternative Pain Relief
- Transcutaneous Electrical Nerve Stimulation (TENS)

2a Complementary Therapies for Pain Relief
- Acupuncture
- Biofeedback
- Relaxation
- Distraction
- Hypnotism
- Cutaneous Stimulation
  - Table 8-5 Methods of Cutaneous Stimulation

Suggestions for Classroom Activities

Have students research alternative or complementary therapies of pain relief. Present the findings to the class.

Suggestions for Clinical Activities

Assign students to attend a pain management clinic and have them observe the types of pain management used with the clients.

Learning Outcome 9

Identify several myths and misconceptions about pain and pain management.

Concepts for Lecture

1. Numerous misconceptions about pain and its management exist among clients and health care professionals. The nurse must understand these misconceptions before appropriate nursing care can be delivered.

PowerPoint Lecture Slides

1 Box 8-3 Misconceptions about Pain Management

Suggestions for Classroom Activities

Discuss the misconceptions of pain management. Ask each student to relate personal and familial misconceptions about pain management.

Learning Outcome 10

Use the nursing process in care of clients experiencing pain.

Concepts for Lecture

1. All pain relief measures must incorporate an individualized and preventive approach.

PowerPoint Lecture Slides

1 Nursing Process in Pain Management
- Assessment of pain and client's perception of pain
  - Use pain-rating scale

PowerPoint Lecture Slides *continued*

- Diagnosing, Planning, and Implementing
  - Explore misconceptions
  - Consider priorities of care
  - Prevent side effects
- Evaluating
  - Determine effectiveness of pain management strategies
  - Give teaching points in writing to client
  - Make referrals as needed

Suggestions for Classroom Activities

Using the nursing process, discuss the nurse's role as caregiver in pain relief.

Suggestions for Clinical Activities

Have students develop a plan of care for pain management for assigned clients.

© 2007 Pearson Education, Inc.

CHAPTER 9
CARING FOR CLIENTS HAVING SURGERY

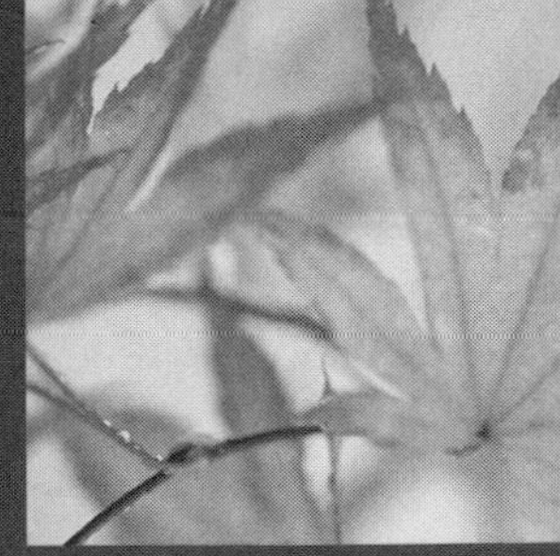

RESOURCE LIBRARY

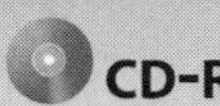

CD-ROM

Video: Preoperative and Postoperative Care
Video: Blood Test Basics
Diazepam
Video: Assisting the Client to Use a Bed Pan

IMAGE LIBRARY

Figure 9-1 Informed consent to operation, administration of anesthetics, and the rendering of other medical services.
Figure 9-2 A scrub nurse in the operating room.
Figure 9-3 (A) Surgical attire. (B) Sterile surgical attire.
Figure 9-4 Surgical areas to be scrubbed. (A) Head surgery. (B) Abdominal surgery. (C) Thoracoabdominal surgery. (D) Gynecologic surgery. (E) Genitourinary surgery. (F) Forearm, elbow, or hand surgery. (G) Hip surgery. (H) Lower leg or foot surgery.
Figure 9-5 Wound healing by primary, secondary, and tertiary intention.
Figure 9-6 Wound complications. (A) Dehiscence. (B) Evisceration.
Figure 9-7 Outpatient care plan form.

LEARNING OUTCOME 1

Describe the classifications of surgical procedures.

CONCEPTS FOR LECTURE

1. Surgical procedures can be classified according to purpose, risk factor, and urgency.
2. Two types of surgeries are performed: inpatient or outpatient.
3. Perioperative nursing includes care of the client through three phases: preoperative, intraoperative, and postoperative.

POWERPOINT LECTURE SLIDES

1 Classification of Surgical Procedures
- Purpose
- Risk factors
- Urgency
- Table 9-1 Classification of Surgical Procedures

2 Types of Surgeries
- Inpatient
  - Admitted to hospital before and after surgery
- Outpatient
  - Performed outside of the hospital
  - Under local or general anesthesia

3 Phases of Perioperative Nursing
- Preoperative phase
- Intraoperative phase
- Postoperative phase

SUGGESTIONS FOR CLASSROOM ACTIVITIES

Describe the classifications of surgical procedures.

SUGGESTIONS FOR CLINICAL ACTIVITIES

Assign the students to the preoperative intake room, the operating room, and the postanesthesia care unit. Have the students write their observations of the events occurring in these units. Also ask the students to identify the health care professionals that work within these units and their duties.

LEARNING OUTCOME 2

Identify laboratory and diagnostic tests used in the perioperative period.

CONCEPTS FOR LECTURE

1. Laboratory and diagnostic tests are performed prior to surgery to provide baseline data and to detect problems that may place a client at risk during and after surgery.

POWERPOINT LECTURE SLIDES

1 Laboratory and Diagnostic Studies Used in the Preoperative Period
- Complete blood count (CBC)
- Serum electrolytes
- Coagulation studies
- Urinalysis
- Chest x-ray
- Electrocardiogram (ECG)

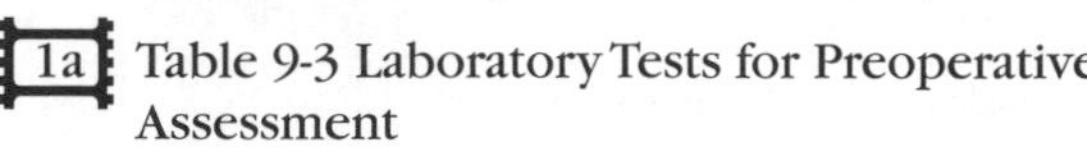

1a Table 9-3 Laboratory Tests for Preoperative Assessment

SUGGESTIONS FOR CLASSROOM ACTIVITIES

Divide the class into small groups. Assign each group to present the laboratory and diagnostic tests performed preoperatively. Discuss the nursing implications for each examination.

SUGGESTIONS FOR CLINICAL ACTIVITIES

Assign students to look up the laboratory and diagnostic studies of a perioperative client. Have them identify parameters that need to be reported to the health care provider.

LEARNING OUTCOME 3

Describe nursing implications for medications prescribed for the surgical client.

CONCEPTS FOR LECTURE

1. The nurse is responsible for administering preoperative medications at the time ordered or when called for by the operative personnel so that desired effects can be obtained.
2. Anesthesia is the use of chemical substances to produce loss of sensation, reflex loss, or muscle relaxation during a surgical procedure, with or without loss of consciousness.

POWERPOINT LECTURE SLIDES

1 Table 9-4 Preoperative Medications and Nursing Implications

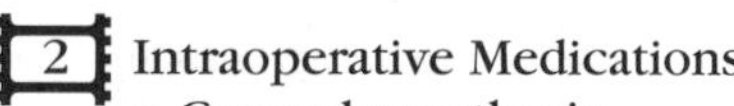

2 Intraoperative Medications
- General anesthesia
- Regional anesthesia
- Conscious sedation
- Antidotes for reversal of effects

SUGGESTIONS FOR CLASSROOM ACTIVITIES

Divide the class into small groups. Assign the students to research the types of anesthesia used for different surgical procedures.

SUGGESTIONS FOR CLINICAL ACTIVITIES

Have the students review the client's operative record and postanesthesia record for the types of medications used. Have them make drug cards of these medications.

LEARNING OUTCOME 4

Discuss appropriate nursing care for the client in the preoperative, intraoperative, and postoperative phases of surgery.

CONCEPTS FOR LECTURE

1. Care of the surgical client should focus on psychologic as well as physiologic risk factors.
2. Thorough nursing assessment is key to identifying potential risk factors that may lead to perioperative complications.

POWERPOINT LECTURE SLIDES

1 Physical Preparation of the Client for Surgery
- Skin preparation
- Insertion of indwelling urinary catheter
- Bowel preparation
- Withholding of food and fluids

© 2007 Pearson Education, Inc.

CONCEPTS FOR LECTURE *continued*

3. All surgical team members have a vital role in the success of the surgery, but nurses are responsible for maintaining the safety of the client and the environment and for providing physiologic monitoring and psychologic support.
4. Nursing interventions are developed to prevent development of perioperative complications.
5. Nursing care of the postoperative client focuses on preventing and monitoring for complications.

POWERPOINT LECTURE SLIDES *continued*

1a Psychological Preparation of the Client and Family for Surgery
- Significant and stressful event that produces anxiety
- Listen actively to verbal and nonverbal communication
- Establish trusting relationship
- Use of therapeutic communication

1b Informed Consent
- Legal document required for procedures or therapeutic measures
- Protects the client, nurse, physician, health care facility
- Most states require 18 years of age or older to sign
- Married minors and emancipated minors may sign consent
- Spouses, children, significant other cannot sign instead of a capable adult

2 Table 9-2 Nursing Implications for Surgical Risk Factors

2a Preoperative Assessment
- Medical history
- Accurate height and weight
- Assistance after the surgical procedure
- Understanding of surgical procedure
- Informed consent
- Vital signs

3 Surgical Team
- Surgeon
- Surgical assistant
- Anesthesiologist
- Circulating nurse
- Scrub nurse

4 Nursing Interventions to Prevent Perioperative Complications
- Surgical attire
- Surgical scrub
- Client preparation
- Table 9-5 Common Surgical Positions

5 Nursing Interventions to Promote Wound Healing
- Wounds heal by primary, secondary, and tertiary intention
- Monitor for wound drainage
  - Serous drainage
  - Sanguineous drainage
  - Purulent drainage
- Teach client wound care
- Box 9-4 Wound Drainage Devices

© 2007 Pearson Education, Inc.

SUGGESTIONS FOR CLASSROOM ACTIVITIES

Divide the class into small groups. Assign the groups to present the common risk factors and the nursing interventions for the client undergoing surgery.

SUGGESTIONS FOR CLINICAL ACTIVITIES

1. Assign the students to work with a nurse who is preparing a client for surgery. Have the students observe preoperative client teaching and review the laboratory and diagnostic tests, informed consent form, preoperative medications, and the items on the preoperative checklist. Have the students share their observations in postconference.
2. Arrange for the students to follow a client to surgery, observe the surgery, and stay with the client in the postanesthesia unit. Have them review the surgeon's operative note, postoperative orders, and the postanesthesia recovery record. Have them compare their experiences in postconference.
3. Assign the students to provide nursing care for clients returning to the nursing unit after surgery. Assist them with postoperative assessment and pain management. Have them review postoperative orders.

LEARNING OUTCOME 5

Identify variations in perioperative care for the older adult.

CONCEPTS FOR LECTURE

1. The older adult is at increased risk for postoperative complications because of the physiologic, cognitive, and psychosocial changes associated with the aging process. The nurse must be aware of these normal changes and must modify nursing care accordingly to provide safe, supportive care.

POWERPOINT LECTURE SLIDES

1 Box 9-3 Older Adult Undergoing Surgery

SUGGESTIONS FOR CLASSROOM ACTIVITIES

Identify variations in preoperative, intraoperative, and postoperative care for the older adult. What impact does the client's medical history have on the surgery experience? What risk factors for surgery complications are present in the older adult?

SUGGESTIONS FOR CLINICAL ACTIVITIES

Assign students to care for older adults who have recently had surgery. Assist the students to identify risks for variations in the perioperative experience, based on the client's medical history and type of surgery. What interventions can be performed to decrease the likelihood of complications?

LEARNING OUTCOME 6

Describe principles of pain management for postoperative pain control.

CONCEPTS FOR LECTURE

1. Control of postoperative pain is a major concern of the surgical client.

POWERPOINT LECTURE SLIDES

1 Postoperative Medications
- Opioid analgesics
- Nonsteroidal anti-inflammatory drugs

SUGGESTIONS FOR CLASSROOM ACTIVITIES

Discuss medications used for postoperative pain, dosage, routes, side effects, and nursing implications for administering the medications.

SUGGESTIONS FOR CLINICAL ACTIVITIES

Assign the students to administer pain medications to postoperative clients. Have them make drugs cards on these medications.

© 2007 Pearson Education, Inc.

Learning Outcome 7

Compare and contrast outpatient and inpatient surgery.

Concepts for Lecture

1. Outpatient, ambulatory, or same-day surgery is performed on a nonhospitalized client under local or general anesthesia.
2. Inpatient surgery is performed on a hospitalized client under regional, general, or conscious sedation anesthesia.

PowerPoint Lecture Slides

1 Outpatient Surgery

- Nonhospitalized client
- Administered local or general anesthesia
- Discharged immediately after procedure or short time after procedure
- More cost effective than inpatient care
- Physical care same as inpatient surgery
- Teaching and emotional support differ from inpatient surgery

2 Inpatient Surgery

- Hospitalized client
- Administered regional, general, or conscious sedation anesthesia
- Costly
- Teaching and emotional support differ from outpatient surgery

Suggestions for Classroom Activities

Ask students to volunteer to role-play a health care professional and a client who is undergoing inpatient surgery, and a client who is undergoing outpatient surgery. Compare and contrast the preparation needed for each type of surgery. Compare the psychologic impact of a client undergoing inpatient versus outpatient surgery.

Suggestions for Clinical Activities

1. Arrange for students to attend an outpatient surgery unit. Have the students assist with the preoperative checklist, preoperative teaching, and preparing the client for surgery. Have the students observe during the surgical procedure and in the postoperative unit. In postconference, have students compare this experience with a surgical rotation in the health care setting.
2. Arrange for students to have a clinical experience in a surgeon's office. Have them follow several clients through the office visit, observing preoperative and postoperative visits. What assessment data do the office personnel obtain? What teaching is completed and what educational materials are made available for the clients?

Learning Outcome 8

Use the nursing process to provide care for the client undergoing surgery.

Concepts for Lecture

1. Patient education is a critical tool to prepare the client for the perioperative experience. Inclusion of family members and caregivers is essential for success of the nursing plan of care.
2. Major postoperative complications include respiratory and cardiovascular disorders, infection, hemorrhage, and elimination disorders.
3. Because the postoperative phase does not end until recovery is complete, the nurse's role is to prepare the client to recuperate at home.

PowerPoint Lecture Slides

1 Preoperative Teaching

- Laboratory and diagnostic tests
- Prescribed preparations
- Time to arrive at the hospital
- Preparations for day of surgery
- Medication taken night before
- Informed consent
- Timetable for surgery and recovery room
- Location of waiting area
- Procedure for transfer to recovery room

© 2007 Pearson Education, Inc.

PowerPoint Lecture Slides *continued*

- Anticipated postoperative routine and devices or equipment
- Postoperative pain control

1a Box 9-1 Client Teaching: Preoperative Exercises

1b Box 9-2 Nursing Care Checklist: Day of Surgery

2 Postoperative Complications
- Cardiovascular complications
  - Shock
  - Hemorrhage
  - Deep venous thrombosis
  - Pulmonary embolism

2a Postoperative Complications
- Respiratory complications
  - Pneumonia
  - Atelectasis
- Elimination complications
  - Urinary retention
  - Altered bowel elimination

2b Postoperative Complications
- Wound complications
  - Infection
  - Dehiscence
  - Evisceration

3 Postoperative Teaching
- Wound care
- Manifestations of a wound infection
- How and when to take a temperature
- Limitations or restrictions on activities
- Control of pain

Suggestions for Classroom Activities

Divide students into small groups and assign them a case study of a surgical client. Have them develop a plan of care based on the nursing process.

Suggestions for Clinical Activities

Have the students formulate a nursing care plan or a concept map using the nursing process for an assigned perioperative client in the health care setting.

© 2007 Pearson Education, Inc.

CHAPTER 10
CARING FOR CLIENTS WITH INFLAMMATION AND INFECTION

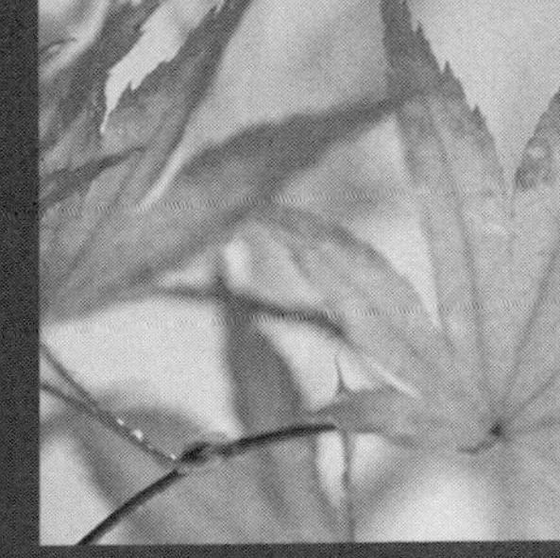

RESOURCE LIBRARY

CD-ROM

Video: Decubitus Ulcers
Penicillin

IMAGE LIBRARY

Figure 10-1 (A) Leukocytes in the circulation. (B) Diapedesis, the process of leukocytes moving from inside the capillary to injured tissue.
Figure 10-2 The process of phagocytosis. (A) Opsonization coats the surface of the bacterium with IgG (an antibody) and complement. (B) The bacterium is bound to and engulfed by the phagocyte. (C) The phagosome is ingested into the cytoplasm of the phagocyte. (D) Lysosomes fuse with the phagosome, releasing digestive enzymes and destroying the antigen.
Figure 10-3 Lymph nodes that may be assessed by palpation.
Figure 10-4 The chain of infection.
Figure 10-5 Neutrophils by stage of maturity and normal distribution in the blood versus shift to left caused by severe infection.

LEARNING OUTCOME 1

Explain the steps of the inflammatory process.

CONCEPTS FOR LECTURE

1. Inflammation is a "nonspecific" response to an injury that develops as soon as one or more harmful invaders injure the body's cells.
2. The body is protected from microorganisms by the skin, physical barriers such as coughing, and chemical defenses.
3. Three steps are involved in the inflammatory response: vascular response, cellular response, and healing and tissue repair.

POWERPOINT LECTURE SLIDES

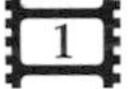

1 Inflammation
- "Nonspecific" response to an injury
  - Same sequence of events regardless of the cause
- Fluid, dissolved substances, and blood cells enter interstitial tissues of injury.
- Purpose is to:
  - Destroy the harmful agent
  - Limit spread to other tissue
  - Begin healing process

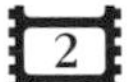

2 Causes of Inflammation
- Mechanical causes
- Physical damage
- Chemical injury
- Microorganisms
- Extremes of heat or cold
- Immunologic responses
- Ischemic damage or trauma

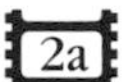

2a Factors to Help Host Resist Infection
- Physical barriers
- Hostile environment
- Antimicrobial factors
- Coughing, sneezing, cilia in respiratory tract
- Neutrophils and macrophages

POWERPOINT LECTURE SLIDES *continued*

3 Three Steps of Inflammatory Response
- Vascular response
- Cellular response
- Healing and tissue repair

3a Box 10-1 Inflammatory Changes in the Older Adult

SUGGESTIONS FOR CLASSROOM ACTIVITIES

1. Discuss the pathophysiology of the inflammatory response. Explain the three steps involved in the inflammatory response. Ask the students to identify the assessment data that can be collected at each step.
2. Divide the class into three groups. Assign the students to one of the following scenarios. Ask the students to describe the inflammatory response in each of the scenarios. If applicable, explain how to prevent transmission of microorganisms. Have groups present the information to the class.
   Scenario A: A 43-year-old female accidentally burns herself while cooking steamed vegetables.
   Scenario B: A 35-year-old male with compound fracture of the left femur has been placed in traction with wound care prescribed. Three days later, signs of infection appear.
   Scenario C: A 25-year-old female employee reports signs and symptoms of a cold. About 72 hours later, two other employees report signs and symptoms of a cold.

LEARNING OUTCOME 2

State the five cardinal manifestations of acute inflammation.

CONCEPTS FOR LECTURE

1. Acute inflammation is a short-term reaction of the body to any tissue damage.
2. Cardinal manifestations of local inflammation are redness, warmth, pain, edema, and loss of function.
3. Management of the client with an inflammation focuses on promoting healing.

POWERPOINT LECTURE SLIDES

1 Acute Inflammation
- Short-term reaction of the body to any tissue damage
- Lasts less than 1 to 2 weeks
- Produces local and systemic manifestations
- Subsides when harmful agent is removed

2 Cardinal Manifestations of Acute Inflammation
- Redness
- Warmth (fever)
- Pain
- Edema
- Loss of function

3 Box 10-2 Manifestations of Inflammation

4 Management of Acute Inflammation
- Wound care
- Encourage rest
- Eat a well-balanced diet, high in carbohydrates and protein with vitamin supplements and extra fluids
- Receive anti-inflammatory medications, antibiotics, corticosteroids
- Apply cold or heat therapy
- Elevate inflamed area

5 Table 10-2 Nursing Implications for Pharmacology: Clients Receiving Anti-Inflammatory Drugs

© 2007 Pearson Education, Inc.

Suggestions for Classroom Activities

1. Discuss the five cardinal manifestations of acute inflammation.
2. Discuss the alterations in the body systems of the elderly that result in a decrease in the inflammatory response time. Explain how the cardinal manifestations may be diminished or absent in the elderly.

Suggestions for Clinical Activities

Have students administer anti-inflammatory drugs in the clinical setting. Discuss implications for giving the medications and nursing interventions to perform related to anti-inflammatory drugs.

Learning Outcome 3

State the purpose of diagnostic tests used to diagnose inflammation and infection.

Concepts for Lecture

1. Fever and WBC count greater than 10,000/mm^3 may indicate a generalized infection.

PowerPoint Lecture Slides

1 Diagnostic Tests to Diagnose Inflammation and Infection
- WBC count with differential
- Erythrocyte sedimentation rate
- C-reactive protein (CRP)
- Cultures of wound, blood, or other infected body fluids
- Sensitivity studies
- Lumbar puncture
- Ultrasound examination

1a Table 10-1 White Blood Cell Count and Differential

Suggestions for Classroom Activities

Discuss the use of laboratory tests to diagnose inflammation and infection.

Suggestions for Clinical Activities

1. Review proper techniques and instruction for obtaining cultures and other laboratory tests. Have students obtain tests when available in the clinical setting.
2. Assign students to clients diagnosed with wound infection. Ask them to review laboratory tests and antibiotic therapy. Ask the students to present the progress of the infection based on the laboratory tests. What were the presenting symptoms and is there improvement in symptoms after beginning antibiotics?

Learning Outcome 4

Describe the chain of infection.

Concepts for Lecture

1. The chain of infection includes a microorganism, a reservoir, a portal of exit from the reservoir, a mode of transmission from the reservoir, and an entry point into a susceptible host.
2. Infectious disease usually follows a predictable course through five stages as it develops.

PowerPoint Lecture Slides

1 Chain of Infection
- Microorganism
- Reservoir
- Portal of exit from reservoir
- Mode of transmission from reservoir to host
- Entry point into a susceptible host

1a Box 10-4 Pathogenic Organisms

1b Table 10-3 Common Infectious Diseases and the Causative Organism

© 2007 Pearson Education, Inc.

PowerPoint Lecture Slides *continued*

2 Stages of the Infectious Process
- Initial stage is incubation period
- Prodromal stage is symptom stage
- Acute stage is pathogen reproduction and increasing manifestations
- Convalescent stage is pathogen destruction and tissue repair
- Resolution is healing of infection

Suggestions for Classroom Activities

Describe the chain of infection.

Suggestions for Clinical Activities

Arrange for students to attend a Wound Care Clinic or to spend time with an enterostomal therapist to see wounds in different stages of the infectious process. Discuss various treatments used to promote wound healing. Discuss the educational needs of the client.

Learning Outcome 5

Identify common nosocomial infections.

Concepts for Lecture

1. Nosocomial infections are infections acquired in a health care setting, such as a hospital or long-term facility.
2. Antibiotic-resistant microorganisms have developed that make common antibiotics ineffective for treating infections.
3. Community-acquired infections are usually referred to as communicable diseases, because they can be transmitted to other people, and are monitored by the World Health Organization (WHO).

PowerPoint Lecture Slides

1 Nosocomial Infections
- Infection acquired in a health care setting
- Two million clients a year develop a nosocomial infection
- Increase hospital stays
- Costly in terms of diagnosis and treatment

1a Box 10-5 Risk Factors for Nosocomial Infections

2 Antibiotic-Resistant Microorganisms
- Methicillin-resistant *Staphylococcus aureus* (MRSA)
- Vancomycin-resistant enterococcus (VRE)
- Penicillin-resistant *Streptococcus* pneumococci (PRSP)
- *Clostridium difficile*-associated diarrhea (CDAD)

Community-Acquired Infections
- Communicable diseases
- Emerging infectious diseases
- Biologic threat infections

Suggestions for Classroom Activities

Discuss the risk factors in the hospital for acquiring a nosocomial infection, such as exposure to infectious microorganisms, invasive procedures, indwelling tubes, nutritional status, and medications that lower immunities.

Suggestions for Clinical Activities

1. Arrange for students to work in an immunization clinic or a nursing home. Have them administer vaccines for influenza and pneumonia to the clients. Review contraindications for not receiving immunizations.
2. Assign students to perform an assessment on patients who are at risk for nosocomial infections, and review principles that will help prevent nosocomial infections.

© 2007 Pearson Education, Inc.

LEARNING OUTCOME 6

Explain age-related changes in older adults that increase their risk for infection.

CONCEPTS FOR LECTURE

1. Older adults are at greater risk for developing pneumonia, influenza, and urinary tract and skin infections.

POWERPOINT LECTURE SLIDES

1 Table 10-5 Special Population: Common Infectious Diseases in Older Adults, Age-Related Changes, and Nursing Implications

2 Age-Related Factors that Increase Risk of Infectious Disease
- Decreased activity
- Poor nutrition and risk for dehydration
- Chronic diseases
- Chronic medication use
- Lack of recent influenza and pneumococcal vaccinations
- Altered mental status and dementias
- Hospitalization or residence in a long-term facility

SUGGESTIONS FOR CLASSROOM ACTIVITIES

Discuss the risk factors for developing infections in the older adult.

SUGGESTIONS FOR CLINICAL ACTIVITIES

Assess nutrition in an older adult. Is the older adult getting the proper nutrition to prevent infections? What teaching needs to be done to promote good nutrition?

LEARNING OUTCOME 7

Identify the common antimicrobial medications, nursing implications, and client teaching guidelines.

CONCEPTS FOR LECTURE

1. Antibiotics, antiviral, antifungal, and antiparasitic medications are the common medications used to manage infections.
2. Antibiotic peak and trough levels monitor therapeutic blood levels of prescribed medications.

POWERPOINT LECTURE SLIDES

1 Antimicrobial Therapy
- Drugs that are capable of killing or incapacitating pathogens
- Includes antibiotic, antifungal, antiviral, and antiparasitic drugs
- Bacteriostatic drugs: inhibit growth of microorganism
- Bactericidal drugs: kill the microorganism
- Narrow-spectrum drugs: act against limited number of pathogens
- Broad-spectrum drugs: act against wide variety of pathogens

1a Routes of Administration
- Topical
- Oral
- Intramuscular
- Intravenous
- Interperitoneal
- Intrathecal

1b Factors to Consider
- History of allergic reactions
- Client's age and childbearing status
- Client's present health status
- Renal and hepatic function

© 2007 Pearson Education, Inc.

POWERPOINT LECTURE SLIDES *continued*

- Site and extent of the infection
- History of chronic diseases and other drug therapy

1c Table 10-6 Nursing Implications for Pharmacology: Clients Receiving Antibiotic Therapy

1d Table 10-7 Nursing Implications for Pharmacology: Clients Receiving Antifungal and Antiviral Drugs

2 Laboratory Studies
- Culture and sensitivity prior to administering antimicrobial
- Peak and trough after a specified number of doses of antimicrobial

SUGGESTIONS FOR CLASSROOM ACTIVITIES

Using the tables in the chapter, discuss the different categories of anti-infective medications, emphasizing the purposes, nursing implications, and client teaching needed for each medication.

SUGGESTIONS FOR CLINICAL ACTIVITIES

1. In the clinical setting, have students review the medical history of their clients for immunization status. Have them ask their clients if they know why immunizations are important.
2. Assess laboratory studies for antibiotic peak and trough levels. Discuss what to do if the levels are too high or too low.

LEARNING OUTCOME 8

Describe the guidelines for Standard and Transmission-based Precautions.

CONCEPTS FOR LECTURE

1. Hand washing is the most important measure in preventing nosocomial infections.
2. Two tiers of isolation are (1) Standard Precautions, and (2) Transmission-based Precautions.

POWERPOINT LECTURE SLIDES

1 Prevention of Nosocomial Infections
- Hand washing
  - Most important measure in infection control
  - For at least 15 seconds
  - Use friction
  - Use antimicrobial soap
- Clean clothing and good hygiene
- Current immunizations
- No illness or open skin lesions when caring for clients
- Follow infection control policies, CDC and OSHA guidelines

2 Isolation Precautions
- Standard Precautions
- Transmission-based Precautions

2a Standard Precautions
- Protect health care worker and client
- Use barrier protection for direct client care and exposure to body fluid
  - Box 10-6 Standard Precaution Guidelines

© 2007 Pearson Education, Inc.

POWERPOINT LECTURE SLIDES *continued*

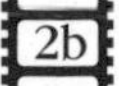
2b Transmission-based Precautions
- Airborne Precautions
- Droplet Precautions
- Contact Precautions
- Table 10-4 Transmission-based Precautions

SUGGESTIONS FOR CLASSROOM ACTIVITIES

Discuss the differences in the two tiers of isolation precautions: Standard and Transmission-based Precautions.

SUGGESTIONS FOR CLINICAL ACTIVITIES

Discuss the importance of hand washing and have students teach clients the importance of hand washing.

LEARNING OUTCOME 9

Use the nursing process to collect data, establish outcomes, provide individualized care, and evaluate responses for clients with inflammation and infections.

CONCEPTS FOR LECTURE

1. Nursing management of clients with an inflammation or infectious disease focuses on prevention, health promotion, and health maintenance. The nursing process is utilized to guide the nurse in client care.

POWERPOINT LECTURE SLIDES

1 Box 10-3 Assessing Clients with Inflammation

1a Box 10-7 Assessing Clients with Infection

1b Nursing Diagnoses
- Risk for Infection
- Imbalanced Nutrition
- Ineffective Thermoregulation

1c Evaluation of Effectiveness of Nursing Care
- Temperature remains normal for 24 hours
- No signs of dehydration
- Clear breath sounds
- Cultures negative for pathogens
- Client takes precautions to prevent spread of infection
- Client completes antibiotic therapy
- Teaching focuses on promoting client recovery, preventing spread of infection to others, and preventing potential complications

SUGGESTIONS FOR CLASSROOM ACTIVITIES

Review the steps of the nursing process and how it can be utilized for the client with an inflammation or infection.

SUGGESTIONS FOR CLINICAL ACTIVITIES

Assign students to clients with an inflammation or infectious process. Have them develop an appropriate nursing care plan for this client.

© 2007 Pearson Education, Inc.

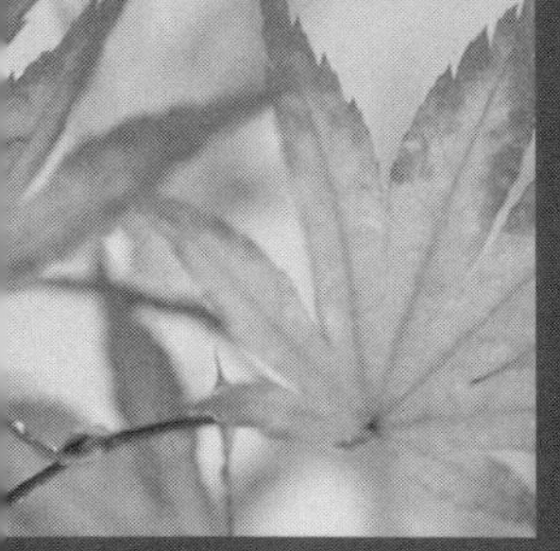

Chapter 11
Caring for Clients with Altered Immunity

Resource Library

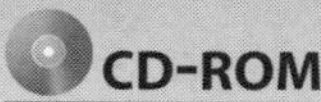

Lymphocytes
B Cells
T Cells
Diphenhydramine
Methotrexate
HIV
Video: AIDS
Zidovudine

IMAGE LIBRARY

Figure 11-1 The development and differentiation of lymphocytes from the lymphoid stem cell (lymphoblasts).

Figure 11-2 The lymphoid system: the central organs of the thymus and bone marrow, and the peripheral organs, including the spleen, tonsils, lymph nodes, and Peyer's patches.

Figure 11-3 Humoral immunity. *Primary response:* During first exposure to an antigen, B cells are stimulated to become plasma cells and produce antibodies or memory cells. *Secondary response:* With reexposure to the same antigen, the memory cells respond rapidly with antibody production.

Figure 11-4 Cellular immunity. (**A**) An infected cell with an antigen on its surface binds with a receptor site on a cytotoxic T or a helper T cell. The cytotoxic T cell produces memory cells or mature cytotoxic cells. (**B**) The helper T cell assists the cytotoxic activity of the cytotoxic cells and stimulates B cells to produce antibodies.

Figure 11-5 Skin testing on the forearm showing induration (hardness) and erythema (redness) typical of a positive response to an antigen.

Figure 11-6 How HIV infects and destroys CD4 cells.

Figure 11-7 The progression of HIV infection. The primary infection begins shortly after contracting the virus, corresponding with a rapid rise in viral levels. Antibodies are formed and remain throughout the infection. Late in the disease, viral activity increases destroying CD4 (T4) cells. Antibody levels gradually decrease as immune function is impaired.

Figure 11-8 Wasting syndrome in a client with AIDS.

Learning Outcome 1

Describe the functions of the lymphoid organs and tissues.

Concepts for Lecture

1. The immune system consists of leukocytes, lymphoid organs (bone marrow, thymus, spleen, lymph nodes), and peripheral lymph tissues such as the tonsils and appendix.
2. The immune system protects the body against infection-causing microorganisms, foreign substances, and cancerous cells.
3. When antigens enter the body, a specific immune response occurs.

PowerPoint Lecture Slides

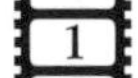

1 Immune System Components

- Leukocytes
    - Table 11-1 Cells of the Immune System
    - Natural killer cells
- Lymphoid Organs and Tissues
    - Bone marrow
    - Thymus
    - Spleen
    - Lymph nodes
    - Lymphatic system

PowerPoint Lecture Slides *continued*

2 Defense Mechanisms that Provide Protection
- First line of defense: skin
- Second line of defense: body's inflammatory response
- Third line of defense: immunity

3 Immune Responses
- Humoral immunity
  - Table 11-2 Immunoglobulin Characteristics and Functions
- Cell-mediated immunity
  - T lymphocytes (T cells)

Suggestions for Classroom Activities

1. Using transparencies, discuss the structure and function of the lymphoid organs and tissues.
2. Discuss the different cells of the immune system and their functions.

Learning Outcome 2

Compare natural and acquired immunity and active and passive immunity.

Concepts for Lecture

1. Natural or acquired immunity is a person's resistance to foreign substances.
2. Active immunity provides long-term immunity either by developing the disease or by an immunization. Passive immunity is short term and involves injecting serum with ready-made antibodies for other humans or animals.

PowerPoint Lecture Slides

1,2 Types of Immunity
- Natural immunity
- Active immunity
  - Naturally acquired—having disease
  - Artificially acquired—immunizations
- Passive immunity
  - Naturally acquired—neonates receive antibodies from mothers
  - Artificially acquired—injecting serum with antibodies

Suggestions for Classroom Activities

Discuss the various types of immunity. Compare acquired immunity with active and passive immunity. Give examples of each type. Describe the types of immunizations or vaccines that are required for prevention.

Learning Outcome 3

List recommended immunizations for adult clients.

Concepts for Lecture

1. Immunizations or vaccines are suspensions of live, attenuated, or killed microorganisms that promote active immunity against a specific organism.

PowerPoint Lecture Slides

1 Types of Immunizations or Vaccines
- Inactivated vaccines
- Live, attenuated vaccines
- Toxoids

1a Table 11-3 Recommended Immunizations for Adults

© 2007 Pearson Education, Inc.

Suggestions for Classroom Activities

Divide the class into two groups. Assign one group to perform the role of a nurse who is assigned to give immunizations in a community health clinic. The other group would be the clients receiving the immunizations. The nursing process should be incorporated into the role-playing.

Suggestions for Clinical Activities

Assign students to clinics where allergy shots and immunizations are administered. Have students administer allergy shots and immunizations. Have them fill out drug cards on the ones they administered.

Learning Outcome 4

Identify laboratory and diagnostic tests used to diagnose and monitor immune response.

Concepts for Lecture

1. Laboratory and diagnostic tests can measure the level of immunity in the body.
2. Several tests may be ordered to diagnose hypersensitivity reactions.
3. Serum assays are used to identify increased levels of antibodies to diagnose specific autoimmune disorders.
4. Basic laboratory and diagnostic tests are performed prior to any surgery but additional studies are performed before organ or tissue transplant.
5. Diagnostic studies are performed to provide evidence of tissue rejection.

PowerPoint Lecture Slides

1 Laboratory/Diagnostic Tests to Measure Level of Immunity

- Serum immunoglobulins
  - Measure levels of immunoglobulins
  - Table 11-2 Immunoglobulin Characteristics and Functions
- Antibody titer testing
  - Identify antibody titer levels
- Skin testing
  - Detect impaired cell-mediated immunity

2 Laboratory/Diagnostic Tests to Detect Hypersensitivity

- Radioallergosorbent test (RAST)
  - Measure IgE to specific allergens
- Skin tests
  - Identify specific allergens
- Prick test
  - To determine possibility of systemic reaction
- Intradermal
  - To determine reaction to allergen
- Patch
  - To determine allergy to allergen

3 Serum Assays to Identify Levels of Antibodies Specific to Autoimmune Disorders

- Antinuclear antibody (ANA) test
  - Specific to screen for systemic lupus erythematosis
- Rheumatoid factor (RF)
  - Specific to screen for rheumatoid arthritis

4 Laboratory/Diagnostic Tests Required for Transplantation

- Blood type and Rh Factor
- Cross-matching
- HLA histocompatibility testing
- Mixed lymphocyte culture

5 Diagnostic Studies to Detect Tissue Rejection

- Ultrasound
- Magnetic resonance imaging
- Tissue biopsies

© 2007 Pearson Education, Inc.

Suggestions for Classroom Activities

Review laboratory and diagnostic tests used to diagnose and monitor immune response. Give examples of results for increased or decreased levels of the studies.

Suggestions for Clinical Activities

Assign students to care for clients in a nursing home or hospital who have autoimmune disorders. Review the client's history, signs and symptoms, medications, and diagnostic test results. The tests should include WBC counts, differentials, and serologic assay tests, including ANA, RA factor, and LE prep. Assist the students to assess the assigned clients' learning needs.

Learning Outcome 5

Describe the nursing implications for medications ordered for clients with altered immunity.

Concepts for Lecture

1. Hypersensitivity reactions range from mild such as hay fever to severe (e.g., blood transfusion reactions, anaphylaxis, and organ transplant rejections).
2. Before administering immunizations, the nurse should collect assessment data to determine whether the immunization is appropriate.
3. Medications can provide symptomatic relief for reaction to a medication.
4. Treatment of autoimmune disorders focuses on medications that relieve symptoms.
5. Specific medications are given pre- and post-transplantation to prevent tissue rejection.

PowerPoint Lecture Slides

1 Altered Immune Responses
- Hypersensitivity
  - Table 11-4 Types of Hypersensitivity Reactions
- Latex allergy
  - Box 11-2 Natural Rubber Latex Products

1a Hypersensitivity Reactions to Medications
- Local reaction
  - Redness, swelling, tenderness, muscle ache
- Systemic reaction
  - Fever, malaise
- Anaphylactic reaction
  - Acute, allergic reaction

2 Box 11-1 Assessing Clients: Immune Status

3 Medications to Relieve Reactions to Medications
- Epinephrine
- Antihistamines
  - Table 11-5 Nursing Implications for Pharmacology: Clients Receiving Antihistamines
- Nasal decongestants
- Glucocorticoids
- Desensitization

4 Medications to Relieve Symptoms of Autoimmune Disorders
- Anti-inflammatory medications
- Antirheumatic medications
- Cytotoxic medications
  - Table 11-7 Nursing Implications for Pharmacology: Clients Receiving Immunosuppressive Agents

5 Medications to Prevent Tissue Rejection
- Preoperative medications
  - Antibiotics
  - Antiviral agents

© 2007 Pearson Education, Inc.

POWERPOINT LECTURE SLIDES *continued*

- Postoperative medications
  - Immunosuppressive drugs
  - Corticosteroids
  - Cytotoxic agents
  - Monoclonal antibodies
  - Antilymphocyte globulins
  - Table 11-7 Nursing Implications for Pharmacology: Clients Receiving Immunosuppressive Agents

SUGGESTIONS FOR CLASSROOM ACTIVITIES

1. Identify products that can be used as alternatives to latex products for clients with latex allergies.
2. Discuss the nursing implications for medications ordered for clients with altered immunity.

SUGGESTIONS FOR CLINICAL ACTIVITIES

1. Interview clients who have had a reaction to medications or blood transfusions or have had organ transplant rejections. Find out what reactions they had and the treatment that was given.
2. Have students administer medications to assigned clients with altered immunity. Discuss the use, dosage, route, side effects, and nursing implications for administering medications. Have students complete drug cards for the medications administered.

LEARNING OUTCOME 6

Teach clients with altered immune responses and their families.

CONCEPTS FOR LECTURE

1. Autoimmune disorders develop when the body fails to identify self from nonself (e.g., rheumatoid arthritis).
2. Because autoimmune disorders are chronic, the client and family need to understand care for the client and the long-term effects of the disorder.

POWERPOINT LECTURE SLIDES

1 Box 11-3 Autoimmune Disorders

2 Client Teaching for Clients with Autoimmune Disorders
- Stress reduction techniques
- Good nutrition
- Medication use and side effects
- Remission of the disorder
- Referrals to support groups or agencies

SUGGESTIONS FOR CLASSROOM ACTIVITIES

Compare and contrast the signs and symptoms, treatment, and nursing interventions for clients with autoimmune disorders.

SUGGESTIONS FOR CLINICAL ACTIVITIES

Assign students to care for clients with autoimmune disorders. Have them develop a discharge teaching plan for the assigned client.

LEARNING OUTCOME 7

Use the nursing process to collect data, establish outcomes, provide individualized care, and evaluate responses for the client experiencing altered immunity.

CONCEPTS FOR LECTURE

1. Nursing care is individualized for the client with an autoimmune disorder.
2. The client who has undergone an organ or tissue transplant has immediate and long-term nursing care needs. Pre- and post-transplant care focuses on reducing the risk of tissue rejection.

POWERPOINT LECTURE SLIDES

1 Use of the Nursing Process
- Assessment data provides the basis for managing a chronic disorder
- Nursing diagnoses and outcomes identify the problems of the client
- Interventions are individualized for client care
- Evaluation is ongoing due to the chronic disorder

© 2007 Pearson Education, Inc.

PowerPoint Lecture Slides *continued*

2 Types of Transplants
- Autograft—client's own tissue
- Autologous—client's own bone marrow and blood
- Isograft—twin transplant
- Allograft—graft between members of same species
- Xenograft—transplant from animal to human
- Histocompatibility—compatibility of transplant

2a Transplant Rejection
- Hyperacute rejection
- Acute rejection
- Chronic rejection
- Graft-versus-host disease
- Table 11-6 Transplant Rejection Episodes

Suggestions for Classroom Activities

1. Discuss the nursing process to collect data, establish outcomes, provide individualized care, and evaluate responses for clients experiencing altered immunity.
2. Divide the students into groups of four. Have the groups design care plans for clients with altered immunity.

Suggestions for Clinical Activities

Arrange for students to have a clinical experience in a hospital with a transplant program. Arrange for students to observe transplant surgeries, and for students to participate in the care of clients during the first few days post-transplant. Have them develop a teaching plan for discharge.

Learning Outcome 8

Identify three ways to prevent the transmission of HIV infection.

Concepts for Lecture

1. The human immunodeficiency virus (HIV) is the cause of acquired immunodeficiency syndrome (AIDS).
2. HIV attacks helper T4 lymphocytes, which decrease a person's ability to remain immunocompetent, and increases the risk for developing opportunistic infections.
3. Education and counseling are the key elements for HIV prevention.

PowerPoint Lecture Slides

1 Routes of Transmission
- Direct person to person through sexual contact
- Direct injection with contaminated blood, blood products, needles
- Mother to fetus

2 Opportunistic Infections
- Respiratory System
  - *Pneumocystis carinii* pneumonia
  - Tuberculosis
  - *Mycobacteria avium* complex
- Gastrointestinal system
  - Candidiasis
  - Cryptosporidiosis
  - Wasting syndrome
- Neurologic System
  - Toxoplasmosis and cryptococcis
- Other Infections
  - Herpes simplex 1 and 2
  - Cytomegalovirus
  - Human papillomavirus
  - Pelvic inflammatory disease

2a AIDS Dementia Complex

2b Secondary Cancers
- Kaposi's sarcoma
- Lymphomas

© 2007 Pearson Education, Inc.

PowerPoint Lecture Slides *continued*

3 Prevention of Transmission of HIV Infection
- Educating about safer sexual practices
  - Box 11-5 Guidelines for Safer Sex
- Educate injection drug users
- Screen voluntary blood donors and donated blood supplies
- Use Standard Precautions

Suggestions for Classroom Activities

Initiate a discussion on HIV infection; emphasize transmission, prevention of transmission, laboratory tests used for diagnosis and treatment, infections associated with HIV, and the treatment modalities.

Suggestions for Clinical Activities

1. Have students review the infection control policy of their facility.
2. Have students observe how the staff institutes infection control on the unit and report their observations in postconference.
3. Assign students the task of contacting the employee health department in the hospital. Review the follow-up protocol for health care workers who have experienced needle sticks. What is the policy about HIV testing on hospital clients and the employees involved in needle sticks? What blood tests are drawn? What medical protocols are prescribed?

Learning Outcome 9

Identify laboratory tests used to diagnose HIV and to monitor HIV progression.

Concepts for Lecture

1. The ELISA and Western blot tests detect antibodies to identify if a person is infected with HIV.

PowerPoint Lecture Slides

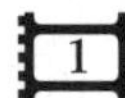

Laboratory Tests to Diagnose HIV and Monitor HIV Progression
- Enzyme-linked immunosorbent assay (ELISA)
- Ora Quick Rapid HIV-1 Antibody Test
- Western blot assay
- HIV viral load test
- CD4 + cell count
- CD4 + CD8 + ratio
- CBC
- Tuberculin skin test
  - Cultures—blood, urine, stool, spinal fluid, sputum

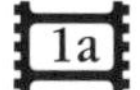

Diagnostic Studies to Diagnose HIV and Monitor HIV Progression
- Magnetic resonance imaging
- Computed tomography

Suggestions for Classroom Activities

Discuss use of each laboratory and diagnostic test for HIV. Review nursing implications for performing these tests.

Suggestions for Clinical Activities

Arrange for students to have clinical experience in a specialist's office or in specialty clinics. Arrange for students to follow clients undergoing allergy testing treatment or clients who are HIV positive or have AIDS.

© 2007 Pearson Education, Inc.

Learning Outcome 10

Provide the nursing management of a client with AIDS, including medications and diet therapy.

Concepts for Lecture

1. Health teaching focuses on safer sex practices, adverse drug reactions, nutrition, and ways to reduce opportunistic infection, to prevent transmission, and to maintain self-care.
2. The client with HIV is managed with a combination of antiretroviral medications, such as zidovudine (AZT) and medications that treat opportunistic infections and malignancies.

PowerPoint Lecture Slides

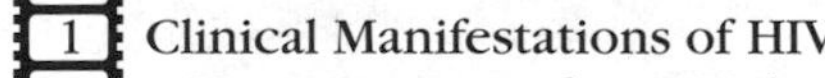

1 Clinical Manifestations of HIV
- No symptoms after initial mononucleosis-like onset
- Severe immunodeficiency with multiple opportunistic infections and cancers
- Box 11-4 Manifestations of HIV Infection

1a Box 11-6 Assessing Clients with HIV Infection and AIDS

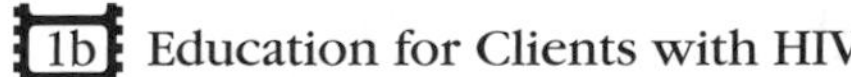

1b Education for Clients with HIV
- Understand HIV infection and AIDS
- How to maintain optimal health
- Use of hand washing and disinfection procedures
- Use of gloves and Standard Precautions
- Strategies to avoid opportunistic infections and signs and symptoms of opportunistic infections
- Stop smoking and eliminate alcohol and recreational or illicit drugs
- Use of prescribed medications
- Use of referrals and support groups

2 Medications Used for HIV Infections
- Antiretroviral Medications
  - Table 11-8 Nursing Implications for Pharmacology: Clients Receiving Antiretroviral Agents

2a Medications Used to Treat Opportunistic Infections and Malignancies
- Table 11-9 Pharmacologic Treatment of Opportunistic Infections and Malignancies

Suggestions for Classroom Activities

1. Ask the students to explore their feelings about taking care of the client with an HIV infection. Ask them to describe how they would dispel any negative feelings they may have toward the client.
2. Discuss medications used for clients with HIV; include the use, dosage, route, side effects, and nursing implications of each medication.

Suggestions for Clinical Activities

1. Assign students to care for clients using Isolation Precautions. In postconference, ask the students to describe their feelings and thoughts while caring for the client.
2. Assign students to administer medications to clients with HIV infections. Have students make drug cards on each of the medications they administer.

© 2007 Pearson Education, Inc.

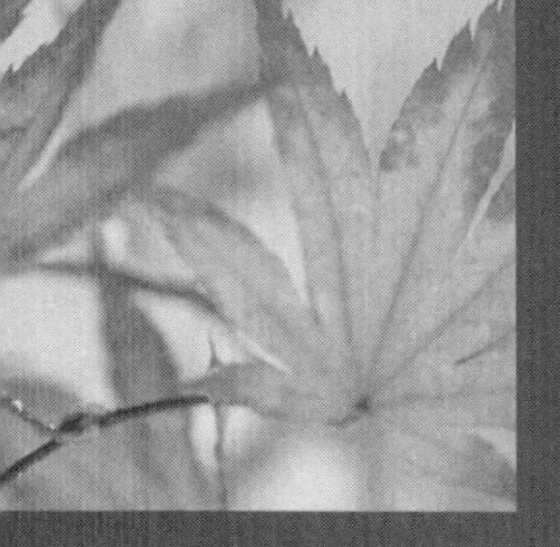

CHAPTER 12
CARING FOR CLIENTS WITH CANCER

RESOURCE LIBRARY

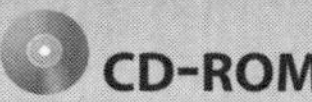

CD-ROM

Video: Skin Cancer
Video: Terminally Ill Patients

IMAGE LIBRARY

Figure 12-1 Metastasis through the bloodstream. Cancer cells disrupt the basement membrane in the blood vessel and gain access into the circulation. Once in the blood, only about 1 cell in 1,000 escapes immune detection, but that can be enough. Undetected cells move out of the blood, entering new tissue. Once in the new site, the malignant cells multiply and establish a metastatic tumor.

Figure 12-2 Cachexic person with cancer. Cancer robs its host of nutrients and increases body catabolism of fat and muscle to meet its demands. Also note alopecia (hair loss) related to chemotherapy.

Figure 12-3 A tunneled vascular access device (VAD) for long-term chemotherapy.

LEARNING OUTCOME 1

Define cancer and differentiate benign from malignant neoplasms.

CONCEPTS FOR LECTURE

1. Cancer is a disease that results when normal cells mutate into abnormal, deviant cells and continue to reproduce within the body. Cancer can affect people of any age, gender, ethnicity, or geographic region.
2. Neoplasms are masses of abnormal cells that grow at a rate uncoordinated with the needs of the body, do not benefit the host, and may be harmful.

POWERPOINT LECTURE SLIDES

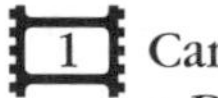

1 Cancer
- Disease that results when normal cells mutate into abnormal, deviant cells
- Abnormal deviant cells reproduce within the body
- Affects people of any age, gender, ethnicity, or geographic region

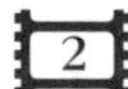

2 Neoplasms
- Mass of abnormal cells that grows independently of its surroundings
- Two types of neoplasms:
  - Benign
  - Malignant
  - Table 12-1 Comparison of Benign and Malignant Neoplasms

SUGGESTIONS FOR CLASSROOM ACTIVITIES

Discuss the different types of cancer, and explain the difference between benign and malignant neoplasms.

LEARNING OUTCOME 2

Discuss the pathophysiology of cancer and factors associated with carcinogenesis.

CONCEPTS FOR LECTURE

1. Pathophysiology of cancer is a disruption in the genetic information coded in the DNA of genes that can produce abnormal cells, which may become cancerous.
2. Metastasis is the spread of malignant cells in the blood or lymph or shed into body cavities. An impairment or alteration of the immune system is a major factor in the establishment of metastatic lesions.
3. Causal factors may act together or in sequence to initiate or promote carcinogenesis. Factors are both external and internal.
4. Many cancer risk factors are controllable; prevention is key.

POWERPOINT LECTURE SLIDES

1 Pathophysiology of Cancer
- Change or disruption in a gene can result in:
  - Inaccurate blueprint coding in DNA
  - Production of abnormal cells that become cancerous

2 Metastasis
- Spread of malignant cells
- Impairment or alteration of the immune system contributes to metastatic lesions
- Common sites of metastasis
  - Table 12-2 Various Cancers and Sites of Metastases

3 Causal Factors of Cancer
- External
  - Chemicals
  - Radiation
  - Viruses
- Internal
  - Hormones, chemotherapeutic drugs, recreational drugs
  - Immune conditions
  - Inherited mutations

4 Risk Factors of Cancer
- Uncontrollable risk factors
  - Heredity, age, gender, poverty
  - Box 12-1 Cancer and the Older Adult
- Controllable risk factors
  - Emotion, diet, weight, occupation, infection, drug and alcohol use, sun exposure, continued stress
  - Occupational risks
  - Infections
  - Cigarette smoking

SUGGESTIONS FOR CLASSROOM ACTIVITIES

Discuss the pathophysiology of cancer and the factors associated with carcinogenesis.

SUGGESTIONS FOR CLINICAL ACTIVITIES

1. Assign a group of students to show poster presentations on risk factors and guidelines to prevent the different categories of cancer.
2. Assign students to care for clients who will undergo surgery or have had surgery to treat cancer in the surgical unit of a hospital. Assist students to correlate the specific type of cancer with this individual client in regard to risk factors, why the client sought medical attention, and associated signs and symptoms. What additional types of treatment are planned for the client after discharge from the hospital?

LEARNING OUTCOME 3

Describe the effects of cancer on the body.

CONCEPTS FOR LECTURE

1. Early detection and treatment are the factors that most influence the prognosis of people with cancer.
2. Clients with cancer need a great deal of emotional support because fear and anxiety are common responses to a diagnosis of cancer.
3. Routine cancer checkups should include counseling to improve health behaviors, physical examination, and instructions for self-examination.

POWERPOINT LECTURE SLIDES

1 Physiologic Manifestations Characteristic of Cancer
- Box 12-2 American Cancer Society Caution Model
- Acute or chronic pain
- Disruption of function
- Hematologic alterations
- Infection
- Hemorrhage
- Anorexia-cachexia syndrome
- Creation of ectopic sites of hormone production
- Physical stress

2 Psychologic Manifestations Characteristic of Cancer
- Stress
- Grief
- Guilt
- Fear and anxiety
- Powerlessness
- Isolation
- Concern for body image
- Sexual dysfunction

3 Routine Cancer Checkups
- Box 12-3 American Cancer Society Guidelines for Cancer Screening

SUGGESTIONS FOR CLASSROOM ACTIVITIES

1. Discuss the effects of cancer on the body, including physiologic and psychologic manifestations.
2. Have students develop posters to demonstrate how to perform self-examinations for cancers.

SUGGESTIONS FOR CLINICAL ACTIVITIES

1. Have students attend a health fair to educate people on how to perform self-examinations for cancer.
2. Have students teach assigned clients how to perform self-examinations for cancers.

LEARNING OUTCOME 4

Describe the laboratory and diagnostic tests used for cancer diagnosis.

CONCEPTS FOR LECTURE

1. Early detection and treatment have the most influence on the prognosis of people with cancer.
2. Tumor identification provides some standardization in diagnosis and treatment protocols.

POWERPOINT LECTURE SLIDES

1 American Cancer Society Goals of Medical Treatment
- To eliminate the tumor or malignant cells
- To prevent metastasis
- To reduce cellular growth and tumor burden
- To promote functional abilities and provide pain relief to those whose disease does not respond to treatment

1a Procedures used to Diagnose Cancer
- X-ray imaging
- Computed tomography
- Ultrasonography

 © 2007 Pearson Education, Inc.

POWERPOINT LECTURE SLIDES *continued*

- Magnetic resonance imaging
- Microscopic histologic examination
- Cytologic examination
- Radioisotope scans
- Angiography
- Monoclonal antibodies
- Direct visualization

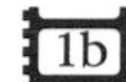
Laboratory Tests Used to Diagnose Cancer
- Blood, urine, and other body fluid tests
- Liver enzymes (ALT), (LDH)
- Tumor markers

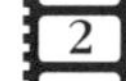
Tumor Identification
- Classification
    - Classified and named by the tissue or cell of origin
- Grading
    - Evaluates the amount of differentiation of the cell and estimates the rate of growth
- Staging
    - Relative size of the tumor and extent of the disease
- Table 12-3 TNM Staging Classification System

SUGGESTIONS FOR CLASSROOM ACTIVITIES

1. Discuss the laboratory and diagnostic tests used to diagnose cancer. Identify tissue markers that are specific to certain types of cancers. What are the treatment options for positive markers?
2. Look at tumor identification systems and discuss what the grading and staging mean.

SUGGESTIONS FOR CLINICAL ACTIVITIES

Assign students to care for clients on an oncology unit. Have the students look at the laboratory and diagnostic studies that were performed of assigned clients. Discuss the findings in postconference.

LEARNING OUTCOME 5

Discuss the use of surgery, radiation therapy, chemotherapy, and biotherapy in the treatment of cancer.

CONCEPTS FOR LECTURE

1. Cancer treatment is aimed at cure, control, or palliation of symptoms. Cancer may be treated through surgery, radiotherapy, chemotherapy, and biotherapy.

POWERPOINT LECTURE SLIDES

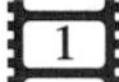
Cancer Treatments
- Surgery
- Radiation therapy
    - Internal radiation
    - External radiation
    - Box 12-6 Nursing Care Checklist: Clients Receiving Radiation Therapy
- Chemotherapy
    - Table 12-4 Nursing Implications for Pharmacology: Chemotherapeutic Drugs
- Biotherapy or immunotherapy
    - Box 12-7 Nursing Care Checklist: Immunotherapy
- Bone marrow transplant
- Complementary therapies
    - Box 12-8 Common Complementary Therapies for Cancer

Suggestions for Classroom Activities

1. Compare and contrast the use of surgery, radiation therapy, chemotherapy, biotherapy, and complementary therapies in the treatment of cancer.
2. Assign groups of students to present a paper on the chemotherapeutic drugs, emphasizing target malignancies, adverse or side effects, and nursing implications for each category.

Suggestions for Clinical Activities

1. Assign students to observe an oncology nurse administering chemotherapy to a client. Have students report observations on the protocol for administering chemotherapeutic drugs. What safeguards are in place to protect the nurses who administer the medications? What side effects are associated with the specific chemotherapeutic drugs? What collaborative interventions are used to minimize these side effects? Review with the students the client's blood counts during the hospitalization noting the effects of chemotherapy.
2. Arrange for students to have clinical experience in an outpatient oncology clinic or in an oncologist physician's office. Assign students to observe the administration of intravenous fluids and chemotherapy to clients who have various types of venous access devices. How are the venous access devices maintained? Are any premedications given to minimize side effects for the clients? Have the students describe the care done to maintain the devices outside the office. What educational literature is available to clients and families?

Learning Outcome 6

Provide teaching for the client and family experiencing cancer.

Concepts for Lecture

1. Nurses should educate all clients about preventive strategies and lifestyle.

PowerPoint Lecture Slides

1 Teaching for Discharge
- Box 12-9 Client Teaching: When to Call for Help

1a Prevention Teaching
- Avoid tobacco, secondhand smoke, alcohol
- Avoid obesity
- Eat a low-fat, high-fiber diet and antioxidant foods; avoid foods with carcinogenic additives, dyes, chemicals
- Take medications as ordered
- Limit exposure to radiation, sun exposure
- Use caution with carcinogenic chemicals or airborne particles
- Protect against viral disease
- Improve immunity by maintaining healthy lifestyle and managing stress

1b Rehabilitation
- Assist with lifestyle changes and emotional support
- Attendance at self-help support groups

1c Home Care
- Teach client and family how to manage at home
  - Wound care
  - Diet
  - Medications and treatments
  - Equipment and supplies
  - Follow-up care

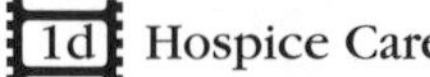

1d Hospice Care
- Assisting with decisions
- Interdisciplinary care

 © 2007 Pearson Education, Inc.

Suggestions for Classroom Activities

1. Discuss the client teaching needed for the client and family experiencing cancer.
2. Compare and contrast needs of the client in rehabilitation care, home care, and hospice care.

Suggestions for Clinical Activities

1. Arrange for students to attend a meeting of a cancer support group. Who is attending the meetings: clients, family members, or both? What are the concerns brought by group participants? What advice is given by group members? How does the group leader facilitate meaningful discussions?
2. Arrange for students to accompany a hospice nurse on client rounds or to visit an inpatient hospice unit. Discuss the needs of these clients and the support given to the client and families as death approaches.

Learning Outcome 7

Use the nursing process as a framework for providing individualized care for the client with cancer.

Concepts for Lecture

1. Nurses have the responsibility of assisting and supporting clients during their treatment, recovery, and rehabilitation for cancer.
2. Evaluating the effectiveness of nursing care for the client with cancer requires ongoing assessment through the nursing process.
3. In caring for clients with cancer, nurses may encounter a number of emergency situations in which their role may be crucial to the client's survival.

PowerPoint Lecture Slides

1 Assessment of the Client with Cancer

1a Diagnosing, Planning, and Implementing Care for the Client with Cancer
- Give psychologic support
  - Anxiety
  - Disturbed Body Image
  - Anticipatory Grieving
- Teach areas of knowledge deficit
- Monitor for risk for infection, risk for injury, impaired tissue integrity
- Monitor nutrition
- Treat pain management

2 Evaluation of Care for the Client with Cancer
- Monitor for exacerbation or remission of the disease process
- Make changes in nursing care as indicated
- Utilize interdisciplinary care and referrals as needed

3 Oncologic Emergencies
- Pericardial effusion and neoplastic cardiac tamponade
- Superior vena cava syndrome
- Sepsis and septic shock
- Spinal cord compression
- Obstructive uropathy
- Hypercalcemia
- Hyperuricemia
- Tumor lysis syndrome

Suggestions for Classroom Activities

1. Discuss the baseline physical assessment needed for a client experiencing cancer who is admitted to a health service facility.
2. Using the nursing process case study in the chapter, initiate a discussion on the nursing diagnoses used in the care of the client experiencing cancer.

Suggestions for Clinical Activities

Invite an oncology nurse and/or a hospice nurse to talk about their careers in caring for clients experiencing cancer. Ask them to explain how they keep physically and psychologically fit when caring for these clients.

© 2007 Pearson Education, Inc.

3. Initiate a discussion by asking the students to explore their thoughts and feelings about cancer. How would they feel if a family member or friend had cancer? Ask them to think about all the serious illnesses, and compare experiencing one of those illnesses with cancer. Discuss all the breakthroughs in cancer treatment.
4. Assign groups of students to present nursing care plans on clients experiencing cancer pain and nutritional deficiencies.

© 2007 Pearson Education, Inc.

Chapter 13
Caring for Clients Experiencing Shock, Trauma, or Critical Illness

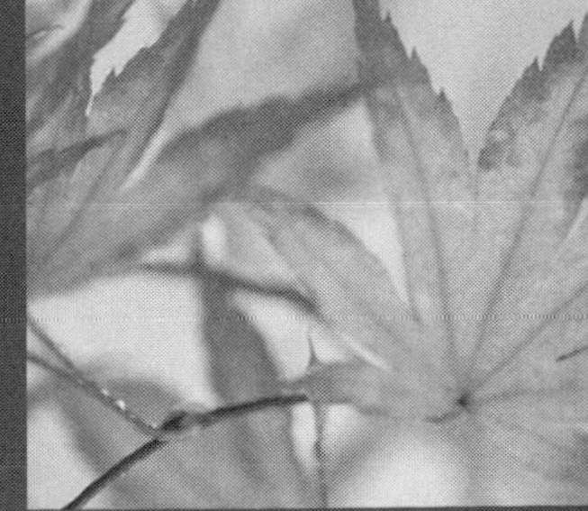

Resource Library

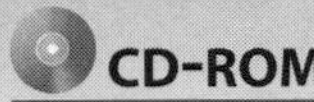

CD-ROM

Shock
Hypovolemic Shock
Video: Bleeding Control/Shock Management
Video: Spinal Immobilization
Video: Administration of Oxygen

IMAGE LIBRARY

Figure 13-1 Multisystem effects of shock.
Figure 13-2 The pathophysiology of hypovolemic shock.
Figure 13-3 Pneumatic antishock garments provide rapid, emergency treatment of shock.
Figure 13-4 Modified Trendelenburg position. Position the client with the lower extremities elevated approximately 20 degrees (knees straight), trunk horizontal, and the head elevated about 10 degrees.
Figure 13-5 Intubation with insertion of an endotracheal tube (ETT). When a client is experiencing respiratory distress, oxygen can be given into the external opening of the tube.
Figure 13-6 The major pressure points used to control bleeding.
Figure 13-7 (**A**) Contusions (bruises) do not cause a break in the skin. (**B**) Abrasions (scrapes) occur when a partial layer of skin is removed. (**C**) Puncture wounds occur when the integument is penetrated by a sharp or blunt object. (**D**) Lacerations are irregular tears in the skin.
Figure 13-8 Application of a cervical collar at an accident scene immobilizes the cervical spine and prevents further injury to the spinal cord.
Figure 13-9 A kinetic continuous rotation bed reduces complications of immobility for a client with multiple injuries.

Learning Outcome 1

Identify the three stages of shock.

Concepts for Lecture

1. Shock is a life-threatening condition, characterized by inadequate blood flow and oxygen to the tissues and cells.
2. There are three stages of shock: compensated, progressive, and irreversible.

PowerPoint Lecture Slides

1 Shock
- Life-threatening condition
- Inadequate blood flow and oxygen to tissues and cells

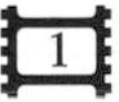

2 Stages of Shock
- Compensated
- Progressive
- Irreversible

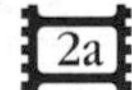

2a Compensated Stage of Shock
- Decreased blood volume reduces cardiac output or vasodilation occurs
- Blood pressure drops and normal tissue perfusion is not maintained
- Baroreceptors stimulate the sympathetic nervous system to release epinephrine and norepinephrine

PowerPoint Lecture Slides *continued*

- Arterial blood vessels constrict, heart rate and strength of heart to contract increases, venous return increases
- Renin–angiotensin system is activated, increasing blood pressure and circulating blood volume
- Antidiuretic hormone is released to increase blood pressure
- Box 13-1 Manifestations Found in Each Stage of Shock

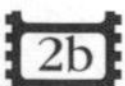

Progressive Stage of Shock

- Compensatory mechanisms fail and organ functions deteriorate
- Effects on body organs:
  - Cardiovascular—decreased cardiac output causes muscle ischemia
  - Respiratory—increased carbon dioxide results in respiratory acidosis
  - Gastrointestinal system—ulceration of mucosa results in stress ulcers and sepsis, paralytic ileus
  - Liver—failure leads to hypoglycemia, bacterial infections
  - Neurologic—decreased blood flow leads to decreased level of consciousness, coma, cerebral edema, and brain damage
  - Renal—reduced blood flow causes oliguria and failure
  - Skin and temperature—vasoconstriction leads to pale skin and mucous membranes, activation of sweat glands produces cool and clammy skin, body temperature decreases
- Box 13-1 Manifestations Found in Each Stage of Shock

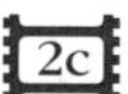

Irreversible Stage of Shock

- Multiple organ dysfunction syndrome (MODS)—tissue and cellular death
- Box 13-1 Manifestation Found in Each Stage of Shock

Suggestions for Classroom Activities

1. Compare and contrast the three stages of shock. What clinical manifestations are exhibited at each stage? What nursing care measures are appropriate for each stage?
2. Divide students into three groups, assigning each group a different stage of shock. Have each group present the clinical manifestations and nursing care for their stage of shock.

Learning Outcome 2

Identify the common causes for each type of shock: hypovolemia, anaphylactic, cardiogenic, septic, and neurogenic.

Concepts for Lecture

1. The five types of shock are hypovolemic, anaphylactic, cardiogenic, septic, and neurogenic.
2. Shock is identified according to its underlying cause.

PowerPoint Lecture Slides

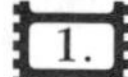

Types of Shock

- Hypovolemic
- Anaphylactic
- Cardiogenic
- Septic
- Neurogenic

© 2007 Pearson Education, Inc.

PowerPoint Lecture Slides *continued*

2 Causes of Hypovolemic Shock
- Decrease in circulating blood volume due to:
  - Hemorrhage due to trauma, surgery, GI bleeding, and hemophilia, and postpartum hemorrhage
  - Internal fluid shifts due to cirrhosis with ascites, pleural effusion, pancreatitis, intestinal obstruction
  - Loss of body fluids due to vomiting, diarrhea, nasogastric suctioning, diuretics, diabetes insipidus
  - Loss of fluids through skin due to diaphoresis or burns

2a Causes of Anaphylactic Shock
- Immunologic reaction from antigens due to:
  - Food allergies
  - Stings and bites from insects
  - Snake venom
  - Substances used to diagnose and treat disease
  - Latex, pollen, molds, food additives

2b Causes of Cardiogenic Shock
- Failure of heart's pumping action or other cardiac disorders
  - Myocardial infarction

2c Causes of Septic Shock
- Overwhelming infection produced by toxins due to:
  - Age <1 year, >65 years
  - Debilitating disease processes
  - Surgery, invasive lines or tubes
  - Drug therapy

2d Causes of Neurogenic Shock
- Changes in sympathetic tone of blood vessels duc to:
  - Spinal cord injury above T_6 level
  - Head injury
  - Spinal anesthesia
  - Opiate drug overdose
  - Insulin reaction

Suggestions for Classroom Activities

Compare and contrast different types and causes of shock.

Learning Outcome 3

Describe the pathophysiology and manifestations of the five types of shock.

Concepts for Lecture

1. Discuss the different types of shock, explaining the manifestations at each stage; explain the effects on the body systems as the shock progresses.
2. The most common complications of shock are adult respiratory distress syndrome and disseminated intravascular coagulation.

PowerPoint Lecture Slides

1 Pathophysiology of Shock
- Alteration in one or more factor:
  - Adequate blood flow
  - Correct heart pumping action
  - Normal blood vessel diameter to maintain tissue perfusion

© 2007 Pearson Education, Inc.

POWERPOINT LECTURE SLIDES *continued*

- Disruption of normal cell function
- Inadequate tissue perfusion to sustain normal cellular metabolism
- Prolonged shock results in hypoxia and cell death, then organ failure and death

1a Pathophysiology and Manifestations of Hypovolemic Shock

- Box 13-2 Initial Manifestations of Hypovolemic Shock

1b Pathophysiology and Manifestations of Anaphylactic Shock

- Antigen–antibody reaction stimulates mast cells to release histamine and other mediators, causing vasodilation, hypotension, and hypovolemia
- Inflammation, bronchoconstriction, and cutaneous reactions occur, causing a life-threatening event
- Box 13-3 Manifestations of Anaphylactic Shock

1c Pathophysiology and Manifestations of Cardiogenic Shock

- Ventricles fail to pump blood into the circulatory system, leading to decreased stroke volume
- Blood backs up in lungs causing pulmonary edema, hypotension, and cardiac failure
- Box 13-4 Manifestations of Cardiogenic Shock

1d Pathophysiology and Manifestations of Septic Shock

- As bacteria are destroyed, endotoxins are released that damage tissues and starve cells of oxygen and nutrients
- Histamine and other chemicals are released, causing vasodilation and increased capillary permeability and hypovolemia occurs
- Microemboli form in capillaries causing cell damage and death
- Box 13-5 Manifestations of Septic Shock

1e Pathophysiology and Manifestations of Neurogenic Shock

- Blood vessels dilate, leading to peripheral vasodilation; blood pools, leading to inadequate tissue perfusion
- Thermoregulation is impaired; organ failure and death occur
- Box 13-6 Manifestations of Neurogenic Shock

2 Complications of Shock

- Adult respiratory distress syndrome (ARDS)
- Disseminated intravascular coagulation (DIC)

SUGGESTIONS FOR CLASSROOM ACTIVITIES

Compare and contrast the pathophysiology and manifestations of each type of shock. Discuss how to minimize complications of shock.

SUGGESTIONS FOR CLINICAL ACTIVITIES

Assign students to care for clients in an intensive care or an emergency department. Have them perform physical assessments and help them to identify signs of shock in their assigned clients.

© 2007 Pearson Education, Inc.

LEARNING OUTCOME 4

Explain the nursing care of the client in shock.

CONCEPTS FOR LECTURE

1. Nursing management of shock includes performing diagnostic tests and providing oxygen therapy, intravenous fluids, blood or blood products, cardiac support, and client support.
2. Shock must be fully resolved before a client can be discharged. Teaching the family to care for the client is needed to provide the client with a supportive and nurturing environment after discharge.

POWERPOINT LECTURE SLIDES

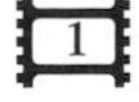

Diagnostic Tests to Identify Type of Shock

- CBC, especially hemoglobin and hematocrit
- Arterial blood gases
- Electrolytes, especially serum sodium and potassium
- Blood glucose levels
- Blood urea nitrogen and creatinine
- Blood cultures
- White blood cell count
- Serum cardiac markers (creatine kinase, CK-MB, troponins)
- X-rays, computerized tomography (CT) scans, magnetic resonance imaging (MRI), peritoneal lavage

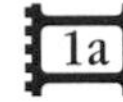

Oxygen Therapy in Shock

- Maintain patent airway
- Administer oxygen via nonbreather mask at 12 to 15 L/min
- Maintain $Pao_2 > 90$ mm Hg
- Monitor for respiratory distress and anticipate endotracheal intubation and mechanical ventilation

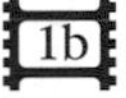

Nursing Management of Client with Hypovolemic Shock

- Box 13-7 Prehospital Emergency Care of the Client Experiencing Hemorrhage
- Initiate intravenous fluids
- Apply pneumatic antishock garments (PASG)
  - To raise blood pressure and stabilize pelvic and femoral fractures

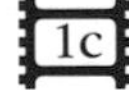

Nursing Management of Client with Anaphylactic Shock

- Maintain patent airway and administer oxygen
- Administer epinephrine subcutaneously or intravenously
- Administer antihistamines
- Administer corticosteroids
- If respiratory distress continues, administer aminophylline or nebulized albuterol

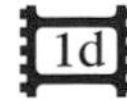

Nursing Management of Client with Cardiogenic Shock

- Administer oxygen
- Administer vasopressor drugs and positive inotropic drugs
- Administer diuretic drugs
- Administer antidysrhythmic drugs
- Monitor mechanical devices
  - Intra-aortic balloon pump (IABP)
  - Ventricular assist device (VAD)

© 2007 Pearson Education, Inc.

PowerPoint Lecture Slides *continued*

1e Nursing Management of Client with Septic Shock
- Obtain blood, urine, wound, sputum cultures
- Administer intravenous fluids
- Administer antibiotic drugs

1f Nursing Management of Client with Neurogenic Shock
- Administer intravenous fluids
- Administer analgesic drugs

1g Client and Family Support in Shock
- Acknowledge anxiety and fear
- Provide comfort measures
- Provide time, space, and privacy
- Provide anticipatory guidance
- Keep family informed

2 Discharge Teaching
- Avoid known allergens
- Notify health care professionals of allergens
- Avoid wearing bright colors, perfumes, and scented hair sprays if allergic to insect stings
- Read package labels if allergic to foods
- Wear Medic-Alert bracelet or necklace
- Advise to carry an emergency kit for anaphylaxis
- Review manifestations of anaphylaxis
- Seek medical attention immediately when symptoms occur

Suggestions for Classroom Activities

1. Invite an emergency room nurse or technician to class to discuss their experiences with treating clients experiencing shock and trauma.
2. Divide students into groups. Give each group a case scenario of a different type of shock. Have them develop a plan of care or concept map for the case scenario and share these with the other groups.
3. Have students develop a discharge teaching plan for clients and families who have experienced a type of shock.

Suggestions for Clinical Activities

Arrange for students to have a clinical experience in the emergency department. Assist the students to view the trauma room and observe how supplies, equipment, and medications are arranged. Review the documentation forms used with trauma cases. If possible, have the students follow a client in shock or with a trauma through the admission and treatment procedure.

Learning Outcome 5

State the nursing implications for administering fluid replacement solutions.

Concepts for Lecture

1. Intravenous fluids are administered alone or in combination with colloids, blood, or blood products. Fluid replacements are given in a 3:1 ratio (300 mL fluid for every 100 mL of fluid loss.

PowerPoint Lecture Slides

1 Intravenous Fluids Administered in Shock
- Replace fluids in a 3:1 ratio (300 mL for every 100 mL fluid loss)
- Crystalloid solutions
- Colloid solutions
  - Table 13-1 Nursing Implications for Pharmacology: Clients Receiving Colloid Solutions
- Blood and blood products
  - Table 13-2 Blood and Blood Products
  - Table 13-3 Blood Group and Rh Types and Compatibilities

© 2007 Pearson Education, Inc.

PowerPoint Lecture Slides *continued*

- Table 13-4 Nursing Implications for Pharmacology: Clients Receiving Blood Transfusions
- Autotransfusion

Suggestions for Classroom Activities

1. Assign groups of students to present on the following subjects: nursing implications for clients receiving colloid solutions and blood transfusions, and the types of blood and blood products.
2. Discuss amount of fluid losses and have students calculate the amount of fluid replacement to administer based on fluid losses.

Suggestions for Clinical Activities

Assign students to observe a client receiving a blood or blood product transfusion. Have them discuss the responsibilities of the nurse in administering blood and blood products. What are the different blood products that are transfused to clients? What is the procedure for obtaining blood from the blood bank? What are the steps to perform when the client has a reaction to the blood or blood product?

Learning Outcome 6

Identify common traumatic injuries.

Concepts for Lecture

1. Trauma is the leading cause of death in young people. It can be prevented by following common safety guidelines such as wearing a seat belt or helmet when riding a bicycle.
2. A variety of medical emergencies can result from environmental injuries.

PowerPoint Lecture Slides

1 Causes of Trauma
- Injury caused by physical force
  - Motor vehicle crashes
  - Falls
  - Drowning
  - Gunshots
  - Burns
  - Stabbing
  - Physical assaults, contact sports
  - Box 13-8 Geriatric Risks for Trauma

1a Common Traumatic Injuries
- Minor trauma
  - Fractures to collarbone
  - Small second-degree burn
  - Cut requiring stitches
- Major or multiple trauma
  - Amputation
  - Multiple-system injuries

1b Common Traumatic Injuries
- Blunt trauma
  - Internal damage that does not break skin
- Penetrating trauma
  - Foreign object that pierces body
  - External appearance of wound does not determine internal damage

2 Common Environmental Injuries
- Hyperthermia
  - Heat exhaustion
  - Heat stroke
- Hypothermia
- Poisonings

Suggestions for Classroom Activities

1. Define and discuss trauma focusing on the following aspects: the populations at risk for trauma, common causes of trauma, types of trauma, and safety guidelines to decrease the risk for trauma.
2. Assign a group of students to show a poster presentation on guidelines to prevent trauma or poisonings.

Suggestions for Clinical Activities

Have students participate in a health or safety fair and educate participants in safety issues.

Learning Outcome 7

Describe emergency management of clients with traumatic injuries.

Concepts for Lecture

1. Clients experiencing a traumatic accident are assessed in the field and in the emergency department for airway, breathing, circulation, disability, and exposure. Traumatic injuries have serious consequences that must be treated rapidly.
2. Injuries that involve criminal activity require legal investigation, including forensic testing.

PowerPoint Lecture Slides

1 Effects of Traumatic Injury
- Airway obstruction
- Pneumothorax
- Hemorrhage
- Hypovolemic shock
- Neurologic injuries
- Gastrointestinal and genitourinary injuries
- Musculoskeletal injuries
- Integumentary injuries
- Psychologic effects on client
- Psychosocial effects on family

1a Emergency Treatment of Traumatic Injury
- Assess to identify extent of injuries
- Provide life support
- Immobilize
- Administer oxygen
- Control bleeding
- Start IV fluids
- Transport
- Emergency Surgery

1b Box 13-7 Prehospital Emergency Care of the Client Experiencing Hemorrhage

1c Diagnostic Tests for Traumatic Injuries
- Tests to rule out shock
- Blood alcohol levels
- Urine drug screen
- Pregnancy test
- Diagnostic peritoneal lavage
- Computerized tomography (CT scan)
- Magnetic resonance imaging (MRI)

2 Legal Investigation of Injuries Related to Criminal Activity
- Identify, store, and properly transfer potential evidence
- Do not cut through clothing containing blood stains or bullet holes
- Place clothing in individual breathable containers and label
- Label bullets or knives

© 2007 Pearson Education, Inc.

POWERPOINT LECTURE SLIDES *continued*

- Record entrance and exit wounds in chart
- Photograph wounds
- Place paper bag over hands if presence of evidence in suspected

SUGGESTIONS FOR CLASSROOM ACTIVITIES

1. Divide student into groups. Assign them to develop a plan of care for the prehospital emergency care of the client experiencing hemorrhage, loss of consciousness, impending respiratory or cardiac arrest, severe burn, or multiple fractures.
2. Have students examine the crash cart and explain the use of the equipment and medications used to treat shock.

SUGGESTIONS FOR CLINICAL ACTIVITIES

Arrange for students to spend time with an ambulance service. Have them compare the role of the emergency technician or paramedic with the role of the nurse in a prehospital emergency situation.

LEARNING OUTCOME 8

Use the nursing process to collect data, establish outcomes, provide individualized care, and evaluate responses for the client experiencing shock or trauma.

CONCEPTS FOR LECTURE

1. Nursing care of the client with a traumatic injury starts with primary assessment, including collaborative interventions, and prepares the client and family for discharge.

POWERPOINT LECTURE SLIDES

1 Assessment of the Client in Shock
- Perform head-to-toe assessment
- Obtain brief history, allergies, past medical history
- Assess vital signs every 5–10 minutes to hourly, to every 2–4 hours
- Assess for early signs of shock
  - Restlessness
  - Tachycardia
  - Slight anxiety
- Assess late signs of shock
  - Hypotension
- Assess urine output

1a Interventions for the client in shock
- Insert nasogastric tube if risk of aspiration
- Apply cardiac monitor to assess cardiac status
- Insert intravenous lines and administer medications as indicated
- Monitor for hypothermia
- Administer tetanus prophylaxis if penetrating wound
- Maintain strict aseptic technique

1b Evaluation of Care
- Absence of infection
- Preventing complications from immobility
- Document healing of injuries

1c Discharge Teaching
- Determine potential home modifications
- Review medication administration
- Give information about diets
- Discuss rehabilitation plan
- Emphasize need for follow-up care
- Discuss emotional changes

© 2007 Pearson Education, Inc.

PowerPoint Lecture Slides *continued*

- Provide referrals as needed
- Provide preventive education
  - Box 13-8 Geriatric Risks for Trauma
  - Box 13-9 Home Safety Tips

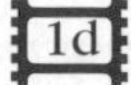 Interventions for Environmental Injuries

- Hyperthermia
  - Move to cool place
  - Loosen clothing
  - Apply cool, wet towels
  - Apply cooling blanket and oxygen for heat stroke
  - Monitor for renal failure and seizures
- Hypothermia
  - Move to warm place
  - Remove wet clothing
  - Apply warm blankets, radiant heat lamp, warming blanket
  - Administer warm intravenous fluids and warm peritoneal lavage
  - Administer warm, humidified oxygen
  - Observe for cardiac arrest

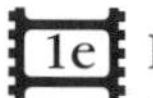 Interventions for Environmental Trauma

- Poisonings
  - Identify the poison
  - Call the local poison control center
  - Assess airway, breathing, and circulation
  - Assist with administration of antidote or elimination method
  - Administer oxygen for inhaled poisons
  - Cleanse contaminated skin with water
- Teaching for Poisoning
  - Box 13-10 Guidelines to Prevent Poisoning

Suggestions for Classroom Activities

1. Using the nursing process, initiate a discussion on nursing care for the client with septic shock, multiple injuries, or poisoning.
2. Assign groups of students to write and present to the class nursing care plans or case studies for clients experiencing each type of shock or trauma.

Suggestions for Clinical Activities

Arrange for students to have clinical experience in the critical care step-down unit and assign the care of clients who were hospitalized because of trauma and/or because they experienced shock. Have the students talk to the clients about their experience. Review the chart to identify the trauma or cause of shock and the care provided and to identify if safety measures were in place.

Learning Outcome 9

Describe the effects of a critical care unit on the client and family.

Concepts for Lecture

1. The critical care unit is overwhelming to clients and families. The nurse plays an important role in reducing the psychosocial effects while caring for the acutely ill client.

PowerPoint Lecture Slides

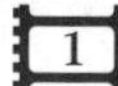 ICU Psychosis in Clients

- Acute confusion after 2 to 3 days in ICU
- Manifestations:
  - Altered attention span
  - Memory loss
  - Confusion
  - Visual and auditory hallucinations

© 2007 Pearson Education, Inc.

PowerPoint Lecture Slides *continued*

1a ICU Psychosis in Clients
- Treatment:
  - Administer sedative or psychotropic drugs
  - Decrease client's sensoriperceptual problems
  - Decrease client's sleep deprivation

1b ICU Effects on Family
- Fear of death of loved one
- Anxious about equipment
- Anxious about client's potential for pain
- Worry about finances and changes in family roles

1c Nurse's Interventions with Family
- Give status reports
- Get involved in client's care
- Assess for signs of exhaustion
- Obtain resources and referrals as needed

Suggestions for Classroom Activities

Discuss the psychosocial effects of the intensive care unit on the client and family. What interventions can the nurse provide to help alleviate these effects?

Suggestions for Clinical Activities

Have students interview clients or families about their intensive care unit experience. Ask what the client or family feels could have made the experience less anxious for them.

Learning Outcome 10

Discuss the legal and ethical considerations of organ donation.

Concepts for Lecture

1. Under the Uniform Anatomical Act, consent for organ donation may be given not only by the donor but also by a spouse, adult child, parent, adult sibling, or guardian. Nurses should know their hospital's organ and tissue donation policies.

PowerPoint Lecture Slides

1 Organ Donation
- Consent may be given by client, spouse, adult child, parent, adult sibling, guardian
- Organs that can be donated: kidneys, heart, lungs, pancreas, intestines, liver, corneas, bones, bone marrow, skin
- Encourage client and family to ask questions and express feelings
- Provide support by a grief counselor or clergy
- Signature must be obtained for organ donation
- Client must be brain dead
  - Box 13-11 Brain Death Criteria
- Notify Organ Procurement Organization with decision to proceed

Suggestions for Classroom Activities

Initiate a discussion on organ donation by asking the students to explore their thoughts and feelings about donating their organs and by discussing organ donations with family and friends.

Suggestions for Clinical Activities

Arrange for students to spend clinical time with the nurses who work in the community's tissue and organ donation organization. Have students review the literature used in recruiting persons to sign organ donor cards. What policies are in place to assist families of persons who are organ donors?

© 2007 Pearson Education, Inc.

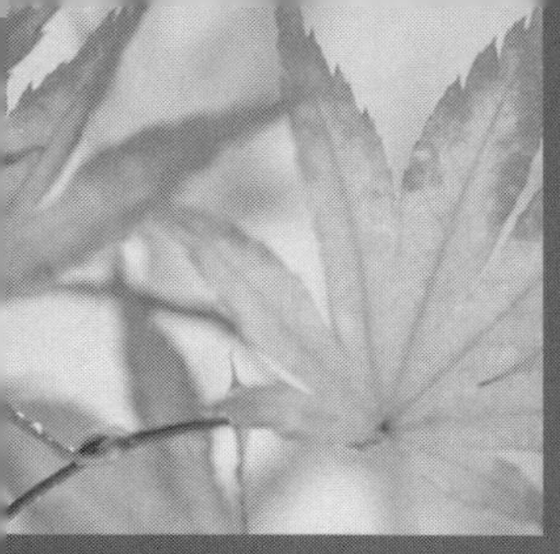

CHAPTER 14
LOSS, GRIEF, AND END-OF-LIFE CARE

RESOURCE LIBRARY

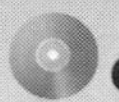 **CD-ROM**

Video: Emotional, Social, & Spiritual Needs

IMAGE LIBRARY

Figure 14-1 Nurses who work with dying clients need support from their colleagues to work through their often overwhelming feelings of grief.

Figure 14-2 The nurse establishes a trusting nurse-client relationship through therapeutic communications and by demonstrating respect for the person's age, culture, religion, race, and values.

LEARNING OUTCOME 1

Define loss, grief, and death.

CONCEPTS FOR LECTURE

1. The stress of loss may initiate physical or emotional changes in a person or family. To deal with the resulting changes, people must resolve their feelings about the loss, through a process called grief work.
2. Death is an irreversible cessation of body functions, an inevitable part of life, and is the most critical loss of all.

POWERPOINT LECTURE SLIDES

 1 Loss

- Valued object, person, body part, or situation is lost or changed
- Can no longer be seen, felt, heard, known, or experienced
- May be temporary or permanent, complete or partial
- May be subjective, physical, symbolic
- May be as painful as death
- Box 14-1 The Most Common Fears of Loss

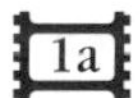 1a Grief

- Emotional response to loss and its accompanying changes
- Internal process used to work through response to loss
- Mourning describes the actions or expressions of the bereaved

 2 Death

- Irreversible cessation of circulatory and respiratory functions
- Irreversible cessation of all functions of the entire brain
- An inevitable part of life
- May be accidental, result of terminal illness, or purposeful
- An immensely difficult loss for dying person and loved ones

SUGGESTIONS FOR CLASSROOM ACTIVITIES

Have students write their own definitions of loss, grief, and death. Have them compare their own definitions with the text definitions.

LEARNING OUTCOME 2

Explain the stages of loss, with commonly experienced emotional responses.

CONCEPTS FOR LECTURE

1. When a valued object, person, body part, or situation is lost or changed, the experience of loss occurs. Grief is the emotional response to loss. Grieving responses are individualized to each person, but commonly include the stages of denial, anger, bargaining, depression, and acceptance.

POWERPOINT LECTURE SLIDES

1 Kubler-Ross's Stages of Death and Dying
- Denial
  - Shock and disbelief
- Anger
  - Resists the loss
- Bargaining
  - Attempts to delay reality of the loss
- Depression
  - Prepares for impending loss by working through struggle of separation
- Acceptance
  - Comes to terms with the loss and resumes activities

1a Table 14-1 Development of the Concept of Death

SUGGESTIONS FOR CLASSROOM ACTIVITIES

Initiate discussion of the chapter by asking students if they have had to deal with the loss of someone close to them, or how they have coped with any loss such as a job or a social relationship. Ask if they remember if and how they proceeded through Kubler-Ross's grieving stages.

SUGGESTIONS FOR CLINICAL ACTIVITIES

Arrange for clinical experience in a nursing home. Assist the students to identify the losses that each of their assigned clients has experienced within the last several years. Losses may be death, health, functionalities, or loss of extremity. Assist the students to identify behaviors of grieving.

LEARNING OUTCOME 3

Discuss factors that influence responses to loss and reflect on one's own responses to loss.

CONCEPTS FOR LECTURE

1. Death is an immensely difficult loss for both the person who is dying and for his or her loved ones. Family, friends, and spiritual practices often facilitate grief work.
2. Rituals of mourning are an important part of the work of mourning and grieving a loss. Culture dictates the rituals of mourning.
3. To give effective nursing care, nurses need to take time to analyze their own feelings and values related to loss and the expression of grief.
4. End-of-life nursing care that ensures a peaceful death was mandated by the International Council of Nurses and supported by the American Association of Colleges of Nursing.

POWERPOINT LECTURE SLIDES

1 Factors that Interfere with Successful Grieving
- Perceived inability to share the loss
- Lack of social recognition of the loss
- Ambivalent relationships prior to the loss
- Traumatic circumstances of the loss

1a Spirituality
- Integrating and transcending the physical, emotional, intellectual, and social dimensions
- Principles, values, personal philosophy, and meaning of life
- Spiritual beliefs provide comfort, help to find meaning in loss
- Nurse provides support by developing a trusting relationship and listening to the client.

2 Rituals of Mourning
- Culture dictates rituals of mourning
  - Table 14-2 Cultural Aspects of Dying and Death
- Funeral ceremony serves needs of bereaved
  - Symbolically express triumph over death
  - Deny fear of death
- Adaptation to the loss

© 2007 Pearson Education, Inc.

POWERPOINT LECTURE SLIDES *continued*

3 Nurse's Response to Client's Loss
- Need to analyze own feelings and values
- Conscious or unconscious reactions influence the outcome of interventions
- Self-reflection helps to approach interactions more objectively.

4 End-of-Life Care
- Client's wishes about death should be respected
- Principles of hospice care
  - People live until the moment they die
  - Care until death may be offered by a variety of health care providers
  - Care is coordinated, sensitive to diversity, offered around the clock
  - Incorporates physical, psychologic, social, and spiritual concerns of the client and client's family
- American Association of Colleges of Nurses defined competencies to provide high-quality end-of-life care

SUGGESTIONS FOR CLASSROOM ACTIVITIES

Ask students to role-play how they would interact with the family of the dying client using verbal and nonverbal communication.

SUGGESTIONS FOR CLINICAL ACTIVITIES

Arrange for students to have a clinical experience in an inpatient hospice or to accompany a hospice nurse making home visits. Assist the students to identify methods of therapeutic communication used by nurses to facilitate clients and families verbalizing concerns and spiritual beliefs.

LEARNING OUTCOME 4

Discuss legal and ethical issues of dying, including advance directives, living wills, do-not-resuscitate orders, and euthanasia.

CONCEPTS FOR LECTURE

1. The dying person may control his or her own care through advance directives, living wills, and a durable power of attorney for health care. The client and family may request that the physician write a do-not-resuscitate (DNR) order.
2. Euthanasia signifies a killing that is prompted by some humanitarian motive. Natural death laws seek to preserve the notion of voluntary versus involuntary euthanasia.
3. Two models of care that focus on the dying client's quality of life are hospice and palliative care.

POWERPOINT LECTURE SLIDES

1 Advance Directives
- Legal documents that allow a person to plan for health care and/or financial affairs in the event of incapacity
  - Box 14-2 Types of Advance Directives
- Durable power of attorney for health care
- Living will

1a Do-Not-Resuscitate Orders
- Written by the physician for the client who is near death
- Based on wishes of the client and family
- No cardiopulmonary resuscitation for respiratory or cardiac arrest
- Provide comfort measures only
- Goal of care is a comfortable, dignified death

2 Euthanasia
- Killing that is prompted by some humanitarian motive

© 2007 Pearson Education, Inc.

PowerPoint Lecture Slides *continued*

- Considered malpractice to participate in a "slow code"
- Voluntary versus involuntary euthanasia

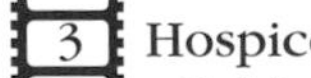

Hospice
- Initiated for clients as they near the end of life
- Emphasizes quality of life
- Client and family are included in plan of care
- Provides support for a dignified and peaceful death
- Palliative rather than curative

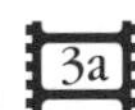

Palliative Care
- Goal is improving the quality of life
- Focused on relief of physical, mental, and spiritual distress
- Involves single person or interdisciplinary team
- Outcomes of care are interventions to manage current manifestations of illness and to prevent new manifestations

Suggestions for Classroom Activities

1. Discuss the types of end-of-life considerations. Assign the students to write their advance directive and/or living will. Explain that this exercise is to help the student to explore his or her own fears, thoughts, and beliefs about dying.
2. Discuss the ethical and legal considerations involved with euthanasia. Compare and contrast voluntary euthanasia and involuntary euthanasia.

Suggestions for Clinical Activities

1. Have students review the advance directives and living wills used in their facility. Have students discuss their findings at a postconference.
2. Arrange for students to attend a team meeting for a hospice client. Assist the students to identify the role of different members of the interdisciplinary team. What common client problems are identified? How do members of the interdisciplinary team support the clients and family members through the grief process?

Learning Outcome 5

Assess physiologic changes in the dying client and signs of death.

Concepts for Lecture

1. As death nears, specific physiologic changes take place. These changes result in manifestations that indicate impending death. Death is pronounced when respiratory and circulatory functions stop or when all brain function ceases.

PowerPoint Lecture Slides

1 Physiologic Changes in the Dying Client
- Weakness and fatigue
- Anorexia and decreased food intake
- Fluid and electrolyte imbalances
- Hypotension and renal failure
- Neurologic dysfunction
- Respiratory changes
- Bowel and bladder incontinence
- Pain
- Box 14-3 Manifestations of Impending Death

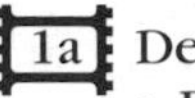

Death
- Box 14-4 Manifestations of Death

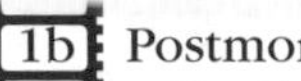

Postmortem Care
- Document time of death
- Notify physician
- Assist family
- Remove jewelry and give to family
- Complete required paperwork

© 2007 Pearson Education, Inc.

Suggestions for Classroom Activities

1. Divide the students into groups of four and assign each group to write a nursing care plan for physiologic changes in the dying client such as anorexia, pain, incontinence, and fatigue.
2. Role-play the death of a client. What are the responsibilities of the nurse? How does the nurse interact with the family? How does the nurse deal with the death of a client?

Suggestions for Clinical Activities

If a death occurs during the clinical rotation, assign a student to assist with the postmortem care. Have the student discuss the procedure and the student's feelings about the experience in postconference.

Learning Outcome 6

Use the nursing process to collect data and provide interventions for the client who is experiencing loss and is at the end of life.

Concepts for Lecture

1. Nursing care for clients who experience loss, grief, or death is implemented to meet the physical, emotional, and spiritual needs of the client and family.
2. Nurses must also be aware of their own responses to these experiences to provide care more effectively.

PowerPoint Lecture Slides

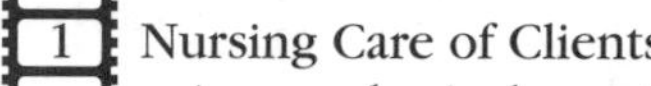

1 Nursing Care of Clients
- Assess physical, emotional, cultural, and spiritual needs
- Provide comfort
  - Box 14-5 Providing Physical Comfort for the Client Nearing Death
- Provide anticipatory grieving interventions
- Explore death anxiety with the client
- Evaluate if client has a comfortable and dignified death
- Teach client care to family
  - Box 14-6 Nursing Care Checklist: End-of-Life Checklist
  - Box 14-7 Client Teaching: Teaching for Clients Experiencing a Loss

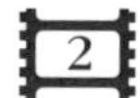

2 Nurse's Grief
- Crying with family is expression of empathy and caring
- Sharing grief with the family
- Reflect on responses to own losses
- Obtain support from peers
- Obtain counseling as needed

Suggestions for Classroom Activities

1. Divide the class into four groups. Assign each to explore the elements of each component of the nursing process as it relates to the grieving and dying process. Have each group present its findings to the class.
2. Divide the class into groups of four. Have each group research the nursing interventions from the "Nursing Interventions Classification Project" and present their findings to the group. Ask the students to explore how the interventions might help in planning and implementing client care. What method can he or she use to help when providing care for the dying client?

Suggestions for Clinical Activities

Arrange for students to have a clinical experience in caring for clients in a palliative care unit or a hospice unit. Assist the students to identify how the nurses assess for pain and evaluate pain relief. What comfort measures are commonly employed? How are nutritional, fluid, and elimination needs addressed?

© 2007 Pearson Education, Inc.

CHAPTER 15
THE ENDOCRINE SYSTEM AND ASSESSMENT

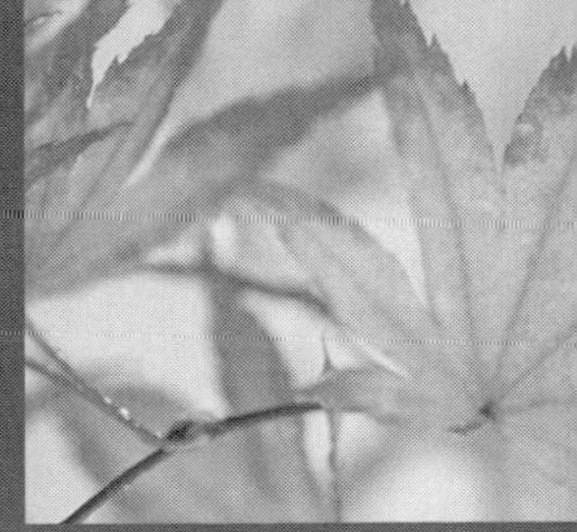

RESOURCE LIBRARY

CD-ROM

Endocrine System

IMAGE LIBRARY

Figure 15-1 Location of the major endocrine glands.
Figure 15-2 Actions of the major hormones of the anterior pituitary.
Figure 15-3 Action of insulin and glucagon on blood glucose levels. (**A**) High blood glucose is lowered by insulin release. (**B**) Low blood glucose is raised by glucagon release.
Figure 15-4 Palpating the thyroid gland from behind the client.

LEARNING OUTCOME 1

Describe the structure and function of the organs of the endocrine system, including the pancreas.

CONCEPTS FOR LECTURE

1. Primary function of the endocrine system is to regulate the body's internal environment.

POWERPOINT LECTURE SLIDES

1 Major Endocrine Organs (Figure 15-1)
- Hypothalamus
- Pituitary gland
- Thyroid gland
- Parathyroid gland
- Adrenal glands
- Pancreas
- Gonads (reproductive glands)

1a Table 15-1

1b Hypothalamus
- Sits between the cerebrum and brainstem
- Houses the pituitary gland and hypothalamus
- Regulates temperature, fluid volume, growth, pain response, pleasure response, hunger, and thirst

1c Pituitary Gland
- Sits beneath the hypothalamus
- Termed the "master gland"
- Has two parts

1d Anterior Pituitary Gland
- Promotes growth
- Stimulates the secretion of six hormones
- Controls pigmentation of the skin

1e Posterior Pituitary Gland
- Stimulates the secretion of two hormones
- Promotes water retention

1f Thyroid Gland
- Butterfly shaped
- Sits on either side of the trachea
- Has two lobes connected with an isthmus

PowerPoint Lecture Slides *continued*

- Functions in the presence of iodine
- Stimulates the secretion of three hormones
- Involved with metabolic rate management and serum calcium levels

1g Parathyroid Glands
- Embedded within the posterior lobes of the thyroid gland
- Secretion of one hormone
- Maintenance of serum calcium levels

1h Adrenal Glands
- Pyramid-shaped organs that sit on top of the kidneys
- Each has two parts:

1i Adrenal Cortex
- Secretion of two hormones
- Involved with blood glucose level, anti-inflammatory response, blood volume, and electrolyte maintenance

1j Adrenal Medulla
- Secretion of two hormones
- Involved with the stress response

1k Pancreas
- Located behind the stomach between the spleen and duodenum
- Has two major functions

Suggestions for Classroom Activities

Provide the students with a schematic drawing of the cerebrum and ask them to identify the location of the pituitary gland. Once identified, ask the students to list disease processes that might adversely affect the function of this gland.

Suggestions for Clinical Activities

Assign students to a client with an endocrine disorder. Have the students assess the client's thyroid gland.

Learning Outcome 2

Explain the functions of hormones secreted by the endocrine glands.

Concepts for Lecture

1. Hormones secreted by endocrine glands regulate growth, reproduction, sex differentiation, metabolism, and fluid and electrolyte balance.
2. Pancreatic hormones—insulin and glucagons—are responsible for maintaining blood glucose levels.

PowerPoint Lecture Slides

1 Definition of Hormones
- Chemical messengers of the body
- Act on specific target cells
- Regulated by negative feedback
- Too much hormone, then hormone release reduced
- Too little hormone, then hormone release increased

1a Pituitary Gland (Figure 15-2)

1b Anterior Pituitary Gland Hormones
- GH: growth hormone
- TSH: thyroid-stimulating hormone
- ACTH: adrenocorticotropic hormone

© 2007 Pearson Education, Inc.

PowerPoint Lecture Slides *continued*

- Melanocyte-stimulating hormone
- FSH: follicle-stimulating hormone
- LH: Luteinizing hormone
- Prolactin

1c Posterior Pituitary Gland Hormones
- ADH: antidiuretic hormone
- Oxytocin

1d Thyroid Gland Hormones
- TH: thyroid hormone
- Calcitonin

1e Parathyroid Gland Hormone
- PTH: parathyroid hormone

1f Adrenal Cortex Hormones:
- Glucocorticoids: cortisol
- Mineralocortocoids: aldosterone

1g Adrenal Medulla Hormones
- Epinephrine
- Norepinephrine

2 Insulin
- Produced by beta cells in the islets of Langerhans

2a Insulin Release
- Increases with rising blood glucose levels
- Decreases when blood glucose levels fall

2b Glucagon
- Produced by the alpha cells in the islets of Langerhans

2c Glucagon Release
- When blood glucose falls below 70 mg/dL

Suggestions for Classroom Activities

After the students are placed in small groups, assign each group to one endocrine gland/organ. Each group is to create a list of activities/functions in which the hormone either is increased or decreased. Multiple groups can work with the anterior pituitary gland/hormones.

Suggestions for Clinical Activities

Assign students to clients with an alteration in hormone levels. Ask the students to identify which hormones are imbalanced and then list the care provided to aid in the imbalance.

Learning Outcome 3

Describe the actions of insulin and glucagon.

Concepts for Lecture

1. Insulin has a specific role in the maintenance of blood glucose levels.
2. Glucagon has a specific role in the maintenance of blood glucose levels.

PowerPoint Lecture Slides

1 Figure 15-3

1a Insulin
- Function is to regulate blood glucose levels

1b Mechanisms
- Eases the active transport of glucose into muscle and fat cells
- Facilitates fat formation

PowerPoint Lecture Slides *continued*

- Inhibits the breakdown and movement of stored fat
- Helps with protein synthesis

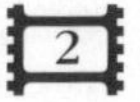
Glucagon
- Prevents blood glucose from decreasing below a certain level

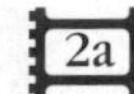
Functions:
- Makes new glucose
- Converts glycogen into glucose in the liver and muscles
- Prevents excess glucose breakdown
- Decreases glucose oxidation and increases blood glucose

Suggestions for Classroom Activities

Provide the students with the following case: Karl Sutherland is a 45-year-old male with the diagnosis of type 2 diabetes mellitus. Explain the mechanism of action behind the development of this type of diabetes. List the possible symptoms this client might demonstrate. Name the hormones that would play the largest role in maintaining his blood glucose level.

Suggestions for Clinical Activities

Assign the students to a client with diabetes. After finding the client's most recent blood glucose levels, have the students diagram the functions of insulin and glucagon to maintain this client's blood glucose level.

Learning Outcome 4

Identify subjective and objective assessment data to collect for clients with endocrine disorders.

Concepts for Lecture

1. Subjective assessment data is collected during the health interview.
2. Objective assessment data is collected during the physical assessment.
3. Specific differences might be seen in the older adult.

PowerPoint Lecture Slides

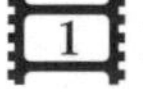
During the Health Interview, Ask the Client:
- Energy level
- Fatigue
- Maintenance of ADLs
- Sensitivity to heat or cold
- Weight level
- Bowel habits
- Level of appetite
- Urination, thirst, salt craving
- Cardiovascular status: blood pressure, heart rate, palpitations, SOB
- Vision: changes, tearing, eye edema
- Neurologic: numbness/tingling lips or extremities, nervousness, hand tremors, mood changes, memory changes, sleep patterns
- Integumentary: hair changes, skin changes, nails, bruising, wound healing

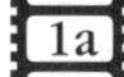
Include Past Medical History:
- Hormone replacement therapy
- Surgeries, chemotherapy, radiation
- Family history: diabetes mellitus, diabetes insipidus, goiter, obesity, Addison's disease, infertility
- Sexual history: changes, characteristics, menstruation, menopause

© 2007 Pearson Education, Inc.

PowerPoint Lecture Slides *continued*

2 Physical Assessment
- General appearance: vital signs, height, weight
- Integumentary: skin color, temperature, texture, moisture, bruising, lesions, wound healing, hair and nail texture, hair growth
- Face: shape, symmetry, eyes, visual acuity, neck (Figure 15-4)
- Extremities: hand and feet size, trunk, muscle strength, deep tendon reflexes, sensation to hot and cold, vibration
- Thorax: lung and heart sounds, extremity edema

3 Relationship between Aging and Endocrine Function:
- Unclear
- Aging causes fibrosis of thyroid gland
- Reduces metabolic rate
- Contributes to weight gain
- Cortisol level unchanged in aging

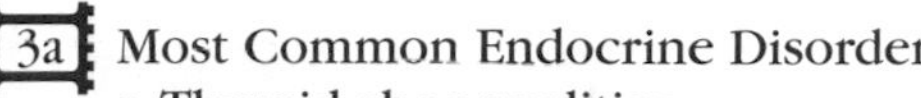

3a Most Common Endocrine Disorders:
- Thyroid abnormalities
- Risk for diabetes mellitus

Suggestions for Classroom Activities

Have the students create a template to use for collecting subjective and objective data on a client with an endocrine disorder.

Suggestions for Clinical Activities

Have the students complete a subjective and objective assessment for a client's endocrine system.

Learning Outcome 5

Identify nursing responsibilities for common diagnostic tests for clients with endocrine disorders.

Concepts for Lecture

1. There are a variety of nursing responsibilities for clients undergoing laboratory tests for endocrine disorders.
2. There are a variety of nursing responsibilities for clients undergoing imaging studies for endocrine disorders.

PowerPoint Lecture Slides

1 Table 15-2

1a Diagnostic Test and Nursing Responsibility:
- GH: fasting, well rested, not physically stressed
- Water deprivation: fasting for 12 hours, no fluids/smoking after midnight
- T_3/T_4: no specific preparation
- Serum calcium/phosphate: fasting may or may not be required
- Cortisol/aldosterone level: two blood samples, client to be up for at least 2 hours before test is drawn
- Urine 17-ketosteroids: 24-hour urine collection that needs to be iced or refrigerated
- FBS: fast before the test
- HbA1c: No fasting required
- OGTT: drink 75 g of glucose and do not eat anything until blood is drawn
- Urine glucose/ketones: fresh urine specimen
- Urine microalbumin: fresh urine specimen

2 Table 15-3

POWERPOINT LECTURE SLIDES *continued*

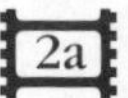
Imaging Studies:

- MRI: metallic implants, lie motionless during test; remove all metal objects
- CT Scan: assess for allergies to iodine and seafood; lie immobile during the test
- Thyroid scan: allergies to iodine and seafood; hold thyroid drugs containing iodine for weeks before the study
- RAI: fast for 8 hours before; can eat 1 hour after radioiodine capsule/liquid taken; hold thyroid drugs with iodine for weeks before the study

SUGGESTIONS FOR CLASSROOM ACTIVITIES

Create a tool that identifies all of the laboratory tests and normal levels. Create a column for abnormal values and the symptoms of each.

SUGGESTIONS FOR CLINICAL ACTIVITIES

Analyze the laboratory findings for a client with an endocrine disorder. Compare the findings with the laboratory tool created in class. Document the client's symptoms for each abnormal value.

© 2007 Pearson Education, Inc.

CHAPTER 16
CARING FOR CLIENTS WITH ENDOCRINE DISORDERS

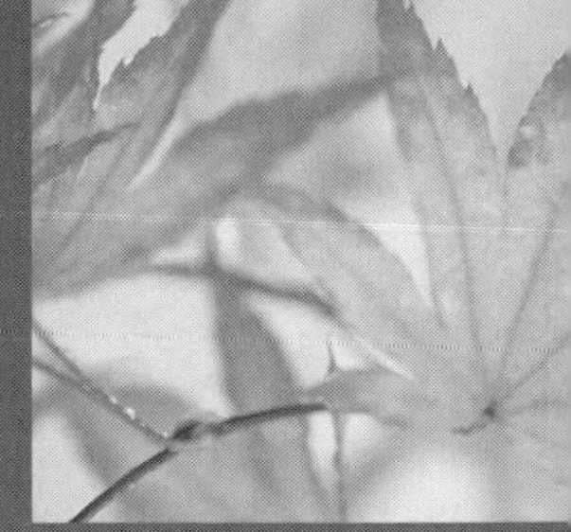

RESOURCE LIBRARY

CD-ROM

Endocrine System
Propranolol

IMAGE LIBRARY

Figure 16-1 Multisystem effects of hyperthyroidism.
Figure 16-2 Individual with enlargement of the thyroid gland (goiter).
Figure 16-3 Exophthalmos in a client with Graves' disease. This is caused by enlargement of muscle and fatty tissue surrounding the eye, which pushes the eyes outward.
Figure 16-4 Multisystem effects of hypothyroidism.
Figure 16-5 A woman before and after developing Cushing's syndrome. In the photo at right, notice the swollen facial features.
Figure 16-6 Major clinical manifestations of Cushing's syndrome.

LEARNING OUTCOME 1

Describe the pathophysiology of the common disorders of the pituitary, thyroid, parathyroid, and adrenal glands.

CONCEPTS FOR LECTURE

1. Disorders within the pituitary, thyroid, parathyroid, and adrenal glands are the result of hyper- or hyposecretion of the associated hormones.

POWERPOINT LECTURE SLIDES

[1] Anterior Pituitary Gland Disorder
- Can be caused by a pituitary tumor

[1a] Disorders with the Anterior Pituitary Gland
- Growth hormone: gigantism, dwarfism, acromegaly

[1b] Posterior Pituitary Gland
- Too much or too little ADH
- Too little ADH: diabetes insipidus
- Too much ADH: SIADH

[1c] Thyroid Gland
- Too much thyroid hormone: hyperthyroidism, Graves' disease, thyrotoxic crisis
- Figure 16-1
- Figure 16-2
- Figure 16-3
- Too little thyroid hormone: hypothyroidism, goiter, Hashimoto's thyroiditis, myxedema coma
- Figure 16-4

[1d] Thyroid Cancer
- Rare but rate is increasing
- Treatment is a subtotal or total thyroidectomy

[1e] Parathyroid Glands
- Hyperparathyroidism leading to hypercalcemia and hypophosphatemia
- Hypoparathyroidism, hypocalcemia, hyperphosphatemia, tetany

POWERPOINT LECTURE SLIDES *continued*

1f Adrenal Glands
- Adrenal cortex: Cushing's syndrome, Addison's disease,
- Figure 16-5
- Figure 16-6
- Adrenal medulla: pheochromocytoma

SUGGESTIONS FOR CLASSROOM ACTIVITIES

Have the students create a grid/table that identifies the endocrine organ, hormone secreted, and condition that develops with either hypo- or hypersecretion.

SUGGESTIONS FOR CLINICAL ACTIVITIES

Assign the students to a client with an endocrine disorder. Once assigned, have the students prepare a report identifying the pathophysiology of the disorder with symptoms.

LEARNING OUTCOME 2

Contrast the manifestations resulting from hypersecretion and hyposecretion of the hormones from the pituitary, thyroid, parathyroid, and adrenal glands.

CONCEPTS FOR LECTURE

1. Clients will present with different manifestations in the presence of hypo- or hypersecretion of the hormones within the endocrine system.

POWERPOINT LECTURE SLIDES

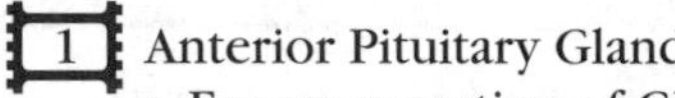

1 Anterior Pituitary Gland
- Excess secretion of GH before puberty results in gigantism
- Excess secretion of GH after puberty results in acromegaly
- Undersecretion of GH before puberty leads to dwarfism

1a Posterior Pituitary Gland
- Too little ADH leads to diabetes insipidus
- Box 16-1
- Too much ADH leads to SIADH
- Box 16-2

1b Thyroid Gland
- Too much thyroid hormone leads to hyperthyroidism, manifested as Graves' disease or thyrotoxic crisis
- Manifestations of hyperthyroidism (Figure 16-1)
- Manifestations of thyrotoxic crisis include high fever, tachycardia, hypertension, restlessness, tremors, progression to confusion, delirium, coma, seizures
- Too little hormone leads to hypothyroidism, manifested as goiter, Hashimoto's thyroiditis, or myxedema coma
- Manifestations of hypothyroidism (Figure 16-4)
- Goiter (Figure 16-2)

1c Parathyroid Glands
- Too much parathyroid hormone leads to hyperparathyroidism
- Manifestations (Box 16-6)
- Too little parathyroid hormone leads to hypoparathyroidism
- Manifestations (Box 16-7)

© 2007 Pearson Education, Inc.

PowerPoint Lecture Slides *continued*

1d Adrenal Gland
- Excess production of cortisol leads to Cushing's syndrome
- Figure 16-6
- Too little production from the adrenal cortex can lead to Addison's disease
- Box 16-9
- Pheochromocytoma, a benign tumor found in the adrenal medulla
- Manifestations include dramatically high blood pressure, pounding headache, tachycardia, profuse sweating, flushing, palpitations

Suggestions for Classroom Activities

Review the grids created for the hypo- and hyper-secreted hormones. Add a column for manifestations for each of the disorders.

Suggestions for Clinical Activities

Assign the students to a client with an endocrine disorder. Have the students identify the manifestations of the disorder with supporting evidence.

Learning Outcome 3

Identify laboratory and diagnostic tests used to diagnose endocrine disorders.

Concepts for Lecture

1. A variety of laboratory tests are available to aid in the diagnosis of an endocrine disorder.
2. A variety of diagnostic tests are available to diagnose an endocrine disorder.

PowerPoint Lecture Slides

1 Posterior pituitary gland
- To aid in the diagnosis of diabetes insipidus, a urine specific gravity is often used

1a Hyperthyroidism
- Laboratory tests used to diagnose this condition include T_3 and T_4 levels and TSH level

1b Hypothyroidism
- Low T_4 level is seen in this condition

1c Hyperparathyroidism
- Blood tests used to diagnose this condition include serum calcium (elevated) and serum phosphorus (low)

1d Hypoparathyroidism
- Blood tests used to diagnose this condition include serum calcium (low) and serum phosphorus (high)

1e Adrenal Cortex
- Tests used to diagnose Cushing's syndrome include plasma cortisol level (increased), 24-hour urine for 17-ketosteroids and 17-hydroxy-corticosteroids (elevated), plasma ACTH level (elevated), serum sodium (elevated), and serum glucose (elevated)
- Tests used to diagnose Addison's disease include serum cortisol (decreased), serum aldosterone (decreased), urinary 17-ketosteroids (decreased), serum potassium (increased), and decreased serum sodium and glucose

PowerPoint Lecture Slides *continued*

1f Adrenal Medulla
- Pheochromocytoma is diagnosed by elevated catecholamine levels in the blood or urine

2 Anterior Pituitary Gland
- MRI and CT scan are used to diagnose an enlarged pituitary gland

2a Hyperthyroidism
- Radioactive iodine (RAI) uptake test is often used to diagnose this condition

2b Adrenal Cortex
- CT and MRI can be used to help diagnose Addison's disease; findings will be atrophy of the adrenal glands

2c Adrenal Medulla
- Pheochromocytoma is diagnosed by CT scan and MRI

Suggestions for Classroom Activities

Have the students divide into small groups. Each group is to be assigned an endocrine organ. Once assigned, the students should create a spreadsheet listing the diagnostic and laboratory tests used to diagnose the endocrine disorder(s) including expected value levels or findings. After completion, all of the spreadsheets can be merged into one document for all of the students to use as a reference.

Suggestions for Clinical Activities

Assign the students to a client with an endocrine disorder. Have the students accompany the client to any scheduled diagnostic tests. Have the students identify laboratory tests (on the medical record) that were done to aid in the diagnosis of the disorder.

Learning Outcome 4

Discuss the nursing implications for medications and treatments ordered for clients with endocrine disorders.

Concepts for Lecture

1. Medications used to treat an endocrine disorder are varied.
2. Treatments for endocrine disorders will depend on the organ involved.

PowerPoint Lecture Slides

1 Anterior Pituitary Gland
- Bromocriptine mesylate (Parlodel) decreases GH production but will not reduce tumor size

1a Posterior Pituitary Gland
- DI: 0.45% normal saline infusion; ADH replacement therapy (Pitressin or DDAVP)
- SIADH: Lasix and fluid restriction; possibly IV hypertonic solution

1b Thyroid Gland
- Thyroid crisis: administer propylthiouracil, acetaminophen
- Hyperthyroidism: Table 16-2
- Hypothyroidism: thyroid hormone replacement therapy
- Thyroid cancer: levothyroxine, chemotherapy

1c Parathyroid Glands
- Hyperparathyroidism: Fosamax, Aredia, Mithracin

© 2007 Pearson Education, Inc.

POWERPOINT LECTURE SLIDES *continued*

- Hypoparathyroidism: IV calcium gluconate; supplemental calcium, oral calcium salts, vitamin D therapy

1d Adrenal Cortex
- Cushing's syndrome: Lysodren, Cytaden
- Addisonian crisis: IV fluids, glucose, sodium, and glucocorticoids
- Addison's disease: hydrocortisone, Florinef
- Table 16-3

1e Adrenal Medulla
- Pheochromocytoma: postop medication therapy includes antihypertensives and/or adrenal hormone replacements

2 Anterior Pituitary Gland
- Removal of pituitary tumor via transsphenoidal hypophysectomy

2a Thyroid Gland
- Hyperthyroidism: treat with radioactive iodine (I-131)
- Hyperthyroidism: subtotal or total thyroidectomy
- Thyroid cancer: sub- or total thyroidectomy, radioactive iodine therapy, external radiation

2b Parathyroid Glands
- Hyperparathyroidism: increase fluid intake to 2 L/day, surgery to remove the parathyroid glands
- Hypoparathyroidism: ensure a patent airway; rebreathing technique

2c Adrenal Cortex
- Cushing's syndrome: adrenalectomy; hypophysectomy; radiation therapy; implant radioactive isotopes

2d Adrenal Medulla
- Pheochromocytoma: adrenalectomy is treatment of choice

SUGGESTIONS FOR CLASSROOM ACTIVITIES

Have the students prepare medication cards for each of the medications used to treat endocrine disorders. Have the students identify postoperative complications for each of the surgical procedures for endocrine disorders.

SUGGESTIONS FOR CLINICAL ACTIVITIES

Assign the students to a client with an endocrine disorder. Have the students research the medications and treatments prescribed to treat the disorder.

LEARNING OUTCOME 5

Identify the preoperative and postoperative nursing care for a client undergoing either a subtotal thyroidectomy or an adrenalectomy.

CONCEPTS FOR LECTURE

1. Preoperative care of a client undergoing a subtotal thyroidectomy or adrenalectomy.
2. Postoperative care of a client undergoing a subtotal thyroidectomy or adrenalectomy.

POWERPOINT LECTURE SLIDES

1 Subtotal Thyroidectomy
- Partial removal of the thyroid gland
- Leaves enough gland tissue to produce an adequate amount of thyroid hormone

POWERPOINT LECTURE SLIDES *continued*

- Provide antithyroid medications and iodine preparations

1a Adrenalectomy
- Stabilize blood pressure

2 Subtotal Thyroidectomy (Box 16-4)

2a Adrenalectomy
- Adrenal hormone replacement therapy
- Continuous treatment for hypertension

SUGGESTIONS FOR CLASSROOM ACTIVITIES

Have the students prepare a plan of care for a client undergoing a subtotal thyroidectomy.

SUGGESTIONS FOR CLINICAL ACTIVITIES

Assign the students to a client with a thyroid disorder. If the client is scheduled for surgery, have the student accompany the client to surgery and participate/observe in the postoperative care.

LEARNING OUTCOME 6

Use the nursing process to care for clients with disorders of the pituitary, thyroid, parathyroid, and adrenal glands.

CONCEPTS FOR LECTURE

1. The nursing process is used to assess, diagnose, plan, implement, and evaluate care provided to clients with endocrine disorders.

POWERPOINT LECTURE SLIDES

1 Anterior Pituitary Disorder
- Help client cope with body image changes and anxiety

1a Diabetes Insipidus
- Manage fluid and electrolyte imbalances
- Nursing Diagnosis: Deficient Fluid Volume related to deficiency of ADH

1b SIADH
- Nursing Diagnoses: Excess Fluid Volume related to excess production of ADH

1c Hyperthyroidism
- Focus on multisystem effects to include altered nutrition, fatigue, cardiovascular problems, visual deficits, and body image disturbance
- Nursing Diagnoses:
  - Risk for Imbalanced Nutrition: Less than Body Requirements
  - Fatigue
  - Risk for Decreased Cardiac Output
  - Risk for Injury: corneal abrasion
  - Disturbed Body Image

1d Hypothyroidism
- Focus on hypothermia, constipation, activity, and altered through processes
- Nursing Diagnoses:
  - Hypothermia
  - Constipation
  - Activity Intolerance
  - Disturbed Thought Processes

© 2007 Pearson Education, Inc.

PowerPoint Lecture Slides *continued*

1e Hyperparathyroidism
- Focus on impaired physical mobility, risk for injury, pain, altered nutritional intake

1f Hypoparathyroidism
- Focus on risk for injury, altered thought processes, personality changes, impaired memory, diet

1g Cushing's Syndrome
- Manage fluid and electrolyte balance, injury, infection, body image
- Nursing Diagnoses:
    - Excess Fluid Volume
    - Risk for Injury
    - Risk for Infection
    - Risk for Impaired Skin Integrity
    - Disturbed Body Image

1h Addison's Disease
- Manage fluid and electrolyte imbalances, activity intolerance, and altered nutrition
- Nursing Diagnoses:
    - Deficient Fluid Volume
    - Activity Intolerance
    - Imbalanced Nutrition: Less than Body Requirements

1i Pheochromocytoma
- Stabilize blood pressure
- Hemodynamic monitoring
- Intravenous antihypertensive medication

Suggestions for Classroom Activities

Divide the students into groups. Have them prepare a plan of care for a client with a specified endocrine disorder.

Suggestions for Clinical Activities

Assign the students to a client with an endocrine disorder. Part of the care of this client includes the creation of a care plan to address the client's needs caused by the endocrine disorder.

Learning Outcome 7

Reinforce teaching guidelines for clients receiving long-term hormonal replacement therapy.

Concepts for Lecture

1. Clients with hypothyroidism or postoperative total thyroidectomy will be prescribed long-term thyroid replacement therapy.
2. Clients with Addison's disease will be prescribed long-term thyroid replacement therapy.

PowerPoint Lecture Slides

1 Table 16-2

1a Teaching associated with thyroid replacement therapy:
- Take every day before breakfast
- Take pulse daily, report resting rate >100 to MD
- Do not take medication with antacids or iron
- Take medication for rest of life
- Report unusual weight loss, nervousness, bleeding, chest pain, or SOB
- Clients with diabetes need to monitor blood glucose levels; insulin may need to be adjusted
- Teach client to carry Medic-Alert card

PowerPoint Lecture Slides *continued*

2 Table 16-3

2a Teaching Associated with Replacement Therapy:
- Take medications with foods
- Report gastric distress or dark stools
- Never abruptly stop the medication
- Take medications for the rest of life
- Eat a diet high in potassium, low in sodium
- Daily weight; report weight gain, edema, or round face
- Avoid accidents
- Wear a Medic-Alert bracelet
- Avoid exposure to infection; wash hands frequently
- Report dizziness upon sitting or standing, nausea and vomiting, pain, thirst, feelings of anxiety, malaise, infection

Suggestions for Classroom Activities

Have the students research new hormone replacement medications and prepare a 10-minute presentation to be shared in class.

Suggestions for Clinical Activities

Assign the student to a client with an endocrine disorder. Ensure the student comprehends the medications prescribed for this disorder.

© 2007 Pearson Education, Inc.

CHAPTER 17
CARING FOR CLIENTS WITH DIABETES MELLITUS

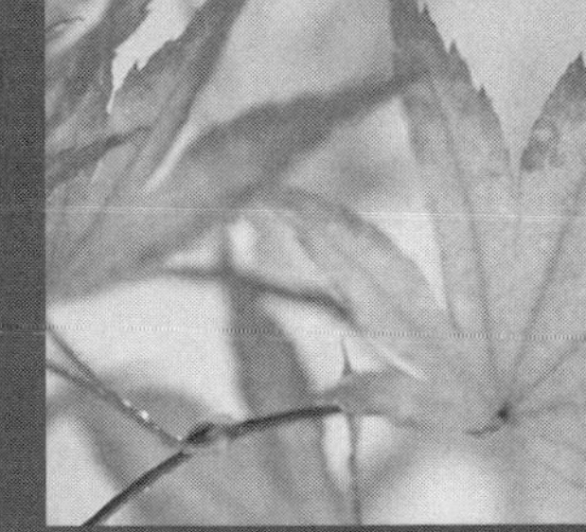

RESOURCE LIBRARY

CD-ROM

Diabetes
Glipizide

IMAGE LIBRARY

Figure 17-1 Sites of insulin injection.
Figure 17-2 Multisystem effects of diabetes mellitus.
Figure 17-3 Pathophysiology of diabetic ketoacidosis.
Figure 17-4 Ulceration following trauma to the foot of a person with diabetes.

LEARNING OUTCOME 1

Define diabetes mellitus, and explain the pathophysiology of Type 1 and Type 2 diabetes mellitus with the related manifestations.

CONCEPTS FOR LECTURE

1. Definition of diabetes mellitus.
2. Pathophysiology and manifestations of type 1 diabetes mellitus.
3. Pathophysiology and manifestations of type 2 diabetes mellitus.

POWERPOINT LECTURE SLIDES

1 Diabetes Mellitus
- Chronic disease of adults
- Not a single disorder
- Group of metabolic disorders
- Characteristics:
  - Hyperglycemia

1a Overview
- Large number of individuals are not diagnosed
- Cannot be cured
- Can be controlled in efforts to control complications

1b Complications:
- Affects:
  - Eyes
  - Kidneys
  - Nervous system
  - Cardiovascular system

2 Occurrence
- Children and adolescents
- Results from an autoimmune disorder that destroys the beta cells

2a Results
- Insulin no longer produced
- Leads to hyperglycemia and breakdown of body fat and protein
- Cells starve
- Burning of fat leads to "ketosis"
- Ketone bodies accumulate

PowerPoint Lecture Slides *continued*

2b Pathophysiology
- Elevated blood glucose
- Excess spills into the urine leading to glycosuria
- Once hyperglycemia and glycosuria occur, three manifestations of diabetes are seen:
  - Polyuria
  - Polydipsia
  - Polyphagia

2c Pathophysiology (continued)
- Manifestations (Box 17.1)

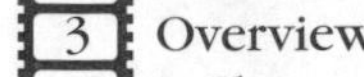

3 Overview
- Characterized by hyperglycemia due to insufficient insulin production and insulin resistance
- Not enough insulin to lower blood glucose levels
- Enough insulin to prevent the breakdown of fats; ketosis does not develop
- Risk factors:
  - Heredity
  - Obesity
  - Increasing age
  - High-risk ethnic group

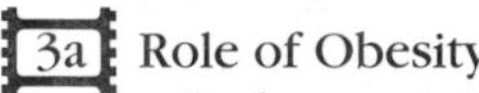

3a Role of Obesity
- Reduces available insulin receptor sites, leading to insulin resistance
- Three-quarters of older adults with type 2 are overweight
- All older adults develop insulin resistance
- Weight loss through diet and exercise can reduce insulin resistance
- With enough weight loss, may not need oral medications

3b Diagnosis
- Often undiagnosed for years
- Less severe hyperglycemia
- Only polyuria and polydipsia are present
- Breeding ground for bacterial infections
- Cloudiness of eye lens leading to blurred vision
- Destruction of peripheral nerves leading to paresthesias
- Fatigue due to tissue starvation

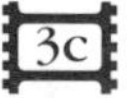

3c Manifestations
- Box 17-1

Suggestions for Classroom Activities

1. Diagram the pathophysiology of type 1/type 2 diabetes mellitus.
2. Based on the diagram, identify the cause of the signs and symptoms of the disease.

Suggestions for Clinical Activities

Assign the students to a client with either type 1 or type 2 diabetes mellitus. Have the students find out from the client:
- The time of diagnosis
- The presenting s/s upon diagnosis
- Current manifestations of the disease

© 2007 Pearson Education, Inc.

Learning Outcome 2

Identify the laboratory and diagnostic tests used to diagnose and monitor self-management of diabetes mellitus.

Concepts for Lecture

1. Laboratory tests used to diagnose and monitor self-management of diabetes mellitus
2. Diagnostic tests used to diagnose and monitor self-management of diabetes mellitus.

PowerPoint Lecture Slides

1 Laboratory Tests to Diagnose
- Plasma glucose (PG) level
- Fasting blood glucose level (FBG)
- Oral glucose tolerance test (OGTT)

1a Routine Screening Tests Should Be Done If:
- Obese
- First-degree relative with DM
- High-risk ethnic population
- Delivered baby > 9 lb or gestational diabetes history
- Hypertensive
- HDL < 35 mg/dL
- Triglycerides > 250 mg/dL
- Impaired glucose tolerance or fasting glucose in the past

1b Self-Monitoring Blood Glucose
- Monitor and achieve metabolic control
- Useful if ill or pregnant
- Useful if symptomatic with hypo- or hyperglycemia
- On insulin: three or more times per day
- Not on insulin: two to three times per week

1c Equipment
- Lancet
- Blood glucose monitoring machine
- Test strips
- Follow manufacturer's instructions for use

1d Noninvasive Blood Glucose Monitoring
- GlucoWatch Biographer: worn as a watch
- Measures glucose value in perspiration

1e Urine Testing for Ketones and Glucose
- Has unpredictable results
- Should be done with type 1 diabetes
- Either Acidtest tablets or Ketostix
- Normal result is no glucose in urine

2 See Chapter 15, Table 15-2

Suggestions for Classroom Activities

Provide a variety of self-monitoring blood glucose meters. Have the students practice using the monitors on each other.

Suggestions for Clinical Activities

Assign the students to a client with diabetes. Have the student measure the client's blood glucose level with a glucometer. Have the student measure the client's urine ketones and glucose with either the tablets or strips. Document the values in the medical record.

© 2007 Pearson Education, Inc.

LEARNING OUTCOME 3

Discuss the nursing implications for insulin and oral antidiabetic agents ordered for clients with diabetes mellitus.

CONCEPTS FOR LECTURE

1. Nursing implications for clients prescribed insulin for diabetes mellitus.
2. Nursing implications for clients prescribed oral antidiabetic agents for diabetes mellitus.

POWERPOINT LECTURE SLIDES

1 Insulin
- Pork or synthetic
- Strengths: rapid-acting, short-acting, intermediate-acting, long-acting
- See Table 17-2 for onset, peak, duration of action

1a Insulin Strengths
- 100 U per mL or 500 U per mL
- Administered in a sterile, single-use, disposable syringe
- All insulin given parenterally
- Regular insulin: either subcutaneous or intravenous

1b Alternative Delivery Methods
- Insulin pen
- Jet injector
- Continuous subcutaneous infusion pump

1c Injection Sites
- See Figure 17-1
- Process: pinch skin, inject needle at 90-degree angle
- Do not inject into muscle; do not massage after injecting
- Rotate injection sites
- Minimize painful injections; see Box 17-2

1d Problems with Insulin Injections:
- Lipodystrophy
- Lipoatrophy

1e Mixing Insulin
- See Procedure 17-1
- See Table 17-3

1f Insulin Regimen
- Individualized
- Mix short and longer acting
- Timing depends on feed, exercise, glucose level, type of insulin
- Tight glucose control results in fewer long-term complications (see Table 17-4)

2 Oral Antidiabetic Agents
- See Table 17-5

SUGGESTIONS FOR CLASSROOM ACTIVITIES

1. Provide students with a variety of insulin vials, syringes, needles. Provide classroom time for the students to practice filling, fixing, and mock-administering insulin.
2. Practice locating anatomic areas for insulin injections.

SUGGESTIONS FOR CLINICAL ACTIVITIES

Assign the students to a client with diabetes mellitus. Have the students prepare/study medication administration card. Have the students prepare and administer the medication.

© 2007 Pearson Education, Inc.

Learning Outcome 4

Compare and contrast the manifestations and interdisciplinary care of hypoglycemia, diabetic ketoacidosis (DKA), and hyperglycemic hyperosmolar nonketotic syndrome (HHNS).

Concepts for Lecture

1. Care of hypoglycemia.
2. Care of diabetic ketoacidosis (DKA).
3. Care of hyperglycemic hyperosmolar nonketotic syndrome (HHNS).

PowerPoint Lecture Slides

1 Hypoglycemia
- Type 1 or type 2 diabetes
- Causes: too much insulin, overdose of oral antidiabetic agents, too little food, excess physical activity
- Sudden onset; blood glucose < 50 mg/dL

1a Manifestations
- See Box 17-5
- Hypoglycemia unawareness: no symptoms of hypoglycemia in the presence of a low blood glucose level

1b Treatment
- Mild: immediate treatment; 15 g rapid-acting sugar
- Severe: hospitalized, intravenous glucose

2 DKA
- Life-threatening illness in type 1
- Characteristics: hyperglycemia, dehydration, coma
- Excess glucose leads to dehydration, sodium and potassium loss
- Burning of fat leads to ketosis
- Kidneys unable to excrete ketones, leads to ketoacidosis

2a Manifestations
- See Box 17-4

2b Treatment
- Hospital admission
- Treatment: fluids, insulin, electrolytes

3 HHNS
- Seen in type 2 diabetes
- Characteristics: elevated blood glucose, extreme dehydration, altered LOC
- Develops slowly over hours to days

3a Manifestations
- See Box 17-4

3b Treatment
- Correct fluid and electrolyte imbalances; provide insulin

Suggestions for Classroom Activities

Have the students diagram the pathophysiology of DKA, HHNS, and/or hypoglycemia. Identify the role of each of the treatments.

Suggestions for Clinical Activities

Assign the students to a client with diabetes mellitus. Assess the client for any history of DKA, HHNS, or hypoglycemia.

© 2007 Pearson Education, Inc.

Learning Outcome 5

Describe the pathophysiology and interdisciplinary care of chronic complications for clients with Type 1 and Type 2 diabetes mellitus.

Concepts for Lecture

1. Pathophysiology and care of macrovascular complications.
2. Pathophysiology and care of microvascular complications.

PowerPoint Lecture Slides

1 Macrovascular Complications:
- Macrocirculation: large blood vessels undergo changes due to atherosclerosis
- Complications: coronary artery disease, stroke, peripheral vascular disease

1a Complication: CAD
- Risk factor for an MI
- High cholesterol and high triglycerides

1b Complication: Stroke
- Two to six times more likely to occur in type 2
- Hypertension plays a role

1c Complication: Peripheral Vascular Disease
- Greater in type 2
- Diabetes-induced arteriosclerosis
- Can lead to leg ulcers and gangrene
- Manifestations
  - See Box 17-6

2 Microvascular Complications:
- Microcirculation: eyes, kidneys, nerves

2a Complication: Diabetic Retinopathy
- Changes in the retinal capillaries; lead to retinal ischemia, retinal hemorrhage, or detachment
- Retinopathy stages: nonproliferative and proliferative
- Leading cause of blindness in people ages 20 to 74
- Yearly eye exams are recommended

2b Complication: Diabetic Nephropathy
- Disease of the kidneys
- Characterized by albumin in the urine, hypertension, edema, renal insufficiency
- Most common cause of renal failure
- First indication: microalbuminuria
- Treatment: ACE inhibitors

2c Complication: Diabetic Neuropathy
- Disorder of the peripheral nerves and autonomic nervous system
- Results: sensory and motor impairments, postural hypotension, delayed gastric emptying, diarrhea, impaired genitourinary function
- Result from the thickening of the capillary membrane and destruction of myelin sheath
- Bilateral sensory disorders; appear first in toes, feet, and progress upward to fingers and hands
- Treatment: none specific; focus on controlling neuropathic pain with tricyclic antidepressants or topical cream capsaicin (Zostrix)

© 2007 Pearson Education, Inc.

PowerPoint Lecture Slides *continued*

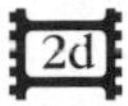 Complication: Autonomic Neuropathy
- Involves numerous organs such as cardiovascular, gastrointestinal, genitourinary

Suggestions for Classroom Activities

Have the students divide into groups. Assign each group a long-term complication. Have each group create a presentation about the complication that includes pathophysiology, presenting signs and symptoms, recommended treatments/therapies.

Suggestions for Clinical Activities

Assign the students to a client with diabetes. Have the students complete an assessment for the presence of any long-term complications.

Learning Outcome 6

Reinforce teaching guidelines to clients with diabetes mellitus regarding self-management of medications, diet, exercise, and foot care.

Concepts for Lecture

1. The teaching plan for a client with diabetes mellitus should include self-management of medications, diet, exercise, and foot care.

PowerPoint Lecture Slides

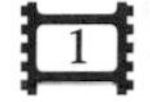 Teaching Plan Contents
- Medications
- Diet
- Exercise
- Foot care

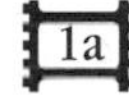 Medications
- Type of medication: oral or insulin
- Insulin: type, dosage, mixing instructions, times of onset and peak, obtaining and care of equipment, self-injections, locations for injections, timing of injections with meals

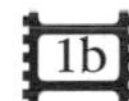 Diet
- Role of diet with control of blood glucose levels
- Complex carbohydrates and food high in fiber
- Limit sugar, fat, sodium, alcohol
- How to read food labels
- Personal food preferences
- Eating away from home
- Relationship between diet, exercise, medication

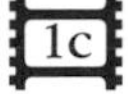 Exercise
- Purpose
- Importance
- Types
- Personal exercise choices

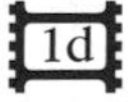 Foot Care
- See Box 17-8
- Wash feet daily; inspect feet daily

Suggestions for Classroom Activities

Have the students create a teaching plan for self-management of medications, diet, exercise, or foot care.

Suggestions for Clinical Activities

Assign the students to a client with diabetes. Implement the teaching plan created in the classroom to instruct the client in one aspect of self-management.

© 2007 Pearson Education, Inc.

Learning Outcome 7

Identify specific concerns for young, middle-aged, and older adults with diabetes mellitus.

Concepts for Lecture

1. Concerns for young adults with diabetes mellitus.
2. Concerns for middle-aged adults with diabetes mellitus.
3. Concerns for older adults with diabetes mellitus.

PowerPoint Lecture Slides

1 Concerns for Young Adults
- Assess the young adult's lifestyle including eating habits/patterns, exercise
- Provide teaching to address the need for scheduled eating patterns and exercise regime

2 Concerns for Middle-Aged Adults
- Assess the client's lifestyle to include eating habits/patterns, exercise
- Provide teaching to address the need for scheduled eating patterns and exercise regime.
- See Table 17-6

3 Concerns for Older Adults
- If obese, might need diet, exercise, and weight reduction program
- Consider: dietary likes/dislikes, eating habits, meal preparation, age-related changes in taste and smell, dental health
- Consider: age-related decline in calorie needs and reduced physical activity
- Might be on a fixed income
- Coexisting illnesses and multiple medications can decrease appetite and reduce energy to plan, cook, or eat
- Dietary restrictions can lead to avoidance of social gatherings
- Decreased thirst mechanism can lead to dehydration
- Exercise should be individualized depending on physical limitations
- Withdrawal from social situations can lead to depression
- Visual and fine motor skill deficits can make insulin administration, glucose monitoring, food preparation, exercise and foot care difficult or impossible.

Suggestions for Classroom Activities

Have the students create a plan of care for an elderly client with type 2 diabetes.

Suggestions for Clinical Activities

Assign the students to clients with diabetes mellitus. Have the students conduct an assessment, provide medications, teach one aspect of self-management, and document all care provided and responses to care for this client.

© 2007 Pearson Education, Inc.

LEARNING OUTCOME 8

Use the nursing process to collect data, establish outcomes, provide individualized care, and evaluate responses for the client with diabetes mellitus.

CONCEPTS FOR LECTURE

1. Nursing process steps for the care of a client with diabetes mellitus.

POWERPOINT LECTURE SLIDES

1 The Nursing Process
- Used to assess, diagnose, plan, implement, and evaluate care for the client with diabetes mellitus.

1a Assessment
- Subjective data
- Objective data

1b Nursing Diagnoses
- Imbalanced Nutrition
- Impaired Skin Integrity
- Risk for Infection
- Risk for Injury
- Ineffective Coping

1c Evaluation
- Collect data related to chronic complications
- Identify frequency of DKA, HHNS, hypoglycemia
- Document VS, LOC, skin integrity, complications
- Notify MD of client's response to treatment
- Reinforce teaching related to medications, diet, and self-care
- Document

SUGGESTIONS FOR CLASSROOM ACTIVITIES

Have the students create plans of care for clients with type 1 and type 2 diabetes.

SUGGESTIONS FOR CLINICAL ACTIVITIES

Assign the students to a client with diabetes. Have the students implement the plan of care created in the classroom. Conclude the clinical experience with a review of the evaluation findings from the plan of care.

© 2007 Pearson Education, Inc.

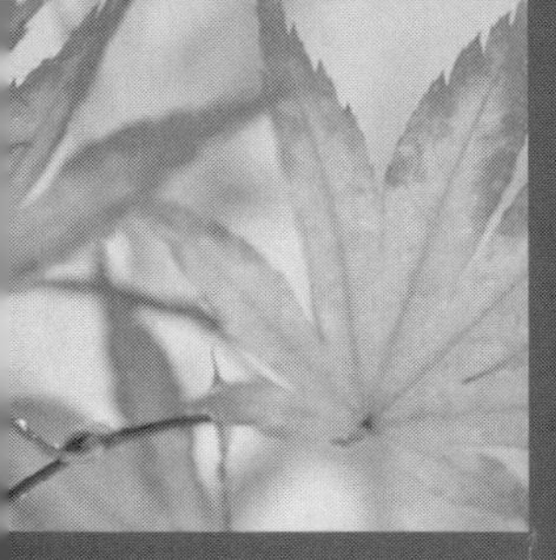

CHAPTER 18
THE GASTROINTESTINAL SYSTEM AND ASSESSMENT

RESOURCE LIBRARY

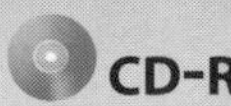

CD-ROM

Digestive System

IMAGE LIBRARY

Figure 18-1 Organs of the gastrointestinal tract and accessory digestive organs.
Figure 18-2 Structures of the stomach and duodenum, including the common bile duct, pancreatic duct, pancreas, and gallbladder.
Figure 18-3 Anatomy of the large intestine.
Figure 18-4 Structure of the rectum and anus.
Figure 18-5 A section of a liver lobule with plates of hepatocytes, the central vein, bile duct, portal vein, and hepatic artery.
Figure 18-6 The gallbladder, common bile duct, and sphincter of Oddi.
Figure 18-7 The four quadrants of the abdomen, with the organs located within each quadrant.

LEARNING OUTCOME 1

Describe the structure and function of the gastrointestinal (GI) tract and accessory organs of digestion (liver, gallbladder, and pancreas).

CONCEPTS FOR LECTURE

1. Organs of the GI tract with primary functions.
2. Organs of the GI tract with accessory functions.

POWERPOINT LECTURE SLIDES

1 Major GI Function Organs Include (Figure 18-1):
- Mouth
- Pharynx
- Esophagus
- Stomach
- Small intestine
- Large intestine

1a Accessory GI Organs Include:
- Liver
- Gallbladder
- Pancreas

1b Mouth
- Teeth chew and grind food into smaller parts
- Moistened with saliva for tasting, chewing, and swallowing

1c Pharynx
- Muscles that propel the food from the mouth

1d Esophagus
- Carries food through peristalsis
- Cardiac/lower esophageal sphincter: closes after food leaves the esophagus

1e Stomach (Figure 18-2)
- Holds the food
- Pyloric sphincter: controls the emptying of the stomach

PowerPoint Lecture Slides *continued*

1f Small Intestine (Figure 18-2)
- 20 feet long, 1 inch in diameter
- Hangs in coils
- Digests food
- Has three regions
  - Duodenum
  - Jejunum
  - Ileum

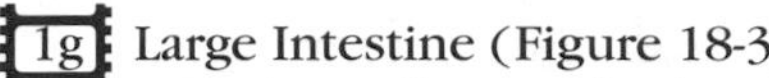

1g Large Intestine (Figure 18-3)
- Begins at ileocecal valve, terminates at the anus
- 5 feet long
- Includes the appendix
- Nutrients absorbed and indigestible materials eliminated
- Parts:
  - Ascending
  - Transverse
  - Descending
    - Sigmoid colon
    - Rectum

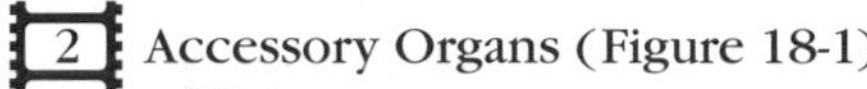

2 Accessory Organs (Figure 18-1)
- Liver
- Gallbladder
- Pancreas

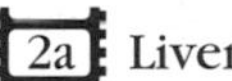

2a Liver
- Largest gland in the body
- Located in the right side of the abdomen (Figure 18-1)
- Has four lobes
- Encased in a fibrous capsule
- Hepatocytes produce bile, which aids in digestion

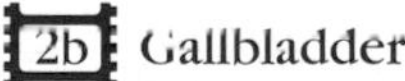

2b Gallbladder
- Stores extra bile
- Located on the inferior surface of the liver (Figure 18-6)

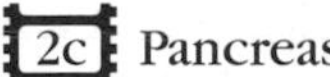

2c Pancreas
- Gland located between the stomach and small intestines
- Figure 18-1
- Exocrine and endocrine functions
- Produce pancreatic juice to neutralize food
- Produce enzymes to digest food

Suggestions for Classroom Activities

1. Have the students study the anatomy and location of the organs of digestion.
2. Have the students study the techniques of inspection, auscultation, percussion, and palpation.
3. Review the contents of the website http://digestive.niddk.nih.gov/ddiseases/pubs/yrdd/.

Suggestions for Clinical Activities

Assign the students a client to auscultate bowel sounds.

© 2007 Pearson Education, Inc.

Learning Outcome 2

Describe the physiologic processes involved in ingestion, digestion, and elimination of foods and nutrients.

Concepts for Lecture

1. Physiologic process with ingestion.
2. Physiologic process with digestion.
3. Physiologic process with elimination.

PowerPoint Lecture Slides

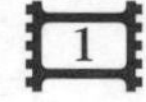
1 The Mouth
- The upper opening of the GI tract
- Is lined by mucous membranes
- The teeth chew and grind food into smaller parts
- *Saliva* (produced by the salivary glands) moistens food for tasting, chewing, and swallowing

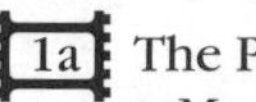
1a The Pharynx
- Muscles here move the food into the esophagus

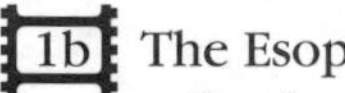
1b The Esophagus
- Carries the food to the stomach through peristalsis

2 Mouth
- Digestive process starts here
- Enzymes in the saliva begin the food breakdown
- Enzymes: amylase, lysozyme

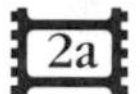
2a Stomach
- Mechanical digestion in the stomach mixes partially digested food with gastric juices to produce *chyme*
- Cells within the stomach lining produce:
  - *Parietal cells* secrete hydrochloric acid and intrinsic factor; hydrochloric acid used to digest protein; intrinsic factor helps with vitamin B_{12} absorption
  - *Chief cells* produce pepsin, which digests protein.
  - *Mucous cells* produce alkaline mucus to protect the lining of the stomach from gastric juices
  - *Enteroendocrine cells* secrete hormones that help regulate digestion

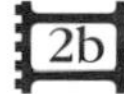
2b Nervous System
- Parasympathetic nervous system signals vagus nerve to increase gastric secretions in response to food
- Emotions (anxiety/stress) reduce gastric secretions and motility

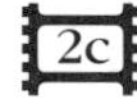
2c Small Intestines
- Location where food is chemically digested and most absorbed
- Enzymes break down carbohydrates, proteins, and fats
- Pancreatic buffers neutralize the stomach acid
- Microvilli enhance absorption
- Most of food, water, vitamins, and minerals are absorbed here into the blood or lymph

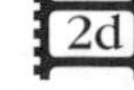
2d Liver
- Digestive functions:
  - Metabolize carbohydrates, proteins, and fats

© 2007 Pearson Education, Inc.

PowerPoint Lecture Slides *continued*

- Synthesize plasma proteins and enzymes
- Store blood, vitamins, and minerals
- Produce and secrete bile

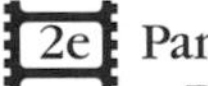 Pancreas
- Produces enzymes for digestion
- Secretion is controlled by the vagus nerve and the hormones secretin and cholecystokinin
- *Lipase* promotes fat breakdown and absorption
- A*mylase* digests starch
- T*rypsin, chymotrypsin,* and *carboxypeptidase* digest protein
- *Nucleases,* which digest nucleic acids, are also present

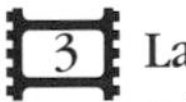 Large Intestine
- Major function: eliminate indigestible food
- Absorbs water, salts, and vitamins forming it into feces or stool
- Feces move with peristalsis
- Goblet cells secrete mucus to aid with defecation
- Defecation reflex: sigmoid colon walls contract and anal sphincter relaxes

Suggestions for Classroom Activities

Track the process of food digestion, beginning with intake through the mouth up to and including defecation. Refer to http://digestive.niddk.nih.gov/ddiseases/pubs/yrdd/ for assistance.

Suggestions for Clinical Activities

Assign the students to a client with a digestive disorder. Have the students prepare a teaching plan to include the organs of ingestion, digestion, and defecation. Utilize this teaching plan for the client.

Learning Outcome 3

Identify sources of various nutrients, including vitamins.

Concepts for Lecture

1. Sources of nutrients and vitamins.

PowerPoint Lecture Slides

1 Nutrients
- Carbohydrates
- Proteins
- Fats
- Vitamins
- Minerals
- Water

1a Carbohydrates
- Simple sugars: milk, sugar cane, sugar beets, honey fruits
- Complex starches: grains, legumes, root vegetables

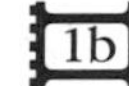 Proteins
- Complete proteins (all essential AA): eggs, milk, milk products, meat, fish, poultry
- Plant proteins: legumes, nuts, grains, cereals, vegetables

POWERPOINT LECTURE SLIDES *continued*

1c Fats
- Saturated fats: animal fats, cocoa butter, palm/coconut oil, hydrogenated vegetable fats
- Unsaturated fats: vegetable oils, soft margarines

1d Vitamins
- Found in fruits, vegetables, grains, and animal products

1e Minerals
- Found in fruits, vegetables, grains, and animal products

1f Water
- Found in fruit juices, milk, coffee, tea, soft drinks, gelatin

SUGGESTIONS FOR CLASSROOM ACTIVITIES

Have the students keep a food journal for 3 days. After the third day, have the students complete a nutritional study of all of the foods in the journal. Website resources include:
www.healthalternatives2000.com/fruitchart.htm
www.lifeclinic.com/focus/nutrition/nutritionview.asp?artId=1023
www.ext.colostate.edu/pubs/foodnut/09306.html

SUGGESTIONS FOR CLINICAL ACTIVITIES

Assign the students to a client and have them conduct the classroom activity with the client.

LEARNING OUTCOME 4

Collect assessment data related to digestion and nutritional status.

CONCEPTS FOR LECTURE

1. Assessment data on digestion and nutritional status.

POWERPOINT LECTURE SLIDES

1 Health History
- Current complaints, food intolerance
- Appetite, heartburn, nausea, vomiting
- Abdominal discomfort, diarrhea, constipation
- Weight changes
- Food allergies
- Pattern and amount of daily food intake
- Teeth, mouth, ability to chew, swallow, dentures
- Change in stool frequency, amount, color, caliber
- Medications
- Chronic diseases
- Previous surgeries

1a Physical Examination
- Overall health status
- Skin color, hair, nails
- Height and weight
- Inspect mouth, teeth, tongue
- Swallow
- Inspect abdomen, observe skin, peristalsis
- Auscultate bowel sounds
- Percuss the abdomen
- Palpate the abdomen
- Box 18-1

© 2007 Pearson Education, Inc.

Suggestions for Classroom Activities

Have the students conduct a nutritional/digestion assessment on each other. Websites to assist in this activity include:
www.jr2.ox.ac.uk/bandolier/band27/b27-8.html
www.nutritionalquotient.com/v2/index.htm

Suggestions for Clinical Activities

Have the students conduct a nutritional/digestion assessment for a client.

Learning Outcome 5

Discuss the nursing implications of diagnostic tests and treatment for clients with disorders of nutrition or affecting the GI tract or accessory organs.

Concepts for Lecture

1. Nursing implications of diagnostic tests.
2. Nursing implications for treatments.

PowerPoint Lecture Slides

1 Diagnostic Tests:
- Gastric analysis
- Urea breath test
- Ambulatory pH monitoring
- Esophageal manometry
- Paracentesis

1a Gastric Analysis
- Instruct client to abstain from food, fluids, smoking, chewing gum, and some medications for 8 to 12 hours before the test
- Insert NG tube and collect samples

1b Urea Breath Test
- Instruct client to abstain from food and fluids for 4 hours prior to the test
- Instruct client to abstain from antacids, bismuth sulfate, antibiotics, and Prilosec for 2 weeks prior to the test

1c Ambulatory pH Monitor
- Instruct client how to care for the electrode and data recorder

1d Esophageal Manometry
- Instruct client to abstain from food and fluids up to 8 hours prior to the test
- Assist with insertion of the tube

1e Paracentesis
- Refer to Chapter 20 for more information

1f Diagnostic Imaging Procedures
- Table 18-5

1g Laboratory tests
- Table 18-3

Suggestions for Classroom Activities

Access the website www.mydna.com/health/digestive. Select one digestive disorder. Prepare a 10-minute presentation on the disorder.

Suggestions for Clinical Activities

Assign the students to a client with a GI disorder. Have the student accompany the client to any diagnostic tests.

© 2007 Pearson Education, Inc.

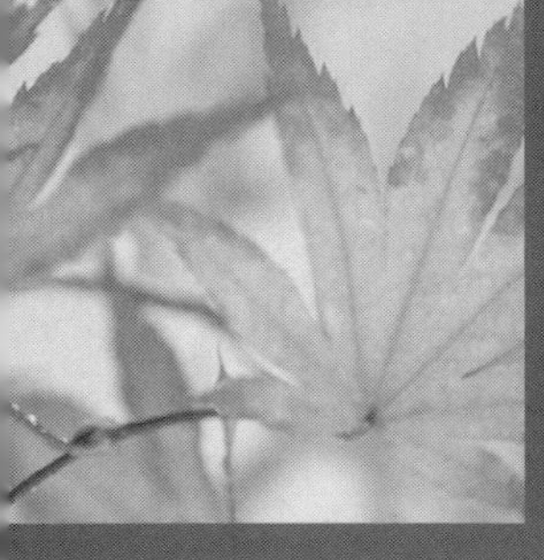

CHAPTER 19
CARING FOR CLIENTS WITH NUTRITIONAL AND UPPER GASTROINTESTINAL DISORDERS

RESOURCE LIBRARY

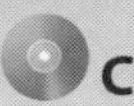 **CD-ROM**

Video: Nasogastric Tube
Video: Anorexia
Video: Bulemia
Video: Eating Disorders
Video: GERD
Video: Gastric Lavage
Video: Ranitidine

IMAGE LIBRARY

Figure 19-1 With calipers, measure the thickness of a fold of skin on the back of the arm or below the shoulder blade.

Figure 19-2 The USDA Food Guide Pyramid.

Figure 19-3 Surgical procedures to treat obesity. **(A)** Vertical banding. **(B)** Gastric bypass.

Figure 19-4 Oral cancer.

Figure 19-5 Hiatal hernias. **(A)** Sliding. **(B)** Paraesophageal.

Figure 19-6 The gastric mucosa and the mucosal barrier. The mucous gel and bicarbonate of the mucosal barrier protect the gastric mucosa from damage by gastric secretions.

Figure 19-7 Sites commonly affected by peptic ulcer disease.

Figure 19-8 A large gastric ulcer.

Figure 19-9 Gastric cancer as seen through an endoscope.

Figure 19-10 Partial and total gastrectomy procedures. **(A)** Partial gastrectomy with anastomosis to the duodenum. **(B)** Partial gastrectomy with anastomosis to the jejunum. **(C)** Total gastrectomy with anastomosis of the esophagus to the jejunum.

Figure 19-11 **(A)** Gastrostomy tube placement. **(B)** The tube is held in place by cross bars.

LEARNING OUTCOME 1

Describe the causes, pathophysiology, and manifestations of common nutritional and upper GI disorders.

CONCEPTS FOR LECTURE

1. Causes of common nutritional and upper GI disorders.
2. Pathophysiology of common nutritional and upper GI disorders.
3. Manifestations of common nutritional and upper GI disorders.

POWERPOINT LECTURE SLIDES

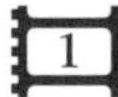 Obesity
- Excess adipose tissue or fat
- Body weight > than ideal for height
- Occurs when excess calories are stored as fat
- Nearly 1/3 of all Americans are obese

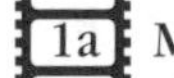 Malnutrition
- Inadequate nutrient intake
- Effects all body systems
- Increases risk of disease and death
- Poor wound healing; lower resistance to infection
- At-risk groups: young, poor, elderly, homeless, low-income women, ethnic minorities
- Disorders (bulimia, anorexia nervosa), fad diets, GI problems
- Box 19-3

PowerPoint Lecture Slides *continued*

1b Eating Disorders
- Anorexia nervosa and bulimia
- Characterized by disturbed eating behavior and weight management

1c Disorders of the Mouth: Stomatitis
- Inflammation of the oral mucosa
- Develops secondary to another condition

1d Disorders of the Mouth: Oral Cancer
- 30,000 new cases of oral cancer are diagnosed annually
- Incidence is twice as high in men as in women
- Seen more often in men over 40
- Major risk factor for oral cancer: smoking and smokeless tobacco
- Alcohol consumption and prolonged exposure to sunlight

1e Disorders of the Esophagus: GERD
- Gastroesophageal reflux: backward movement of gastric contents into the esophagus
- Affects 15% to 20% of adults

1f Disorders of the Esophagus: Hiatal Hernia
- Usually occur with aging or because of increased intra-abdominal pressure

1g Disorders of the Esophagus: Esophageal Cancer
- Mostly uncommon
- Smoking and alcohol use linked to the development

1h Disorders of the Stomach/Intestines: Gastroenteritis
- Inflammation of stomach and intestines
- Caused by viral, bacterial, or parasitic infection
- Food poisoning

1i Disorders of the Stomach/Intestines: Gastritis
- Inflammation of the stomach lining
- Caused by coffee, aspirin, alcohol, bacteria
- Common in the elderly, chronic alcoholics, cigarette smokers

1j Disorders of the Stomach/Intestines: Peptic Ulcer Disease
- Chronic health problem
- Affects adults
- Causes: *H. pylori* infection, aspirin, NSAIDs, smoking

1k Disorders of the Stomach/Intestines: Cancer of the Stomach
- Less common in the United States; most common in the world
- *H. pylori* major risk factor

2 Obesity
- Appetite, hormones, heredity, and social and cultural influences play a role in body weight
- Appetite regulated by CNS and emotions
- Eat to relieve anxiety or stress

© 2007 Pearson Education, Inc.

PowerPoint Lecture Slides *continued*

- Studies show leptin resistance contributes to the development of obesity
- Strong link between heredity and obesity
- Role of physical activity
- Percentage of fat ingested contributes to obesity
- Environmental and sociocultural influences

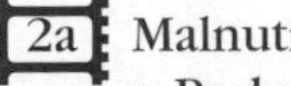

2a Malnutrition

- Body uses stores of glycogen, proteins, and fats to meet metabolic needs
- Size of all compartments reduces and the body is in a state of "wasting" or catabolism
- Leads to protein-calorie malnutrition
- Leads to edema, increased risk of infection, CV and GI system malfunctions

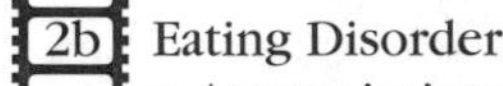

2b Eating Disorders

- Anorexia: intense fear of weight gain; weight less than 85% of normal for height
- Bulimia: normal body weight; more common; binge-purge syndrome

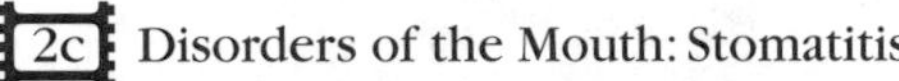

2c Disorders of the Mouth: Stomatitis

- Caused by viral infection (herpes simplex) or fungal infection *(Candida albicans)*
- Prolonged antibiotic therapy; at risk for candidiasis (thrush)
- Mechanical trauma (e.g., cheek biting) and irritants such as tobacco
- Chemotherapy or radiation therapy
- Canker sores are a type of stomatitis; can last weeks to months

2d Disorders of the Mouth: Oral Cancer

- Most are squamous cell
- Damaged cells lining the mouth and oropharynx grow more rapidly to repair damage, increasing the risk for malignancy
- Oral cancer may develop anywhere on the oral mucosa, including the lips, tongue, or pharynx
- Figure 19-4

2e Disorders of the Esophagus: GERD

- Lower esophageal sphincter does not function effectively or gastric emptying is delayed
- Gastric contents may *reflux* (back up) into the lower esophagus
- Factors contributing: increased volume of the stomach following meals, positioning, and increased gastric pressure due to obesity or restrictive clothing.

2f Disorders of the Esophagus: Hiatal Hernia

- Part of the stomach protrudes through the opening of the diaphragm into the chest cavity

2g Disorders of the Esophagus: Esophageal Cancer

- Most tumors affect the middle or lower third of the esophagus

© 2007 Pearson Education, Inc.

PowerPoint Lecture Slides *continued*

2h Disorders of the Stomach/Intestines: Gastroenteritis
- Infection produces inflammation through production of enterotoxins and invasion/ulceration of the mucosa

2i Disorders of the Stomach/Intestines: Gastritis
- Acute gastritis: local irritation to the stomach lining; caused by drugs/medications
- Chronic gastritis: associated with *H. pylori,* alcohol, smoking, toxin exposure

2j Disorders of the Stomach/Intestines: Peptic Ulcer Disease
- Ulcers develop when the mucosal barrier is unable to prevent damage by gastric digestive juices
- Mucosal barrier can be impaired by poor circulation, decreased mucus, or reflux of bile or pancreatic enzymes into the stomach or duodenum
- *H. pylori* infection secretes substances that break down mucous gel and also appears to stimulate acid production in the stomach
- Cigarette smoking contributes by inhibiting bicarbonate secretion

2k Disorders of the Stomach/Intestines: Cancer of the Stomach
- Develop in the distal portion of the stomach
- Lesions spread by direct extension to tissues surrounding the stomach, particularly the liver
- Lymph involvement common
- Metastatic lesions often found in the lung, liver, ovaries, peritoneum

3 Obesity
- Upper body
  - Higher risk of complications
  - More common in men than women
- Lower body:
  - More common in women than men

3a Malnutrition
- Depends on nutrient deficiency
- Table 18-1
- Weight loss, body mass reduced, skinfold reduced, wasted appearance, dry brittle hair, pale mucous membranes, peripheral edema, sore smooth tongue

3b Eating Disorders
- Anorexia: weight < 85% of normal; Disturbed Body Image; fear of weight gain; refusal to eat, excessive exercise; muscle wasting; skin and hair changes; amenorrhea; low blood pressure, slow pulse; low body temperature; constipation; insomnia
- Bulimia: weight normal or greater than normal; binge-purge behavior; scant menses or amenorrhea; lacerations of palate (from induced vomiting); callous on fingers or back of hand

© 2007 Pearson Education, Inc.

PowerPoint Lecture Slides *continued*

3c Disorders of the Mouth: Stomatitis
- Vary, depending on the cause
- Herpes lesions clustered and painful, usually occurring on the lips and oral mucosa
- Candidiasis (thrush) causes painful white patches with a red base
- Other manifestations: red and swollen oral mucosa, pain, and possible ulcerations

3d Disorders of the Mouth: Oral Cancer
- Sore or lesion in the mouth that does not heal
- *Leukoplakia:* irregular white patches on the lips, tongue, gums, tonsil, or oral mucosa
- *Erythroplakia:* slightly raised, irregular red patches that bleed easily when scraped
- Visible or palpable masses of the lips, cheek, or tongue
- Sore throat or a feeling of something caught in the throat
- Difficulty chewing, swallowing, or moving the jaw or tongue
- Asymmetry of the head, face, jaws, or neck
- Loosening of teeth, or dentures that no longer fit properly
- Swollen lymph nodes
- Blood-tinged sputum

3e Disorders of the Esophagus: GERD
- Heartburn: increases after meals, aggravated by bending over or lying down
- Sore throat, pain with swallowing, or chest pain

3f Disorders of the Esophagus: Hiatal Hernia
- Sliding hernia: part of the stomach slides through the opening of the diaphragm when reclining; moves back into place with standing
- Paraesophageal hernia: part of the stomach protrudes through the opening beside the esophagus

3g Disorders of the Esophagus: Esophageal Cancer
- Dysphagia, weight loss, regurgitation, blood loss

3h Disorders of the Stomach/Intestines: Gastroenteritis
- Diarrhea, fluid loss, electrolyte imbalances, dehydration, hypovolemia, acid–base imbalance

3i Disorders of the Stomach/Intestines: Gastritis
- Anorexia
- Nausea and vomiting
- Abdominal pain or discomfort
- Manifestations of acute and chronic gastritis (Box 19-9)

3j Disorders of the Stomach/Intestines: Peptic Ulcer Disease
- Epigastric pain: gnawing, burning, aching, hunger-like
- Occurs when stomach is empty; middle of the night
- Radiates to the middle of the back

© 2007 Pearson Education, Inc.

PowerPoint Lecture Slides *continued*

- Complain of heart burn, regurgitation, vomiting
- Elderly complaints: vague, check pain, dysphagia

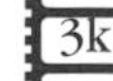 Disorders of the Stomach/Intestines: Cancer of the Stomach

- Early satiety, anorexia, indigestion, vomiting
- Ulcerlike pain unrelieved with antiacids
- Weight loss
- Cachectic

Suggestions for Classroom Activities

Access the website www.nationaleatingdisorders.org/p.asp?WebPage_ID=294. Select one eating disorder and analyze the causes, treatments, and long-term prognosis.

Suggestions for Clinical Activities

Assign the students to a client with an eating disorder or disorder of the small intestine. Conduct a health history for this client.

Learning Outcome 2

Recognize and take appropriate action for common complications of nutritional and upper GI disorders.

Concepts for Lecture

1. Common complications of nutritional and upper GI disorders.

PowerPoint Lecture Slides

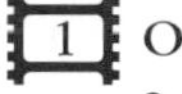 Obesity:

- CV disease: HTN, CAD, HF
- Insulin resistance and type 2 DM
- Reduced hormones in men
- PCOS in women
- See Box 19-1

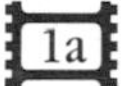 Malnutrition

- Protein-calorie malnutrition: increased risk of skin/tissue breakdown leading to decubitus ulcers, impaired wound healing, drop in serum albumin levels, abdominal edema, diarrhea, increased risk for falls

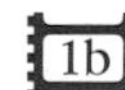 Eating Disorders

- Anorexia: electrolyte and acid-base imbalances; low cardiac output, dysrhythmias; anemia; hypoglycemia; osteoporosis; delayed gastric emptying; abnormal liver function
- Bulimia: enlarged salivary glands; stomatitis; loss of dental enamel; fluid, electrolyte, and acid-base imbalances; dysrhythmias; esophageal tears, stomach rupture

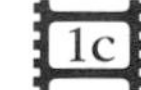 Disorders of the Mouth: Stomatitis

- Weight loss
- Loss of appetite

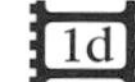 Disorders of the Esophagus: GERD

- Corrosive gastric fluids lead to tissue inflammation
- May cause erosions, ulcers, or *strictures* (narrowing) of the esophagus
- Risk of esophageal cancer is increased in clients with GERD

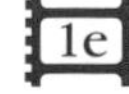 Disorders of the Esophagus: Hiatal Hernia

- Upper GI bleeding or erosive esophagitis

© 2007 Pearson Education, Inc.

POWERPOINT LECTURE SLIDES *continued*

1f Disorders of the Esophagus: Esophageal Cancer
- Weight loss, anorexia

1g Disorders of the Stomach/Intestines: Gastroenteritis
- Metabolic alkalosis
- Metabolic acidosis
- Hyponatremia
- Hypokalemia

1h Disorders of the Stomach/Intestines: Gastritis
- Hematemasis
- Melena

1i Disorders of the Stomach/Intestines: Peptic Ulcer Disease
- Hemorrhage, obstruction, perforation

1j Disorders of the Stomach/Intestines: Cancer of the Stomach
- Metastatic disease

SUGGESTIONS FOR CLASSROOM ACTIVITIES

Use the website www.nedic.ca/ to research one eating disorder. Review the long-term complications of this disorder. Create a teaching plan to aid a client with this eating disorder.

SUGGESTIONS FOR CLINICAL ACTIVITIES

Assign the students to a client with an eating disorder or disorder of the small intestine. Utilizing the teaching plan created in class, have the students review the teaching material with the client.

LEARNING OUTCOME 3

Contribute to assessing, planning, and evaluating care for clients with nutritional and upper GI disorders.

CONCEPTS FOR LECTURE

1. Care for clients with nutritional and upper GI disorders.
2. Assessing clients with nutritional and upper GI disorders.
3. Planning care for clients with nutritional and upper GI disorders.
4. Evaluating care for clients with nutritional and upper GI disorders.

POWERPOINT LECTURE SLIDES

1 Obesity
- Interdisciplinary approach to include behavior modification, diet, and exercise
- Diagnostic tests: height/weight table, BMI, fatfold measure, waist/hip ratio; lab tests, EKG
- Diet: low in calories and fats; high fiber (Figure 19-2)
- Behavior modification: support groups, food records (Box 19-2)
- Medication therapy: appetite suppressants, serotonin reuptake inhibitor, fat absorption inhibitors
- Surgery: gastric banding, gastric bypass

1a Malnutrition
- Laboratory studies: serum albumin, H&H
- Goals of treatment: restore to ideal weight, replace nutrients and minerals
- Types of feedings:
  - Enteral:
    - Tube feedings (Procedure 19-1)
    - Placements of tubes
    - Types of formulas
  - Parenteral
    - Hyperalimentation or TPN
    - Location for infusion

© 2007 Pearson Education, Inc.

   - Types of solutions
   - Nursing care (Box 19-4)

1b Eating Disorders
- Early identification of individuals with an eating disorder to begin treatment/therapy

1c Disorders of the Mouth: Stomatitis
- Focus is on cause and symptoms
- Lesions analyzed to focus treatment

1d Disorders of the Mouth: Oral Cancer
- Biopsy used to diagnose
- Avoid risk factors
- Treatment depends on extent of cancer: surgery, radiation, chemotherapy

1e Disorders of the Esophagus: GERD/Hiatal Hernia
- Diagnostic tests: barium swallow, upper endoscopy, ambulatory pH
- Management: lifestyle changes and medications
- Nursing implications with medications (Table 19-4)

1f Disorders of the Esophagus: Esophageal Cancer
- Treatment: surgery, radiation, chemotherapy
- Control dysphagia with TPN or tube feedings

1g Disorders of the Stomach/Intestines: Gastroenteritis
- Identify cause and treat
- Stool specimens
- Fluid and electrolyte replacement
- Antidiarrheal drugs
- Gastric lavage
- Botulism antitoxin

1h Disorders of the Stomach/Intestines: Gastritis
- Diagnosed by history, physical, symptoms
- Diagnostic tests
- Medications
- GI tract rest
- Complementary therapies: herbal tea, ginger, garlic, mint

1i Disorders of the Stomach/Intestines: Peptic Ulcer Disease
- Relieving symptoms
- Healing ulcers
- Preventing complications
- Preventing reoccurrence
- Diagnosis: diagnostic tests
- Treatment: medications, diet
- Treat complications: surgery

1j Disorders of the Stomach/Intestines: Cancer of the Stomach
- Palpable abdominal mass
- Occult blood in the stool
- Diagnosis: biopsy, endoscopy
- Surgery

© 2007 Pearson Education, Inc.

POWERPOINT LECTURE SLIDES *continued*

- Complications: dumping syndrome
- Radiation
- Chemotherapy

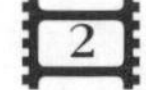

Obesity
- Eating habits
- Exercise
- Prior weight loss efforts
- Changes in appetite or weight
- Medical problems
- Height/weight
- Fatfold measurements
- Waist circumference

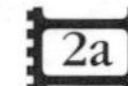

Malnutrition
- Eating habits, typical daily food intake
- Recent weight changes, factors contributing to weight change
- Other factors such as anorexia, nausea, medications, ability to buy and prepare food for meals
- Medical problems
- Psychosocial factors such as body image, loneliness, depression, and economic status
- Food preferences
- Assess height, weight, and fatfold measurements
- Evaluate the mouth for inflammation, gum disease, dental caries, or poorly fitting dentures
- Ability to swallow liquids, semisolid and solid foods

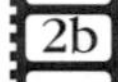

Eating Disorders
- Complaints of being overweight
- History of dieting, laxative use, diuretic use, high amounts of exercise

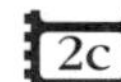

Disorders of the Mouth: Stomatitis
- Inspect mouth and oropharynx
- Complaints of soreness in mouth, tongue
- Teeth/gum condition
- Mouth odor
- Ability to chew/swallow

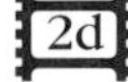

Disorders of the Mouth: Oral Cancer
- Assess for oral lesions
- Assess airway and maintain patency if client postoperative

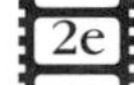

Disorders of the Esophagus: GERD
- Reflux of gastric contents with sleep

Disorders of the Stomach/Intestines: Gastroenteritis
- Onset of diarrhea
- Nausea, vomiting, abdominal pain
- Recent travel
- Changes in water or diet
- Picnics, pot-luck meals
- Other family members experiencing same symptoms
- Frequency/severity of nausea, vomiting, diarrhea

© 2007 Pearson Education, Inc.

- Abdominal pain, cramping
- What was done to aid the symptoms

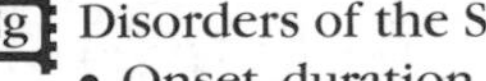

2g Disorders of the Stomach/Intestines: Gastritis
- Onset, duration, and nature symptoms
- Foods, fluids, and other substances (such as aspirin or other drugs)
- Bleeding in emesis or stools
- Vital signs, including orthostatic blood pressures
- Inspect the abdomen and auscultate bowel sounds
- Measure abdominal girth and lightly palpate for tenderness
- Measure and document the color and character of any emesis or stools

2h Disorders of the Stomach/Intestines: Peptic Ulcer Disease
- Subjective and objective data (Box 19-12)
- Pain
- Assess for presence of complications

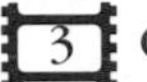

3 Obesity
- Nursing diagnoses:
  - Imbalanced Nutrition: More than Body Requirements
  - Chronic Low Self-Esteem

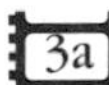

3a Malnutrition
- Nursing diagnoses:
  - Imbalanced Nutrition: Less than Body Requirements
  - Risk for Infection
  - Risk for Deficient Fluid Volume
  - Risk for Impaired Skin Integrity

3b Eating Disorders
- Nursing diagnoses:
  - Imbalanced Nutrition: Less than Body Requirements
  - Disturbed Body Image
  - Ineffective Family Coping

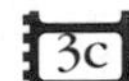

3c Disorders of the Mouth: Stomatitis
- Nursing diagnoses:
  - Depend upon the cause

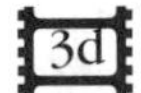

3d Disorders of the Esophagus: GERD/Hiatal Hernia
- Focuses on teaching

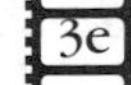

3e Disorders of the Stomach/Small Intestines: Gastritis
- Nursing diagnoses:
  - Deficient Fluid Volume
  - Imbalanced Nutrition: Less than Body Requirements

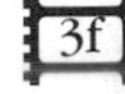

3f Disorders of the Stomach/Small Intestines: Peptic Ulcer Disease
- Nursing diagnoses:
  - Pain
  - Imbalanced Nutrition: Less than Body Requirements
  - Decreased cardiac output

© 2007 Pearson Education, Inc.

POWERPOINT LECTURE SLIDES *continued*

4 Obesity
- Monitor weight
- Eating and exercise patterns
- Sense of success and self-image
- Document weight loss goals and effective interventions

4a Malnutrition
- Collect information about consuming prescribed diet; evidence of weight gain; stable intake and output; laboratory values improving; remains free of infection or skin breakdown
- Document weight, food and fluid intake, and responses to meals and snacks
- Note skin condition, recording and reporting any areas of redness or early tissue breakdown

4b Eating Disorders
- Ongoing treatment is the key to success
- Whole family involvement

4c Disorders of the Mouth: Stomatitis
- Monitor weight, food intake, and healing
- Client's understanding of the treatment

4d Disorders of the Esophagus: GERD/Hiatal Hernia
- Improvement in symptoms

4e Disorders of the Stomach/Small Intestines: Gastritis
- Fluid and electrolyte balance indicators
- Response to treatment

4f Disorders of the Stomach/Small Intestines: Peptic Ulcer Disease
- Pain level
- Weight
- Nutritional status
- Fluid balance
- Circulation
- Complications postoperatively
- Document interventions
- Document teaching provided

SUGGESTIONS FOR CLASSROOM ACTIVITIES

Have the students select one nutritional disorder or disorder of the small intestine. Create a plan to assess an individual with this disorder.

SUGGESTIONS FOR CLINICAL ACTIVITIES

Assign the students to a client with a nutritional disorder or disorder of the small intestine. Assess the client using the tool created in class.

LEARNING OUTCOME 4

Implement client-centered nursing care for clients with nutritional and upper GI disorders.

CONCEPTS FOR LECTURE

1. Implementation of care for clients with nutritional and upper GI disorders.

POWERPOINT LECTURE SLIDES

1 Obesity
- Identification of factors that contribute to excess food intake
- Establish realistic weight-loss goals
- Provide teaching about well-balanced diet plans

© 2007 Pearson Education, Inc.

POWERPOINT LECTURE SLIDES *continued*

- Exercise plan; 30 minutes of sustained activity daily
- Willingness to make changes in daily patterns of diet, exercise, and lifestyle
- Behavior modification strategies and support systems to promote weight loss and maintenance
- Refer to a dietitian, nutritional counselor, or weight-loss support program
- Strategies to deal with "stress" eating or relapses to previous eating patterns
- Goals and offer positive feedback and encouragement
- Psychologic counseling

Malnutrition

- Monitor weight
- Dietary consult
- Mouth care before and after meals
- Small frequent meals
- Rest before and after meals
- Monitor vital signs
- Be alert to S/S of infection
- Good hand washing
- Monitor condition of mucous membranes
- Skin turgor
- Urine output and specific gravity
- Daily weights
- Intake and output
- Skin assessment
- Turn and reposition every 2 hours
- Good skin care

Eating Disorders

- Monitor weight
- Monitor food intake during meals and snacks, recording amount consumed. Continue close observation for at least 1 hour after meals; do not allow to use the bathroom alone
- Serve small, frequent balanced meals, gradually increasing serving size

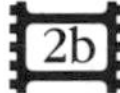

Disorders of the Mouth: Stomatitis

- Assist with mouth care as needed after eating and at bedtime
- Use sponge or gauze toothettes or a water pick with gentle pressure
- Avoid alcohol-based mouthwashes
- Encourage a high-calorie, high-protein diet
- Offer soft, lukewarm, or cool foods or liquids (eggnog, milkshakes, nutritional supplements, popsicles, and puddings) frequently in small amounts
- Avoid spicy or irritating foods
- Use straws or feeding syringes as needed to promote intake

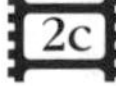

Disorders of the Mouth: Oral Cancer

- Support with enteral or parenteral nutrition

© 2007 Pearson Education, Inc.

POWERPOINT LECTURE SLIDES *continued*

- If able to eat, offer a soft, bland diet with enriched foods or dietary supplements
- Offer small, frequent feedings, making mealtimes pleasant
- Dietary consultation
- Provide a magic slate, flash cards, or picture or alphabet board as needed to facilitate communication
- Allow ample time for communication, and do not answer for the client
- Observe nonverbal communications to supplement verbal efforts
- If unable to speak clearly, use yes/no questions and simple phrases
- Keep the call light within easy reach and respond promptly
- Alert all staff if the client is unable to respond verbally over the intercom system
- Consult with a speech therapist as needed
- Assess coping, self-perception, and responses to surgery
- Encourage to express feelings regarding body image changes
- Provide emotional support

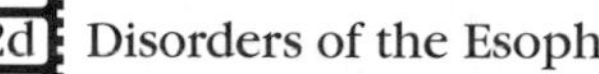
2d Disorders of the Esophagus: GERD

- Avoid lying down within 3 hours after meals
- Elevate the head of the bed on 6-inch blocks or use a foam wedge when sleeping
- Avoid using alcohol and tobacco
- Information about smoking cessation
- Weight loss, smaller meals, and avoiding bending
- Diet changes, such as avoiding acidic foods (such as orange juice), and foods that affect the lower esophageal sphincter or gastric emptying (fatty foods, peppermint, and chocolate)

2e Disorders of the Esophagus: Hiatal Hernia

- Symptoms persist, might need surgery

2f Disorders of the Esophagus: Esophageal Cancer

- Aspiration and airway problems postoperatively
- Assess LOC and respiratory status
- Deep breathing and coughing
- Wound care
- Follow-up
- Referal to hospice

2g Disorders of the Stomach/Intestines: Gastroenteritis

- Fluid and electrolyte replacement
- Hand washing
- Wash contaminated linens
- Maintain good personal hygiene
- Food safety measures

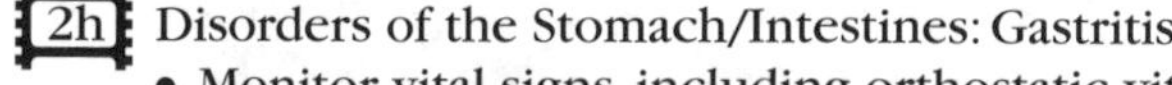
2h Disorders of the Stomach/Intestines: Gastritis

- Monitor vital signs, including orthostatic vital signs

© 2007 Pearson Education, Inc.

POWERPOINT LECTURE SLIDES *continued*

- Monitor and record intake and output
- Provide meticulous skin and mouth care frequently
- Fluids by mouth or enterally
- Monitor lab values
- Administer meds
- Safety
- Measure emesis
- Daily weights
- Dietary consult
- Nutritional supplements prn

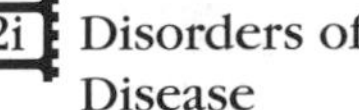

Disorders of the Stomach/Intestines: Peptic Ulcer Disease

- Assess pain; report changes
- Administer medications as prescribed
- Limit food intake
- Assess diet
- Dietary consult prn
- Document/report anorexia, fullness, nausea, vomiting, dumping syndrome
- Monitor and record VS
- Monitor stools and gastric lavage for melena/blood
- IV fluid therapy

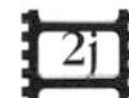

Disorders of the Stomach/Intestines: Cancer of the Stomach

- Depends on the extent of the disease and the treatment plan
- TPN
- Grief counseling

SUGGESTIONS FOR CLASSROOM ACTIVITIES

Access the web site http://digestive-disorders.healthcares.net/. Prepare a plan of care for a client with a nutritional disorder.

SUGGESTIONS FOR CLINICAL ACTIVITIES

Assign the students to a client with a nutritional disorder or disorder of the small intestines. Provide care to this client utilizing the plan of care created in class.

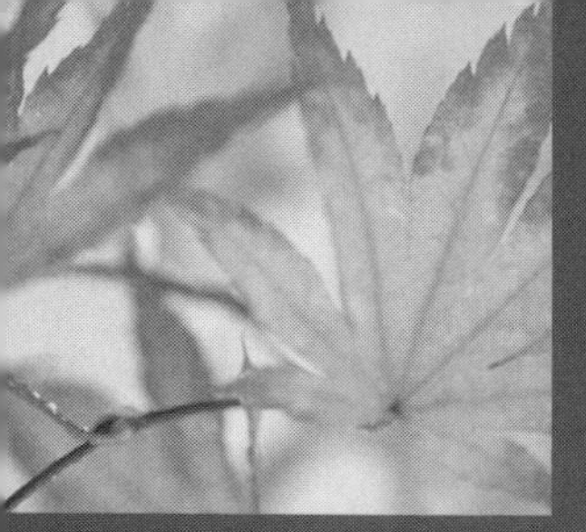

CHAPTER 20
CARING FOR CLIENTS WITH BOWEL DISORDERS

RESOURCE LIBRARY

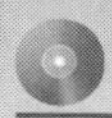

CD-ROM

Enema

IMAGE LIBRARY

Figure 20-1 McBurney's point, located midway between the umbilicus and the anterior iliac crest in the right lower quadrant.
Figure 20-2 An intestinal tube is advanced in increments of 1 to 2 inches every hour. Suction is applied after the balloon or weighted tip passes the pyloric valve.
Figure 20-3 An illustration of the major characteristics of Crohn's disease in the small intestine, and a potential complication (fistula formation).
Figure 20-4 A healthy appearing stoma.
Figure 20-5 Kock's (continent) ileostomy.
Figure 20-6 Ileoanal anastomosis with reservoir.
Figure 20-7 The distribution and frequency of colorectal cancer.
Figure 20-8 The location of different types of colon and small intestinal ostomies.
Figure 20-9 A temporary, double-barrel colostomy. The proximal stoma expels feces; the distal stoma expels mucus from the distal colon.
Figure 20-10 Selected causes of mechanical bowel obstruction. (**A**) Adhesions, (**B**) incarcerated (irreducible) hernia, (**C**) tumor, (**D**) intussusception (telescoping of the bowel), (**E**) volvulus (twisting of the bowel).
Figure 20-11 An abdominal wall (ventral or incisional) hernia and an inguinal hernia.
Figure 20-12 Diverticula of the colon.
Figure 20-13 The location of internal and external hemorrhoids.

LEARNING OUTCOME 1

Discuss the pathophysiology, manifestations, and management of bowel absorption and elimination disorders.

CONCEPTS FOR LECTURE

1. Pathophysiology, manifestations, and management of disorders of intestinal motility and absorption.
2. Pathophysiology, manifestations, and management of inflammatory disorders.
3. Pathophysiology, manifestations, and management of structural and obstructive disorders.
4. Pathophysiology, manifestations, and management of anorectal disorders.

POWERPOINT LECTURE SLIDES

1 Diarrhea—Pathophysiology
- Result from impaired water absorption or increased water secretion into the bowel
- Increased water absorption: increased peristalsis or decreased bowel surface
- Increased water secretion: osmosis, infection, unabsorbed fat, medications

1a Diarrhea—Manifestations
- Depend on the cause, duration, severity, and area of bowel affected

1b Diarrhea—Complications
- Loss of water and electrolytes
- Dehydration, hypovolemic shock
- Potassium, magnesium, and bicarbonate loss can lead to metabolic acidosis

1c Diarrhea—Management
- Identify and treat underlying cause
- Diagnostic tests

POWERPOINT LECTURE SLIDES *continued*

- Dietary management
- Medications

1d Constipation—Pathophysiology
- Organic cause—tumor or partial bowel obstruction
- Lifestyle and psychogenic causes
- Habitual use of laxatives
- Table 20-3

1e Constipation—Manifestations
- Fecal impaction
- Watery mucus
- Full sensation in rectum with abdominal cramping

1f Constipation—Management
- Digital exam of rectum
- Diagnostic tests
- Dietary management
- Medications
- Enemas

1g Irritable Bowel Syndrome—Pathophysiology
- CNS innervation altered
- Affected by eating, hormones, stress, drugs
- Sensory responses increased
- Increase in mucous production

1h Irritable Bowel Syndrome—Manifestations
- Change in frequency, consistency of stools
- Box 20-5

1i Irritable Bowel Syndrome—Management
- Diagnostic tests
- Treatment

1j Fecal Incontinence—Pathophysiology
- Physiologic and psychologic factors
- Box 20-7

1k Fecal Incontinence—Manifestations
- Loss of voluntary control of defecation

1l Fecal Incontinence—Management
- Directed at cause
- Measure to either reduce diarrhea or constipation
- Exercises for pelvic floor muscle tone
- Bowel retraining program
- Establish daily routine for bowel evacuation

1m Malabsorption—Pathophysiology
- Celiac disease, lactose intolerance
- Bowel resection: short bowel syndrome

1n Malabsorption—Manifestations
- Depends on the cause
- Box 20-8

1o Malabsorption—Management
- Find the cause
- Treatment

© 2007 Pearson Education, Inc.

PowerPoint Lecture Slides *continued*

2 Appendicitis—Pathophysiology
- Obstruction with fecalith
- Distention
- Pressure leads to impaired blood supply
- Leads to inflammation, edema, ulceration, infection
- 24–36 hours necrosis
- Classified by stages

2a Appendicitis—Manifestations
- Generalized or upper abdominal pain
- Localizes in right lower quadrant
- Aggravated moving, walking, coughing
- Localized and rebound tenderness
- Right hip extension increases pain
- Low-grade fever, anorexia, nausea, vomiting

2b Appendicitis—Complications
- Perforation

2c Appendicitis—Management
- Prompt diagnosis and management to prevent perforation
- Hospitalization, IV fluids, NPO until diagnosis confirmed
- Diagnostic tests
- Surgery

2d Peritonitis—Pathophysiology
- Bowel contents enter a sterile abdominal cavity
- Generalized inflammation of the abdominal cavity
- Third spacing
- Paralytic ileus

2e Peritonitis—Manifestations
- Depend on severity and extent of the infection
- Box 20-10

2f Peritonitis—Complications
- Life-threatening, localized, systemic
- Abscess formation
- Septicemia
- Shock

2g Peritonitis—Management
- Diagnostic tests
- Intestinal decompression
- Antibiotics
- Surgery

2h Ulcerative Colitis—Pathophysiology
- Inflamed mucous membranes bleed easily
- Mucous membranes ulcerate, slough, get lost in the feces
- Scar tissue forms; bowel thickens and shortens

2i Ulcerative Colitis—Manifestations
- Gradual onset of diarrhea and bleeding
- Intermittent rectal bleeding and mucous
- Dehydration, malnutrition

© 2007 Pearson Education, Inc.

- Urgency, cramps,
- Fatigue, anorexia, weakness

 Ulcerative Colitis—Complications
- Perforated colon
- Toxic megacolon
- High risk for colon cancer

 Crohn's Disease—Pathophysiology
- Inflammatory lesions of bowel mucosa
- Ulcers and deep fissures develop
- Fistula formation
- Scarring, narrowing
- Rubber hose appearance

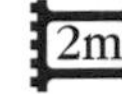 Crohn's Disease—Manifestations
- Diarrhea
- Abdominal pain, palpable mass
- Lesions of the rectum, anus

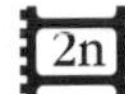 Crohn's Disease—Complications
- Intestinal obstruction, abscess, fistula formation
- Increased risk cancer of colon

 Ulcerative Colitis and Crohn's Disease—Management
- Manage symptoms
- Control disease process
- Supportive care
- Diagnostic tests
- Medications
- Dietary management
- Surgery

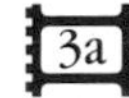 Colorectal Cancer—Pathophysiology
- Begin as benign polyps
- Grows undetected in the colon or rectum (Figure 20-7)
- Direct extension into the bowel wall
- Spread to neighboring organs
- Seed other organs
- Metastasis

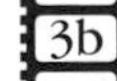 Colorectal Cancer—Manifestations
- Bleeding with defecation
- Change in bowel habits
- Pain, anorexia, weight loss
- Prognosis depends on extent of the disease

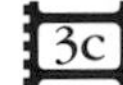 Colorectal Cancer—Complications
- Bowel obstruction
- Perforation into neighboring organs

 Colorectal Cancer—Management
- Annual screening beginning at age 50
- Diagnostic tests
- Surgery
- Adjunctive therapy

3d Bowel Obstruction—Pathophysiology
- Mechanical or functional
- Adhesions, tumors, twisted bowel

© 2007 Pearson Education, Inc.

PowerPoint Lecture Slides *continued*

- Paralytic ileus
- Gas and fluid are trapped in the bowel
- Distention, pressure, ischemia, necrosis, hypovolemia, shock

3e Bowel Obstruction—Manifestations
- Progressive crampy or colicky pain
- Vomiting
- Loud bowel sounds, at first
- Reduced bowel sounds, abdomen distended and tender

3f Bowel Obstruction—Complications
- Hypovolemic shock
- Strangulated colon

3g Bowel Obstruction—Management
- Diagnostic tests
- Gastric decompression
- Surgery

3h Hernia—Pathophysiology
- Protrusion of an organ or structure through the muscular wall of the abdomen
- Described by location
- Pain radiating to groin
- Reducible
- Irreducible
- Incarcerated
- Strangulated

3i Hernia—Management
- Diagnosis made if able to reduce or manipulate
- Surgery

3j Diverticular Disease—Pathophysiology
- Inflammation and perforation of a diverticulum
- Infection, perforation

3k Diverticular Disease—Manifestations
- Pain
- Constipation, diarrhea, nausea, vomiting, low-grade fever

3l Diverticular Disease—Management
- Nothing prescribed prior to surgery
- Diagnostic tests
- High fiber diet
- Bowel rest
- Antibiotics

4 Hemorrhoids—Pathophysiology
- Distended rectal veins caused by straining, pregnancy, prolonged sitting, obesity, chronic constipation, low-fiber diet
- Internal
- External

4a Hemorrhoids—Manifestations
- Pain, rupture, bleeding

© 2007 Pearson Education, Inc.

PowerPoint Lecture Slides *continued*

4b Hemorrhoids—Management
- Conservative
- Diagnostic tests
- Medications
- Sclerotherapy

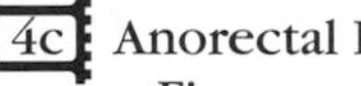
Anorectal Lesions
- Fissures
- Abscess
- Fistula
- Pilonidal disease

Suggestions for Classroom Activities

Access the website www.merck.com/mrkshared/mmanual/section3/chapter32 and research one bowel disorder. Prepare to present the findings about this bowel disorder in class.

Suggestions for Clinical Activities

Review the diagnostic tests, treatments, and prescribed management for a client with a bowel disorder.

Learning Outcome 2

Provide appropriate nursing care and teaching related to measures used to manage bowel disorders.

Concepts for Lecture

1. Nursing care and teaching related to disorders of intestinal motility and absorption.
2. Nursing care and teaching related to inflammatory disorders.
3. Nursing care and teaching related to structural and obstructive disorders.
4. Nursing care and teaching related to anorectal disorders.

PowerPoint Lecture Slides

1 Diarrhea—Nursing Care
- Identify the cause
- Relieve the symptoms
- Prevent complications
- Prevent spread of infection

1a Diarrhea—Teaching
- Teach causes and preventative measure
- Infection control
- Purification of water for travel
- Fluid replacement
- Chronic diarrhea (Table 20-1)

1b Constipation—Nursing Care
- Relieve constipation
- Prevent reoccurrence

1c Constipation—Teaching
- Diet high in natural fiber
- High fluid intake
- Exercise
- Normal bowel habits
- Use of laxatives
- Avoid straining

1d Irritable Bowel Syndrome—Nursing Care
- Same as that for diarrhea and constipation

1e Irritable Bowel Syndrome—Teaching
- Symptoms are real
- Discuss related factors
- Relationship between stress and manifestations
- Stress reduction techniques
- Psychologic factors
- Dietary influences

© 2007 Pearson Education, Inc.

POWERPOINT LECTURE SLIDES *continued*

- Exercise
- Dietary patterns
- Notification of PCP with any changes

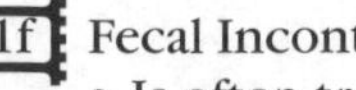 Fecal Incontinence—Teaching
- Is often treatable
- Constipation teaching (Box 20-3)
- Bowel retraining instructions
- Importance of good skin care

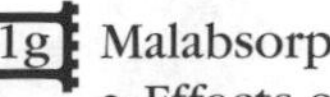 Malabsorption—Nursing Care
- Effects on nutrition and bowel patterns
- Nutritional status
- Weight, fatfold measurements, lab data, dietary intake
- Enteral feeding supplements as prescribed
- Intake/output, daily weights, skin turgor, mucous membranes
- Frequency stools
- Medications
- Skin care

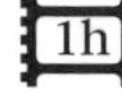 Malabsorption—Teaching
- Daily management
- Diet
- Medication regime
- Reading labels
- Fluid intake
- Exercise
- Daily weights
- Manifestations to report to physician
- Dietician or counselor referrals

 Appendicitis—Nursing Care
- Pain: onset, severity, duration
- Food, fluids, allergies, medications

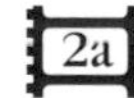 Appendicitis—Teaching
- Preop teaching: turn, coughing, deep breathing, pain management

2b Peritonitis—Nursing Care
- Intensive nursing and medical interventions

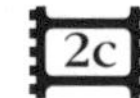 Peritonitis—Teaching
- Wound care, dressing changes
- Needed supplies
- Medications
- S/S further infection
- Activity restrictions

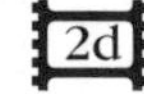 Ulcerative Colitis and Crohn's Disease—Nursing Care
- Manage diarrhea
- Psychosocial effects

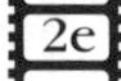 Ulcerative Colitis and Crohn's Disease—Teaching
- Disease process, effects, stress
- Treatment options
- Medications
- Complications, management
- Diet

© 2007 Pearson Education, Inc.

POWERPOINT LECTURE SLIDES *continued*

- Nutritional supplements
- Fluids
- Exercise
- Teaching for surgery

3 Colorectal Cancer—Nursing Care
- Provide emotional support
- Teaching
- Surgical needs

3a Colorectal Cancer—Teaching
- Prevention
- American Cancer Society recommendations
- Regular health examinations
- Tests and procedures
- Ostomy care
- Pain and symptom management

3b Bowel Obstruction—Nursing Care
- Preventing complications from obstruction and surgery

3c Bowel Obstruction—Teaching
- Wound care, activity level

3d Hernia—Nursing Care
- Preoperative assessment
- Postoperative care

3e Hernia—Teaching
- Risk factors
- Surgical intervention
- Pain management
- Activity restrictions

3f Diverticular Disease—Teaching
- Diet
- Food and fluid limitations
- Postoperative instructions as necessary

4 Hemorrhoids—Teaching
- Fiber, fluids, exercise
- Constipation management
- Complications
- Postoperative teaching

4a Anorectal Lesions—Teaching
- Diet
- Fluids
- Prevent constipation
- Postoperative care

SUGGESTIONS FOR CLASSROOM ACTIVITIES

Prepare a teaching plan for a client with chronic constipation.

SUGGESTIONS FOR CLINICAL ACTIVITIES

Provide the teaching plan prepared in class for a client with constipation.

© 2007 Pearson Education, Inc.

Learning Outcome 3

Effectively care for the client undergoing intestinal surgery.

Concepts for Lecture

1. Care of clients having intestinal surgery.

PowerPoint Lecture Slides

1 Bowel Surgery
- Box 20-13

Suggestions for Classroom Activities

Access the website http://healingwell.healthology.com/healingwell/17412.htm and prepare a presentation about the future of at least one intestinal surgical procedure.

Suggestions for Clinical Activities

Observe an abdominal intestinal surgical procedure.

Learning Outcome 4

Discuss the care of clients with a colostomy or ileostomy.

Concepts for Lecture

1. Care of clients with a colostomy or ileostomy.

PowerPoint Lecture Slides

1 Ostomy Care
- Box 20-17
- Procedure 20-1
- Procedure 20-2

Suggestions for Classroom Activities

Create a spreadsheet of the different types of ostomies after accessing the website http://healingwell.healthology.com/healingwell/17412.htm.

Suggestions for Clinical Activities

Provide care to a client with an ostomy.

Learning Outcome 5

Contribute to assessment, planning, and evaluation of nursing care for clients with disorders of bowel absorption and elimination.

Concepts for Lecture

1. Assessment, planning, and evaluation of nursing care for clients with disorders of intestinal motility and absorption.
2. Assessment, planning, and evaluation of nursing care for clients with inflammatory disorders.
3. Assessment, planning, and evaluation of nursing care for clients with structural and obstructive disorders.

PowerPoint Lecture Slides

1 Diarrhea—Assessment
- Box 20-2

1a Diarrhea—Planning
- Nursing diagnoses:
  - Diarrhea
    - Stool count
    - Abdominal girth
    - Medications
    - Food intake
  - Risk for Deficient Fluid Volume
    - I&O; daily weights, skin turgor, mucous membranes, urine specific gravity
    - Vital signs; orthostatic changes
    - Out of bed with assistance
    - Fluid and electrolyte replacements
  - Risk for Impaired Skin Integrity
    - Skin care
    - Frequent position changes
    - Protect pressure areas
    - Perianal cleansing

© 2007 Pearson Education, Inc.

PowerPoint Lecture Slides *continued*

1b Diarrhea—Evaluation
- Stool frequency
- Nutritional status
- Weight
- Fluid volume status
- Skin integrity
- Monitor electrolytes

1c Constipation—Planning
- Nursing diagnoses:
  - Constipation
    - Normal defecation pattern
    - Diet, fluid intake, activity
    - Abdominal shape, girth, bowel sounds, tenderness
    - Warm water
    - Dietary consult
    - Provide stool softeners as prescribed

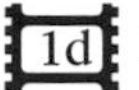

Fecal Incontinence—Planning
- Nursing diagnoses
  - Bowel Incontinence
    - Daily bowel evacuation time
    - Glycerine suppository use
    - Caring, nonjudgmental manner
  - Risk for Impaired Skin Integrity
    - Skin care
    - Frequent change of incontinence pads

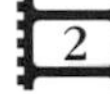

Appendicitis—Planning
- Nursing diagnoses
  - Ineffective Tissue Perfusion: Gastrointestinal
    - Signs of perforation
    - Vital signs
    - IV fluids
    - Postop care
  - Pain
    - Pain assessment
    - Prescribed analgesics
    - Effectiveness of pain medication
    - Alternative methods of pain relief

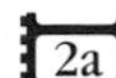

Appendicitis—Evaluation
- Teach wound/incision care
- Wound assessment instructions
- Dressing changes
- Hand washing
- What to report to the physician
- Activity restrictions
- Driving, return to work
- Home care nurses

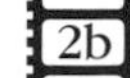

Peritonitis—Assessment
- Monitor current status
- Progress of recovery
- Identify complications
- Box 20-11

© 2007 Pearson Education, Inc.

PowerPoint Lecture Slides *continued*

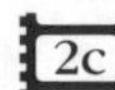
Peritonitis—Planning

- Nursing diagnoses:
  - Pain
    - Positioning
    - Analgesics
    - Pain management techniques
  - Deficient Fluid Volume
    - Vital signs, I&O, weight, skin turgor, mucous membranes
    - Lab values, H&H, specific gravity, serum electrolytes
    - Fluid and electrolyte replacements
    - Good skin care
    - Frequent oral hygiene
  - Ineffective Protection
    - Monitor signs of infection
    - Cultures as ordered
    - Hand washing
    - Fluid balance and nutrition
  - Anxiety
    - Level and coping skills
    - Calm manner
    - Reduce changes in caregiver assignments
    - Explain all procedures
    - Teach and assist with measures to reduce anxiety

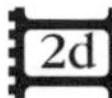
Peritonitis—Evaluation

- Pain level
- Weight
- Urine output
- Documentation
- Wound healing

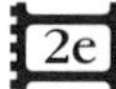
Ulcerative Colitis and Crohn's Disease—Assessment

- Current health status
- Complications
- Psychosocial factors
- Box 20-14

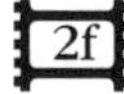
Ulcerative Colitis and Crohn's Disease—Planning

- Nursing Diagnoses
  - Diarrhea
    - Amount and frequency
    - Medications
    - Skin assessment
  - Risk for Deficient Fluid Volume
    - Accurate intake and output
    - VS every 4 hours
    - Daily weights
    - Fluid intake
    - Skin care
  - Imbalanced Nutrition: Less than Body Requirements
    - Food intake
    - Dietary consult
    - Parenteral nutrition
    - Monitor laboratory values

© 2007 Pearson Education, Inc.

- ○ Disturbed Body Image
  - – Encourage exploration of feelings
  - – Discuss treatment options
  - – Teach coping strategies
  - – Nonjudgmental care
  - – Support group?

2g Ulcerative Colitis and Crohn's Disease—Evaluation
- Number of daily stools
- Skin integrity
- Hydration
- Weight
- Diet/intake
- Coping

3 Colorectal Cancer—Assessment
- Effects of the disease
- Treatment
- Client's ability to function and maintain ADLs

3a Colorectal Cancer—Planning
- Nursing diagnoses:
  - ○ Pain
    - – Use pain scale to assess pain level
    - – Effectiveness of pain medication
    - – Abdominal assessment
    - – Administer analgesics
    - – Nonpharmacologic pain measure
    - – Splinting
  - ○ Anticipatory Grieving
    - – Trusting relationship with patient Encourage expression of fears
    - – Coping mechanisms
    - – Support groups
  - ○ Risk for Sexual Dysfunction
    - – Express feelings
    - – Social services
    - – Ostomy society

3b Colorectal Cancer—Evaluation
- Pain levels
- Evaluate pain measures
- Responses to disease and treatments

3c Bowel Obstruction—Assessment
- Assess for bowel sounds, distention
- Assess for complications

3d Bowel Obstruction—Planning
- Nursing diagnoses
  - ○ Deficient Fluid Volume
    - – Monitor vital signs and CVP
    - – Intake and output, urine output, gastric output
    - – Measure abdominal girth
  - ○ Ineffective breathing pattern
    - – Respiratory rate, lung sounds
    - – Respiratory support

© 2007 Pearson Education, Inc.

POWERPOINT LECTURE SLIDES *continued*

3e Bowel Obstruction—Evaluation
- Abdominal girth, bowel sounds, pain, tolerance, fluid volume status, potential complications

3f Hernia—Planning
- Nursing diagnosis:
  - Risk for Ineffective Tissue Perfusion: Gastrointestinal
    - Comfort measures
    - Bowel sounds
    - Signs of strangulation

SUGGESTIONS FOR CLASSROOM ACTIVITIES

Prepare a plan of care for a client with a bowel disorder.

SUGGESTIONS FOR CLINICAL ACTIVITIES

Provide care for a client with a bowel disorder.

 © 2007 Pearson Education, Inc.

CHAPTER 21

CARING FOR CLIENTS WITH GALLBLADDER, LIVER, AND PANCREATIC DISORDERS

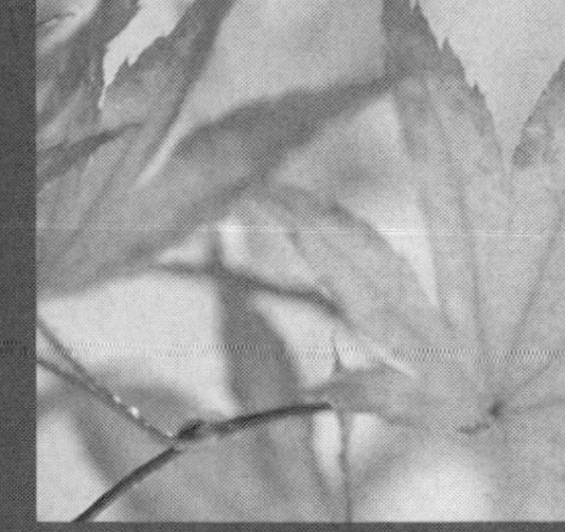

RESOURCE LIBRARY

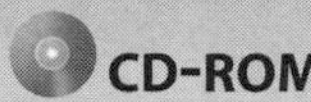

CD-ROM

Video: Fowler's Position

IMAGE LIBRARY

Figure 21-1 Common locations of gallstones.

Figure 21-2 T-tube placement in the common bile duct. Bile flows by gravity into a collection device placed below the level of the abdomen.

Figure 21-3 Portal hypertension in cirrhosis. **(A)** The portal vein, which drains capillaries of the gut, provides the majority of the liver's blood supply. **(B)** In cirrhosis, cellular necrosis leads to fibrosis and scarring. Isolated liver cells continue to regenerate, forming nodules among the fibrous scar tissue. **(C)** The nodules and scar tissue interfere with blood flow through the liver, increasing pressure and congestion in the portal venous system. Shunting of blood into lower pressure vessels leads to esophageal varices, hemorrhoids, and visible surface veins. The increased pressure also contributes to ascites.

Figure 21-4 The multisystem effects of cirrhosis.

Figure 21-5 Liver biopsy. **(A)** The client exhales completely and holds breath, bringing the liver and diaphragm to their highest position. The needle is inserted between the 6th and 7th ribs. **(B)** A small amount of saline is injected to clear the needle of blood and tissue. **(C)** A tissue sample is aspirated into the needle. The needle is then withdrawn and pressure is applied to the site.

Figure 21-6 Position of the client during paracentesis.

Figure 21-7 Transjugular intrahepatic portosystemic shunt (TIPS). **(A)** A catheter inserted via the internal jugular vein is guided into the hepatic vein. From there, a new route connecting the hepatic and portal veins is created through liver tissue. **(B)** An expandable metal stent is positioned between the portal and hepatic veins. **(C)** The catheter and guidewire are removed, leaving the stent in place.

Figure 21-8 A triple-lumen nasogastric (Sengstaken–Blakemore) tube used to control bleeding esophageal varices.

Figure 21-9 Whipple's procedure. **(A)** Areas of resection. **(B)** Appearance following resection.

LEARNING OUTCOME 1

Describe the pathophysiology, manifestations and effects, and management of common disorders of the gallbladder, liver, and exocrine pancreas.

CONCEPTS FOR LECTURE

1. Pathophysiology, manifestations and effects, and management of common gallbladder disorders.
2. Pathophysiology, manifestations and effects, and management of liver disorders.
3. Pathophysiology, manifestations and effects, and management of exocrine pancreatic disorders.

POWERPOINT LECTURE SLIDES

1 Cholelithiasis—Pathophysiology
- Inflammation of the gallbladder
- Stones in the common bile duct
- Figure 21-1
- Bile backs up into the liver

1a Cholelithiasis—Manifestations and Effects
- Asymptomatic
- Vague
- Gastric distress
- Biliary colic

1b Cholelithiasis—Management
- Diagnostic tests
- Medications
- Dietary
- Other: ESWL
- Complementary alternative therapy: herb therapy

PowerPoint Lecture Slides *continued*

1c Cholecystitis—Pathophysiology
- Inflammation of the gallbladder due to stones
- Figure 21-1
- Ischemia of gallbladder
- Edema, necrosis, perforation

1d Cholecystitis—Manifestations and Effects
- Acute: severe epigastric pain radiation to right scapula (Box 21-2)
- 12–18 hours, anorexia, nausea, vomiting
- Chronic (Box 21-2)

1e Cholecystitis—Management
- Surgery: nursing care (Box 21-4)

1f Gallbladder Cancer—Pathophysiology
- Rare
- Over age 65
- Women more than men
- Intense pain, RUQ
- Jaundice, weight loss
- Metastasize
- Death within 1 year

2 Hepatitis—Pathophysiology
- Inflammation, virus, alcohol use, toxins, gallbladder disease
- Viral, six types: A, B, C, D, E (Table 21-1)
- Chronic infection leads to cirrhosis, cancer, or liver failure
- Noninfectious: acute or chronic secondary to alcohol use, medications, toxins

2a Hepatitis—Manifestations and Effects
- Asymptomatic to being fatal
- Three phases: preicteric, icteric, posticteric (Box 21-7)

2b Hepatitis—Management
- No specific treatments (Box 21-9)
- Diagnostic tests
- Prevention, vaccines (Table 21-1)
- Recovery period, 3 to 16 weeks

2c Cirrhosis—Pathophysiology
- Liver cells destroyed
- Scar tissue
- Impaired blood flow
- Increased pressure in liver
- Liver failure

2d Cirrhosis—Manifestations and Effects
- Enlarged liver
- Tender
- RUQ pain
- Weight loss, weakness, anorexia
- Figure 21-4
- Portal hypertension
- Ascites

© 2007 Pearson Education, Inc.

POWERPOINT LECTURE SLIDES *continued*

2e Cirrhosis—Management
- Prevent further damage
- Diagnostic tests
- Medications
- Diet
- Fluids
- Surgery

2f Liver Cancer—Pathophysiology
- Parenchymal cells
- Primary is rare
- Metastasis to lung common

2g Liver Cancer—Manifestations and Effects
- RUQ pain and mass
- Epigastric fullness
- Weight loss
- Anorexia
- Fever

2h Liver Cancer—Management
- Diagnostic tests
- Surgery
- Chemotherapy, radiation

2i Liver Trauma—Pathophysiology
- Causes
- Prevention
- Treat hypovolemic shock
- Fluids
- Surgery to repair if possible

3 Pancreatitis—Pathophysiology
- Acute, damage, blocked ducts
- Types: interstitial edematous and necrotizing

3a Pancreatitis—Manifestations and Effects
- Acute: sudden onset, severe epigastric and abdominal pain radiating to the back (Box 21-17)
- Turner's sign, Cullen's sign, pseudocyst
- Chronic: occurs after acute; cause unknown, irreversible (Box 21-7)

3b Pancreatitis—Management
- Diagnostic tests
- NPO
- NG tube
- TPN
- Analgesics
- Avoid alcohol
- Treat diabetes
- Surgery

3c Pancreatic Cancer—Pathophysiology
- Smoking history
- Poor prognosis

3d Pancreatic Cancer—Manifestations
- Weight loss
- Anorexia

POWERPOINT LECTURE SLIDES *continued*

- Nausea
- Flatulence
- Dull pain

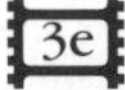
3e Pancreatic Cancer—Management
- Surgery (Figure 21-9)
- Radiation
- Chemotherapy

SUGGESTIONS FOR CLASSROOM ACTIVITIES

Access the website http://digestive.niddk.nih.gov/ and create a teaching plan for a client with a disorder of the gallbladder, liver, or pancreas.

SUGGESTIONS FOR CLINICAL ACTIVITIES

Conduct a health history for a client with a gallbladder, liver, or pancreas disorder.

LEARNING OUTCOME 2

Discuss nursing implications for dietary and pharmacologic interventions related to the gallbladder, liver, and exocrine pancreas.

CONCEPTS FOR LECTURE

1. Nursing implications for dietary and pharmacologic interventions related to the gallbladder.
2. Nursing implications for dietary and pharmacologic interventions related to liver disorders.
3. Nursing implications for dietary and pharmacologic interventions related to pancreatic disorders.

POWERPOINT LECTURE SLIDES

1 Cholelithiasis—Nursing and Dietary
- Low-fat diet
- Box 21-3

1a Cholelithiasis—Nursing and Pharmacology
- Oral bile salts
- Monitor liver enzymes
- Increased risk for diarrhea

2 Cirrhosis—Nursing and Dietary
- No alcohol
- High calories
- Restrict sodium
- Restrict fluids
- Vitamin and mineral supplements

2a Cirrhosis—Nursing and Pharmacology
- Diuretics
- Medications to reduce ammonia (Table 21-2)
- Beta blockers
- Vitamin K
- Platelets
- Histamine antagonists
- Antacids
- Antianxiety medications

3 Pancreatitis—Nursing and Dietary
- Small frequent meals
- High carbohydrates, low protein, low fat
- Avoid caffeine, spices, or gas-producing foods

3a Pancreatitis—Nursing and Pharmacology
- Synthetic hormone
- Enzyme supplements (Table 21-4)
- Control gastric acidity

© 2007 Pearson Education, Inc.

SUGGESTIONS FOR CLASSROOM ACTIVITIES

Access the website http://digestive.niddk.nih.gov/ and create a diet teaching plan for a client with a gallbladder, liver, or pancreas disorder.

SUGGESTIONS FOR CLINICAL ACTIVITIES

Provide diet instruction for a client with a gallbladder, liver, or pancreas disorder.

LEARNING OUTCOME 3

Provide appropriate nursing care for the client who has surgery of the gallbladder, liver, or pancreas.

CONCEPTS FOR LECTURE

1. Nursing care for the client with surgery of the gallbladder.
2. Nursing care for the client with surgery of the liver.
3. Nursing care for the client with surgery of the pancreas.

POWERPOINT LECTURE SLIDES

1 Cholecystitis—Surgical Nursing Care
- Similar to abdominal surgery
- Deep breathing and coughing
- Early ambulation
- T tube (Figure 21-2)
- Box 21-5

1a Gallbladder Cancer—Surgical Nursing Care

2 Cirrhosis—Surgical Nursing Care
- Liver transplant (Box 21-12)
- Paracentesis (Figure 21-6, Box 21-13)
- Transjugular intrahepatic portosystemic shunt (TIPS) (Figure 21-7)
- Esophageal varices procedures

2a Liver Trauma—Surgical Nursing Care
- Prevent respiratory complications
- S/S infection
- S/S bleeding

3 Pancreatitis—Surgical Nursing Care

SUGGESTIONS FOR CLASSROOM ACTIVITIES

Research surgical procedures and provide a 10-minute report on the procedure for the class.

SUGGESTIONS FOR CLINICAL ACTIVITIES

Observe the surgical procedure and postoperative care of a client with a gallbladder, liver, or pancreas disorder.

LEARNING OUTCOME 4

Use the nursing process to assess, plan, provide, and evaluate care for clients with disorders of the gallbladder, liver, or exocrine pancreas.

CONCEPTS FOR LECTURE

1. Assess, plan, provide, and evaluate care for clients with disorders of the gallbladder.
2. Assess, plan, provide, and evaluate care for client with disorders of the liver.
3. Assess, plan, provide, and evaluate care for clients with disorders of the pancreas.

POWERPOINT LECTURE SLIDES

1 Cholelithiasis/Cholecystitis—Assess
- Assessment (Box 21-6)

1a Cholelithiasis/Cholecystitis—Plan and Provide
- Acute Pain:
  - Fat intake (Box 21-3)
  - Pain medications
  - Fowler's position
- Nausea
  - Monitor
  - Antiemetics
  - Avoid noxious foods/odors
  - Oral care
  - NPO as needed

POWERPOINT LECTURE SLIDES *continued*

- Risk for Impaired Gas Exchange
  - Turn, deep breathe, and cough every 2 hours
  - Incentive spirometer
  - Splints
  - Evaluate temperature every 4 hours

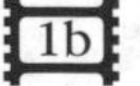

Cholelithiasis/Cholecystitis—Evaluate

- Comfort level
- Intake
- Respiratory status
- Free of infection
- Teaching:
  - Disease, medications, diagnostic procedures, treatment options
  - Food in relation to acute episodes
  - Preop teaching
  - D/C teaching
  - Wound care
  - Pain control
  - Activities
  - Diet
  - Return to work
  - Dietary consult

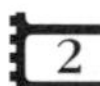

Hepatitis—Assess

- Classic signs and symptoms
- Box 21-10

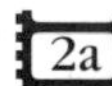

Hepatitis—Plan/Provide

- Risk for Infection (transmission)
  - Universal precautions
  - Hand washing
  - Immunization
- Activity Intolerance
  - Rest
- Imbalanced Nutrition: Less than Body Requirements
  - Small frequent meals
  - High calories
  - Eat when not nauseated
  - IVF as needed

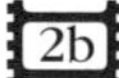

Hepatitis—Evaluate

- No transmission to others
- Universal precautions
- Rest
- Stable weight
- Teaching:
  - Prevent spread of disease
  - Vaccination
  - No sharing personal items
  - No sexual activity until no longer infectious

Cirrhosis—Assess

- Box 21-14

Cirrhosis—Plan/Provide

- Excess Fluid Volume
  - Daily weights
  - Intake and output

© 2007 Pearson Education, Inc.

  - Neck vein distention
  - Peripheral edema
  - Abdominal girth
  - Low sodium diet
- Disturbed Thought Processes
  - No CNS depressant medications
  - Assess LOC
  - Low-protein diet
  - Medications
  - Orient ×3
- Ineffective Protection
  - Vital signs
  - Bleeding precautions (Box 21-5)
  - Lab values
- Risk for Suffocation
  - NG tube care
  - Fowler's position
  - Blakemore tube pressure
- Ineffective Breathing Pattern
  - High-Fowler's position
  - Monitor respiratory rate, oxygen saturation levels
- Impaired Skin Integrity
  - Warm water
  - No soap
  - Prevent scratching
  - Turn every 2 hours

2e Cirrhosis—Evaluate
- Outcomes related to nursing diagnoses
- Teaching
  - Box 21-16
  - Diet
  - Fluid
  - Medications
  - Postop care
  - Hospice referral

3 Pancreatitis—Assess
- Onset of S/S
- Pain
- Previous attacks
- Alcohol use
- Food intake
- Bowel sounds

3a Pancreatitis—Plan/Provide
- Acute Pain
  - Analgesics
  - NPO
  - NG tube
  - Bed rest
  - Comfort measures
- Risk for Imbalanced Nutrition: Less than Body Requirements
  - Daily weights
  - Stool count
  - Bowel sounds
  - IVF, TP\N

© 2007 Pearson Education, Inc.

POWERPOINT LECTURE SLIDES *continued*

- Risk for Injury
  - Vital signs
  - Respiratory status
  - Urine output
  - Assess LOC

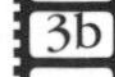

Pancreatitis—Evaluate

- Pain level
- Weight management
- Teaching
  - Avoid further attacks
  - Role of alcohol and smoking
  - Medications
  - Diet therapy
  - S/S infection

SUGGESTIONS FOR CLASSROOM ACTIVITIES

- Access the website http://digestive.niddk.nih.gov/ to research the treatments for a client with a gallbladder, liver, or pancreas disorder.

SUGGESTIONS FOR CLINICAL ACTIVITIES

Provide care to a client with a gallbladder, liver, or pancreas disorder.

© 2007 Pearson Education, Inc.

CHAPTER 22
THE RESPIRATORY SYSTEM AND ASSESSMENT

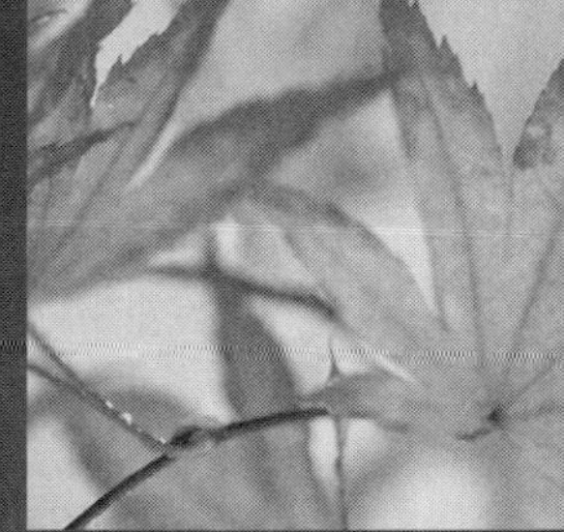

RESOURCE LIBRARY

CD-ROM

Respiratory System
Diaphragm

IMAGE LIBRARY

Figure 22-1 (**A**) Structures of the upper respiratory system. (**B**) The sinuses.
Figure 22-2 The lower respiratory system, showing the lungs and layers of the visceral and parietal pleura.
Figure 22-3 The functional tissue of the lungs, including the respiratory bronchioles and alveoli.
Figure 22-4 (**A**) During inspiration, the diaphragm contracts and flattens, and the intercostals muscles contract, moving the chest wall up and outward. This increases the volume of the chest cavity. (**B**) During expiration, the muscles relax, the diaphragm rises, and the lungs recoil.
Figure 22-5 Sequence for lung auscultation on the back.
Figure 22-6 Sensor probe placed on the finger for oxygen saturation analysis, and a microprocessing unit with digital display.
Figure 22-7 The relationship of lung volumes and capacities. Volumes shown are for an average adult male.

LEARNING OUTCOME 1

Describe the structure and function of the respiratory tract.

CONCEPTS FOR LECTURE

1. Structures of the upper respiratory tract include the nose and sinuses, pharynx, and larynx. Main function is to clean, humidify, and warm air. Upper respiratory tract necessary for effective breathing.
2. Structures of the lower respiratory tract include the lungs, bronchi, alveoli, pulmonary arteries, and pulmonary veins.

POWERPOINT LECTURE SLIDES

1 Nose and Sinuses
- Structure
- Function

1a Pharynx
- Nasopharynx
- Oropharynx
- Laryngopharynx

1b Larynx
- Structure
- Function

1c Lungs
- Structure
- Function

1d Bronchi and Alveoli
- Structure
- Function

1e Pulmonary Circulation
- Pulmonary arteries
- Pulmonary veins
- Pulmonary capillary network

POWERPOINT LECTURE SLIDES *continued*

1f Pleura
- Structure
  - Parietal
  - Visceral
- Function

1g Rib Cage and Intercostal Muscles
- Structure
- Function

2 Lungs
- Structure
- Function

2a Bronchi and Alveoli
- Structure
- Function

2b Pulmonary Circulation
- Pulmonary arteries
- Pulmonary veins
- Pulmonary capillary network

2c Pleura
- Structure
  - Parietal
  - Visceral
- Function

2d Rib Cage and Intercostal Muscles
- Structure
- Function

SUGGESTIONS FOR CLASSROOM ACTIVITIES

1. Have the student identify the anatomy and physiology of the structures in the respiratory system.
2. Have the student identify the position of the diaphragm and the difference in volumes and intrathoracic pressures during inspiration and expiration.

SUGGESTIONS FOR CLINICAL ACTIVITIES

Assign students to complete a respiratory assessment on any of their clinical clients. Assessment findings should be submitted in writing.

LEARNING OUTCOME 2

Explain the mechanics of respiration.

CONCEPTS FOR LECTURE

1. Ventilation is the movement of air into and out of the lungs and has two phases: inspiration and expiration. Two phases make up a breath, which normally occur 12–20 per minute.
2. The phases of respirations are inspiration, during which air flows into the lungs, and expiration, during which gases flow out of the lungs.
3. Factors that affect respirations include the respiratory center in the brain, chemoreceptors in the brain, aortic arch, and carotid arteries. Receptors respond to changes in the amount of oxygen, carbon dioxide, and hydrogen ions in arterial blood. Other factors that

POWERPOINT LECTURE SLIDES

1 Ventilation
- Divided into phases
- Normal breath 12–20 times per minute

2 Inspiration
- Lasts 1–1.5 seconds
- Diaphragm contracts and flattens
- Intercostal muscles contract; increases size of chest cavity
- Lungs stretch and volume increases
- Pressure in lungs slightly less than atmospheric (causes air to rush in)

© 2007 Pearson Education, Inc.

Concepts for Lecture *continued*

affect ventilation and the work of breathing are airway resistence, compliance, elasticity, and surface tension on the walls of alveoli.

4. Aging commonly leads to structural and functional changes of the respiratory system.

PowerPoint Lecture Slides *continued*

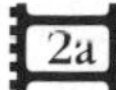

2a Expiration
- Lasts 2 to 3 seconds
- Passive
- Muscles relax
- Diaphragm rises
- Ribs descend
- Lungs recoil
- Pressure in chest cavity increases (compressing alveoli)
- Pressure in lungs higher than atmospheric causes gases to flow out of the lungs

3 Factors Affecting Respirations
- Respiratory center of the brain
- Chemoreceptors in the brain, aortic arch, and carotid arteries
- Airway resistance
- Compliance
- Elasticity
- Surface tension of alveoli

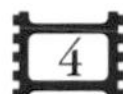

4 Respiratory Changes Associated with Aging
- Cartilage that connects ribs to sternum and spinal cord calcifies
- Anterior-posterior diameter of chest increases
- Respiratory muscles weaker
- Cough and laryngeal reflexes less effective
- Size of lungs decreases
- Alveoli less elastic
- Older client at greater risk for developing respiratory infections

Suggestions for Classroom Activities

1. Have the students measure their own oxygen saturation with a pulse oximeter. Have them identify saturation variations with the probe at different body locations and when they hold their breath.
2. In a laboratory setting, have students perform respiratory assessments and practice client interviews with one another. The students acting as clients should be told to give some answers that would indicate a possible respiratory system disorder. Findings and difficulties encountered while performing the assessments may be discussed by the class.

Suggestions for Clinical Activities

Assign students to perform a respiratory assessment on a client who smokes and one who does not smoke. The students should then compare and contrast their findings.

Learning Outcome 3

Describe assessment and data collection for respiratory function.

Concepts for Lecture

1. Assessment and data collection should include both subjective and objective information.

PowerPoint Lecture Slides

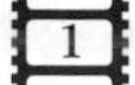

1 Subjective
- Current complaint or existing condition
- Onset or duration of symptoms
- Ability to maintain ADLs
- Nasal congestion, nosebleeds
- Sore throat, difficulty swallowing

© 2007 Pearson Education, Inc.

POWERPOINT LECTURE SLIDES *continued*

- Changes in voice quality
- Difficulty breathing, orthopnea
- Pain on breathing
- Presence of cough frequency, duration, productive or unproductive
- Sputum amount, color, and consistency
- Exposure to infections (colds or influenza)
- History of chronic lung conditions
- Occupational exposure to chemicals, smoke, asbestos
- Hx previous respiratory problems
- Allergies to medication or environmental allergens
- Use of tobacco, chewing tobacco, marijuana, cocaine, injected drugs, and alcohol

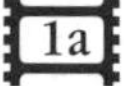
Objective
- Assess state of health
- Color
- Ease of breathing
- Note respiratory rate and pattern
- Observe nasal flaring
- Use of accessory muscles for breathing
- Listen for hoarseness in client's speech
- Inspect mucosa of nose, mouth, and oropharynx
- Inspect neck, position of trachea
- Inspect anterior/posterior diameter of chest
- Palpate lips for nodules, chest for tenderness or swelling
- Auscultate breath sounds, note absence or presence and quality
- Note adventitious breath sounds (wheezing or crackles)

SUGGESTIONS FOR CLASSROOM ACTIVITIES

Assign students to review audiotapes of abnormal breath sounds to become familiar with them.

LEARNING OUTCOME 4

Provide appropriate nursing care and teaching for clients undergoing diagnostic tests and procedures related to the respiratory system.

CONCEPTS FOR LECTURE

1. Diagnostic tests and procedures related to the respiratory tract include pulse oximetry, arterial blood gases, serum alpha$_1$-antitrypsin, sputum and tissue specimens, imaging studies, pulmonary function tests, and direct visualization (laryngoscopy and bronchoscopy).

POWERPOINT LECTURE SLIDES

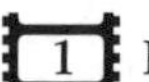
Pulse Oximetry
- Monitors oxygen saturation ($Sa{O_2}$)
- $Sa{O_2}$—amount of arterial hemoglobin that is combined with oxygen
- Nursing Care
  - Apply to fingertip, forehead, earlobe, or nose
  - Remove nail polish when using fingertip

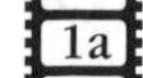
Arterial Blood Gases
- Refer to Table 7-12 and Box 7-13 for normal values and evaluation
- Nursing care
  - Apply pressure to site 2–5 minutes following arterial puncture

© 2007 Pearson Education, Inc.

- Serum alpha$_1$-antitrysin deficiency in this serum protein contributing factor in emphysema and COPD; normal value in adults 150–350 mg/dL
- Nursing care and instructions
  - Fasting specimen obtained in client with elevated cholesterol or triglycerides
- Throat or nose swab
- Nursing care: Refer to Procedure 23-1
- Sputum specimen
- Culture and sensitivity
- Gram's stain
- Acid-fast stain
- Cytology
- Nursing care and client teaching: refer to Table 22-1

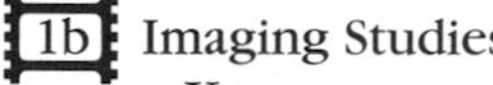

1b Imaging Studies
- X-rays
- CT scans
- Ventilation perfusion scans
- Nursing care and client teaching: refer to Table 22-1
- If contrast used remember to ask about allergies, especially iodine and seafood

1c Pulmonary Function Tests
- Measures lung volume and capacity
- Factors that affect PFTs
- Smoking, caffeine, and bronchodilators also interfere with results
- Total lung capacity (TLC) = (VT) tidal volume + (IRV) inspiratory reserve volume + (ERV) expiratory reserve volume + (RV) reserve volume
- (VC) vital capacity = VT + IRV + ERV
- VC normal value in adults 4,500–4,800 mL
- Nursing care and client teaching
  - Instruct client to stop bronchodilators 4–6 hours prior to test
  - Instruct client not to smoke or drink caffeinated drinks prior to test

1d Direct Visualization
- Direct or indirect laryngoscopy—used to identify and evaluate laryngeal tumors
- Nursing care and client teaching:
  - Make sure consent form has been signed
  - Remove dentures, partial plates, bridges prior to procedure
  - NPO before procedure
  - NPO after procedure until gag reflex returns

1e Bronchoscopy
- Used to visualize trachea, bronchi and bronchioles for:
  - Tumors and structural disorders
- Obtain tissue biopsy

© 2007 Pearson Education, Inc.

POWERPOINT LECTURE SLIDES *continued*

- Obtain sputum specimen
- Removal of foreign body
- Nursing and teaching for bronchoscopy: refer to Box 24-2

SUGGESTIONS FOR CLASSROOM ACTIVITIES

Practice sputum collection methods.

SUGGESTIONS FOR CLINICAL ACTIVITIES

1. Assign students to perform a respiratory assessment on a young adult and an older adult. The clients chosen should have no history of respiratory abnormalities. Instruct the students to identify nonpathologic variations in the assessment.
2. Assign students to perform a respiratory assessment on a client with a respiratory disorder. Have the student identify the abnormalities.

© 2007 Pearson Education, Inc.

CHAPTER 23
CARING FOR CLIENTS WITH UPPER RESPIRATORY DISORDERS

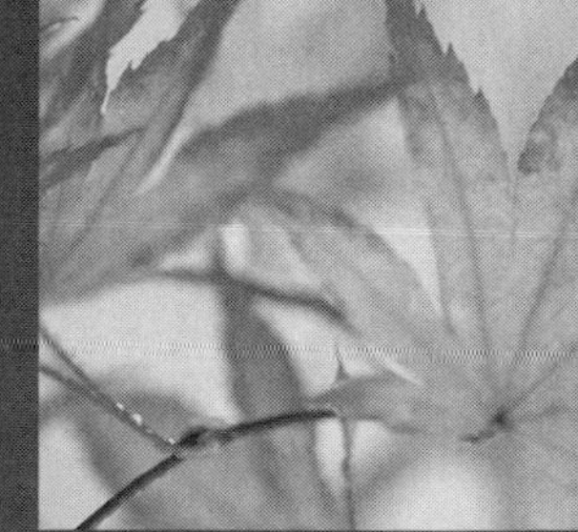

RESOURCE LIBRARY

IMAGE LIBRARY

Figure 23-1 Posterior nasal packing. Ties exiting through the nose and mouth are used to stabilize the packing in position and remove it when it is no longer needed.
Figure 23-2 **(A)** The Heimlich maneuver performed on a conscious victim who is sitting or standing. **(B)** The Heimlich maneuver performed on an unconscious victim.
Figure 23-3 In obstructive sleep apnea, the pharynx is obstructed by the soft palate and tongue.
Figure 23-4 Cancer of the larynx. Most lesions form along the edges of the glottis.
Figure 23-5 Following a total laryngectomy, the client has a permanent tracheostomy. No connection between the trachea and esophagus remains.
Figure 23-6 The tracheoesophageal prosthesis allows air from the trachea to be diverted through the prosthesis into the esophagus and oropharynx, producing speech when the tracheostomy stoma is occluded. A one-way valve prevents food from entering the trachea.
Figure 23-7 **(A)** The client holds the vibrating tip of the speech generator against the throat, using the mouth to form words. **(B)** A plastic tube on the handpiece of the speech aid device produces an audible tone. The client holds the tube against the roof of the mouth when forming words.

LEARNING OUTCOME 1

Describe common disorders affecting the upper respiratory tract and their manifestations.

CONCEPTS FOR LECTURE

1. Upper respiratory infections may affect the nose, sinuses, pharynx, tonsils, and larynx. Most upper respiratory infections are minor illnesses; however, life-threatening complications can result, especially in the frail older adult. Most URIs are caused by viruses or allergens that enter the airway, causing acute inflammation of the sinuses, pharynx, or larynx. Mucosa swells and secretes clear, yellow, or greenish exudates. Bacterial infections may develop following a viral infection.

POWERPOINT LECTURE SLIDES

1 **Rhinitis**—Inflammation of Nasal Cavities
- Types
  - Acute viral rhinitis
  - Allergic rhinitis
- Manifestations (Table 23-1)

1a Influenza
- Mode of transmission
- Complications
- Manifestations (Table 23-1)

1b Sinusitis
- Manifestations
- Complications

1c Acute Epiglottis—Medical Emergency
- Manifestations
- **Clinical alert:**
  - Monitor clients with epiglottitis for signs of respiratory distress
    - Nasal flaring
    - Restlessness
    - Stridor
    - Use of accessory muscles
    - ↓ oxygen saturation
  - Don't insert nasal or oral airway (may cause spasm and airway obstruction)

PowerPoint Lecture Slides *continued*

- Nasotracheal intubation may be necessary; be prepared for intubation

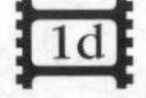 Laryngitis
- Manifestations
- Interdisciplinary care

Learning Outcome 2

Discuss the nursing implications for diagnostic tests, medications, and treatments ordered for clients with upper respiratory disorders.

Concepts for Lecture

1. Most acute URIs are self-limiting. Medical management focuses on accurate diagnosis, providing symptomatic relief, and preventing complications.
2. Education is the primary nursing role in caring for most clients with acute or chronic URIs. Clients need to be able to recognize the difference between acute, self-limiting disorders and those that require medical attention.

PowerPoint Lecture Slides

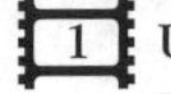 URIs
- Control of URIs in long-term care facilities
- Refer to Box 23-3

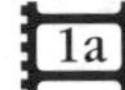 **Diagnostic Tests**
- Throat swab for streptoccocal pharyngitis (Procedure 23-1)
- LA antigen and ELISA rapid identification of strep
- CBC
- Nasal swabs
- X-ray
- CT scan

1b Medications (Table 23-2)

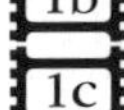 Polyvalent Influenza Vaccine
- 85% effective in preventing influenza
- Criteria for clients who should receive vaccine
- Should not be given to clients with allergy to eggs
- Serious adverse reactions to vaccine

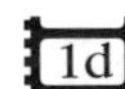 **Antibiotics**
- Treatment for bacterial infections
- Use for up to 10 days
- Client no longer contagious after 24 hours of antibiotic therapy
- Antibiotics may be used up to 2 weeks for sinusitis
- Medications used to treat rhinitis are:
  - Mild decongestants
  - Topical decongestant nasal sprays or drops (refer to Box 23-4 for administration)
- Clinical alert for nasal decongestants
- Clinical alert for pseudoephedrine
- Antihistamines

1e **Sore Throat**
- Warm saltwater gargles
- Throat lozenges
- Mild analgesics

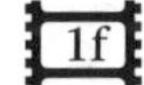 **Cough**
- Antitussives
- Systemic mucolytic agents (guaifenesin)

© 2007 Pearson Education, Inc.

PowerPoint Lecture Slides *continued*

1g Complementary Therapies
- Herbal remedies
- Aromatherapy

1h Surgical Interventions
- Endoscopic sinus surgery; relieves obstruction of opening to sinus and restores ventilation and drainage of sinus
- Nasal packing left in place 24–48 hours postop
- Discharge instructions

1i Tonsillectomy
- Postop complications
- Postop care

1j Peritonsillar Abscess
- Treatment: I&D needle aspiration followed by tonsillectomy

2 Nursing Care for URIs:
- Education main focus

2a Nursing Process
- **Assessment:**
  - Determine effect of URI on client's life
  - Identify risk factors for complications
  - Determine whether problem will require medical treatment or self-care appropriate

2b Diagnosis, Planning, and Implementation for Clients with Significant Manifestations or Complications
- Maintain airway clearance
- Effective breathing patterns
- Adequate rest

2c Nursing Diagnoses
- Ineffective Breathing Pattern
- Ineffective Airway Clearance
- Disturbed Sleeping Pattern
- Impaired Verbal Communication

2d Implementation: Ineffective Breathing Pattern
- Monitor respiratory rate and pattern
- Auscultate lungs
- Pace activities
- Elevate head of bed

2e Implementation: Ineffective Airway Clearance
- Monitor effectiveness of cough
- Note whether cough is productive or nonproductive
- Auscultate lungs

2f Implementation: Disturbed Sleep Pattern
- Assess sleep pattern
- Place in semi-Fowler's or Fowler's position
- Provide antipyretics and analgesics
- Cough suppressant at nighttime

© 2007 Pearson Education, Inc.

PowerPoint Lecture Slides *continued*

 **Implementation: Impaired Verbal Communication—Laryngitis**

- Encourage client to rest voice; use alternative method to communicate (writing pad)
- Comfort measures: lozenges, gargle, or sprays
- Encourage client to quit smoking

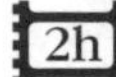 **Evaluation and Documentation**

- Document initial assessment
- Teaching important since most URIs treated at home
- Encourage rest
- Adequate hydration
- Hand washing after coughing
- Avoid exposure to crowds
- Avoid physical or psychologic stress
- Prevention for influenza—vaccine for high-risk groups
- Discuss OTC medications for relief of symptoms
- Assist client to identify possible allergens for allergic rhinitis
- Stress importance of completing entire course if on antibiotics
- Teach complications of influenza and URIs

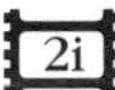 **Pertussis (Whooping Cough)**

- Pathophysiology and manifestations
- Interdisciplinary care
- Nursing care: promoting immunization of vulnerable group
- Clinical alert

Learning Outcome 3

Provide care for clients having surgery involving the upper respiratory system.

Concepts for Lecture

1. Upper respiratory trauma or obstruction includes epistaxis, nasal trauma or deviated septum, nasal fractures, laryngeal obstructions or trauma. Surgeries performed to correct these conditions include rhinoplasty, septoplasty. Severe epitaxis may be treated with nasal packing or surgery.
2. Tumors of the upper respiratory tract are relatively uncommon. However, they can obstruct the airway and interfere with breathing. The larynx is the upper airway structure most affected by tumors.

PowerPoint Lecture Slides

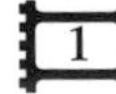 **Epistaxis**

- Pathophysiology and manifestations
- Interdisciplinary care
- Medications:
    - Topical vasoconstrictors
    - Cauterization with silver nitrate or gelfoam
- **Nasal packing**
    - Anterior packing left in place 24–72 hours
    - Posterior packing left in place up to 5 days; uncomfortable (refer to Figure 23-1)
    - Supplemental oxygen given with posterior packing
    - Complications with posterior packing
    - Foley catheter may be used as alternative to posterior packing
- **Surgery**—procedure to ligate artery in posterior bleed
- Postop—monitor for bleeding or respiratory complications

 © 2007 Pearson Education, Inc.

POWERPOINT LECTURE SLIDES *continued*

- Nursing care for epistaxis:
  - Main goals:
    - Reduce anxiety
    - Maintain open airway
- Assessment:
  - Subjective
  - Objective
- **Nursing diagnoses and Interventions**
  - Anxiety
  - Interventions
  - Risk for Aspiration
  - Interventions
- Evaluation and documentation
- Continuing care

1a **Nasal Trauma or Deviated Septum**

- Pathophysiology and manifestations (refer to Box 23-6)
- Interdisciplinary care—main goals to maintain patent airway and prevent deformity
- If CSF leak suspected, CT scan performed
- More complex fractures require surgery:
  - **Rhinoplasty**—done to relieve airway obstruction and repair visible deformity
  - **Septoplasty or submucosal resection (SMR)**—done to correct septal deviation
- **Nursing care**
  - Airway management
  - Control of bleeding, pain & swelling
  - Provide necessary teaching
  - Assessment: for pain, swelling, bleeding, difficulty breathing, deformities, ecchymosis and crepitus
- **Nursing Diagnoses**
  - Ineffective Airway Clearance
  - Interventions
  - Risk for Infection
  - Interventions
    - Evaluating and documenting
    - Continuing care

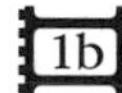

Laryngeal Obstruction or Trauma—Life-Threatening Emergency

- **Pathophysiology and manifestations**
- Obstruction can be caused by:
  - Laryngospasms
  - Laryngeal edema
  - Aspirated food or foreign object
  - Trauma to larynx
- **Manifestations** of laryngeal obstruction
- **Manifestations** of laryngeal trauma
- **Interdisciplinary care**
  - X-rays, diagnostic tests, or ultrasound to locate obstruction
  - Insertion of endotracheal tube
  - For laryngeal edema due to anaphylaxis, epinephrine given

© 2007 Pearson Education, Inc.

POWERPOINT LECTURE SLIDES *continued*

- **Clinical alert:** complete airway obstruction; Heimlich maneuver performed (refer to Figure 23-2)
- **Nursing care**
  - Closely monitor clients at risk for laryngeal obstruction
  - Suction airway
  - Be prepared for endotracheal intubation or tracheotomy
  - Be prepared to initiate CPR
  - Teach prevention

1c **Sleep Apnea**

- Types
- Risk factors
- Manifestations
- Treatments: CPAP therapy
- Nursing care: focus on teaching use of respiratory equipment and avoidance or correction of risk factors

2 **Benign Laryngeal Tumors**

- Common in clients who chronically shout, project, or vocalize in very high or low tone
- Manifestations
- Treatment
- Surgery
- Voice rest

2a **Laryngeal Cancer**

- Risk factors
- Pathophysiology and manifestations
  - Leukoplakia
  - Erythroplakia
  - Refer to common manifestations (Box 23-8)
  - Interdisciplinary care: determined by stage of cancer
- **Diagnostic tests**
  - Laryngoscopy
  - CT scan
  - MRI
  - Needle biopsy
  - Barium swallow
- **Treatment**
  - Radiation
  - Chemotherapy
  - Surgery: type determined by size, site, and invasiveness of tumor
  - Carcinoma *in situ* and vocal polyps treated with laser on outpatient basis
  - Laryngectomy: removal of larynx
- **Total laryngectomy**
  - Entire larynx removed
  - Normal speech lost
  - Permanent tracheostomy
- **Modified or radical neck dissection** in addition to total laryngectomy if cervical lymph nodes are cancerous
- Nursing care of total laryngectomy (Box 23-9)

© 2007 Pearson Education, Inc.

PowerPoint Lecture Slides *continued*

- Clinical alert for laryngectomies
- **Nursing care of clients with laryngeal cancer**
  - Assessment (Box 23-10)
  - Nursing diagnoses
    - Impaired Verbal Communication
    - Interventions
    - Imbalanced Nutrition: Less than Body Requirements
    - Interventions
    - Anticipatory Grieving
    - Interventions
  - Evaluation
  - Documentation
  - Continuing care
  - Assessment for discharge (Box 23-11)

Learning Outcome 4

Identify nursing care needs for the client with a tracheostomy.

Concepts for Lecture

1. A tracheostomy (surgical opening into the trachea) may be inserted to maintain the airway in the early postoperative period following a partial laryngectomy. It is usually removed within a week postop and the stoma is allowed to heal. In the total laryngectomy a permanent tracheostomy is created. The tracheostomy tube inserted during surgery may be left in place for several weeks and then removed, leaving a natural stoma, or it may be left in place permanently. Because the trachea and the esophagus are permanently separated there is no risk of aspiration during swallowing.

PowerPoint Lecture Slides

1 Tracheostomy Care Checklist (Procedure 23-2)

Suggestions for Classroom Activities

1. Discuss the pathophysiology and assessment of each upper respiratory disorder.
   - Have students identify the populations at risk for upper respiratory disorders and discuss ways to prevent the transmission of upper respiratory infections.
   - Review Table 23-1 comparing rhinitis and influenza. Ask students to discuss the differences in methods of transmissions, clinical manifestations, and nursing interventions for each disorder.
2. Initiate a discussion on the use of pharmacologic/nonpharmacologic comfort measures, and complementary therapies in the treatment of upper respiratory disorders.
3. List the nursing diagnoses, goals, and interventions on transparencies. Ask the students to prioritize the nursing diagnoses, goals, and interventions for each disorder and give the rationale for each selection.
   - Summarize the nursing responsibilities in caring for clients with acute or chronic upper respiratory infections.

Suggestions for Clinical Activities

1. In the clinical lab setting have students demonstrate the ability to:
   - Administer nasal drops.
   - Obtain a throat swab.
   - Administer a vaccine injection.
2. In clinical lab setting have students demonstrate tracheostomy care and suctioning.
3. Assign students to care for clients with laryngectomies. Discuss the risk factors of laryngeal cancer and methods of preventing laryngeal cancer. Have the students describe the multiple needs of the clients in postconference. Discuss the nursing diagnoses, goals, and nursing interventions for the clients.

© 2007 Pearson Education, Inc.

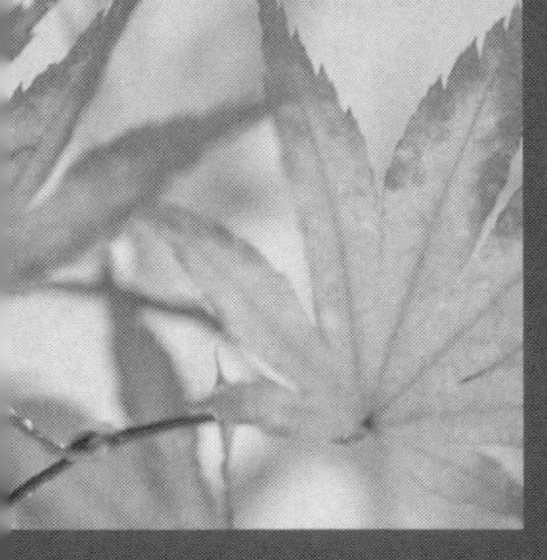

CHAPTER 24
CARING FOR CLIENTS WITH LOWER RESPIRATORY DISORDERS

RESOURCE LIBRARY

CD-ROM

Video: Nasal Cannula
Video: Nonrebreather Mask
Video: Oxygen Mask
Asthma
Salmeterol
Video: Nebulizer Treatment
Video: Humidifier
Video: Metered-Dose Inhaler
ARDS

IMAGE LIBRARY

Figure 24-1 Fiberoptic bronchoscopy.
Figure 24-2 (**A**) Nasal cannula. (**B**) Simple face mask. (**C**) Nonrebreather mask.
Figure 24-3 Percussing the upper posterior chest. Note the cupped position of the nurse's hands.
Figure 24-4 Positions for postural drainage.
Figure 24-5 The pathogenesis of tuberculosis.
Figure 24-6 (**A**) Intradermal injection of PPD. (**B**) A local inflammatory response to PPD. (**C**) Measuring induration produced by the inflammatory response.
Figure 24-7 The sequence of an acute episode of asthma.
Figure 24-8 The process of COPD.
Figure 24-9 Typical appearance of a client with emphysema.
Figure 24-10 (**A**) A normal lung scan showing perfusion of all areas of the lungs. (**B**) A lung scan showing impaired blood flow to the right lung due to pulmonary embolus.
Figure 24-11 Example of a vena caval filter to prevent emboli from reaching the lungs.
Figure 24-12 Thoracentesis. A needle is inserted between the ribs into the pleural space to withdraw excess pleural fluid.
Figure 24-13 A closed chest drainage system.
Figure 24-14 Flail chest with paradoxic chest movement.
Figure 24-15 Nasal endotracheal intubation.

LEARNING OUTCOME 1

Describe the pathophysiology, manifestations and interdisciplinary care of infectious and inflammatory disorders of the lower respiratory tract.

CONCEPTS FOR LECTURE

1. Impairment of normal respiratory defenses increases risk for infection of the lower respiratory tract and can result in infection and inflammation of the bronchi or pneumonias that invade the alveoli of the lung.
2. Interdisciplinary care is directed to maintaining a patent airway and normal respiration and treating the underlying cause.
3. Other primary infections of the lower respiratory tract that occur with less frequency are tuberculosis, lung abscesses, empyema, and other emerging respiratory infections.
4. The diagnosis, treatment, and nursing care are directed to maintaining a patent airway, normal respiration, and treating the underlying cause when possible and preventing the spread of infection to others.

POWERPOINT LECTURE SLIDES

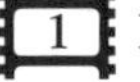

1 Infections of the Lower Respiratory Tract
- Impairment of the normal defenses
  - Cilia
  - Mucus
- Types
  - Acute bronchitis
    - Inflammation of the bronchi
    - Acute or chronic
    - Acute common among adults
    - Chronic in clients with COPD
    - Pathophysiology and manifestations:
      - Follows an upper respiratory infection
      - People at risk—smokers, impaired defense mechanisms
      - Viruses, bacteria, toxic gases
      - Inflammation causing increased mucous production and cough

POWERPOINT LECTURE SLIDES *continued*

    - Paroxysms (uncontrollable bursts)
    - Substernal chest pain
    - Fever, malaise
- Pneumonia
  - Inflammation of respiratory bronchioles and alveoli
  - Leading cause of death in U.S. among older adult and people with debilitating disease
  - Infectious
    - Bacteria
    - Viruses
    - Fungi
    - Protozoa
    - Other microbes
  - Noninfectious
    - Aspiration of gastric contents
    - Inhalation of toxic or irritating gases
  - Pathophysiology and Manifestations
    - Classified as bacterial or viral
    - Colonize the nasal and oral pharynx
    - Enter the lungs when secretions are aspirated
    - *Streptococcus pneumoniae* (pneumococcal pneumonia)
    - *Haemophilus influenzae*
  - Types of Pneumonia
    - Acute bacterial
    - *Pneumocystis carinii* pneumonia
    - Legionnaire's disease
    - Atypical
    - Viral
    - Aspiration

2 Interdisciplinary Care

- Diagnosis
  - Sputum Gram stain
  - CBC
  - ABG
  - Pulse oximetry
  - Chest x-ray
  - Fiberoptic bronchoscopy
- Immunization and prevention
- Medications
  - Antibiotics
  - Bronchodilators
  - Expectorants
- Oxygen therapy
- Other therapies
- Nursing care
  - Ineffective Airway Clearance
  - Ineffective Breathing Pattern
  - Activity Intolerance
- Continuing care
  - Teaching focused on prevention
  - Immunizations
  - Taking medications
  - Limit activities to conserve energy
  - Maintain nutrition and fluid intake

© 2007 Pearson Education, Inc.

POWERPOINT LECTURE SLIDES *continued*

3 Other Primary Infections

- Tuberculosis
  - Chronic recurrent infection of the lungs
  - *Myobacterium tuberculosis*
  - Health problem worldwide
  - Pathophysiology
    - Slow-growing organism
    - Transmitted by droplet nuclei
  - Types
    - Pulmonary tuberculosis
      - Alveolus or respiratory bronchiole
      - Upper lobe
      - WBCs phagocytize and isolate bacteria
      - Sealed off colony of bacilli (tubercle)
      - Scar tissue forms around tubercle
      - Reactivation tuberculosis
      - Manifestations
        - Fatigue
        - Fever
        - Weight loss
        - Night sweats
        - Cough
    - Extrapulmonary tuberculosis
      - Develop in other organs active or dormant
      - Kidney or GU tract
      - Large weight-bearing joints
      - Miliary tuberculosis
      - Tuberculosis meningitis
      - Manifestations
        - Vary depending on organ involved
- Lung abscess and empyema
  - Potential complication of pneumonia and other respiratory infections
  - Local lung destruction or necrosis and pus formation
  - Aspiration pneumonia common cause
  - Empyema
    - Pus in the pleural cavity
    - Bacterial pneumonia, rupture of lung abscess, infection from chest trauma are causes
  - Manifestations
    - Two weeks after initiating event
    - Signs of acute infection
  - Treatment with antibiotics
- Emerging respiratory infections
  - Severe acute respiratory syndrome (SARS)
    - Virus called SARS-associated coronavirus
  - Inhalation anthrax
    - *Bacillus anthracis*

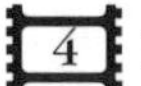

Interdisciplinary Care

- Collaborative focus
  - Early detection
  - Effective treatment
  - Preventing spread
- Screening
  - Tuberculin test
  - Purified protein derivative (PPD)

© 2007 Pearson Education, Inc.

POWERPOINT LECTURE SLIDES *continued*

- Diagnosis
  - Acid-fast bacilli smear and culture
  - Chest x-ray
  - Fiberoptic bronchoscopy
- Medications
  - Drugs to prevent and treat
  - INH (isoniazid)
  - Two antitubercular drugs
  - Treated for a period of 6 months
- Nursing care
  - Assessment
  - Diagnosis, planning, intervention
    - Risk for Infection
      - Negative flow room
      - HEPA-filtered respirator
      - Respiratory isolation
    - Deficient Knowledge
    - Ineffective Therapeutic Regimen Management
  - Continuing care
    - Teaching to reduce spread
    - Regular screening of high-risk individuals
    - Medication administration

SUGGESTIONS FOR CLASSROOM ACTIVITIES

1. Examine CDC website for information on incidence, prevalence, and control of tuberculosis in the United States and other countries.
2. Discuss national practice guidelines for the treatment of pneumonia.
3. Invite infection control surveillance nurse to speak on pneumonia and tuberculosis prevention and precautions.

SUGGESTIONS FOR CLINICAL ACTIVITIES

1. Assign students to clients with pneumonia.
2. Review institutional policies on TB screening, negative flow rooms, HEPA masks, and treatment of TB clients.
3. Arrange for clinical in public health department for treatment of clients with TB.

LEARNING OUTCOME 2

Describe the pathophysiology, manifestations, and interdisciplinary care of obstructive and restrictive disorders of the lower respiratory tract.

CONCEPTS FOR LECTURE

1. Diseases that affect the airways and airflow cause an increase in the work of breathing, air trapping, and decreased oxygenation.
2. Asthma is a common chronic inflammatory disorder that can result in severe airway obstruction and death.
3. Interdisciplinary care of asthma is focused on early recognition, environmental control, airway management, and prevention of complications.
4. Chronic obstructive pulmonary disease is a progressive deterioration of lung tissue and reduction of air flow to the lungs, which results in decreased oxygenation.
5. The two primary conditions include chronic bronchitis and emphysema.

POWERPOINT LECTURE SLIDES

1 Diseases of the Airway and Airflow

- Airflow decreases
  - Secretions obstruct airway
  - Airway walls are edematous or swollen
  - Smooth muscle of airways constricts
  - Lungs lose elasticity
  - Supportive tissue lost
- Result in:
  - Increased work of breathing
  - Air trapping
  - Less oxygen for gas exchange in the alveoli

2 Asthma

- Chronic inflammatory disorder
  - Recurrent episodes of
    - Wheezing
    - Breathlessness

© 2007 Pearson Education, Inc.

Concepts for Lecture *continued*

6. Interdisciplinary care of chronic obstructive pulmonary disease is directed toward early detection, reducing symptoms, and maintaining optional function.
7. Other disorders can occur that damage lung tissue and reduce the capacity of the lungs to maintain oxygenation.
8. Interdisciplinary care of other disorders is directed toward treatment and management of underlying causes and to maintain adequate oxygenation.

PowerPoint Lecture Slides *continued*

- Chest tightness
- Coughing

◦ Common in children and adults

• Pathophysiology
  ◦ Triggered by:
    - Tobacco smoke
    - Smog
    - Workplace pollutants
    - Respiratory infection
    - Exercise
    - Stress
    - Drugs
  ◦ Early response
    - Inflammatory mediators
      ▪ Bronchoconstriction
      ▪ Increased capillary permeability
      ▪ Edema and narrowing of airways
      ▪ Figure 24-7
  ◦ Late-phase response
    - 4–12 hours after exposure
    - Activation of inflammatory cells
    - Air is trapped distal to narrow airways
    - Blood flow is reduced to distended alveoli
    - Hypoxemia develops
• Manifestations
  ◦ Abrupt or develop slowly
  ◦ Chest tightness, difficulty breathing, wheezing, cough
  ◦ Prolonged expiration
  ◦ Increased heart rate and respiratory rate
  ◦ Anxiety
• Status asthmaticus
  ◦ Severe prolonged asthma that does not respond to routine treatment

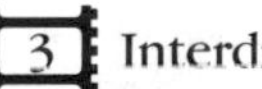

Interdisciplinary Care

• Diagnosis by history and manifestations
  ◦ Peak expiratory flow rate
  ◦ Pulse oximetry and arterial blood gases
• Treating and controlling symptoms to prevent acute attacks
• Preventive measures
  ◦ Avoid allergens
    - Pets
    - Tobacco
    - Air filtering systems
    - Other
• Medications
  ◦ Anti-inflammatory agents
  ◦ Rapid and long-acting bronchodilators
  ◦ Leukotriene modifiers
  ◦ Anticholinergic drugs
• Complimentary therapy
• Nursing care
  ◦ Assessment of airway
  ◦ Diagnosing, planning, and implementing
    - Ineffective Airway Clearance
    - Fatigue

© 2007 Pearson Education, Inc.

POWERPOINT LECTURE SLIDES *continued*

- – Anxiety
- – Ineffective Therapeutic Regimen Management
- ◦ Continuing care
  - – Teaching PEFR monitoring
  - – Use of short-acting inhalers
  - – Medications
  - – Prevention

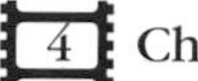

Chronic Obstructive Pulmonary Disease (COPD)

- Progressive obstruction of airflow in the lungs
- Middle to older adults
- Smoking most common cause of COPD
- Second leading cause of disability and lost work time
- Pathophysiology
  - ◦ Airways are narrowed and gradually obstructed by
    - – Inflammation
    - – Excess mucous production
    - – Loss of elastic tissue and alveoli
    - – Two processes
      - ▪ Chronic bronchitis
      - ▪ Emphysema
    - – Alveolar ventilation is impaired as is gas exchange

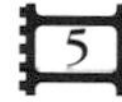

COPD Diseases

- Chronic bronchitis
  - ◦ Chronic inflammatory airway disorder
    - – Excessive secretion of thick tenacious mucus
    - – Productive cough lasting 3 or more months
    - – Narrowed airways due to mucosal edema and excess secretions
    - – Expiratory airflow affected
    - – Ciliary function impaired
- Emphysema
  - ◦ Destruction of alveolar walls
  - ◦ Large abnormal airspaces
  - ◦ Deficiency of alpha$_1$-antitrypsin
  - ◦ Surface area for gas exchange decreases
  - ◦ Alveoli become less elastic
  - ◦ Air trapping
  - ◦ Barrel chest (Figure 24-9)
  - ◦ Expiration prolonged

Interdisciplinary Care

- Diagnosis
  - ◦ Pulmonary function
  - ◦ Serum alpha$_1$-antitrypsin levels
  - ◦ ABGs
  - ◦ Pulse oximetry
- Treatment
  - ◦ Medications
  - ◦ Oxygen therapy
  - ◦ Smoking cessation
  - ◦ Fluid and nutritional support
  - ◦ Airway clearance procedures

© 2007 Pearson Education, Inc.

- Breathing exercises
- Lung transplant or lung reduction surgery

- Nursing care
  - Assessment of airway
  - Diagnosis, planning, and implementation
    - Ineffective Airway Clearance
    - Imbalanced Nutrition: Less than Body Requirements
    - Ineffective Coping
    - Decisional Conflict: Smoking
  - Continuing care
    - Effective coughing and breathing exercises
    - Nutrition and fluid intake
    - Exercise and activity
    - Avoid crowds and infection exposure risks
    - Stress reduction
    - Recognition of symptoms
    - Medication administration

7 Other Obstructive Disorders of the Lung

- Cystic fibrosis
  - Heredity disorder of childhood
  - Causes excess mucous secretion
  - Thick mucus plugs small airways and impairs normal airway clearing mechanisms
  - Leads to atelectasis, infection, bronchiectasis, and airway dilation
  - COPD, pulmonary hypertension develop over time
  - Dyspnea, chest congestion, and chronic cough of thick sticky sputum
- Atelectasis
  - Partial or total lung collapse and airlessness
  - Acute or chronic
  - Small or large segment of lung
  - Compression or inability to keep alveoli open
  - Prevention is primary treatment
- Bronchiectasis
  - Permanent dilation of large airways
  - Repeated respiratory infections
  - Secretions pool in dilated bronchial walls
  - Chronic cough and production of large amounts of sputum
  - Treatment similar to COPD
- Interstitial lung disorders
  - Inflammation damages alveoli and interstitial tissue
    - Occupational lung disease
      - Exposure to inhaling noxious substances at work
        - Pneumoconiosis
        - Hypersensitivity pneumonitis
    - Sarcoidosis
      - Chronic systemic disease
      - Affects lungs, lymph nodes, liver, eyes, skin, and other organs
      - As lesions heal, scarring develops

 © 2007 Pearson Education, Inc.

PowerPoint Lecture Slides *continued*

8 Interdisciplinary Care
- Diagnosis
  - Pilocarpine iontophoresis sweat chloride test for CF
  - Chest x-ray
  - Pulmonary function testing
- Treatment
  - Dornase alfa enzyme to liquefy secretions in CF
  - Chest physiotherapy
  - Medications to reduce inflammation and treat infection
- Nursing care
  - Assessment of airway and airway clearance
  - Diagnosis, planning, and implementation
    - Ineffective airway clearance
    - Similar to COPD
  - Continuing care
    - Teaching respiratory care techniques

Suggestions for Classroom Activities

1. Present asthma and COPD in a comparison and contrast so that students can differentiate symptoms and disease management.
2. Discuss smoking cessation techniques and their effectiveness.
3. Invite speaker from Cystic Fibrosis Foundation.

Suggestions for Clinical Activities

1. Arrange for clinical experience in public health department clinics for occupational respiratory diseases.
2. Arrange for clinical experience in emergency department to care for clients with asthma or acute respiratory problems.
3. Assign students to work with respiratory therapist.

Learning Outcome 3

Describe the pathophysiology, manifestations, and interdisciplinary care of cancer of the lower respiratory tract.

Concepts for Lecture

1. Leading cause of cancer deaths in the United States with cigarette smoking the primary cause.
2. Cancers arise from cells lining airways and tend to be aggressive, locally invasive, and metastasize widely.
3. Interdisciplinary care is focused toward prevention, early diagnosis, and treatment and maintaining pulmonary function and oxygenation.

PowerPoint Lecture Slides

1 Lung Cancer
- Leading cause of cancer deaths in the United States
- Most die within 1 year of diagnosis
- Cigarette smoking is most important cause—85% related to smoking
- Other risk factors include radiation exposure and inhaled irritants

2 Pathophysiology, Manifestations, and Complications
- Primary tumors arise from cells lining airways
- Differ by cell type (Table 24-7)
- Aggressive and locally invasive
- Metastasize widely vial lymph
- Manifestations of lung cancer (Box 24-11)
- Paraneoplastic manifestations
- Sites for metastasis
  - Brain
  - Bones
  - Liver
  - Other organs
- Superior vena cava syndrome
  - Partial or complete obstruction of superior vena cava

© 2007 Pearson Education, Inc.

POWERPOINT LECTURE SLIDES *continued*

3 Interdisciplinary Care
- Diagnosis
  - Chest x-ray
  - Sputum cytology
  - CT scan
  - Bronchoscopy
  - Percutaneous needle biopsy
- Medications
  - Combination chemotherapy
- Surgery
- Radiation therapy
- Other therapies for symptom management
  - Pleural effusion—thoracentesis
- Nursing care
  - Assessment
    - Smoking history
    - Respiratory and cardiovascular status
  - Diagnosis, planning, and implementation
    - Ineffective Breathing Pattern
    - Activity Intolerance
    - Pain
    - Anticipatory Grieving
  - Continuing care
    - Information about disease and expected outcome
    - Smoking cessation
    - Information on treatment and other services

SUGGESTIONS FOR CLASSROOM ACTIVITIES

Review with class *Healthy People 2010* initiatives and goals for treatment of lung cancer and smoking cessation

SUGGESTIONS FOR CLINICAL ACTIVITIES

1. Assign students to clients who are receiving treatment for lung cancer.
2. Assign students clinical time in cancer treatment center to observe clients receiving radiation or chemotherapy for treatment of lung cancer.

LEARNING OUTCOME 4

Describe the pathophysiology, manifestations, and interdisciplinary care of pulmonary vascular disease of the lower respiratory tract.

CONCEPTS FOR LECTURE

1. Disorders of the pulmonary vasculature result in a disruption of blood flow to the lungs, which reduces oxygenation of the blood.
2. The interdisciplinary care is focused on prevention, treatment of symptoms, and maintaining adequate circulation to the lungs and adequate oxygenation.

POWERPOINT LECTURE SLIDES

1 Pulmonary Vascular Disorders
- Cardiovascular and respiratory systems are closely linked
- Airflow is affected by blockage or conditions that restrict blood flow to the lungs
- Pulmonary embolism
  - Blockage of pulmonary artery
  - Thromboemboli
  - Also tumors, bone marrow fat, amniotic fluid, foreign matter
  - Can be fatal
  - Pathophysiology
    - Begins as clot in deep veins of legs or pelvis

© 2007 Pearson Education, Inc.

- Clot breaks loose and travels to heart and enters the pulmonary artery
- Clot is trapped, obstructing blood flow

∘ Manifestations
- Symptoms depend on size and location
- Fat emboli from long gone fracture

• Pulmonary hypertension and cor pulmonale
∘ Abnormal elevation of pulmonary arterial pressure
∘ Causes can vary
∘ Long-standing can lead to cor pulmonale with right ventricular hypertrophy and failure
∘ Manifestations
- Dyspnea
- Fatigue
- Angina
- Syncope with exertion
- Productive cough
- Dyspnea and wheezing
- Signs of right heart failure

2 Interdisciplinary Care for Vascular Disorders

• Diagnosis
∘ Plasma D-dimer levels
∘ Ventilation-perfusion scan
∘ Pulmonary angiography

• Treatment
∘ Medications
- Thrombolytic drugs
- Anticoagulants

∘ Surgery
- Umbrella-like filter in the inferior vena cava

∘ Treatment of pulmonary hypertension
Oxygen
- Calcium channel blockers
- Rapid-acting direct vasodilators

• Nursing care
∘ Assessment
- Chest pain, shortness of breath
- Identifying clients at risk
- Vital signs, oxygen saturation

∘ Diagnosis, planning, implementation
- Risk for Ineffective Tissue Perfusion: Cardiopulmonary
- Impaired Gas Exchange
- Decreased Cardiac Output
- Anxiety
- Activity Intolerance
- Fatigue

∘ Continuing care
- Anticoagulants
- Precautions to prevent bleeding
- Reduce risk of DVT
- Rest

© 2007 Pearson Education, Inc.

Suggestions for Classroom Activities

Ask students to brainstorm what clients they have cared for in the past who would be at risk for the development of deep vein thrombosis and pulmonary embolisms.

Suggestions for Clinical Activities

Assign students to observe in radiology department for ventilation-perfusion testing.

Learning Outcome 5

Describe the pathophysiology, manifestations, and interdisciplinary care of pleural disorders and trauma of the lower respiratory tract.

Concepts for Lecture

1. Plural disorders result from conditions that cause excess fluid, air, or blood in the pleural space that interferes with lung expansion and breathing.
2. The interdisciplinary care is directed to identifying and treating the cause of pleural disorders, restoring normal respiratory function, and managing associated symptoms.
3. Chest and lung injuries result from penetrating, blunt, or inhalation injuries that interfere with lung expansion and breathing.
4. The interdisciplinary care is directed to identifying the extent of the trauma to the lung and to restore normal respiratory function.

PowerPoint Lecture Slides

1 Pleural Disorders

- Pleuritis
  - Inflammation of the pleura
  - Results from another process
    - Viral infection
    - Pneumonia
    - Rib injury
  - Symptoms
    - Onset abrupt
    - Pleuritic pain is sharp or stabbing and localized
    - Deep breathing, coughing aggravate pain
    - Breathing is rapid and shallow
    - Breath sounds diminished
    - Pleural friction rub
  - Treatment
    - Analgesics
    - Nonsteroidal anti-inflammatory drugs
- Pleural effusion
  - Collection of excess fluid in pleural space
  - Results from respiratory disorders
    - Pneumonia
    - Cancer
    - Trauma
  - Results from systemic disorders
    - Heart failure
    - Kidney disease
  - Symptoms
    - Dyspnea and shortness of breath
    - Diminished breath sounds
    - Limited chest wall movement
  - Treatment
    - Thoracentesis (Figure 24-12)
    - Pain control
    - Maintaining respiratory function
- Pneumothorax
  - Accumulation of air in the pleural space
    - Can occur without cause
    - Due to chronic lung disease
    - Result of trauma
  - Pathophysiology
    - Air enters pleural space
    - Pressure in space is no longer negative and lung collapses

© 2007 Pearson Education, Inc.

- Types
  - Spontaneous
  - Traumatic open pneumothorax
  - Tension pneumothorax
- Manifestations
  - Dependent on the size and extent of lung collapse
  - Primary pneumothorax affects tall, slender, young adult men
  - Secondary pneumothorax occurs in people with preexisting lung disease, usually COPD
  - Both have an abrupt onset if chest pain and shortness of breath present
  - Tachypnea and tachycardia
  - Diminished breath sounds
  - Other
    - Air heard or felt
    - Deviated trachea
- Diagnosis and treatment
  - Chest x-ray
  - Treatment dependent on severity
  - Thoracentesis
  - Chest tubes to reexpand the lungs
- Hemothorax
  - Blood in the pleural space
  - Chest trauma or surgery
  - Symptoms similar to pneumothorax
  - Treatment with thoracentesis or chest tubes

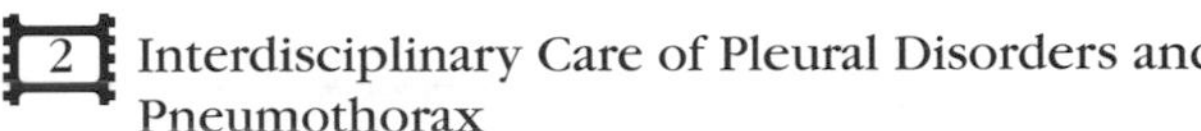

2 Interdisciplinary Care of Pleural Disorders and Pneumothorax
- Chest tubes
  - Treatment for pneumothorax
  - Closed-drainage system
  - One-way valve—water seal prevents air from entering chest cavity
  - Box 24-16 outlines nursing care
- Nursing care
  - Assessment of respiratory status and pain
  - Diagnosis, planning, and implementation
    - Impaired Gas Exchange
    - Risk for Injury
    - Altered Comfort
  - Continuing care
    - Avoid smoking
    - Follow-up care and monitoring

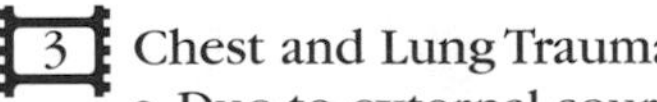

3 Chest and Lung Trauma
- Due to external source that can affect chest wall and lung
- Rib fracture
  - Single rib fracture most common chest wall injury
  - Usually minor
  - Can lead to pneumonia, atelectasis, and respiratory failure
  - If displaced, can cause a tear in the pleura and cause pneumonthorax

© 2007 Pearson Education, Inc.

- Pain on inspiration
- Bruising and crepitus

- Flail chest
  - Two or more adjacent ribs broken
  - Chest wall becomes free floating
  - Paradoxic movement
    - Flail segment moves inward during inspiration and outward during expiration
  - Pain and dyspnea
  - Crepitus and diminished breath sounds
- Pulmonary contusion
  - Chest trauma when chest is rapidly compressed and then decompressed
  - Alveoli and pulmonary vessels rupture
  - Causes tissue hemorrhage and edema
  - Inflammation sets in, which further impairs breathing
  - Symptoms
    - Shortness of breath and restlessness
    - Chest pain
    - Copious blood tinged sputum
    - Tachycardia, cachypnea, dyspnea, and cyanosis
- Smoke inhalation
  - Leading cause of death in burn injury
  - Common when a burn occurs in a closed space
  - Suspected with burns of the face and upper torso
  - Burns airways; carbon monoxide or cyanide poisoning
  - Lung damage from noxious gases
  - Manifestations
    - Dyspnea
    - Wheezes
    - Ashlike material in sputum
    - Carbon monoxide poisoning (Box 24-17)
    - Brochospasm
    - Edema
- Near-drowning
  - Aspiration and oxygen deprivation
    - Immersion of 3–5 minutes can cause significant hypoxemia and loss of consciousness
    - Death occurs within 5–10 minutes
    - Very cold water may prolong survival
    - Aspirates fresh or saltwater; causes pulmonary edema and respiratory failure
    - Manifestations
      - Altered consciousness
      - Restlessness
      - Apprehension
      - Hypothermia
      - Other signs
      - Shock and cardiac arrest

© 2007 Pearson Education, Inc.

PowerPoint Lecture Slides *continued*

4 Interdisciplinary Care
- Diagnosis
  - Serum electrolytes and ABGs
  - Carboxyhemoglogin
  - Chest x-ray
  - Bronchoscopy
- Treatment
  - Analgesia
  - Intercostals nerve block
  - Taping of chest wall—flail chest
  - CPR for drowning victim
- Nursing care
  - Diagnosis, planning, implementation
    - Impaired Airway Clearance
    - Impaired Gas Exchange
    - Pain
    - Ineffective Tissue Perfusion: Cerebral
  - Continuing care
    - Prevention
      - Seat belts
      - Smoke detectors
      - Life preservers and flotation vests
      - Avoid alcohol
      - Know CPR

Suggestions for Classroom Activities

1. Obtain x-ray examples of chest injuries to illustrate pathology to the class.
2. Demonstrate chest tube drainage system.

Suggestions for Clinical Activities

1. Assign students to observe in trauma center.
2. Assign students to pulmonary unit or ICU where they can gain experience with clients who have chest tubes.

Learning Outcome 6

Describe the pathophysiology, manifestations, and interdisciplinary care of critical respiratory conditions.

Concepts for Lecture

1. Critical respiratory conditions include respiratory failure or a severe form of acute respiratory failure. In both cases, the lungs cannot maintain oxygenation without external respiratory support.
2. The pathophysiology differs between the two conditions of respiratory failure.
3. The interdisciplinary care is the same for both conditions and focuses on underlying cause, supportive ventilation, and correcting hypoxemia and hypercapnia.

PowerPoint Lecture Slides

1 Critical Respiratory Conditions
- Respiratory failure
  - Lungs unable to oxygenate blood and remove carbon dioxide
  - COPD is usual cause
  - Other diseases include trauma, neuromuscular disorders, and heart disease
- Acute respiratory distress syndrome (ARDS)
  - Noncardiac pulmonary edema and progressive hypoxemia that does not respond to oxygen therapy
  - Follow direct lung injury
    - Smoke inhalation
    - Near-drowning
  - Indirect lung injury
    - Shock
    - Sepsis

© 2007 Pearson Education, Inc.

POWERPOINT LECTURE SLIDES *continued*

2 Pathophysiology

- Respiratory failure
  - Blood oxygen levels are low: $Po_2 < 50–60$ mmHg
  - Carbon dioxide levels rise
  - Tissue hypoxia
  - Acidosis
- Acute respiratory distress syndrome
  - Massive unregulated systemic inflammatory response
  - Lung damage occurs rapidly within 24 hours
  - Alveolar-capillary membrane allow plasma and blood cells to leak into interstitial space and alveoli
  - Alveolar surfactant is inactivated; cells that produce surfactant are damaged
  - Alveolar collapse
  - Work of breathing increases and gas exchange is impaired
  - Hypoxemia develops

Interdisciplinary Care of Critical Respiratory Conditions

- Treatment is the same for both respiratory failure and ARDS
- Diagnosis
  - ABGs
  - Chest x-ray
  - Ventilation perfusion scan
  - Exhaled carbon dioxide ($ETCo_2$)
- Medications
  - Bronchodilators
  - Corticosteroids
  - NSAIDs
  - Surfactant
  - Sedation during ventilation
- Oxygen therapy
  - COPD clients—1 to 3 liters by nasal cannula
  - Avoid high flow rates to prevent oxygen toxicity
  - Continuous positive airway pressure (CPAP)
- Airway management
  - Endotracheal tube
  - Tracheostomy
  - Nasogastric and feeding tubes
- Mechanical ventilation
  - Positive pressure ventilators
  - Types, modes, settings (Table 24-11)
    - Rate
    - Tidal volume
    - Oxygen percentage
    - Positive end expiratory pressure (PEEP)
  - Complications
    - Pressure necrosis of nose, lip, trachea
    - Less saliva is produced
    - Dislodgement of tube
    - Infection
    - Barotraumas

© 2007 Pearson Education, Inc.

POWERPOINT LECTURE SLIDES *continued*

- Weaning processes
  - Terminal weaning
- Other therapies
  - Pulmonary artery catheter
  - Fluid replacement

- Nursing care
  - Assessment and monitoring frequently
  - Diagnosis, planning, and implementing
    - Impaired Spontaneous Ventilation
    - Ineffective Airway Clearance
    - Risk for Injury
    - Decreased Cardiac Output
    - Anxiety

SUGGESTIONS FOR CLASSROOM ACTIVITIES

1. Obtain sample endotracheal and tracheostomy tubes and suctioning materials to demonstrate to the class their use and management.
2. Invite respiratory therapist to speak to class on mechanical ventilation. Request that the speaker bring a ventilator to demonstrate if possible.

SUGGESTIONS FOR CLINICAL ACTIVITIES

Assign students to clients in an ICU or respiratory care unit that has clients requiring mechanical ventilation.

© 2007 Pearson Education, Inc.

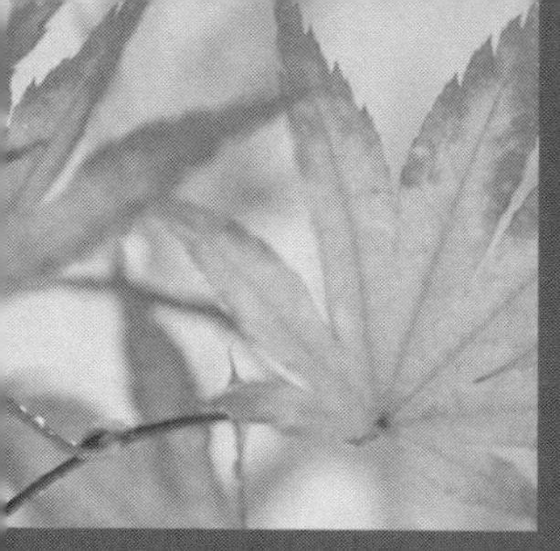

Chapter 25
The Cardiovascular System and Assessment

Resource Library

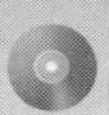
CD-ROM

Heart
Chambers of the Heart
Ventricular Contraction
Blood Pressure
Video: Apical
Video: ECG

IMAGE LIBRARY

Figure 25-1 Location of the heart within the chest cavity.
Figure 25-2 The internal anatomy of the heart.
Figure 25-3 Pulmonary and systemic circulation.
Figure 25-4 The coronary arteries.
Figure 25-5 The cardiac conduction system.
Figure 25-6 The cardiac cycle. Ventricular filling occurs during diastole (**1**); blood is pumped out of the heart to the pulmonary and systemic circulation during ventricular systole (**2**).
Figure 25-7 Structure of arteries, veins, and capillaries.

Learning Outcome 1

Describe the structure and function of the heart and vascular systems.

Concepts for Lecture

1. Structure of the heart and vascular systems.
2. Function of the heart and vascular systems.

PowerPoint Lecture Slides

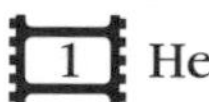

Heart—Structure
- Covered by pericardium; two layers
  - Parietal
  - Visceral (epicardium)
- Outer heart layer: epicardium
- Middle heart layer: myocardium
- Inner layer: endocardium (Figure 25-2)
- Four hollow chambers: two upper, atria; two lower, ventricles
- Divided by septum and valves

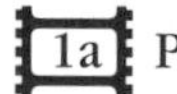

Peripheral Vascular System—Structure
- Aorta, arteries, arterioles, capillaries
- Venules, veins, superior and inferior vena cava
- Three layers: intima, media, adventitia (Figure 25-7)

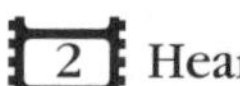

Heart—Function
- Right atrium, receives deoxygenated blood
- Right ventricle pumps blood to lungs (Figures 25-3)
- Left atrium receives oxygenated blood
- Left ventricle pumps oxygenated blood to body
- AV valve closure: S_1 heart sound
- Semilunar valve closure: S_2 heart sound
- Coronary circulation (Figure 25-4)

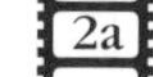

Peripheral Vascular System—Function
- Circulation
- Peripheral vascular resistance: viscosity, length, diameter
- Blood pressure control

SUGGESTIONS FOR CLASSROOM ACTIVITIES

Access the website www.innerbody.com/image/cardov.html to review an interactive demonstration of the heart.

SUGGESTIONS FOR CLINICAL ACTIVITIES

Listen to the heart sounds of a client. Analyze the quality of the heart sounds.

LEARNING OUTCOME 2

Discuss the mechanical and electrical properties of the heart.

CONCEPTS FOR LECTURE

1. Mechanical and electrical properties of the heart.

POWERPOINT LECTURE SLIDES

1 Heart—Mechanical
- Conduction system (Figure 25-5)
- SA node: pacemaker
- Cardiac output
- Stroke volue
- CO = HR × SV
- Cardiac reserve
- Heart rate
- Preload
- Starling's law
- Afterload
- Contractility

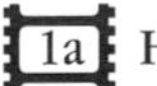

1a Heart—Electrical
- Action potential
- Polarization
- Depolarization
- Repolarization
- Refractory period
- Cardiac cycle (Figure 25-6)
- Diastole
- Systole

SUGGESTIONS FOR CLASSROOM ACTIVITIES

Access the website http://cardiovascular.cx/ and view the video for more information on determining cardiac output.

SUGGESTIONS FOR CLINICAL ACTIVITIES

Collect information regarding a client's heart rate. Determine the client's cardiac output.

LEARNING OUTCOME 3

Identify subjective and objective assessment data to collect for clients with cardiovascular disorders.

CONCEPTS FOR LECTURE

1. Subjective and objective assessment data.

POWERPOINT LECTURE SLIDES

1 Assessment—Subjective
- Health history
- Chest pain
- SOB
- Leg pain
- Pillows to sleep
- Medications
- Lifestyle: diet, alcohol use, exercise, smoking, drugs

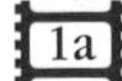

1a Assessment—Objective
- General appearance
- Skin

PowerPoint Lecture Slides *continued*

- Wounds
- Pulses
- Jugular vein distention
- Edema
- Breathing

Suggestions for Classroom Activities

Practice assessing the cardiovascular and peripheral vascular status of a classmate.

Suggestions for Clinical Activities

Collect subjective and objective data for a client. Determine if the client is experiencing a cardiovascular or peripheral vascular disorder.

Learning Outcome 4

Identify nursing responsibilities for common diagnostic tests and monitors for clients with cardiovascular disorders.

Concepts for Lecture

1. Diagnostic tests and monitors.

PowerPoint Lecture Slides

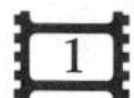

Nursing—Diagnostic Tests

- Lipid profile: instruct to fast, no alcohol, 24 hours
- C-reactive protein: no nursing implications
- Serum cardiac monitors: no nursing implications
- Serum cardiac hormones: instruct to fast, no cardiac medications for 24 hours after test
- 12-lead ECG: instruct to hold still during the tracing
- Stress ECG: physician available, emergency cart available
- TTE: conductive is cold; wash the gel off the client after the exam is over
- TEE: monitor breathing, cough, gag reflex; keep NPO until gag reflex returns
- Dopplers: monitor BP, wash extremities to remove gel after test completed
- X-rays/CT scan/EBCT: document client allergy to fish or shellfish; pregnancy risk
- Angiography/cardiac catheterization: See Chapter 26
- MRI: document presence of implanted electronic devices
- Radionuclear scans: increase fluids after the test

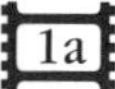

Nursing—Monitors

- Telemetry/Holter:
  - Teach about purpose
  - Dry skin
  - Remove hair
  - Avoid getting unit wet
  - When to phone the MD

Suggestions for Classroom Activities

Review the various types of diagnostic tests and monitors used to assess the cardiovascular and peripheral vascular systems. Practice applying the leads for an ECG on a classmate.

Suggestions for Clinical Activities

Review the different diagnostic tests prescribed for a client with a cardiovascular or peripheral vascular disorder. Provide appropriate nursing care for the client undergoing diagnostic tests.

© 2007 Pearson Education, Inc.

CHAPTER 26
CARING FOR CLIENTS WITH CORONARY HEART DISEASE AND DYSRHYTHMIAS

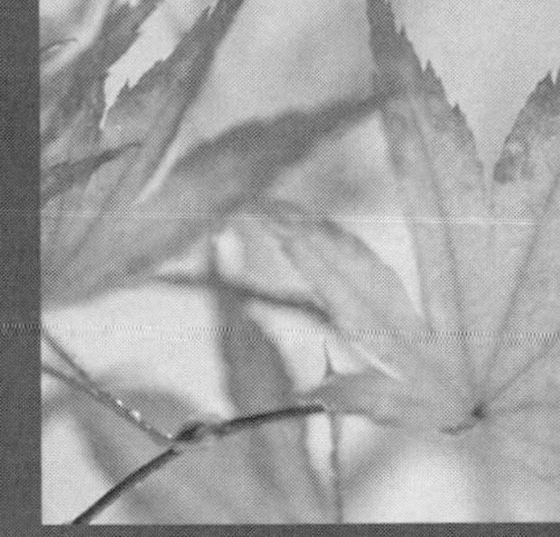

RESOURCE LIBRARY

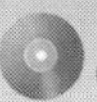 **CD-ROM**

Video: CHD
Atorvastatin
Angina
Video: Administering Nitroglycerin
Nifedipine
Video: Dysrhythmia
Lidocaine
Amiodarone
Digoxin
Defibrillation

IMAGE LIBRARY

Figure 26-1 Coronary heart disease.
Figure 26-2 ECG changes during an episode of angina. Note the ST-segment depression and T-wave inversion characteristic of myocardial ischemia.
Figure 26-3 PTCA. **(A)** The balloon catheter is threaded into the affected coronary artery. **(B)** The balloon is positioned across the area of obstruction. **(C)** The balloon is then inflated, flattening the plaque against the arterial wall **(D)**.
Figure 26-4 Placement of an intracoronary stent. **(A)** The stent is fitted over the balloon-tipped catheter. **(B)** The stent is positioned in the area of narrowing and expanded with balloon inflation. **(C)** The balloon is deflated and removed, leaving the stent in place.
Figure 26-5 CABG using the internal mammary artery and a saphenous vein graft.
Figure 26-6 A diagram of a cardiopulmonary bypass pump. Venous blood is removed from the venae cavae, pumped through the oxygenator, and returned to the body via the ascending aorta.
Figure 26-7 ECG changes noted with acute myocardial infarction. Note the deep Q wave and significant elevation of the ST segment characteristic of AMI.
Figure 26-8 The intra-aortic balloon pump. **(A)** The balloon inflates during diastole to help perfuse coronary, renal, and cerebral arteries. **(B)** During systole, the balloon is deflated, allowing blood to freely flow past it.
Figure 26-9 Placement of paddles or pads for defibrillation.
Figure 26-10 A permanent pacemaker with a transvenous electrode into the right ventricle.
Figure 26-11 Ventricular pacing. Note the presence of pacer spikes prior to the wide, ventricular QRS complexes, and the absence of spikes when the client's natural rhythm resumes.
Figure 26-12 An automatic external defibrillator for emergency resuscitation.

LEARNING OUTCOME 1

Describe the causes, pathophysiology, effects, and manifestations of coronary heart disease and heart rhythm disruptions.

CONCEPTS FOR LECTURE

1. Causes, pathophysiology, effects, and manifestations of coronary artery disease.
2. Causes, pathophysiology, effects, and manifestations of heart rhythm disruptions.

POWERPOINT LECTURE SLIDES

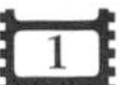 CHD—Causes
- Narrowing coronary arteries
- Risk factors (Table 26-2)
  - Age, gender, race, heredity
  - Lifestyle: smoking, obesity, exercise
  - High blood pressure
  - Hyperlipidemia
  - Metabolic syndrome

POWERPOINT LECTURE SLIDES *continued*

1a CHD—Pathophysiology
- Atherosclerosis causing occlusions
- Leads to ischemia

1b Angina Pectoris—Pathophysiology
- Obstructed coronary artery
- Increased myocardial oxygen demand
- Lactic acid release
- Leads to pain
- Three types:
  - Stable
  - Unstable
  - Prinzmetal's

1c Angina Pectoris—Manifestations
- Chest pain
- Radiates
- Onset with exercise, etc.
- Relieved by rest, NTG
- SOB, pallor, fear

1d Acute Myocardial Infarction (AMI)—Pathophysiology
- Occluded coronary artery stops blood flow to part of cardiac muscle
- Cellular death
- Tissue necrosis
- Description—heart area affected
- Classification

1e AMI—Manifestations
- Pain
- Radiates to shoulder, neck, jaw, arms
- Lasts >15–20 minutes
- Not relieved with NTG
- Box 26-6
- Women and elderly S/S (Box 26-7)

1f AMI—Complications
- Related to size and location of infarct
- Dysrhythmias (Table 26-6)
- Pump failure
- Cardiogenic shock
- Other: pericarditis

2 Cardiac Dysrhythmias—Pathophysiology
- Due to altered formation of impulses or altered conduction of the impulse through the heart
- Ectopic beats
- Heart block
- Reentry phenomenon
- Classified to the site of impulse formation or the site and degree of conduction block
- Types
  - Supraventricular
    - Sinus tachycardia
    - Sinus bradycardia
    - PAC
    - A flutter
    - A fib
    - Junctional

© 2007 Pearson Education, Inc.

POWERPOINT LECTURE SLIDES *continued*

- Ventricular dysrhythmias
  - PVCs
  - Ventricular tachycardia
  - Ventricular fibrillation
- AV conduction blocks
  - First degree
  - Second degree
  - Third degree

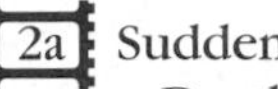
Sudden Cardiac Death
- Death within 1 hour after onset of cardiac S/S
- V-fibrillation and cardiac arrest
- CPR started within 2 to 4 minutes
- Procedure 26-2
- Automated external defibrillator (Figure 26-12)

SUGGESTIONS FOR CLASSROOM ACTIVITIES

Review the signs and symptoms of coronary artery disease and dysrhythmias. Using the website www.diagnose-me.com/cond/C495951.html, analyze the pathophysiological basis for the signs and symptoms.

SUGGESTIONS FOR CLINICAL ACTIVITIES

Review the medical record for a client with coronary artery disease or a dysrhythmia. Assess the ECG for evidence of the disorder.

LEARNING OUTCOME 2

Discuss nursing implications for drugs commonly prescribed for clients with coronary heart disease or dysrhythmias.

CONCEPTS FOR LECTURE

1. Nursing implications for drugs prescribed for coronary artery disease or dysrhythmias.

POWERPOINT LECTURE SLIDES

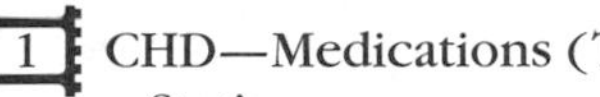
CHD—Medications (Table 26-3)
- Statins:
  - Teach common side effects: headache, gastrointestinal upset
  - Muscle aches, skin rashes
  - Liver function tests and muscle enzymes are monitored
- Nicotinic acid:
  - Flushing, pruritis
- Cholesterol binding:
  - Gastrointestinal side effects

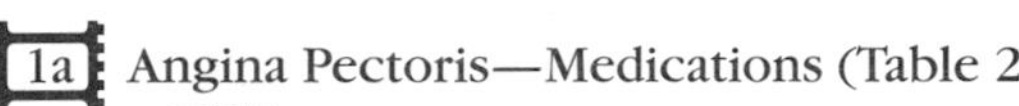
Angina Pectoris—Medications (Table 26-4)
- NTG
- Beta blockers
- Low-dose aspirin

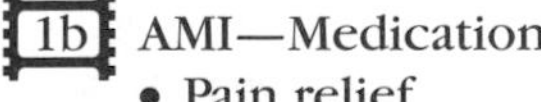
AMI—Medications
- Pain relief
- Antianxiety
- Thrombolytics: nursing care
  - Bleeding disorders
  - Care during infusion
  - Care postinfusion
- Aspirin
- Heparin
- Antidysrhythmic medications
- Beta blockers
- ACE I
- IV NTG

© 2007 Pearson Education, Inc.

POWERPOINT LECTURE SLIDES *continued*

1c Cardiac Dysrhythmias—Medications
- Antidysrhythmics (Table 26-7)

SUGGESTIONS FOR CLASSROOM ACTIVITIES

Create a spreadsheet listing all of the medications used to treat coronary artery disease in order of priority of symptoms. Use the website www.nlm.nih.gov/medlineplus/ency/article/001101.htm for more information.

SUGGESTIONS FOR CLINICAL ACTIVITIES

Provide medications for a client with coronary artery disease or a dysrhythmia. Determine the reason to assess vital signs before administering these medications.

LEARNING OUTCOME 3

Describe nursing care for clients undergoing invasive procedures or surgery of the heart.

CONCEPTS FOR LECTURE

1. Nursing care for invasive procedures or cardiac surgery.

POWERPOINT LECTURE SLIDES

1 Angina Pectoris—Management
- Diagnostic tests:
  - Coronary angiogram and PTCA
- Nursing:
  - Reinforce teaching
  - Preoperative care
  - Medications
  - Allergies
  - Procedure takes 1–2 hours
  - Height/weight
  - Vital signs
  - Feel warmth, metal taste in mouth
  - Postoperative nursing care
    - VS, pulses
    - Cardiac monitoring
    - Bed rest
    - Pressure dressing
    - Fluid intake
    - Medications
    - Intake and output
    - Labs

1a Angina Pectoris—Surgery
- PTCA—same as coronary angiogram
- CABG: Preop teaching
  - Tubes, drains, monitoring equipment, respiratory equipment, incisions, dressing, activity, diet
- CABG: postoperative
  - VS, oxygen saturation, cardiovascular status, respiratory status, cardiac rhythm, intake and output, chest tube, rewarming, PCA, endotube, ventilator, incentive spirometer, dressing changes, labs, family involvement

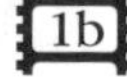

AMI—Revascularization
- Angioplasty with STENT
- IABP
- VADs

© 2007 Pearson Education, Inc.

POWERPOINT LECTURE SLIDES *continued*

1c Cardiac Dysrhythmias—Management/Treatment
- Cardioversion/defibrillation
  - Electrical shock
  - Synchronized
  - Premedicate with anticoagulants
- Automatic implantable cardioverter-defibrillator
- Pacemakers: temporary, permanent

1d Cardiac Dysrhythmias—Nursing Care Permanent Pacemaker
- Before procedure: preoperative teaching
- After procedure: CXR, pain medications, ROM exercises after 24 hours

1e Cardiac Dysrhythmias—Surgery
- Surgical ablation
- Ectopic focus

SUGGESTIONS FOR CLASSROOM ACTIVITIES

Prepare a preoperative teaching plan for a client planning to undergo cardiovascular surgery. Use the website www.frankfordhospitals.org/healthinfo/t_and_p/heart/TP128.html for more information.

SUGGESTIONS FOR CLINICAL ACTIVITIES

Using the teaching plan created in class, provide the instruction to a client planning to undergo cardiovascular surgery. Document the client's comprehension in the medical record.

LEARNING OUTCOME 4

Use the nursing process to collect assessment data, contribute to care planning, and provide individualized nursing care for clients with coronary heart disease and dysrhythmias.

CONCEPTS FOR LECTURE

1. Nursing process to provide care for clients with coronary artery disease and dysrhythmias.

POWERPOINT LECTURE SLIDES

1 CHD—Management
- Diagnostic tests
- Manage risk factors: low-fat, low-cholesterol diet, complementary therapies

1a Angina Pectoris—Assessment
- Risk factors
- Pain
- Focused assessment (Box 26-5)

1b Angina Pectoris—Diagnosis, Planning, Implementation
- Ineffective Tissue Perfusion: Cardiopulmonary
  - NTG at bedside
  - Oxygen
  - Rest between activities
  - Manage risk factors
  - Exercise
  - Smoking cessation
- Risk for Ineffective Therapeutic Regimen Management
  - Angina teaching
  - Medications
  - Cardiac rehabilitation program

1c Angina Pectoris—Evaluation
- Management of anginal episodes

© 2007 Pearson Education, Inc.

POWERPOINT LECTURE SLIDES *continued*

- Teaching: NTG before activities; 1 every 15–20 minutes ×3; NTG storage

1d AMI—Management
- Early recognition
- Lab tests
- Diagnostic tests
- Medical management:
  - Monitoring
  - IVF
  - Oxygen
  - Bed rest with bedside commode
  - Quiet calm environment

1e AMI—Assessment
- Immediate and hourly
- ECG
- Labs
- Box 26-9

1f AMI—Diagnosis, Planning, Intervention
- Pain
  - Sign of pain
  - Oxygen
  - Physical and psychologic rest
  - Morphine
  - Ongoing chest pain
- Ineffective Tissue Perfusion
  - Change in heart rate, rhythm
  - LOC
  - UOP
  - Skin appearance
  - Heart and breath sounds
  - ECG
  - Antidysrhythmics as prescribed
- Ineffective Coping
  - Trust
  - Denial
  - Anger
  - Coping skills
  - Privacy
- Fear
  - Client's perception
  - Encourage questions
  - Antianxiety medications
  - Stress reduction

1g AMI—Evaluating
- Pain
- Evidence of adequate tissue perfusion
- Physical assessment findings

1h Cardiac Dysrhythmias—Management
- Diagnostic tests
- Cardiac monitoring
- Telemetry

1i Cardiac Dysrhythmias—Assessment
- Assess before treating with dysrhythmia medications

© 2007 Pearson Education, Inc.

POWERPOINT LECTURE SLIDES *continued*

- Chest pain
- SOB
- Palpitations
- VS
- Skin color
- LOC, mental status
- Heart sounds, peripheral pulses
- Respiratory status
- Anxiety

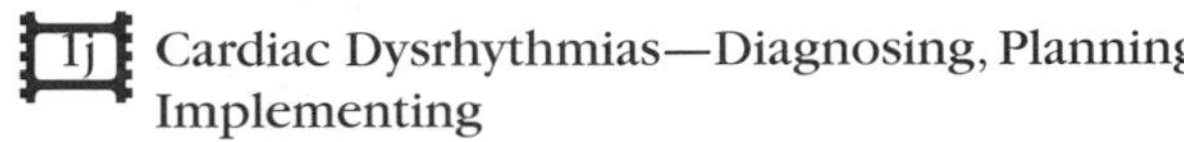

1j Cardiac Dysrhythmias—Diagnosing, Planning, Implementing

- Decreased Cardiac Output
  - Assess for manifestations of decreased cardiac output
  - ECG
  - VS
  - Lab values
  - IV access
  - Emergency procedures prn
- Risk for Ineffective Tissue Perfusion: Cerebral
  - LOC, orientation ×3
  - Neurologic status
  - Oxygen therapy
  - HOB 15-degree angle
  - Rest
- Anxiety
  - Keep family and client informed

1k Cardiac Dysrhythmias—Evaluation

- Cardiac output
- Cerebral perfusion
- Cardiac rhythm
- Lab data

SUGGESTIONS FOR CLASSROOM ACTIVITIES

Practice conducting a cardiovascular assessment on a classmate. Document the findings. Use the website www.clevelandclinicmeded.com/diseasemanagement/cardiology/cad/cad.htm for more information or assistance.

SUGGESTIONS FOR CLINICAL ACTIVITIES

Conduct an assessment of a client with coronary artery disease or a dysrhythmia. Document your findings in the medical record.

LEARNING OUTCOME 5

Provide and reinforce appropriate teaching for clients with coronary heart disease or dysrhythmias and their families.

CONCEPTS FOR LECTURE

1. Teaching for clients/families with coronary artery disease or dysrhythmias.

POWERPOINT LECTURE SLIDES

1 CHD—Nursing Care

- Teach smoking cessation
- Healthy weight
- Exercise
- Control high blood pressure, diabetes, lipid levels
- Reduce stress

1a AMI—Cardiac Rehabiliation

- Improve the quality of life

PowerPoint Lecture Slides *continued*

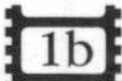
AMI—Teaching
- Reduce risk of future events
- Diet
- Activity
- Medications
- Refer to cardiac rehabilitation
- Community resources
- Learn CPR

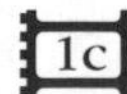
Cardiac Dysrhythmias—Teaching
- Coping strategies
- Medications
- Follow up MD visits
- Teach about implanted devices
- Activities
- Safety
- Driving
- Learn CPR

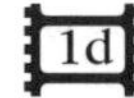
Advanced Directives
- All measures used to treat cardiac arrest
- Advance directives—treatment decisions

Suggestions for Classroom Activities

Divide the class into two groups. The first group is to prepare discharge instructions for a client with coronary artery disease. The second group is to prepare discharge instructions for a client with a dysrhythmia. Each group is to present their discharge plan for the entire class. Use the website community.nursingspectrum.com/MagazineArticles/article.cfm?AID=1300 for more information.

Suggestions for Clinical Activities

Provide care to a client with coronary artery disease or a dysrhythmia. Begin discharge planning with the client. Incorporate content from the classroom discharge planning exercise into these instructions.

 © 2007 Pearson Education, Inc.

CHAPTER 27
CARING FOR CLIENTS WITH CARDIAC DISORDERS

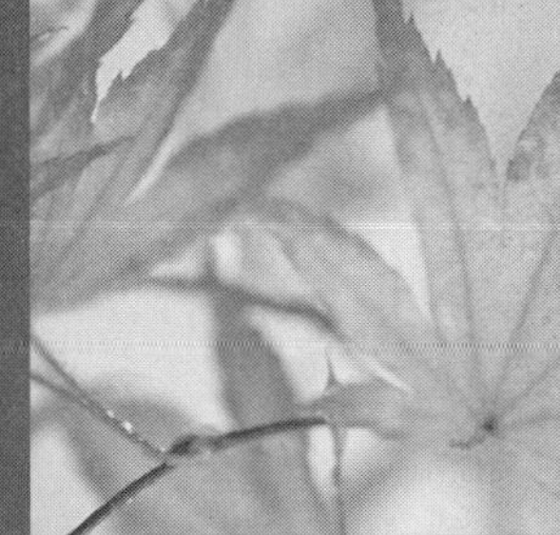

RESOURCE LIBRARY

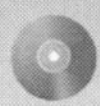 **CD-ROM**

Lisinopril
Dopamine
Congenital Heart Defects

IMAGE LIBRARY

Figure 27-1 The forward and backward effects of left-sided heart failure.
Figure 27-2 The effects of right-sided heart failure.
Figure 27-3 A hemodynamic monitoring setup.
Figure 27-4 Cardiac transplantation. **(A)** The heart is removed, leaving the posterior walls of the atria intact. The donor heart is sutured to the atria **(B)** and the great vessels **(C)**.
Figure 27-5 Pericardiocentesis.
Figure 27-6 Mitral stenosis.
Figure 27-7 Mitral regurgitation.
Figure 27-8 Aortic stenosis.
Figure 27-9 Aortic regurgitation.
Figure 27-10 Balloon valvuloplasty. The balloon catheter is positioned across the stenosed valve. The balloon is then inflated to increase the size of the valve opening.
Figure 27-11 Prosthetic heart valves. **(A)** Carpentier-Edwards biologic aortic valve prosthesis. **(B)** Medtronic Hall prosthetic valve.

LEARNING OUTCOME 1

Compare and contrast the causes, pathophysiology, effects, and manifestations of common cardiac disorders.

CONCEPTS FOR LECTURE

1. Pathophysiology, effects, and manifestations of common cardiac disorders.

POWERPOINT LECTURE SLIDES

1 Heart Failure—Conditions
- Impaired contractions
- Increased workload of the heart
- Leading causes: HTN, CHD, AMI
- Classified as A, B, C, or D

1a Heart Failure—Pathophysiology
- Cardiac output drops
- Compensatory mechanisms activated
- Sympathetic nervous system stimulated
- Arteries and veins constrict
- Venous return increases to the heart
- Increase in preload
- Renin-angiotensin-aldosterone system activated
- Salt and water retention
- Heart chambers dilate
- Ventricular hypertrophy
- Reduced cardiac reserve
- Classifications: left sided or right sided

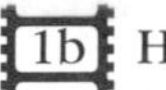 Heart Failure—Manifestations
- Left sided:
  - Pulmonary congestion
  - Reduced cardiac output
  - Fatigue, activity intolerance

POWERPOINT LECTURE SLIDES *continued*

- DOE
- Orthopnea

- Right sided:
  - Fatigue
  - Activity intolerance
  - JVD
  - Peripheral edema
  - Anorexia, nausea
  - Abdominal distention
  - Ascites
  - Liver/spleen enlarged and tender

1c Heart Failure—Complications

- Acute pulmonary edema
  - Dyspnea
  - SOB
  - Anxiety
  - Cough and pink frothy sputum
  - Client drowning
- Right-sided heart failure
- Biventricular failure
- Acute and chronic failure

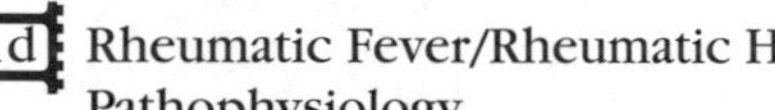

1d Rheumatic Fever/Rheumatic Heart Disease—Pathophysiology

- Streptococcus bacteria
- Valves swollen and red
- Scarring of valves
- RHD: scarring leads to valve stenosis and regurgitation

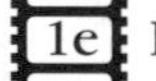

1e RF/RHD—Manifestations

- Box 27-3
- Fever
- Migratory joint pain and inflammation
- Rash on trunk or extremities
- Chest pain/discomfort
- Tachycardia
- SOB
- Heart sound changes
- Muscle spasms

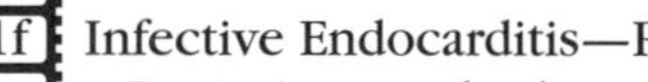

1f Infective Endocarditis—Pathophysiology

- Bacteria enter body and settle in mitral valve
- Onset and disease course (Table 27-3)
- Organisms attach to endocardial heart lining
- Vegetations develop on heart valve leaflets
- Vegetations prevent normal valve closure leading to regurgitation

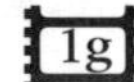

1g IE—Manifestations

- Elevated temperature
- Flu-like S/S
- Cough
- SOB
- Joint pain
- Petechiae
- Splinter hemorrhages

© 2007 Pearson Education, Inc.

POWERPOINT LECTURE SLIDES *continued*

1h Myocarditis—Pathophysiology
- Causes: infection, immunity, radiation, poisons, drugs, burns

1i Myocarditis—Manifestations
- Asymptomatic or fever, fatigue, malaise, dyspnea
- Heart failure manifestations

1j Pericarditis—Pathophysiology
- Damaged pericardial tissue
- Fluid and exudates in pericardial space

1k Pericarditis—Manifestations
- Chest pain, sharp
- Pericardial friction rub
- Fever
- Pericardial effusion
- Cardiac tamponade

1l Valvular Heart Disease—Pathophysiology
- Stenosis: valve leaflets fuse
- Regurgitation: valves do not close
- Heart muscle atrophy
- Pulmonary complications
- Heart failure
- Table 27-5

1m Valvular Heart Disease—Manifestations
- Mitral stenosis (Figure 27-6)
- Mitral regurgitation (Figure 27-7)
- Mitral valve prolapse
- Aortic stenosis (Figure 27-8)
- Aortic regurgitation (Figure 27-9)

1n Cardiomyopathy—Pathophysiology
- Group of disorders
- Categorized by effects on heart, Table 27-6
- Types
  - Dilated
  - Hypertrophic
  - Restrictive

SUGGESTIONS FOR CLASSROOM ACTIVITIES

Review the physiology of heart failure, explaining the difference between systolic and diastolic heart failure. Refer to the website www.chfpatients.com/faq/dhf.htm.

SUGGESTIONS FOR CLINICAL ACTIVITIES

Analyze the prescribed medical care for a client with heart disease. Compare the prescribed treatment with the physiology of the disorder.

LEARNING OUTCOME 2

Identify nursing responsibilities for common diagnostic tests and monitors for clients with heart disease.

CONCEPTS FOR LECTURE

1. Nursing care for common diagnostic tests and monitors.

POWERPOINT LECTURE SLIDES

1 Heart Failure—Diagnostic Tests
- Cardiac hormones, atrial natriuretic factor, and B-type natriuretic peptide
- Serum electrolytes
- Chest x-ray

PowerPoint Lecture Slides *continued*

- Echocardiogram
- ECG

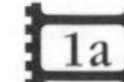 Heart Failure—Hemodynamic Monitoring

- Assess cardiovascular function
- Multilumen catheter inserted through central vein in right side of the heart
- Pulmonary artery used to measure central venous pressure, pulmonary artery pressures, and cardiac output
- Arterial blood pressure measured using a peripheral arterial line
- Figure 27-3

Suggestions for Classroom Activities

Create a spreadsheet listing all of the diagnostic tests available to aid in the diagnosis, treatment, and prognosis for a client with heart disease. Refer to the website http://heart-disease.health-cares.net/heart-diagnostic-tests.php.

Suggestions for Clinical Activities

Provide care to a client undergoing hemodynamic monitoring.

Learning Outcome 3

Discuss nursing implications for drugs commonly prescribed for clients with heart disease.

Concepts for Lecture

1. Nursing implications for providing medications.

PowerPoint Lecture Slides

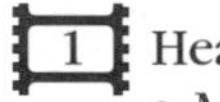 Heart Failure—Medications

- Morphine sulfate: pulmonary edema treatment
- Digitalis: positive inotropic effect on heart; narrow therapeutic index; easy digitalis toxicity

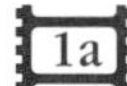 Cardiomyopathy—Pharmacology

- Positive inotropic agents
  - Digoxin
    - Take pulse, hold for <60 bmp
    - Contact MD with S/S side effects, toxicity
- Sympathomimetic agents
  - Dopamine
    - Notify MD with abdominal pain, rash, or burning
- ACE I
  - Vasotec, Prinivil
    - Change position slowly
    - Report bruising
    - Report weight gain
- Diuretics
  - Abdominal pain, jaundice
  - Electrolyte imbalances
  - Blood pressure changes

Suggestions for Classroom Activities

Categorize specific types of medications used to treat heart disorders. Identify which medications are most commonly prescribed and the effect on the heart's function. Refer to the website www.nhlbi.nih.gov/actintime/hdm/hdm.htm.

Suggestions for Clinical Activities

Provide medications to a client with a heart disorder.

© 2007 Pearson Education, Inc.

Learning Outcome 4

Describe nursing care for clients undergoing invasive procedures or surgery of the heart.

Concepts for Lecture

1. Nursing care for invasive procedures or surgery.

PowerPoint Lecture Slides

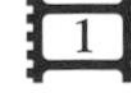
Heart Failure—Surgery

- Heart transplant
  - Nursing care
    - Infection and rejection main concerns
    - Immunosuppressive drugs
- Dynamic cardiomyoplasty
  - Skeletal muscle graft around heart to support myocardium
  - No real success

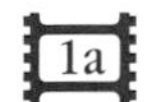
Pericarditis—Pericardiocentesis

- May be done to remove fluid from the pericardial sac (Figure 27-5)
- Large (16- to 18-gauge) needle inserted into the pericardial sac
- Excess fluid taken out
- May be done as an emergency procedure for cardiac tamponade
- Nursing care (Box 27-9)

Valve Disease—Percutaneous Balloon Valvuloplasty

- Balloon catheter inserted into the femoral vein or artery and advanced to the stenotic valve.
- Balloon inflated for approximately 90 seconds to divide the fused leaflets and enlarge the valve opening
- Figure 27-10
- Nursing care similar to that for the client with percutaneous coronary revascularization (Box 26-3)

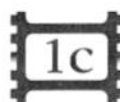
Cardiomyopathy—Nursing Care

- Open heart/cardiac surgery
- (Box 26-4)

Suggestions for Classroom Activities

Review the nursing care involved in various heart procedures. Refer to the website www.ncbi.nlm.nih.gov/.

Suggestions for Clinical Activities

Assist with care needed for a client undergoing an invasive cardiac procedure.

Learning Outcome 5

Use the nursing process to collect assessment data, contribute to care planning, and provide individualized nursing care for clients with disorders of the heart.

Concepts for Lecture

1. Nursing process to provide care.

PowerPoint Lecture Slides

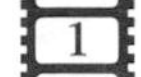
Heart Failure—Management

- Diagnostic tests
- Hemodynamic monitoring
- Medication therapy
  - ACE I
  - Diuretics
  - Inotropic medications

© 2007 Pearson Education, Inc.

PowerPoint Lecture Slides *continued*

  - Vasodilators
  - Table 27-2
- Hawthorn therapy

1a Heart Failure—Diet and Activity
- Low-sodium diet
- Bed rest during acute phase
- Activity gradually increased

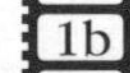

Heart Failure—Assessment
- Subjective
  - SOB
  - Activity intolerance
  - Pillows
  - Edema
  - Weight gain
- Objective
  - VS
  - DOE

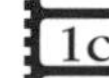

Heart Failure—Diagnosis, Planning, and Implementation
- Decreased Cardiac Output
  - Heart and breath sounds
  - Mental status
  - UOP
  - Oxygen
  - Medications
  - Rest
  - Quiet
- Excess Fluid Volume
  - Panic
  - I&O
  - Daily weights
  - Fowler's position
  - Diuretics/medications
  - Fluid restriction
- Activity Intolerance
  - VS
  - Rest periods
  - Assist with care
  - Progressive activity plan
  - Small frequent meals

1d Heart Failure—Evaluation
- VS
- UOP
- DOE
- Heart sounds
- Tolerance activity

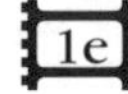

RF/RHD—Management
- Lab tests
- Treat infection
- Manage manifestations
- Prevent complications
- Prevent recurrence
- Medications:
  - Antibiotics
  - Aspirin
  - Ibuprofen

© 2007 Pearson Education, Inc.

- NSAIDs
- Steroids

1f RF/RHD—Assessment
- Recent sore throat
- Chest pain
- SOB
- Fatigue
- Weakness
- Fever
- Joint pain
- Rash

1g RF/RHD—Diagnosis, Planning, and Implementation
- Pain
  - Report increased chest pain
  - Administer medications as prescribed
  - Compresses prn
- Activity Intolerance
  - To reduce stress on the heart
  - Diversional activities
  - Monitor activity intolerance

1h RF/RHD—Evaluation
- Degree of pain
- VS
- Response to activity

1i IE—Management
- Prevention
- Risks of IV drug use
- No definitive tests
- Antibiotics (Table 27-4)
- Surgery: replace damaged valves

1j IE—Assessment
- Risk factors
- Recent surgery or dental work
- IV drug use
- Current S/S
- VS
- Heart and breath sounds

1k IE—Diagnosis, Planning, and Implementation
- Risk for Imbalanced Body Temperature
  - Temperature every 2 to 4 hours
  - Blood cultures
  - Anti-inflammatory/antipyretic medications
  - Antibiotics
- Risk for Ineffective Tissue Perfusion
  - Review of systems

1l IE—Evaluation
- Reduction in symptoms

1m Myocarditis—Management
- Treat inflammatory process
- Bed rest
- Oxygen
- Antibiotics
- Steroids
- Digoxin

© 2007 Pearson Education, Inc.

POWERPOINT LECTURE SLIDES *continued*

1n Myocarditis—Diagnosis, Planning, and Implementation
- Decreased Cardiac Output
- Fatigue
- Anxiety
- Excess Fluid Volume

1o Pericarditis—Management
- Self-limiting
- Will resolve
- ASA, Tylenol, NSAIDs
- Pericardiocentesis (Figure 27-5), Nursing care (Box 27-9)

1p Pericarditis—Diagnosis, Planning, and Implementation
- Pain
  - Pain scale
  - NSAIDs
  - Calm/quiet environment
- Ineffective Breathing Pattern
  - Respiratory rate
  - Incentive spirometer
  - Oxygen
- Risk for Decreased Cardiac Output
  - VS
  - Heart sounds
  - Prepare for pericardiocentesis as necessary

1q Valvular Heart Disease—Management
- Echocardiogram
- Cardiac catheterization
- Percutaneous balloon valvuloplasty (Figure 27-10)
- Surgery: valvuloplasy, resection, commissurotomy, replacement (Figure 27-11)

1r Valvular Heart Disease—Diagnosis, Planning, and Implementation
- Decreased Cardiac Output
  - VS
  - Hemodynamic measures
  - Cardiac output every 8 hours
  - I&O
  - Daily weights
  - Fluid restriction
  - Elevate HOB
  - Oxygen
  - Medications
- Activity Intolerance
  - VS
  - Gradually increase activity
  - Assist as needed
- Ineffective Protection
  - Stools for occult blood
  - Avoid ASA/NSAIDs

1s Cardiomyopathy—Management
- Prevent heart failure
- Treat dysrhythmias
- Prevent sudden cardiac death

© 2007 Pearson Education, Inc.

Suggestions for Classroom Activities

Create a plan of care for a client with a heart disorder. Include at least three nursing diagnoses, interventions, and data needed to evaluate the success of nursing care. Refer to the NIH website at www.nih.gov/.

Suggestions for Clinical Activities

Implement the plan of care created in class for a client with a heart disorder.

Learning Outcome 6

Provide and reinforce appropriate teaching for clients with heart disorders and their families.

Concepts for Lecture

1. Teaching for clients and families with hearts disorders.

PowerPoint Lecture Slides

1 Heart Failure—Teaching
- Understanding of HF
- Medications
- Diet
- Activities
- What to report to MD
- Low salt intake
- Exercise
- Box 27-6

1a RF/RHD—Teaching
- Antibiotic therapy
- Antibiotic prophylaxis
- Low salt intake

1b IE—Teaching
- Education and support
- Teaching to prevent recurrence
- Teaching plan (Box 27-8)

1c Pericarditis—Teaching
- Stay on medications
- Medication teaching
- Fluid intake
- Activity restrictions

1d Valvular Heart Disease—Teaching
- Prevent rheumatic fever
- Explain all tests and procedures
- Diet
- Medications
- Rest
- Evaluate for edema

Suggestions for Classroom Activities

Identify one heart disorder. Create a discharge teaching plan for this disorder. Refer to the NIH website www.nih.gov/.

Suggestions for Clinical Activities

Implement the discharge teaching plan for a client with a heart disorder.

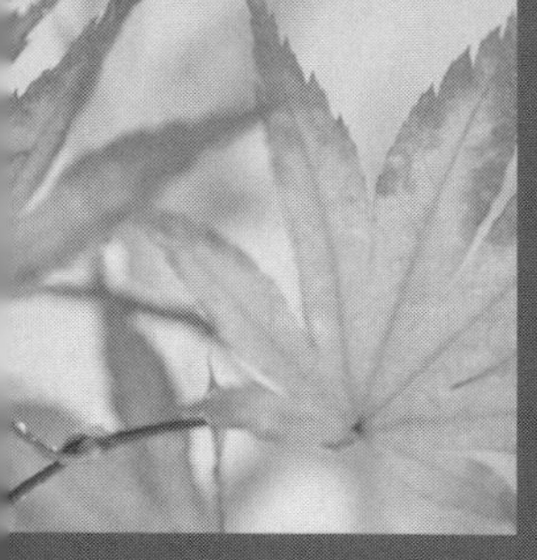

CHAPTER 28
CARING FOR CLIENTS WITH PERIPHERAL VASCULAR DISORDERS

RESOURCE LIBRARY

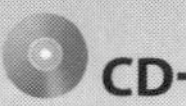 **CD-ROM**

Doxazosin
Video: Measuring BP
Video: Radial
Warfarin

IMAGE LIBRARY

Figure 28-1 Aortic aneurysms. **(A)** Fusiform aneurysm of the abdominal aorta. **(B)** Saccular aneurysm of the descending thoracic aorta. **(C)** Dissecting aneurysm of the ascending thoracic aorta.
Figure 28-2 Repair of an abdominal aortic aneurysm. **(A)** The aneurysm is exposed and clamped above and below the vessel dilation. **(B)** A synthetic graft is used to replace the aneurysm. The arterial wall is then sutured around the graft.
Figure 28-3 A Doppler (ultrasound) stethoscope.
Figure 28-4 Common locations of deep venous thrombosis.
Figure 28-5 Chronic venous insufficiency. Note the discoloration of the ankle and the stasis ulcer.
Figure 28-6 A vena caval filter to trap emboli from the pelvis and lower extremities.
Figure 28-7 **(A)** Normal leg veins. **(B)** Varicose veins.

LEARNING OUTCOME 1

Relate the physiology of the peripheral vascular system to common disorders affecting the peripheral vascular system.

CONCEPTS FOR LECTURE

1. Common disorders of the peripheral vascular system.

POWERPOINT LECTURE SLIDES

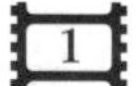

Hypertension
- Blood pressure higher than 140 mm Hg systolic or 90 mm Hg diastolic on three separate readings several weeks apart
- Very common in people over age 40
- Hypertension in the elderly (Box 28-1)
- Often called the silent killer
- Classified by cause and course
- Primary: has no identified cause, risk factors (Box 28-2)
- Secondary: known cause

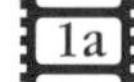

Secondary Hypertension
- Elevated blood pressure related to another disorder
- Kidney disease, coarctation of the aorta, pregnancy, endocrine, neurologic disorder, use of stimulants
- Diagnostic tests: blood, urine tests

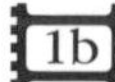

Aneurysms—Thoracic Aortic
- Often asymptomatic
- Might have substernal (anginal), neck, or back pain
- Pressure on thoracic structures might cause SOB, stridor, cough, swallowing difficulties, facial edema, JVD
- Enlarge, rupture, leading to death

PowerPoint Lecture Slides *continued*

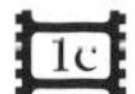
Aneurysm—Abdominal Aortic
- Associated with HTN, smoking, advancing age
- Found in adults over age 70
- Asymptomatic; might have a pulsating mass in the mid/upper abdomen with a bruit
- Complaints of mild to severe midabdominal/lower back pain
- Pain an indication of pending rupture

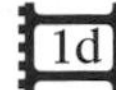
Aortic Dissection
- Life-threatening emergency
- Tear in the inner layer of aorta with bleeding into middle layer
- Vessel wall splits
- Common in the ascending aorta
- HTN, Marfan syndrome at higher risk (Box 28-7)
- Symptoms:
  - Ripping pain
  - High blood pressure followed by a sudden drop
  - Absent peripheral pulses

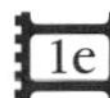
Buerger's Disease—Manifestations
- Pain in the involved extremity
- Cramping in the instep of the foot or leg calves, relieved by rest
- Rest pain in fingers and toes
- Smoking, cold, emotional distress trigger burning pain
- Pale, cool/cold to touch
- Skin shiny, thin; nails thick and malformed
- Pulses difficult to obtain or absent (Figure 28-3)
- Intense rubor

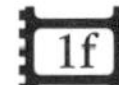
Raynaud's Phenomenon
- Spasms of the small arteries of extremities
- Spasms limit blood flow
- Manifestations
  - S/S occur after exposure to cold or work-related vibration
  - Blue-white-red syndrome
  - Numbness, stiffness, decreased sensation, aching pain

Suggestions for Classroom Activities

Assign the students to small groups and have them select one disorder. Using the Internet, research the disorder and prepare a 10-minute presentation about the disorder for the rest of the class. See www.reference.com/Dir/Health/Conditions_and_Diseases/Vascular_Disorders/.

Suggestions for Clinical Activities

Assign the students to a client with a peripheral vascular disorder. Have the students assess the client in an effort to identify any manifestations of the disorder.

© 2007 Pearson Education, Inc.

Learning Outcome 2

Describe the pathophysiology of common peripheral vascular disorders.

Concepts for Lecture

1. Common peripheral vascular disorders.

PowerPoint Lecture Slides

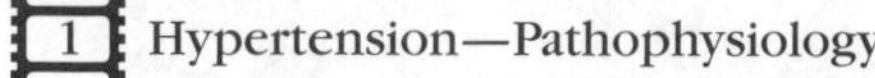

1 Hypertension—Pathophysiology
- Peripheral vascular resistance primary factor determining blood pressure
- Hypertension, increased resistance to blood flow
- Disrupted physiologic mechanisms:
  - Overactive sympathetic nervous system
  - Overactive rennin-angiotensin-aldosterone system
  - Atrial natriuretic peptide participates
  - Insulin resistance plays a role
- Blood volume and peripheral vascular resistance increase
- Workload of left ventricle increases
- Left ventricular muscle mass increases

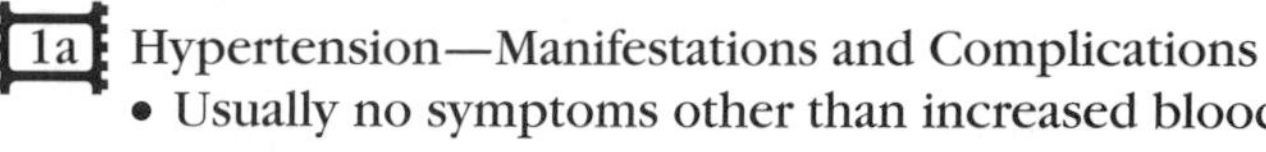

1a Hypertension—Manifestations and Complications
- Usually no symptoms other than increased blood pressure
- Complaints of vague headache or dizziness
- Morning headache, blurred vision, unsteadiness, depression, nocturia

1b Hypertensive Crisis
- Rapid increase in systolic pressure 240 mm Hg or diastolic pressure 120 mm Hg
- Malignant hypertension: diastolic pressure > 130 mm Hg
- Immediate treatment
- Headache, confusion, blurred vision, restlessness, motor/sensory deficits

1c Aneurysm—Pathophysiology
- Classified by shape and location (Figure 28-1)
- Types:
  - Fusiform
  - Saccular
  - Berry
  - Aortic dissection
- Often are asymptomatic
- Pressure on adjacent tissues and organs causes manifestations (Table 28-4)

1d Peripheral Atherosclerosis—Pathophysiology
- Thick peripheral arteries, plaque deposits, lumen narrows
- Decreased blood flow and oxygen to distal tissues
- Symptoms after 60% vessel occluded

1e Peripheral Atherosclerosis—Manifestations
- Pain
- Intermittent claudication
- Skin color changes
- Pulse changes
- Bruit
- Complications: gangrene, amputation

© 2007 Pearson Education, Inc.

POWERPOINT LECTURE SLIDES *continued*

1f Arterial Thrombus/Embolism—Pathophysiology
- Occlusion of blood flow through an artery
- Atherosclerotic changes can cause a thrombus or blood clot
- Blood clot breaks away, becomes an embolus
- Lodges in small vessels
- Leads to tissue necrosis, gangrene
- Manifestations (Box 28-12)

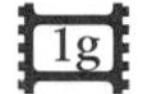

Venous Thrombosis—Pathophysiology
- Risk factors (Box 28-13)
- Small clots develop in veins
- Three pathologic factors: Virchow's triad
  - Venous stasis
  - Increased blood coagulability
  - Vessel wall injury
- Deep venous thrombosis (DVT)
  - Figure 28-4
  - Manifestations:
    - Calf pain, muscle tenderness
    - Dull, aching pain with walking
    - Enlarged calf, cyanotic
    - Positive Homan's sign
  - Complications
    - Pulomary embolism
- Superficial vein thrombophlebitis
  - Trauma to vein wall
  - Manifestations (Box 28-14)
- Venous insufficiency
  - Pathophysiology:
    - Large veins of legs occluded
    - Distends veins
    - Valves damaged
    - Valves fail to close
    - Blood collects and pools in lower extremities
    - Congestion and edema of leg tissue
    - Venous stasis ulcers develop (Figure 28-5)
  - Manifestations
    - Skin shiny, atrophic, cyanotic
    - Skin color brown

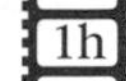

Varicose Veins
- Pathophysiology
  - Figure 28-7
  - Increased pressure stretches the vessel wall
  - Standing increases pressure in the leg veins
  - Decreases venous return to the heart
  - Blood collects in the leg veins
- Manifestations
  - Box 28-16
  - Can lead to venous insufficiency, stasis dermatitis, stasis ulcers
  - Skin above ankles thin and discolored
  - Venous thrombosis may develop

© 2007 Pearson Education, Inc.

Suggestions for Classroom and Clinical Activities

See Learning Outcome 1 activities.

Learning Outcome 3

Identify subjective and objective assessment data to collect for clients with peripheral vascular disorders.

Concepts for Lecture

1. Assessment data for peripheral vascular disorders.

PowerPoint Lecture Slides

1 Hypertension—Nursing Care
- Assessment: accurate blood pressure readings (Box 28-5)

1a Peripheral Atherosclerosis—Nursing Care
- Assessment
  - Chief complaint
  - Box 28-10

1b Acute Arterial Occlusion—Nursing Care
- Care similar to that for peripheral atherosclerosis
- Assessment:
  - Complaints of pain
  - Pulses
  - Teaching

1c Venous Conditions—Nursing Care
- Assessment:
  - Box 28-15
  - Table 28-6

Suggestions for Classroom Activities

Prepare a list of assessment questions and measurements to be used to assess a client with a peripheral vascular disorder. See www.ncbi.nlm.nih.gov/entrez/query.fcgi?cmd=Retrieve&db=PubMed&list_uids=2235633&dopt=Abstract.

Suggestions for Clinical Activities

Using the assessment information prepared in class, assess a client with a peripheral vascular disorder.

Learning Outcome 4

Explain the nursing implications of drugs used to treat clients with peripheral vascular disorders.

Concepts for Lecture

1. Nursing implications of drug therapy.

PowerPoint Lecture Slides

1 Hypertension—Medications
- Diuretics
- Beta blockers
- Sympatholytics
- Vasodilators
- ACE I
- Calcium channel blockers
- Table 28-3

1a Aneurysms—Medication Mangement
- Antihypertensives
- Anticoagulants

1b Peripheral Atherosclerosis—Medications
- Aspirin
- Plavix

© 2007 Pearson Education, Inc.

PowerPoint Lecture Slides *continued*

- Pletal
- Vasodilators

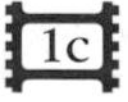
Venous Conditions—Management
- Medications:
  - NSAIDs
  - Anticoagulants
    - Heparin
    - Oral warfarin
    - Table 28-5
    - Thrombolytics

Suggestions for Classroom Activities

Prepare medication provision cards/sheets for the major drug classifications of medications used to treat peripheral vascular disorders. Utilize any medication text for this information.

Suggestions for Clinical Activities

Provide medications to a client with a peripheral vascular disorder.

Learning Outcome 5

Describe pre- and postoperative care for clients having vascular surgery.

Concepts for Lecture

1. Care for clients having vascular surgery.

PowerPoint Lecture Slides

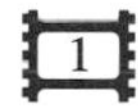
Aneurysms—Surgery
- Repair those that are tender or enlarging
- Excise the aneurysm and replace with graft (Figure 28-2)
- Nursing care
  - Preop
    - Routine care
    - ICU environment
    - Report changes in medical condition
    - Bed rest
    - Avoid Valsalva maneuver
  - Postop
    - General care
    - Chest tube
    - Assess for bleeding
    - Fluid/blood transfusions
    - Complications

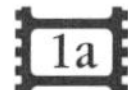
Peripheral Atherosclerosis
- Surgery
  - Revascularization
  - Endarterectomy
  - Box 28-8

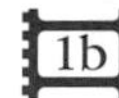
Venous Conditions—Management
- Surgery
  - Venous thrombectomy
  - Umbrella (Figure 28-6)

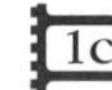
Vericose Veins—Management
- Surgery
  - Sclerotherapy
  - Vein stripping

Suggestions for Classroom Activities

Identify one surgical procedure used to treat a peripheral vascular disorder. Research the extent of surgery. See www1.va.gov/ps_vascularsurgery/.

Suggestions for Clinical Activities

Observe a surgical procedure for a client with a peripheral vascular disorder. Accompany this client into the recovery room.

Learning Outcome 6

Reinforce client and family teaching to promote and maintain health in clients with common peripheral vascular disorders.

Concepts for Lecture

1. Teaching for common peripheral vascular disorders.

PowerPoint Lecture Slides

1 Hypertension—Teaching
- Primary care provider
- Need for home care (Box 28-6)
- Daily medication
- Realistic exercise plan
- Stress reduction
- Regular follow-up care

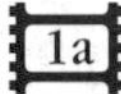

Aneurysms—Ongoing Care
- Control HTN, diet, stress reduction, alcohol, smoking, medications
- Prevent complications
- Postop teaching
- Rest
- Prevent constipation
- Follow up appointments

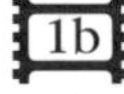

Peripheral Atherosclerosis—Teaching/Continuing Care
- Exercise
- Smoking cessation
- Legs/foot care (Box 28-11)
- Exercise
- Stress reduction
- Medications
- Surgical teaching

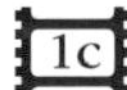

Venous Conditions—Nursing Care
- Teaching
  - Disease process
  - Course of treatment
  - Lab tests
  - Medications
  - Wound care
  - Activity
  - Measures to prevent recurrence
  - Follow-up visits
  - Efforts to avoid complications

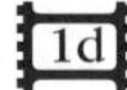

Varicose Veins
- Teaching
  - Daily walks
  - Antiembolic hose
  - Elevate legs
  - Avoid sitting/standing
  - Calf/thigh muscle exercises

© 2007 Pearson Education, Inc.

SUGGESTIONS FOR CLASSROOM ACTIVITIES	SUGGESTIONS FOR CLINICAL ACTIVITIES
Create a teaching plan for a peripheral vascular disorder.	Instruct a client with a peripheral vascular disorder on the content placed in the teaching plan during the classroom activity.

LEARNING OUTCOME 7

Use the nursing process to provide individualized care to clients with peripheral vascular disorders.

CONCEPTS FOR LECTURE

1. Nursing process to provide care.

POWERPOINT LECTURE SLIDES

1 Hypertension—Treatment
- No specific diagnostic tests
- Lab tests done to diagnose secondary hypertension
- Treatment to lower blood pressure
- Reduce the risk of damage to CV system and other target organs
- Control lifestyle variables and medication
- Table 28-2

1a Hypertension—Lifestyle Modifications
- Restrict alcohol use, restrict cigarette smoking, increase physical activity, stress reduction
- Weight loss
- Diet: reduce sodium and fat; promote weight loss; DASH diet (Box 28-3)
- Alcohol and smoking: 1 ounce alcohol per day; smoking cessation
- Physical activity: regular exercise, 30 minutes most days of the week
- Stress reduction: exercise is treatment of choice (Box 28-4)

1b Hypertension—Diagnosis, Planning, and Implementation
- Ineffective Health Maintenance
  - Teaching
  - Prescribed treatment
  - Lifestyle changes
  - Sodium intake
  - Weight loss strategies

1c Hypertension—Evaluation
- Client information
- Response to treatment
- Teaching

1d Aneurysms—Management
- Diagnosis with abdominal or chest x-ray
- Abdominal ultrasound
- CT scan/MRI

1e Aneurysms—Nursing Care
- Manage anxiety
- Nursing diagnoses:
  - Anxiety
  - Pain
  - Ineffective Tissue Perfusion

© 2007 Pearson Education, Inc.

POWERPOINT LECTURE SLIDES *continued*

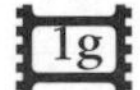

Peripheral Atherosclerosis—Management

- Improve/maintain blood supply and relieve symptoms
- Diagnostic tests
  - Segmented blood pressures
  - Exercise stress testing
  - Doppler ultrasounds (Figure 28-3)
  - Transcutaneous oximetry
  - Angiography

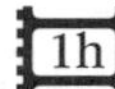

Peripheral Atherosclerosis—Treatment

- Smoking cessation
- Exercise
- Weight reduction
- Complementary therapies (Box 28-9)
- Nonsurgical
  - Percutaneous transluminal angioplasty
  - Stent
  - Atherectomy

Peripheral Atherosclerosis—Nursing Care

- Diagnosis, Planning, and Implementation
  - Ineffective Tissue Perfusion: Peripheral
    - Pulses
    - Warmth
    - Frequent position changes
  - Pain
    - Pain scale
    - Warmth
    - Smoking cessation
    - Stress reduction
  - Impaired Skin Integrity
    - Assess every 8 hours
    - Foot and leg care
    - Foot cradle
- Evaluation
  - Strength/equality of pulses
  - Capillary refill
  - Skin color
  - Temperature
  - Pain
  - Bleeding

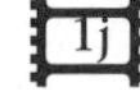

Acute Arterial Occlusion—Management

- Diagnosis and treatment
  - Physical examination
  - Angiography
  - Thrombolytic therapy
  - Anticoagulant therapy
  - Surgery
- Treatment
  - Smoking cessation
  - Exercise
  - Keep extremities warm
  - Amputation might be necessary

1j Acute Arterial Occlusion—Nursing Care

- Nursing Diagnosis
  - Ineffective Protection

© 2007 Pearson Education, Inc.

PowerPoint Lecture Slides *continued*

- Thrombolytic drugs
- Report bleeding
- H&H levels; PT times

 Venous Conditions—Management

- Prevention
- Diagnostic tests, nursing implications (Table 25-3)
  - Duplex venous ultrasound
  - Plethysmography
  - MRI
  - Ascending contrast phlebography or venography
- Conservative therapy
  - Prevention
  - Elastic stockings
  - Pneumatic compression devices
  - Leg exercises
  - Early ambulation
  - No leg crossing
  - Compresses to relieve symptoms
  - Bed rest
  - Elevate legs
  - TED hose
- Stasis dermatitis and stasis ulcer care
  - Wet compresses, boric acid, Burrow's solution, isotonic saline
  - Topical ointments
  - Unna boot

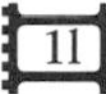 Venous Conditions—Nursing Care

- Diagnosis, Planning, and Implementation
  - Ineffective Tissue Perfusion: Peripheral
    - Peripheral pulses
    - Calf and thigh diameter
    - Elevate legs
    - Antiembolic hose/stockings
    - Frequent position changes
    - Anticoagulants/thrombolytics
    - Lab values
  - Pain
    - Pain scale
    - Warm, moist heat
    - Bed rest
  - Impaired Skin Integrity
    - Assess every 8 hours
    - Mild soap, solutions, lotions
    - Mattress
    - Active/passive ROM
    - Progressive ambulation
- Evaluation
  - Comfort level
  - Peripheral circulation
  - Bruising/bleeding
  - Lab results

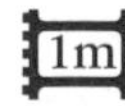 Vericose Veins—Management

- Treatment
  - Conservative

© 2007 Pearson Education, Inc.

PowerPoint Lecture Slides *continued*

- Reduce discomfort
- No real cure

- Diagnostic tests
  - Doppler ultrasound
  - Trendelenburg test
- Conservative therapy
  - Antiembolic stockings
  - Daily walking
  - Avoid prolonged sitting/standing
  - Elevate legs

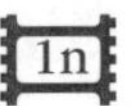 Varicose Veins—Nursing Care

- Nursing diagnosis:
  - Ineffective Tissue Perfusion: Peripheral
    - Assess pulses, capillary refill, skin temperature, edema
    - Antiembolic hose
    - Leg wraps as prescribed
    - Leg exercises
    - Leg positioning

Suggestions for Classroom Activities

Prepare a plan of care for a client with a peripheral vascular disorder.

Suggestions for Clinical Activities

Provide care to a client with a peripheral vascular disorder.

© 2007 Pearson Education, Inc.

CHAPTER 29
THE HEMATOLOGIC AND LYMPHATIC SYSTEMS AND ASSESSMENT

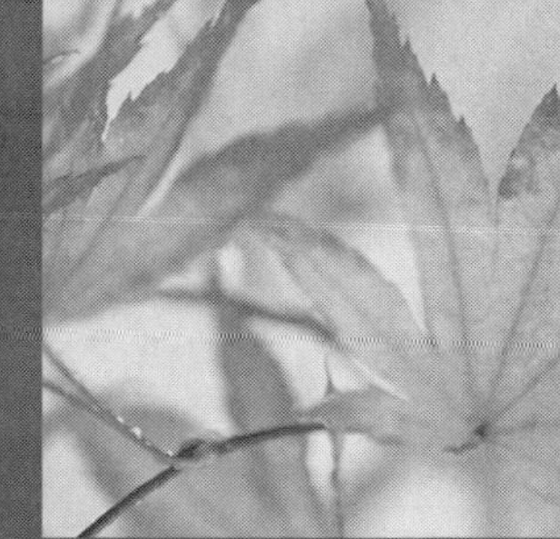

RESOURCE LIBRARY

CD-ROM

Lymphatic System

IMAGE LIBRARY

Figure 29-1 The formation of different types of blood cells from the stem cell. The stem cell differentiates into one of five types of blast (immature) cells, which then mature into red blood cells (erythrocytes), platelets (thrombocytes), or white blood cells (leukocytes).

Figure 29-2 Top and side views of a red blood cell. Note the distinctive concave shape.

Figure 29-3 Both the slower intrinsic pathway (on the left) and the more rapid extrinsic pathway (on the right) are necessary to form a stable blood clot.

Figure 29-4 The lymphatic system.

LEARNING OUTCOME 1

Describe the cells of the hematologic system with their functions.

CONCEPTS FOR LECTURE

1. Hematologic system with the functions.

POWERPOINT LECTURE SLIDES

1 Blood and Blood Cells
- Purpose: transport oxygen removes waste
- Blood components
  - Plasma
  - RBC
  - WBC
  - Platelets
- Formation of blood
  - Liver
  - Bone marrow
  - Stem cells
  - Figure 29-1

1a Red Blood Cells
- Carry oxygen and carbon dioxide
- Shaped: biconcave disks (Figure 29-2)
- Formed in bone marrow via erythropoiesis
- Tissue hypoxia stimulates the kidneys to release erythropoietin to stimulate RBC production in bone marrow
- Figure 29-1
- Contain hemoglobin
- Life span: 120 days
- Old RBCs: destroyed by phagocytes in the spleen, liver, bone marrow, lymph nodes; hemolysis
- Amino acids and iron saved and reused by body, circulates as transferrin; stored as ferritin; heme converted to bilirubin
- Normal lab values differ by gender (Table 29-1)
- Terms used: normocytic, microcytic, macrocytic, normochromic, hypochromic

PowerPoint Lecture Slides *continued*

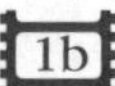
White Blood Cells

- Leukocytes
- 5000 to 10,000; make up 1% of total blood volume
- Leukocytosis: high WBC count
- Leukopenia: low WBC count
- Originate from stem cells in bone marrow (Figure 29-1)
- Move to where they are needed; migrate to other tissues
- Three types: granulocytes, monocytes, lymphocytes
- Three types of granulocytes: neutrophils, eosinophils, basophils
- Monocytes: largest WBC
- Lymphocytes: regulate immune response
- Normal values (Table 29-2)

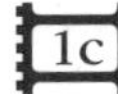
Platelets

- Part of the clotting mechanism
- Fragments of cytoplasm without nuclei
- Most stored in the spleen
- 250,000 to 400,000 in each mL of blood
- Excess termed thrombycytosis
- Live approximately 10 days

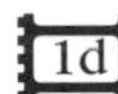
Hemostasis

- Blood clotting to stop bleeding
- Five stages:
    - Vessel spasm
    - Formation of platelet plug
    - Clot formation
        - Intrinsic pathway
        - Extrinsic pathway (Figure 29-3)
    - Clot retraction
    - Clot dissolution (Table 29-3)

Suggestions for Classroom Activities

Divide the students into two groups. Group 1 will focus on the RBCs. Group 2 will focus on the WBCs. Each group is to create a presentation that describes the creation, purpose, and life span of their respective cell type. Present the information to the entire class.

Suggestions for Clinical Activities

On the clinical unit, collect laboratory data about a client's RBC and WBC status. Correlate the findings with the client's primary medical diagnosis.

Learning Outcome 2

Identify and describe the structures and functions of the lymphatic system.

Concepts for Lecture

1. Lymphatic system structures and functions.

PowerPoint Lecture Slides

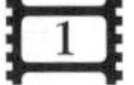
Lymphatic System

- Figure 29-4
- Includes lymph vessels, nodes, organs
- Assist immune system
- Largest organ is the spleen

© 2007 Pearson Education, Inc.

SUGGESTIONS FOR CLASSROOM ACTIVITIES

Trace a drop of lymph fluid through the lymphatic tissue and structures. See www.nlm.nih.gov/medlineplus/ency/article/002247.htm.

SUGGESTIONS FOR CLINICAL ACTIVITIES

Assess a client's lymphatic system.

LEARNING OUTCOME 3

Collect subjective and objective assessment data related to the hematologic and lymphatic systems.

CONCEPTS FOR LECTURE

1. Subjective and objective assessment data.

POWERPOINT LECTURE SLIDES

1 Assessment

- Health History
  - Changes in energy level
  - Usual activities
  - Pain, burning, tingling
  - Changes in skin color or temperature
  - Edema
  - Bruising, dizziness, fatigue
  - Diet
  - Medications
  - Tobacco, alcohol, recreational drugs
  - Medical history
  - Family history

1a Physical Examination

- Inspection:
  - Petechiae
  - Purpura
  - Figures 5-3 and 5-6
  - Documentation (Box 29-1)

SUGGESTIONS FOR CLASSROOM ACTIVITIES

Create a guide sheet for the assessment of a client's hematologic and lymphatic systems.

SUGGESTIONS FOR CLINICAL ACTIVITIES

Utilizing the guide sheet prepared in class, assess a client's hematologic and lymphatic systems.

LEARNING OUTCOME 4

Provide appropriate nursing care for clients undergoing diagnostic tests to evaluate the hematologic and lymphatic systems.

CONCEPTS FOR LECTURE

1. Nursing care associated with diagnostic testing.

POWERPOINT LECTURE SLIDES

1 Diagnostic Tests

- Laboratory
  - CBC (Tables 29-1, 29-2, and 29-3)
  - Clotting/coagulation profile (Table 29-3)
  - Coombs' test
  - Hemoglobin electrophoresis
  - Iron stores (Table 29-3)
  - Schilling's test
- Bone marrow aspiration
  - Nursing care (Box 29-2)
    - Preprocedure: consent, purpose, vital signs
    - Postprocedure: pressure, vital signs, dressing
    - Teaching: 20 minutes, anesthetic, still, ache

© 2007 Pearson Education, Inc.

PowerPoint Lecture Slides *continued*

- Biopsy
  - Lymph tissue
- Imaging studies
  - Lymphangiogram

Suggestions for Classroom Activities

Review the trays used for a bone marrow aspiration and/or lymph node biopsy. See http://medicalcenter.osu.edu/patientcare/healthinformation/otherhealthtopics/HematologyBloodDisorders/BoneMarrowTransplantation4487/.

Suggestions for Clinical Activities

Assist or accompany a client undergoing a bone marrow biopsy or lymph node tissue biopsy.

© 2007 Pearson Education, Inc.

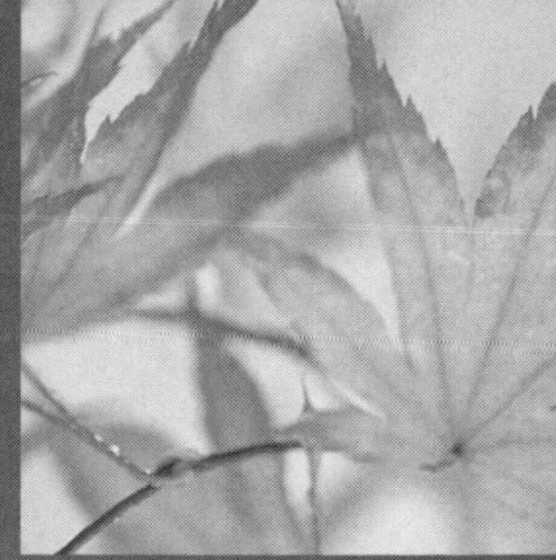

CHAPTER 30
CARING FOR CLIENTS WITH HEMATOLOGIC AND LYMPHATIC DISORDERS

RESOURCE LIBRARY

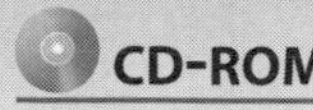

Sickle Cell

IMAGE LIBRARY

Figure 30-1 The multisystem effects of anemia.
Figure 30-2 The inheritance pattern for sickle cell anemia.
Figure 30-3 Pathophysiology illustrated: sickle cell anemia. Sickle cell anemia is caused by an inherited defect in hemoglobin (Hb) synthesis. When sickle cell hemoglobin (HbS) is oxygenated, it has the same globular shape as normal hemoglobin. However, when HbS is not bound with oxygen, it becomes insoluble and crystallizes into rodlike structures. Clusters of these rods form long chains that bend the erythrocyte into the characteristic crescent shape of the sickle cell.
Figure 30-4 The multisystem effects of leukemia.
Figure 30-5 The inheritance pattern for hemophilia A and B. Both are X-linked recessive disorders; females may carry the trait, but only males develop the disorder.
Figure 30-6 Severe lymphedema of the lower extremity.
Figure 30-7 Areas of radiation for total nodal radiation therapy.

LEARNING OUTCOME 1

Describe the pathophysiology and manifestations of common hematologic and lymphatic disorders.

CONCEPTS FOR LECTURE

1. Pathophysiology and manifestations of hematologic disorders.
2. Pathophysiology and manifestations of lymphatic disorders.

POWERPOINT LECTURE SLIDES

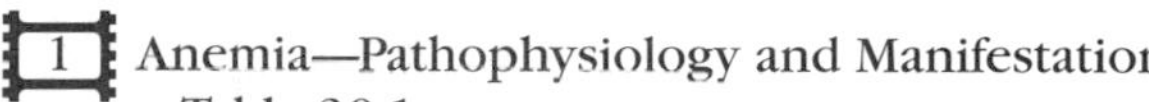

1 Anemia—Pathophysiology and Manifestations
- Table 30-1
- Reduces the oxygen-carrying capacity of the blood
- Causes tissue hypoxia
- Body attempts to restore oxygen delivery
- Leads to pallor, angina, fatigue, DOE, night cramps, bone pain, headache, dizziness, dim vision
- Blood loss anemia:
  - Acute or chronic bleeding
  - Both lead to anemia
- Nutritional anemia
  - Lack of nutrients for RBC formation or development
  - Iron deficiency
    - Cheilosis
    - Smooth, sore tongue
    - Pica
  - Vitamin B_{12}
    - Pernicious anemia
    - Paresthesias

- Folic acid
  - Chronic malnourishment
  - Glossitis
  - Chielosis
  - Diarrhea
- Anemia of chronic disease
  - Seen in AIDs, rheumatoid arthritis, IBD, chronic hepatitis, CRF
  - Severity depends on the severity of underlying disease
  - Manifestations similar to iron deficiency anemia
- Hemolytic anemias
  - Premature destruction of RBCs
  - Intrinsic or acquired causes
  - Sickle cell disorders (Figure 30-2)
    - Abnormal Hgb, changes shape (Figure 30-3)
    - Box 30-1
    - Intense pain, chest, back, joints
  - Thallassemia
    - Inherited caused by abnormal Hgb synthesis
    - Liver and spleen enlarged
    - Target cells
  - Acquired hemolytic anemias
    - Damage by outside factors
      - Mechanical trauma
      - Antibody reactions
      - Immune responses
      - Drugs, toxins, chemical agents, venoms
- Aplastic anemia
  - Bone marrow fails to produce RBCs
  - Cause unknown
  - Pancytopenia
- Myelodysplastic syndrome
  - Group of stem cell disorders
  - Seen in order adults
  - Anemia, enlarged spleen

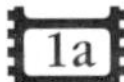

Polycythemia—Pathophysiology and Manifestations
- Erythrocytosis
- Abnormally high RBC count, high Hct
- Blood sticky
- Secondary form is the most common
- Develops due to chronic hypoxemia or excess erythropoietin
- Polycythemia vera: primary type; production of all blood cells increased; cause unknown; insidious onset; gangrene complication

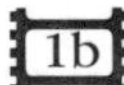

Hemophilia—Pathophysiology and Manifestations
- Group of hereditary clotting factor deficiencies
- Types: hemophilia A and B
- Hemophilia A: most common type, deficiency in Factor VIII
- Hemophilia B (Christmas disease): less common, deficiency in Factor IX
- Transmitted from mother to son, sex-linked recessive disorder on X chromosome (Figure 30-5)

© 2007 Pearson Education, Inc.

- Hemorrhages into body tissues
- Types of hemophilia (Table 30-5)

1c Disseminated Intravascular Coagulation—Pathophysiology and Manifestations
- Simultaneous blood clotting and hemorrhage (Box 30-5)
- Intrinsic and/or extrinsic clotting cascades activated
- Widespread clotting of small vessels
- Clotting factors depleted; leads to bleeding
- Bleeding most obvious manifestations
- Manifestations (Box 30-6)

2 Leukemia—Pathophysiology and Manifestations
- Malignant disorders of WBCs
- Cause of most unknown
- Classified by onset and duration: acute or chronic
- Four types (Table 30-3)
- Malignant transformation of a single stem cell
- Cells proliferate slowly, nonfunctional WBCs
- Bone marrow filled with leukemic cells
- Leave bone marrow and infiltrate other tissues
- Death from hemorrhage or infection
- Manifestations from anemia, infection, bleeding
- Figure 30-4

2a Multiple Myeloma—Pathophysiology and Manifestations
- Myeloma cells replace bone marrow, infiltrate bone
- Bone weakened, pathologic fractures
- Bone/back pain most common symptoms
- Kidney damage

2b Thrombocytopenia—Pathophysiology
- Platelet count less than 100,000 per mL
- Common cause of abnormal bleeding
- Idiopathic thrombocytopenia purpura most common form
  - Platelets destroy more rapidly than normal
  - Autoimmune disorder
  - Manifestations: purpura, ecchymoses, petechiae, epistaxis, menorrhagia, hematuria

2c Lymphangitis and Lymphedema—Pathophysiology and Manifestations
- Lymphangitis: inflammation of lymph vessel
- Lymphedema: obstructed lymph vessel
- Figure 30-6

2d Infectious Mononucleosis—Pathophysiology and Manifestations
- Acute infection caused by Epstein-Barr virus
- Benign and self-limiting
- Kissing disease
- Headache, malaise, fatigue
- Fever, sore throat, enlarged and painful cervical lymph nodes, enlarged spleen

© 2007 Pearson Education, Inc.

POWERPOINT LECTURE SLIDES *continued*

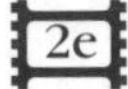 Malignant Lymphoma—Pathophysiology and Manifestations
- Cancer of lymph tissue
- Classified as Hodgkin's or non-Hodgkin's
- Hodgkin's
  - Most curable
  - Painless progressive enlargement of one or more lymph nodes
  - Reed-Sternberg cells
  - Cause unknown
  - Manifestations (Box 30-7)
- Non-Hodgkin's
  - More common
  - Multiple lymph nodes involved

SUGGESTIONS FOR CLASSROOM ACTIVITIES

Have the students research one hematologic or lymphatic system disorder. Include in this research any recent studies or activities to aid in the diagnosis and treatment. See http://medicalcenter.osu.edu/patientcare/healthinformation/otherhealthtopics/HematologyBloodDisorders/BloodDisorders/.

SUGGESTIONS FOR CLINICAL ACTIVITIES

Assign the students to a client with a hematologic or lymphatic disorder. Have the students list/identify the client's signs/symptoms that caused the client to seek medical attention/treatment.

LEARNING OUTCOME 2

Discuss interdisciplinary care of clients with hematologic or lymphatic disorders, including diagnostic tests and commonly prescribed medications.

CONCEPTS FOR LECTURE

1. Care for common diagnostic tests.
2. Care for commonly prescribed medications.

POWERPOINT LECTURE SLIDES

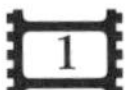 Anemia—Management
- Diagnostic tests
  - CBC
  - Iron levels
  - Serum ferritin
  - Sickle cell screening
  - Hemoglobin electrophoresis
  - Schilling's test
  - Bone marrow aspiration

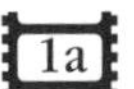 Leukemia—Treatment
- Diagnostic tests
  - CBC with differential and platelet count
  - Bone marrow

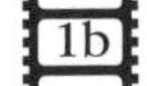 Multiple Myeloma—Treatment
- Diagnostic tests
  - Urine samples
  - CBC
  - Bone marrow
  - Bone x-rays
- No cure; treatment on relieving symptoms; death within 2 to 5 years
- Treatment: chemotherapy, radiation, medications, pain control, blood transfusions

© 2007 Pearson Education, Inc.

POWERPOINT LECTURE SLIDES *continued*

1c Thrombocytopenia—Treatment
- Diagnostic tests
  - CBC, platelet count
  - Bone marrow
  - Antinuclear antibodies

1d Hemophilia—Treatment
- Diagnostic tests
  - Platelet count
  - Coagulation studies
  - Clotting factors

1e DIC—Treatment
- Clotting studies
- Treatment: underlying disease

1f Infectious Mononucleosis—Treatment
- Diagnostic tests
  - Increased lymphocytes and monocytes
  - Increased WBC count
  - Low platelets

1g Malignant Lymphoma—Treatment
- Diagnostic tests
  - Chest x-ray
  - Abdominal CT
  - Biopsy
  - Ann Arbor staging system
  - Cotswold staging classification system

2 Anemia—Medications
- Depends on type and cause
  - Iron replacement
  - Vitamin B_{12}
  - Folic acid
  - Hydroxyurea
  - Immunosuppressive therapy or androgens
  - Nursing implications (Table 30-2); Z-track technique (Procedure 30-1)

2a Leukemia—Treatment
- Chemotherapy
  - Destroy leukemic cells and produce remission

2b Thrombocytopenia—Medications
- Steroids
- Immunosuppressive drugs

2c Hemophilia—Medications
- Replace clotting factors: fresh frozen plasma, cryoprecipitates, concentrates
- DDAVP

2d DIC—Treatment
- Medications
  - Control bleeding: fresh frozen plasma, heparin

2e Infectious Mononucleosis—Treatment
- Recovery in 2 to 3 weeks
- Bed rest, analgesics

© 2007 Pearson Education, Inc.

POWERPOINT LECTURE SLIDES *continued*

2f Malignant Lymphoma—Treatment
- Chemotherapy
  - Combination
  - Remission in >75%
- Radiation
  - Used for both
  - Combined with chemotherapy
  - Figure 30-8

SUGGESTIONS FOR CLASSROOM ACTIVITIES

A variety of medications are available to treat hematologic and lymphatic disorders. Have the students research the most current medications available including the route of administration and side effects. See www.umm.edu/blood/index.htm.

SUGGESTIONS FOR CLINICAL ACTIVITIES

Assign the students to a client with a hematologic or lymphatic disorder. Have the students either administer or observe the administration of the client's medications.

LEARNING OUTCOME 3

Relate the nursing implications for selected treatment measures for clients with hematologic or lymphatic disorders.

CONCEPTS FOR LECTURE

1. Nursing care for selected treatments.

POWERPOINT LECTURE SLIDES

1 Anemia—Dietary Considerations
- Iron that is readily absorbed
- Iron sources (Box 30-2)

1a Anemia—Blood Transfusions
- Replace RBCs
- Whole blood or packed RBCs

1b Polycythemia—Management
- Treatment
  - Reduce blood viscosity and volume
  - Relieve symptoms
  - Phlebotomy to keep blood volumc within normal levels
  - Chemotherapy

1c Leukemia—Treatment
- Achieve remission, cure, relieve symptoms
- Radiation therapy
  - Shrink lymph nodes
- Biologic therapy
  - Interferons, interleukins
  - Colony-stimulating factors (Table 30-4)
- Bone marrow transplantation
  - Types: allogenic, autologous
  - Allogenic: eliminate leukemic cells; donor marrow transfused
  - Autologous: own bone marrow withdrawn, treated, frozen, reinfused later
- Stem cell transplant
  - Donor treated with colony-stimulating factors to increase concentration of stem cells in blood
  - Blood removed from donor, given to patient

© 2007 Pearson Education, Inc.

PowerPoint Lecture Slides *continued*

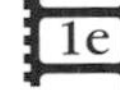
1d Thrombocytopenia—Treatment
- Platelet transfusions
- Plasmapheresis
- Surgery:
  - Splenectomy

1e Lymphangitis and Lymphedema—Treatment
- Relieve edema, maintain skin integrity, prevent/treat infection
- Lymphangitis: moist heat, elevate, immobilize, skin/wound care, antibiotics
- Lymphedema: elevate, elastic stockings, skin care, bed rest, sodium restriction

Suggestions for Classroom Activities

Have the students analyze a drop of blood in the learning lab. Document the characteristics, color, texture, etc., of this blood.

Suggestions for Clinical Activities

Assign the students to observe activities in the organization's blood bank. Ideally, the students should begin with blood donation, processing, and preparation for infusion into a client.

Learning Outcome 4

Provide individualized nursing care for clients with hematologic or lymphatic disorders.

Concepts for Lecture

1. Nursing care for hematologic or lymphatic disorders.

PowerPoint Lecture Slides

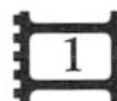
1 Anemia—Nursing Care
- Assessment (Box 30-3)
- Diagnosing, Planning, and Implementation
  - Activity Intolerance
    Vital signs
    - Rest periods
    - Energy conservation
    - Smoking cessation
  - Impaired Oral Mucous Membranes
    - Assess lips and tongue
    - Mouthwash
    - Frequent oral hygiene
    - Avoid alcohol-based mouthwashes
    - Petroleum jelly for lips
    - Avoid spicy foods
    - Encourage soft bland foods
    - Small high-protein balanced meals each day
  - Self-Care Deficit
    - Assist with ADLs
    - Rest periods
    - Concerns about self-care
- Evaluation
  - Independent ADLs
  - Increased level of activity
  - Skin and oral mucous membranes
  - Diet

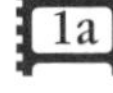
1a Leukemia—Nursing Care
- Assessment (Box 30-4)
  - Recognize manifestations

© 2007 Pearson Education, Inc.

PowerPoint Lecture Slides *continued*

- Diagnosing, Planning, and Implementation
  - Risk for Infection
    - Infection precautions
    - Avoid invasive procedures
    - Report evidence of infection
    - Monitor vital signs
    - Report lab values
    - Explain precautions and restrictions
  - Imbalanced Nutrition: Less than Body Requirements
    - Monitor weight
    - Promote food and fluid intake
    - Avoid procedures around meals
  - Impaired Oral Mucous Membranes
    - Assess mouth
    - 1:1 solution saline/peroxide as mouthwash
    - Soft-bristle toothbrush
    - Medications for infection, pain
    - Avoid alcohol-based mouth washes
  - Ineffective Protection
    - Monitor LOC
    - Report manifestations of bleeding
    - Avoid invasive procedures
    - Apply pressure to puncture sites
    - Avoid straining with bowel movement
  - Anticipatory Grieving
    - Therapeutic communication
    - Manage stressful situations
    - Support groups for the grieving process
- Evaluation
  - Freedom from infection
  - Weight
  - Food intake
  - Oral mucous membranes
  - Bleeding
  - Coping

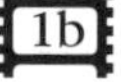

Multiple Myeloma—Nursing Care

- Diagnoses and Implementation
  - Chronic Pain
    - Assess pain
    - Positioning, support with pillows
    - Use of analgesics
    - Nonpharmacology pain control
    - Rest periods
  - Impaired Physical Mobility
    - Reposition
    - Change positions every 2 hours
    - Trapeze
    - Safety measures

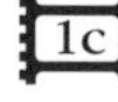

Thrombocytopenia—Nursing Care

- Diagnoses and Implementation
  - Ineffective Protection
    - Monitor LOC
    - Manifestations of bleeding
    - Avoid invasive procedures
    - Pressure dressing to puncture sites
    - Avoid straining at bowel movement

© 2007 Pearson Education, Inc.

POWERPOINT LECTURE SLIDES *continued*

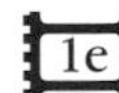

Hemophilia—Nursing Care

- Diagnoses and Implementation
  - Risk for Injury
    - Signs of bleeding
    - Stop bleeding with pressure, ice
    - No IM injections
    - Safety measures
  - Risk for Ineffective Therapeutic Regimen Management
    - Assess knowledge/reinforce teaching
    - Emotional support
    - Opportunities to learn/practice administration clotting factors

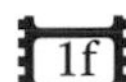

DIC—Nursing Care

- Diagnoses and Implementation
  - Ineffective Tissue Perfusion
    - Assess pulses
    - Turn every 2 hours
    - No knee crossing
    - Minimize tape use
  - Impaired Gas Exchange
    - O_2 saturation levels
    - ABGs
    - Oxygen
    - Fowler's/semi-Fowler's position
    - Bed rest
    - Deep breathing and coughing
  - Pain
    - Pain scale
    - Handle gently
    - Cool compresses to painful joints
  - Fear
    - Verbalize concerns
    - Answer questions
    - Coping strategies
    - Emotional support
    - Calm environment
    - Respond to calls for help
    - Relaxation techniques

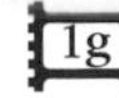

Lymphangitis and Lymphedema—Nursing Care

- Implementation
  - Measure effected extremity
  - I&O
  - Daily weights
  - Sodium restriction
  - Antiembolic stockings/intermittent pressure devices
  - Elevate extremities
  - Skin care
  - Protective devices

1g Malignant Lymphoma—Nursing Care

- Diagnoses and Implementation
  - Risk for Impaired Skin Integrity
    - Measures to reduce itching

© 2007 Pearson Education, Inc.

PowerPoint Lecture Slides *continued*

- ○ Nausea
  - – Antiemetics
  - – Measures to relieve/reduce nausea
- ○ Fatigue
  - – Assess malaise
  - – Encourage talking about disease
  - – Quiet activities
  - – Rest periods
  - – High-carbohydrate diet
  - – Fluids
- ○ Disturbed Body Image
  - – Body image assessment
  - – Objective signs of altered body image
  - – Coping with alopecia
  - – Effects of illness on sexuality
  - – Support groups

Suggestions for Classroom Activities

Have the students prepare a plan of care for a client with nausea and pain. See www.umm.edu/blood/blooddis.htm.

Suggestions for Clinical Activities

Assign the students to a client with a hematologic or lymphatic disorder. Implement the plan of care for nausea and pain.

Learning Outcome 5

Identify continuing care needs for clients with hematologic or lymphatic disorders.

Concepts for Lecture

1. Teaching needs for hematologic or lymphatic disorders.

PowerPoint Lecture Slides

1 Anemia—Continuing Care and Teaching
- Types of anemia
- Diet
- Medications
- Genetic counseling
- Follow-up appointments
- Support groups

1a Polycythemia—Nursing Care
- Teaching
  - ○ Hydration
  - ○ Prevent blood stasis
  - ○ Elevate legs
  - ○ Support stockings
  - ○ Smoking cessation
  - ○ Report S/S thrombosis

1b Leukemia—Teaching
- Diagnosis, treatment, bone marrow, complications
- Cancer as a chronic illness
- Balance activity with rest
- Maintain weight and nutrition
- Hydration
- Prevent infection
- Oral hygiene
- Avoid crowds, sick people
- Avoid immunizations
- Reduce risk of bleeding or injury

© 2007 Pearson Education, Inc.

POWERPOINT LECTURE SLIDES *continued*

- Avoid OTC medications that can cause bleeding
- Refer to social services, support groups, home health

1c Multiple Myeloma—Teaching
- Teach S/S complications
- Hospice

1d Thrombocytopenia—Teaching
- Continue treatment to maintain remission
- Long-term steroid treatment
- Splenectomy

1e Hemophilia—Teaching
- How to prevent bleeding
- Provide medications
- Genetic counseling

1f DIC—Teaching
- Proper foot care
- Heparin home therapy
- When to contact physician

1g Lymphangitis and Lymphedema—Teaching
- Use of pressure devices, elastic stockings
- Skin inspection
- Skin care
- Elevate extremity
- Activity, diet, diuretics

1h Malignant Lymphoma—Teaching
- Treatment and effects of treatment
- Skin care
- New symptoms
- Complementary pain management strategies
- Rest and exercise
- Diet
- American Cancer Society referral

SUGGESTIONS FOR CLASSROOM ACTIVITIES

Have the students prepare a teaching plan for a client with Hodgkin's disease that includes age-related (under age 50 years) considerations, family considerations, and follow-up care.

SUGGESTIONS FOR CLINICAL ACTIVITIES

Assign the students to a client with a hematologic or lymphatic disorder. Determine at least one teaching need for the client and provide appropriate instruction.

© 2007 Pearson Education, Inc.

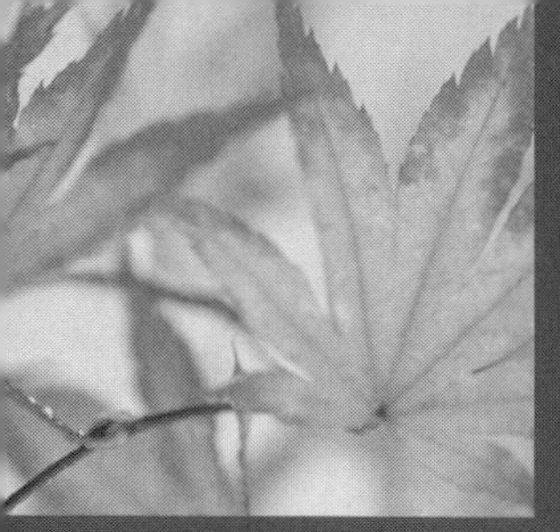

CHAPTER 31
THE URINARY SYSTEM AND ASSESSMENT

RESOURCE LIBRARY

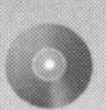 **CD-ROM**

Urinary System
Kidney Structure
Kidney
Urinary Bladder

IMAGE LIBRARY

Figure 31-1 Anterior view of the urinary system.
Figure 31-2 Internal anatomy of the kidney.
Figure 31-3 Structure of a nephron.
Figure 31-4 Structure of the urinary bladder.
Figure 31-5 Percussing the kidney.
Figure 31-6 Inspecting the urinary meatus of the male.

LEARNING OUTCOME 1

Identify and describe the structures and functions of the renal and urinary system.

CONCEPTS FOR LECTURE

1. The urinary system is composed of two kidneys, two ureters, the bladder, and the urethra.
2. The kidney is composed of three distinct regions: cortex, medulla, and pelvis.
3. The outer region contains the glomeruli, small clusters of capillaries that are part of the nephron.
4. The nephron is the functional unit of the kidney, responsible for making urine.
5. Different portions of the nephron are involved in the absorption of water and electrolytes, which concentrate urine.
6. Glomerular filtration is the process in which fluids and solutes pass through the nephron.
7. The kidney is responsible for the regulation of blood pressure via the renin-angiotension-aldosterone system.
8. The renin-angiotension-aldosterone system also regulates the sodium level in the body, which assists with fluid regulation.
9. The kidney also secretes erythropoietin, which is responsible for the formation of RBCs.
10. As adults age, nephrons are lost, resulting in a decrease in the glomerular filtration rate. This can affect medication tolerance.

POWERPOINT LECTURE SLIDES

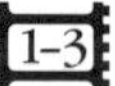

Anatomic review of kidney structure to include visual of kidneys, bladder, and ureters
- In-depth review of kidney structure to include helium, renal cortex, renal medulla, pyramid, renal pelvis, and calyx
- Anatomic review of structures within the nephron
- Anatomic and functional review of ureter, bladder, and urethra

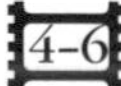

Review the function of the nephron and actions that occur within the nephron
- Glomerular filtration
- Glomerular filtration rate
- Tubular reabsorption
  - Include water and electrolytes
- Tubular secretion
- Urine concentration

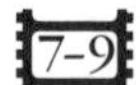

Endocrine Function
- Renin-angiotensin-aldosterone system and its role in blood pressure and sodium reabsorption
- Erythropoietin and its role in RBC production
- Vitamin D and calcium regulation
- Acid-base balance

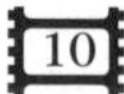

Age-Related Changes
- Changes in nephron and GFR—how this affects medications
- Urine concentration—risk for dehydration

Suggestions for Classroom Activities

1. Trace the flow of urine through the kidney into the bladder.
2. Have the student diagram the formation and concentration of urine.
3. Have students diagram the renin-angiotensin-aldosterone system and apply to assessment findings in clients.
4. Discuss how the flow, concentration of urine, and electrolytes may change with aging.

Suggestions for Clinical Activities

1. Using medications a client may be taking, discuss their effects on the renin-angiotension-aldosterone system.
2. Discuss the purpose of urine.
3. Discuss the importance of GFR in medication excretion/tolerance.
4. Using medications a client may be taking, discuss how medication effects may change with aging and changing GFR.

Learning Outcome 2

Collect subjective information and physical assessment data related to the urinary system and kidney function.

Concepts for Lecture

1. A detailed health history is an important aspect of identifying disorders of the urinary system.
2. Various disease processes and past history may be the cause of present urinary disorders. Ex: diabetes, surgery.
3. Vital signs and other objective findings change with urinary disorders.
4. Normal urine is clear, pale yellow without blood, protein, WBCs, or nitrates.
5. The genital area and urinary meatus should be free of sores, lesions, or tenderness.
6. The costovertebral angle is the area over the kidney; tenderness in this area may indicate a kidney infection.

PowerPoint Lecture Slides

1 Steps in obtaining a urinary history: ask about color, clarity, amount of urine
- Difficulty initiating urination or changes in stream
- Changes in urinary pattern
- Defintions to be reviewed: dysuria, nocturia, hematuria, pyuria; also the presence of these findings

2 History of urinary problems, urinary or abdominal Surgeries, number of children
- Social history that may affect urinary system: smoking, alcohol use, number of sexual partners and type of sexual relationship
- Chance of pregnancy at time of history
- History of diabetes or other endocrine disorders
- History of kidney stones

3 Vital Signs and Skin Assessment
- How vital signs may change in urinary disorders

4 Normal Urine Characteristics
- Color, clarity
- Normal findings on a urine dipstick

5 Normal Findings in Assessing the Genital Area and Urinary Meatus
- May also include abnormal findings, particularly of the urinary meatus, narrowing, strictures, lesions

6 Location of costovertebral angle and how to assess for tenderness

Suggestions for Classroom Activities

1. Present a case study to students and have them identify which areas of the study relate to the urinary system.
2. Using a case study, have students practice documenting a urinary assessment.
3. Using a "Jeopardy" game format, have the students answer questions as to how various disorders may affect the urinary system, review definitions, questions that relate to normal and abnormal findings, subjective and objective findings.

Suggestions for Clinical Activities

1. Have students complete a urinary history in the clinical area.
2. Have students assess their clients for costovertebral tenderness.
3. Allow students to check clients' urine and assess for abnormalities.
4. Allow students to document assessment findings.
5. Discuss how a client's vital signs may be affected by kidney function.

© 2007 Pearson Education, Inc.

LEARNING OUTCOME 3

Provide appropriate nursing care for clients undergoing diagnostic tests to identify disorders of the urinary system or kidneys.

CONCEPTS FOR LECTURE

1. Many diagnostic tests are used to assess the urinary system.
2. Diagnostic tests include blood studies, urine studies, and radiology studies.
3. Testing may be done at the bedside with little to no patient preparation.
4. Testing may be done in the radiology or surgical area and require conscious sedation.
5. Nursing care for urinary studies may include patient teaching, assessments, and patient preparation.

POWERPOINT LECTURE SLIDES

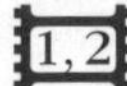

Diagnostic Tests: Indications and Contraindications

- Clean-catch urine
- 24-hour urine
- Culture and sensitivity
- BUN, creatinine and creatinine clearance
- IVP
- CT scan
- Renal scan
- Ultrasound
- Bladder scan
- Cystoscopy
- Uroflowmetry

For each test listed, discuss important preparation and teaching aspects, including the need for sedation and patient consent, NPO status

Discuss important aspects of each procedure: NPO, IV site needs

- Assessment during the procedure if appropriate
- Postprocedure assessment, frequency of VS, intake and output

SUGGESTIONS FOR CLASSROOM ACTIVITIES

1. Give the students various diagnostic studies and have them develop a nursing care plan for a client undergoing that study. This could be done as group or individual work.
2. Have each student pick a diagnostic study and review the study in depth and present to class.

SUGGESTIONS FOR CLINICAL ACTIVITIES

1. Assign students clients undergoing urinary diagnostic studies.
2. Have students visit the radiology department to observe diagnostic studies.
3. Take a client's blood and/or urine studies and have the students identify abnormalities in the studies and discuss what these abnormalities mean to patient care.
4. Have students perform patient teaching for clients undergoing diagnostic studies.

© 2007 Pearson Education, Inc.

CHAPTER 32
CARING FOR CLIENTS WITH RENAL AND URINARY TRACT DISORDERS

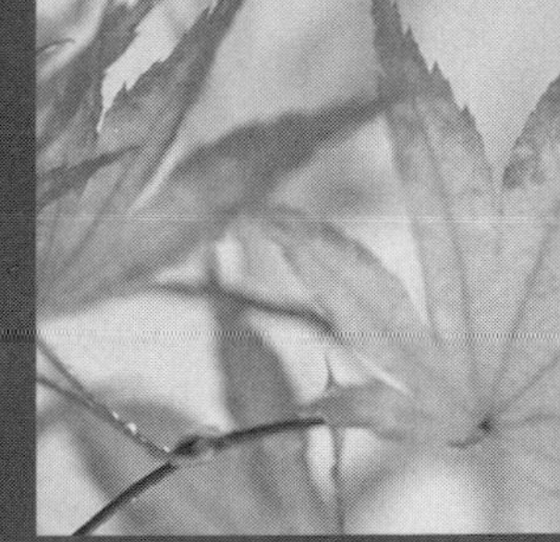

RESOURCE LIBRARY

CD-ROM

Video: Kidney Stones
Video: Renal Failure

IMAGE LIBRARY

Figure 32-1 A sample voiding diary.
Figure 32-2 The pathophysiology of glomerulonephritis.
Figure 32-3 Severe edema in a client with nephrotic syndrome.
Figure 32-4 Potential locations of stones within the urinary tract.
Figure 32-5 Extracorporeal shock-wave lithotripsy. Acoustic shock waves created by the shock-wave generator travel through soft tissue to shatter the urinary stone into fragments, which are then eliminated in the urine.
Figure 32-6 Percutaneous lithotripsy. A nephroscope is inserted through the skin into the renal pelvis, and the stone is fragmented using ultrasonic waves or laser.
Figure 32-7 A ureteral stent.
Figure 32-8 A polycystic kidney and a normal kidney for comparison.
Figure 32-9 A papillary lesion of the bladder wall.
Figure 32-10 Urinary diversion procedures. **(A)** Ileal conduit. **(B)** A continent urinary diversion.
Figure 32-11 Incisions used for kidney surgery. **(A)** flank, **(B)** lumbar, and **(C)** thoracoabdominal.
Figure 32-12 **(A)** In acute tubular necrosis, tubular epithelium is damaged by hypotension and shock or by a toxin. **(B)** As a result, the flow of glomerular filtrate is blocked, and increased pressure in the tubule causes glomerular filtration to slow. The elimination of salt, water, and waste products is impaired.
Figure 32-13 The relationship of renal function to BUN and serum creatinine in the course of chronic renal failure.
Figure 32-14 The multisystem effects of uremia.
Figure 32-15 A hemodialysis system.
Figure 32-16 An arteriovenous fistula.
Figure 32-17 Continuous renal replacement therapy (CRRT) from an artery to a vein.
Figure 32-18 Peritoneal dialysis.
Figure 32-19 Placement of a transplanted kidney.

LEARNING OUTCOME 1

Describe the pathophysiology of common disorders of the kidneys and urinary tract.

CONCEPTS FOR LECTURE

1. Urinary incontinence is involuntary urination. This disorder can affect young and old and is not a normal part of the aging process.
2. Urinary incontinence has many causes.
3. Urinary retention occurs when the bladder cannot empty and may be caused by an obstructive or neurologic cause.
4. Urinary tract infection is a common disorder due to a bacterial process. This disorder is more prevalent in women. UTIs are also a common nosocomial infection.
5. Cystitis is a lower urinary tract infection involving the bladder.
6. Pyelonephritis is an inflammatory disorder of the kidney, usually due to a bacterial process.

POWERPOINT LECTURE SLIDES

1 Bladder sphincter and loss of control

2 Types of urinary incontinence: stress, urge, functional, overflow, and reflex

3 Causes of urinary retention, obstruction vs. neurologic

4 Causes of urinary tract infection and anatomic review for increased incidence in women

5 Cause of cystitis

6 Cause of pyelonephritis

7 How glomerulus is damaged and its associated symptoms

Concepts for Lecture *continued*

7. Glomerulonephritis is a disorder of the glomerulus, which may be acute or chronic and may lead to renal failure.
8. Nephrotic syndrome is a group of symptoms that result from damage to the glomerular membrane.
9. Urinary calculi are small stones that develop anywhere in the urinary system. They may cause blockage, pain, and hematuria.
10. Hydronephrosis is dilation of the renal pelvis and calyces. This dilation may damage the nephron.
11. Polycystic kidney disease is a hereditary disease characterized by cyst formation and kidney enlargement. This disease may affect children and adults.
12. The kidneys are usually protected from trauma by the rib cage. Trauma to the kidneys may result in pain, hemorrhage, and possible shock due the vascular nature of the kidney.
13. Both the bladder and the kidney may be affected by cancerous tumors. These tumors may lead to obstruction, renal failure, hemorrhage, and invasion of other surrounding tissues.
14. Acute renal failure is a rapid abrupt decline in renal function.
15. Acute renal failure may result from prerenal causes such as hypovolemia. Intrarenal causes include inflammation and vascular disorders such as hypertension. Acute tubular necrosis occurs from exposure to nephrotoxins.
16. Acute renal failure can last up to 1 year and is identified by various stages of renal decline.
17. Chronic renal failure is a slow process resulting in kidney destruction.
18. Chronic renal failure may go on for years prior to being recognized, or the client having symptoms.

PowerPoint Lecture Slides *continued*

8 The physiology of nephritic syndrome

9 How urinary calculi develop and how they can cause additional injury within the urinary system

10 The development of hydronephrosis and its affect on kidney function

11 Review of a kidney with polycystic kidney disease and effects on urinary development

12 Types of kidney trauma and the effects on the kidney

13 Review of types of tumors affecting the urinary system, and how these tumors cause ongoing damage, and may affect urine formation

14 The pathophysiology of acute renal failure

15 The types of causes of acute renal failure: prerenal, intrarenal, and acute tubular necrosis

16 The stages of acute renal failure

17 How damage is done in chronic renal failure

18 How chronic renal failure may progress with few clinical signs and symptoms

Suggestions for Classroom Activities

1. Using case studies, have students describe the types of urinary incontinence.
2. Have students describe the formation of urinary calculi.
3. Using various case studies, have students describe the causes of acute renal failure.
4. Using an anatomic model, discuss how hydronephrosis may develop due to obstruction.
5. Have students develop a plan of care for a client with chronic renal failure.

Suggestions for Clinical Activities

1. Have students care for clients experiencing urinary incontinence. Have each student present his or her client and the type of incontinence, and how it varies from other types.
2. In reviewing client histories, have students identify potential causes of acute/chronic renal failure.

Learning Outcome 2

Compare and contrast the manifestations of common disorders of the kidneys and urinary tract.

Concepts for Lecture

1. Incontinence is categorized as stress, urge, overflow, reflex, and functional. Each has a different presentation although all result in involuntary leakage of urine.

PowerPoint Lecture Slides

1 Using visual slides describe the various types of urinary incontinence: stress, urge, reflex, functional, and overflow.

© 2007 Pearson Education, Inc.

CONCEPTS FOR LECTURE *continued*

2. Urinary retention is the inability to empty the bladder completely. Assessment findings may include firm, distended bladder that may be misplaced. The patient may complain of the sensation of needing to void, or may not have any symptoms if the patient is suffering from a neurologic cause.
3. Symptoms of urinary tract infection vary due to location. Cystitis may cause painful urination, urgency, and foul-smelling urine. Pyleonephritis may cause chills, fever, general malaise, and costovertebral tenderness.
4. Glomerulonephritis may cause few clinical symptoms although edema may be seen. The patient may exhibit changes in the urine such as proteinuria, hematuria. Blood studies may include an increase in BUN and creatinine.
5. Acute glomerulonephritis may develop quickly in 10–14 days after initial injury or infection. Hypertension and edema may be seen.
6. Chronic glomerulonephritis may occur over time. Symptoms develop slowly and may not be recognized until renal failure is evident.
7. Urinary calculi may obstruct urine flow. This usually results in pain, hematuria, and may cause symptoms of UTI such as pyelonephritis, depending on stone location.
8. Hydronephritis may develop quickly and cause acute symptoms such as fever, colicky flank pain, hematuria, and nausea and vomiting. Hydronephritis that develops over time may also cause hematuria and fever, yet pain may be dull and intermittent.
9. Polycystic kidney disease occurs over time, and symptoms may not occur until the client is in his thirties or forties. Common symptoms usually include flank pain, hematuria, proteinuria. Renal calculi may also develop and most clients develop hypertension. The kidneys enlarge and may be palpable. Over time, signs of renal failure develop.
10. Kidney trauma may develop from a blunt or penetrating injury. Due to the vascular nature of the kidney, hemorrhage is common. Renal trauma may also include pain, hematuria, oliguria or anuria.
11. Tumors of the urinary system cause symptoms based on their location. Bladder tumors may cause signs of obstruction or UTI.
12. Kidney tumors may disrupt urine formation, leading to proteinuria and hematuria. The patient may exhibit flank pain and signs of pyelonephritis. The patient may also exhibit fatigue, weight loss, and anemia.
13. Renal failure may be acute or chronic. Acute renal failure is manifested by oliguria. Acute renal failure involves three stages.
14. Chronic renal failure is a slow process and is often not identified until uremia develops. Clients may have early signs such as nausea, apathy, weakness and fatigue. As the disease progresses, clients may experience vomiting, lethargy, and confusion. Uremic symptoms may develop and affect all systems.

POWERPOINT LECTURE SLIDES *continued*

2 Using visual slides, show how urinary retention is caused by obstruction. Discuss the assessment findings in urinary retention.

3 Differentiate the signs and symptoms found in lower urinary tract infections vs. pyelonephritis.

4 Show the changes that occur in glomerulonephritis.

5,6 Differentiate the signs and symptoms that occur with acute vs. chronic glomerulonephritis.

7 Review the causes of urinary calculi, and the injury they can cause in the urinary system. Discuss how calculi cause changes in the urine.

8 Using an anatomic visual slide, show the changes in the kidney due to hydronephritis and how this affects urine formation.

9 Review the statistical occurrence of polycystic kidney disease, its presentation, and an anatomic presentation of the changes in kidney function and appearance.

10 Review the types of kidney trauma and signs and symptoms that may develop. Discuss treatment options for kidney trauma.

11,12 Show visuals of the bladder and kidney tumors and how the location of these tumors may affect urine formation and output.

13 Discuss the causes of acute renal failure: prerenal, intrarenal, and acute tubular necrosis. Discuss the signs and symptoms seen in each of the phases of acute renal failure.

14 Review the causes of chronic renal failure and the changes that occur in each body system. Discuss the clinical manifestations that occur and why they affect all body systems.

© 2007 Pearson Education, Inc.

Suggestions for Classroom Activities

1. Using a game format, give students clinical manifestations and have them determine the origin of the problem.
2. Giving the students a case study for acute renal failure, have them identify the cause and phase the client is experiencing.
3. Using patient scenarios, have the student identify risk factors for urinary and kidney disorders.

Suggestions for Clinical Activities

1. With the clients they are assigned, have the students identify risk factors for urinary and kidney disorders.
2. Develop a plan of care for a client with a urinary/kidney disorder.
3. Using laboratory studies, have students identify changes in urinary/kidney function.

Learning Outcome 3

Discuss the nursing implications of medications prescribed for clients with these disorders.

Concepts for Lecture

1. Tolterodine and oxybutynin are anticholinergic medications used to treat urge incontinence. Due to the effects of these medications, they may be contraindicated in other disorders such as glaucoma or urinary retention. Estrogen may also be given to increase urethral resistance.
2. Cholinergic medications may be useful in promoting bladder emptying in urinary retention. Common medications include bethanechol chloride. If bladder retention is due to an enlarged prostrate, medications may be given to help decrease the size of the prostrate and maintain urine flow. Common medications include tamsulosin, finasteride.
3. Urinary tract infections are commonly treated with antibiotics that are affective against gram-negative bacilli. An uncomplicated UTI is treated with a 3–7 to 10-day course of medications such as sulfonamide, trimethoprim-sulfamethoxazole, and fluoroquinolones.
4. No specific medications are available for treating glomerulonephritis. Often glucocorticoids are used along with other immunosuppressive medications to reduce the risk of renal failure. It is important that students recognize the side effects of steroids on other body systems. Antibiotics may be used in clients with poststreptococcal glomerulonephritis.
5. Nephrotic syndrome results from damage to the glomerular membranes and results in severe protein loss in the urine.
6. Medications used in renal calculi are mainly for pain relief. Narcotic analgesics provide analgesia and relieve ureteral spasms. Often analgesics are administered intravenously for rapid pain relief. Respiratory rate and depth along with level of consciousness are important assessment parameters when administering IV narcotics.
7. In polycystic kidney disease, medications are given to control symptoms associated with the disease. These include ACE inhibitors and other antihypertensive agents.

PowerPoint Lecture Slides

1 Review cholinergic and anticholinergic effects.

- Discuss the indications for medications such as tolterodine and oxybutynin and their common side effects.
- Review contraindications to these medications.

2 Using an anatomic visual, show how cholinergic medications may increase bladder emptying.

- The prostrate may be the cause of the obstruction. Therefore, medications such as tamsulosin and finasteride may be used to promote urinary excretion.
- Discuss the side effects of these medications and precautions with their administration.
- Monitoring urine flow will assist in determining the effectiveness of the medications.

3 Using an anatomic review, discuss the pathophysiology of UTI and how *Escherichia coli* is introduced into the urinary system.

- Review the antibacterial properties of common antibiotics used to treat UTI.
- Show a visual slide on obtaining a urine culture.
- Antibiotic resistance is of great concern; clients should complete all their medications. Patient teaching will help prevent any confusion regarding medication administration.
- Pyelonephritis may require antibiotics for up to 21 days.
- The patient may go home with a PICC (peripherally inserted central catheter) for IV antibiotics. Care of the PICC line is similar to that of other central lines. Discuss flushing, dressing changes, and important patient teaching.

4 Glomerulonephritis is often seen following an infection of Group A beta-hemolytic streptococcus. In this instance, antibiotics are used to treat the infections.

- Glucocorticoids are used for their anti-inflammatory response to assist in decreasing the effects of glomerulonephritis.

© 2007 Pearson Education, Inc.

Concepts for Lecture *continued*

8. Tumors of the kidney and bladder may be malignant and need chemotherapeutic agents to treat the tumor. These agents may be instilled in the bladder for local action. Other medications may include BCG live to cause a local inflammatory action to reduce superficial tumors.
9. During acute renal failure, all nephrotoxic medications are avoided or used with great caution. All drug dosages need to be adjusted due to slowed excretion and prolonged half-life. The same is true with chronic renal failure.
10. Often in chronic renal failure, diuretics such as furosemide (Lasix) are used to reduce fluid volume. Daily weight and intake and output will assist in monitoring fluid status. Other antihypertensive agents, particularly ACE inhibitors, are used to lower blood pressure.
11. Care must be taken to know the type of dialysis the patient with chronic renal failure is having. Many medications are excreted during the dialysis treatment and their doses need to be adjusted when the patient is receiving dialysis.

PowerPoint Lecture Slides *continued*

- Glucocorticoids have a number of side effects: poor glucose tolerance, often elevating blood glucose levels; poor wound healing; decreased immune response. Long-term use can lead to cataracts and osteoporosis.

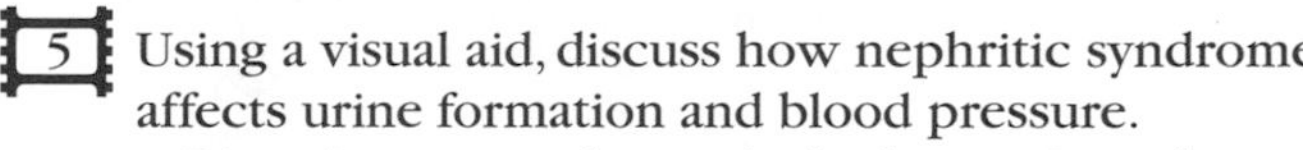

5 Using a visual aid, discuss how nephritic syndrome affects urine formation and blood pressure.

- Diuretics are used to assist in decreasing edema by increasing urine output. Various types of diuretics are available.
- Common side effects of diuretics include electrolyte imbalance and weight loss. Monitoring daily weights and electrolyte studies will assist in recognizing complications.
- Discuss the angiotensin–aldosterone system. Angiotensin converting enzyme (ACE) inhibitors assist in preventing the conversion of angiotensin I to angiotensin II, which is a potent vasoconstrictor. This assists in lowering blood pressure and helps with protein loss through the urine.
- Glucocorticoids such as prednisone may be used. Review common side effects.

6 Discuss the formation of urinary calculi and how they may cause discomfort.

- Narcotics are often used intravenously to decrease pain. Common important assessments with narcotics include respiration and level on consciousness.
- Patient teaching is important to assure understanding in the administration of medications and to prevent side effects.
- Clients should be made aware that they should not drive or operate machinery while taking narcotics, and also the expectations of the progression of the stone.
- After the stone is passed, it may be analyzed. If it is a calcium stone, thiazide diuretics are used to decrease the formation of calcium stones.
- Discuss patient teaching so the client knows how to obtain the stone by straining the urine, and why stone analysis may assist in the prevention of further stone formation.

7 Polycystic kidney disease affects blood pressure. Medications used to treat this disorder are aimed at treating the symptoms.

- Actions of antihypertensive agents may vary. Discuss their use and potential side effects.

8 With tumors of the kidney and bladder, chemotherapeutic agents are often used.

- Chemotherapeutic agents may be given into the bladder (intravesical) to assist in decreasing tumor size. Side effects often include frequency, dysuria, and contact dermatitis due to bladder irritation.

PowerPoint Lecture Slides *continued*

- As always, caution must be used when handling chemotherapeutic agents.
- Common side effects of chemotherapeutic agents include immunosuppression. Discuss how to assess for immunosuppression and common precautions taken to prevent infections.
- Analgesia may also be used to promote comfort in clients with bladder or kidney tumors.

9 Review common nephrotoxic medications. Ex: NSAIDs.

- Discuss the half-life of medications and why this is affected in acute renal failure.

10 Furosemide (Lasix) may be used in chronic renal failure for the following indications: reduce fluid volume, lower blood pressure, and lower serum potassium levels.

- ACE inhibitors are also used to control blood pressure.
- Acidosis may occur in renal failure; sodium bicarbonate or calcium carbonate help to manage acidosis.
- Serum potassium levels may rise in chronic renal failure due the inability to excrete potassium. Potassium binding exchange resins may be given orally or rectally to promote potassium excretions. Discuss the indications and administration of these medications.
- Glucose and insulin may be used to drive potassium back into the cell until a more definitive treatment can be used.
- Anemia is common in these clients. Nutritional supplements may help to combat nutritional deficiencies.

11 The various types of dialysis may affect medication administration and excretion. Review the types of dialysis: hemodialysis, peritoneal dialysis.

- Hemodialysis alters medication levels in the blood. The nurse needs to know what medications to give prior to dialysis and which ones to hold. Due to the potential of hypotension during the treatment, antihypertensives are often held.

Suggestions for Classroom Activities

1. Using a case study approach, have students identify medication classes that may be beneficial in each disorder.
2. Have students discuss the angiotensin–aldosterone system and determine where various medications act to cause therapeutic results.
3. Give students the names of various medications and have them discuss the major side effects in small groups.

Suggestions for Clinical Activities

1. Using assigned clients, have students identify potential nephrotoxic medications.
2. Have students discuss medications clients are taking and determine their use in urinary and kidney disorders.
3. Identify common side effects of medications that clients may be taking for urinary or kidney disorders.

© 2007 Pearson Education, Inc.

4. Using medications clients may be taking, have students discuss the medication and its effects during hemodialysis. Also, should the medication be held prior to hemodialysis.

LEARNING OUTCOME 4

Provide appropriate nursing care for the client having surgery of the kidneys or urinary tract.

CONCEPTS FOR LECTURE

1. Urinary incontinence is commonly not treated with surgery. If the incontinence is due to urethrocele bladder, neck suspension may be done. If urinary incontinence or retention is due to an enlarged prostrate, a prostatectomy may be performed.
2. The patient with glomerulonephritis may undergo a kidney biopsy to determine the extent of kidney damage and to identify any causative factors. The patient will need adequate teaching and NPO status 8 hours prior to the procedure. Following the biopsy, close assessment of the site for bleeding is important for the first 24 hours. Frequent vital signs along with assessment of hemoglobin and hematocrit are important. Urine output is monitored, and initial hematuria is common.
3. Urinary calculi may require surgical intervention if the stones are too large to pass spontaneously. Lithotripsy, which is the crushing of renal calculi with sound or shock waves, is commonly used. For the patient undergoing lithotripsy, adequate preprocedure teaching is needed. Following the procedure, frequent vital sign monitoring is needed. The urine output is monitored for amount, color, and clarity.
4. Hydronephritis may develop from a renal calculi. To assist in keeping the ureters open, a ureteral stent may be placed. These stents may be temporary or permanent and are placed during cystoscopy or during a surgical incision.
5. Kidney trauma may necessitate surgical intervention to stop bleeding and/or remove a damaged kidney. Ensuring the patient is hemodynamically stable postoperatively is essential. Adequate vital sign monitoring, hemoglobin and hematocrit, and intake and output are essential to ensure adequate circulation and prevent complications. As with other surgical procedures, the surgical site is monitored for bleeding and drainage.
6. Tumor of the kidney and urinary tract may necessitate surgical intervention. Surgical procedures may range from simple resection of the tumor to removal of the bladder and surrounding structures.
7. The patient with chronic renal failure will need a dialysis access. This involves the creation of an arteriovenous fistula. Preoperative teaching is similar to other surgical procedures. Postoperatively, assessment of vital signs, laboratory studies, and patency of the graph is essential. The graph is assessed for a palpable bruit or thrill and an audible bruit to assure functioning.

POWERPOINT LECTURE SLIDES

- General Pre/Postoperative Guidelines
  - Review common preoperative guidelines that apply to preoperative patients:
    - Preoperative teaching—expectations, procedure, and postoperative course
    - Consent form
    - Respiratory function—incentive spirometry
    - Equipment seen postoperatively: indwelling urinary catheter, nephrostomy tubes, nasogastric tube if needed, intravenous lines
    - NPO status
    - Activity level; when expected to get out of bed
    - Pain management, the need for patient-controlled analgesia or other pain control methods
- Review common postoperative care that may apply to all patients having surgical procedures of the urinary system:
  - Frequent vital sign monitoring and the signs of hemorrhage
  - Monitor urine for amount, color, clarity
  - Accurate intake and output
  - Care of indwelling catheters and nephrostomy tubes
  - Monitor dressing
  - Pain management
  - Patient teaching to ensure understanding of activity level, potential complications, and when to notify health care provider once discharged

1 Using an anatomic visual, discuss the bladder neck suspension procedure.

- Review the care of a suprapubic and/or urethral catheter.
- Using an anatomic visual, discuss the various types of prostate surgery.
- Using a visual slide, review the use of continuous bladder irrigation, rationale, length of use, expected outcomes, and accurate intake and output.

2 Review the anatomy of the kidney and how a renal biopsy is obtained.

- Discuss the highly vascular nature of the kidney and the importance of monitoring for hemorrhage.
- Review the occurrence of hematuria and that it should clear in about 24 hours.

© 2007 Pearson Education, Inc.

POWERPOINT LECTURE SLIDES *continued*

- Discuss activity restrictions such as coughing, straining for 24 hours postoperatively.

3 Discuss the signs of a urinary calculi and the importance of pain management.

- Review the lithotripsy procedure both noninvasive and invasive.
- Discuss normal urine color and clarity postprocedure.
- Review the care of urethral catheters and nephrostomy tubes including irrigation.
- Discuss potential complications.
- Review the common incisional sites for a nephrectomy.
- Discuss the importance of pulmonary hygiene.
- Review the importance of monitoring the dressing and adequate intake and output.
- Force fluids to 2,000–2,500 mL/day.
- Label and secure all catheters, nephrosotomy tubes.

4 Review the indications for a urethral stent and common anatomic placement.

- Discuss the types of procedures used for placing a urethral stent.
- Discuss the signs of infection and/or bleeding.

5 With renal trauma, surgery is often needed. Review trauma with kidney surgery (discussed in Slide 3). When discussing renal trauma, reviewing the vascular nature of the kidney may be beneficial.

6 Review the origin of kidney tumors. A nephrectomy may be done (discussed in Slide 3).

- Using an anatomic slide, discuss the cystectomy procedure.
- Review the origin of a stoma.
- Show the students a normal postoperative stoma, red and edematous.
- Review potential stoma emergencies, cyanosis and gray.
- Discuss the various appliances to maintain continence.
- Review the procedure to change a urinary appliance on a stoma; include measuring and fitting the appliance.
- Review irrigation or catheterization of the stoma.
- Discuss the importance of skin care and method to foster self-esteem.

7 Using an anatomic slide, review the formation of an arteriovenous fistula.

- Adding sounds, review assessing for a bruit.
- Review the placement of a catheter for peritoneal dialysis and the care involved in the catheter.
- Discuss the indications for a renal transplant.
    - Review the requirements for transplant, blood typing, ability to comply with medical regimen.

© 2007 Pearson Education, Inc.

PowerPoint Lecture Slides *continued*

- Using an anatomic slide, discuss the surgical procedure including the presence of the diseased kidney.
- Review the signs and types of rejection.
- Discuss the process of organ donation.

Suggestions for Classroom Activities

1. Using a case study format, have students identify potential complications for clients undergoing surgical procedures of the urinary system.
2. Divide the students into small groups. Have each group develop a teaching plan for a client undergoing various surgical procedures. Have each group present to the class.
3. Have a volunteer wear a urinary diversion device for one day. Allow that student to discuss his or her feelings and how nurses can assist in this lifestyle change.

Suggestions for Clinical Activities

1. If feasible, have students spend time with an enterostomal nurse and identify potential stoma sites.
2. Have students care for clients undergoing surgical procedures of the urinary system.
3. Discuss laboratory findings and how they may relate to disorders and complications of the urinary system.
4. Allow students to assess a postoperative client.
5. Have students share information about their client and the client's urinary system.

Learning Outcome 5

Use the nursing process as a framework for providing individualized care to clients with disorders of the kidneys or urinary tract.

Concepts for Lecture

1. Applying the nursing process to clients with disorders of the kidneys or urinary tract is similar for many of the disorders.
2. Client-centered goals assist in providing care to clients with kidney and urinary disorders. Goals may be short term or long term depending on the disease process. Goals assist in planning nursing care.
3. Many nursing interventions are common for clients with kidney and urinary disorders. Interventions are numerous and expand to include all systems.
4. Evaluation of the client includes ensuring the client remains free of discomfort. Client should exhibit normal vital signs, stable weight, and laboratory studies that are normal for the client and her disease process. The client demonstrating adequate care of equipment and remaining free of infection are also part of the evaluation phase.
5. Discuss the different disorders of the kidneys and urinary tract.

PowerPoint Lecture Slides

1 Review the nursing process.

2 Assessment: Questions

- Subjective data: onset, duration of symptoms, other diseases, medications, changes in fluid intake or urine output.
- Objective data: vital signs, urine and laboratory studies, weight changes, presence of edema.
  - Questions to ask to elicit a voiding history.
  - How to assess level of comfort, both verbal and nonverbal, along with common symptoms associated with various disorders, e.g., retention, discomfort; calculi, pain.
  - Assessing level of knowledge and support systems.
  - Interpretation of laboratory studies, normal/abnormal findings on urinalysis, blood work.
  - Correlation of vital signs with renal disorders.

3 Review appropriate goals for the client with renal, urinary disorder. Differentiate short-term and long-term goals for various disorders.

4 Review the procedure for monitoring intake and output. Discuss the importance of daily weights. Review the care of indwelling catheters and other urinary equipment. Discuss the proper procedure to obtain various urine cultures. Review the procedure for insertion of a catheter. Discuss patient teaching methods.

© 2007 Pearson Education, Inc.

POWERPOINT LECTURE SLIDES *continued*

5 Disorders of the urinary tract:

- Urinary Incontinence—obtaining subjective and objective information in reference to incontinence episodes
  - How to implement a toileting schedule
  - Teaching Kegel exercises
- Urinary Retention—obtaining a history for urinary retention.
  - Using the bladder scan
  - Straight catheterization techniques
  - Palpation of the bladder
  - Applying pressure to ensure bladder emptying (Crede maneuver)
- Urinary Tract Infections—obtaining subjective and objective information.
  - How various diseases may increase the incidence of UTI
  - Assessing for costovertebral angle tenderness
  - Patient teaching to force fluids, what types of fluids may irritate the bladder
  - Patient teaching for female clients
- Glomerulonephritis—assessment of edema and rating scale
  - Where to assess for edema
  - Instituting a fluid restriction
    - Low sodium diet
- Nephrotic Syndrome—as glomerulonephritis
- Urinary Calculi
  - Review assessing the urine with a dipstick to determine hematuria
  - Address the quality of pain in renal calculi
  - Review the procedure for screening urine to detect stones
- Hydronephritis
  - Review the causes and monitoring of intake and output
  - Discuss the care of indwelling catheters, ureteral stents, and nephrostomy tubes
- Polycystic Kidney Disease
  - Review the sequelae of the disease and important patient teaching aspects, increased fluid, avoidance of nephrotoxic medications
  - Discuss genetic counseling and the possibility of renal transplant
- Kidney Trauma
  - Discuss how the kidney is protected by the ribs
  - Review the signs of hemorrhage and shock that may occur
  - Assess vital signs, skin color, and temperature
- Tumors of the Kidney and Urinary Tract
  - Provide the client with information regarding the types of surgery and changes in lifestyle
  - Encourage early self-care of urinary diversion device to promote well-being
  - Force fluids

 © 2007 Pearson Education, Inc.

POWERPOINT LECTURE SLIDES *continued*

- Allow the client to ventilate feelings due to changes in lifestyle and unknown course of the disease
- Refer to support groups for ongoing support and services if needed

- Renal Failure
  - Discuss the signs of renal failure, acute and chronic, and obtaining a history
  - Cardiovascular function may affect renal perfusion
  - Excess fluid balance may include intake and output, vital signs, auscultation of lungs, assessment of edema monitoring of electrolytes and BUN and creatinine, maintaining a fluid restriction
  - Nutrition—review diet and the importance of maintaining adequate nutritional status
  - Risk for Infection—hand washing, skin care, mouth care monitoring of the CV = BC
  - Anxiety—changes in lifestyle, adhering to medical regimen and dialysis schedule, support services available to the client and family
  - Deficient Knowledge—care of dialysis graph

SUGGESTIONS FOR CLASSROOM ACTIVITIES

1. Using a case study approach, have students develop a plan of care and a teaching plan for a client with a renal or urinary disorder.
2. Give students various measurements and have them determine the amount of intake in milliliters, and then determine how to construct this information for a client with a fluid restriction.
3. Have students keep a voiding diary, which may assist them in teaching clients.
4. Have students develop goals for clients with urinary disorders.

SUGGESTIONS FOR CLINICAL ACTIVITIES

1. Have students care for clients with kidney and urinary disorders and develop a plan of care.
2. Allow students to assess clients with AV fistulas in the clinical setting.
3. If feasible, have students observe hemodialysis.
4. Have students participate in client/family teaching for clients with renal disorders.
5. Have students participate in intake and output and fluid restrictions.
6. Give students clients that need daily weights. Allow the students to assess fluid status based on weight changes.

© 2007 Pearson Education, Inc.

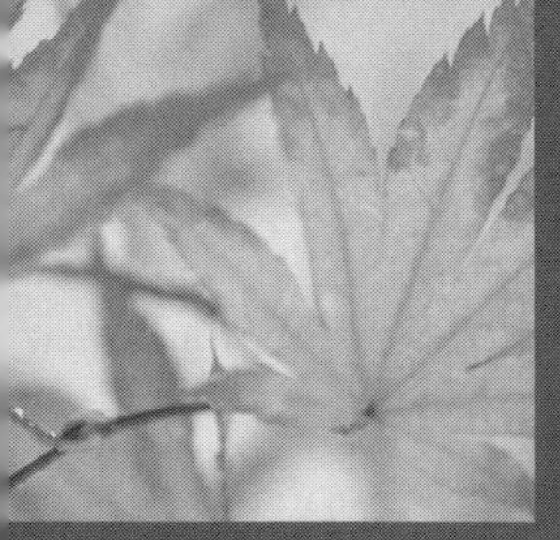

CHAPTER 33
THE REPRODUCTIVE SYSTEM AND ASSESSMENT

RESOURCE LIBRARY

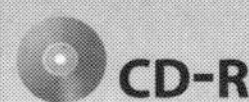

CD-ROM

Male Pelvis
Male Reproductive System
Female Pelvis
Female Reproductive System

IMAGE LIBRARY

Figure 33-1 The male reproductive system.
Figure 33-2 The internal organs of the female reproductive system.
Figure 33-3 (**A**) Changes in ovarian follicles during the 28-day ovarian cycle. (**B**) Corresponding changes in the endometrium during the menstrual cycle.
Figure 33-4 The female external genitalia.
Figure 33-5 Structure of the female breast.
Figure 33-6 Palpating the male inguinal area for bulges.
Figure 33-7 A suggested pattern for palpating the breast.
Figure 33-8 Laparoscopy. A flexible, lighted instrument (laparoscope) is inserted through a small incision to visualize the abdominal and pelvic cavities.

LEARNING OUTCOME 1

Identify the major structures and functions of the male reproductive system.

CONCEPTS FOR LECTURE

1. Although the structures of the reproductive system in men and women are very different their functions are the same: reproduction, sexual pleasure, and development of secondary sex characteristics. The reproductive organs, in conjunction with the endocrine system, also produce hormones that are important in biologic development and sexual behavior. The male reproductive system includes paired testes, the scrotum, ducts, glands, and penis.

POWERPOINT LECTURE SLIDES

1 Structures and Functions of the Male Reproductive System
- Testes—produce:
  - sperm (spermatogenesis)
  - Testosterone
- Ducts
- Semen
- Prostate gland
- Penis

LEARNING OUTCOME 2

Identify the major structures and functions of the female reproductive system.

CONCEPTS FOR LECTURE

1. The female reproductive system includes the paired ovaries and fallopian tubes, uterus, vagina, and external genitalia. In women the urethra and urinary meatus are separated from the reproductive system; however, they are so close together that a health problem with one also affects the other.

POWERPOINT LECTURE SLIDES

1 Major Structures of the Female Reproductive System and Their Function
- Internal structures include:
  - Ovaries—produce progesterone and estrogen
  - Fallopian tubes—thin tubes attached to the uterus; fertilization usually occurs in outer portion
  - Uterus—receives fertilized ovum
  - Vagina—birth canal; allows excretion of menstrual fluid, organ of sexual response

POWERPOINT LECTURE SLIDES *continued*

- External genitalia include:
  - Mons pubis
  - Labia
  - Clitoris
  - Vaginal opening
  - Urethral opening
  - Glands
  - Breasts

LEARNING OUTCOME 3

Identify and describe the functions of female sex hormones.

CONCEPTS FOR LECTURE

1. The female sex hormones include estrogen, progesterone, and androgens. They are responsible for the menstrual cycle, secondary sex characteristics, and preparation of the uterus for growth of the fetus.

POWERPOINT LECTURE SLIDES

1 Functions of Female Sex Hormones
- Estrogen: essential to development of secondary sex characteristics; levels vary with menstrual cycle
- Progesterone: affects breast glandular tissue and the endometrium; relaxes smooth muscle during pregnancy; ↓ uterine contractions
- Androgens produced in small quantities by adrenal glands and ovaries responsible for normal hair growth patterns at puberty
- FSH (follicle-stimulating hormone) and LH (luteinizing hormone) stimulate maturation of immature ovum

LEARNING OUTCOME 4

Collect subjective and objective assessment data related to the reproductive system.

CONCEPTS FOR LECTURE

1. Assessment of the reproductive system includes both subjective and objective data. This data can be obtained through a health history, physical examination, and diagnostic tests.

POWERPOINT LECTURE SLIDES

1 Subjective Data
- Presenting problem
- Identify onset manifestations and effect on ADLs
- Inquire about contributing factors
- Question if any problems with urination
- Vaginal discharge
- History of chronic diseases
- Family history of cancer
- Exposure to DES
- Current medications
- Physical and/or psychosocial stressors that may contribute to sexual problems
- Use of alcohol tobacco or street drugs
- History of sexual problems

1a Physical Assessment of the Male Includes:
- Inspection and palpation of the breasts, inguinal area, and groin
- Inspect penis, urinary meatus; retract foreskin, check for sores or skin irritations
- Palpate each testes and epidydymis

© 2007 Pearson Education, Inc.

PowerPoint Lecture Slides *continued*

1b Physical Assessment of the Female Includes:
- Inspection and palpation of each breast
- In lithotomy position inspect and palpate:
  - Labia majora and labia minora
  - Inspect the clitoris, vaginal opening, and perineum
  - Instruct client to bear down; check for bulging of vaginal wall, protrusion of cervix or uterus, or urinary incontinence

Learning Outcome 5

Provide appropriate nursing care for clients undergoing diagnostic tests related to the reproductive system.

Concepts for Lecture

1. A variety of diagnostic tests may be used to identify disorders affecting the reproductive system, including diagnostic examinations, laboratory testing, imaging studies, and special procedures. Diagnostic examinations, such as digital prostate exam and clinical breast exam, are discussed in chapters that follow. The following procedures are discussed in this chapter: pelvic examination, mammography, abdominal laparoscopy, and colposcopy.

PowerPoint Lecture Slides

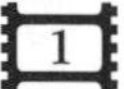
Nursing Care for Diagnostic Procedures
- Nursing Care Checklist: Pelvic Examination (Box 33-2)
- Nursing Care: Mammography (see discussion of mammography—Imaging Studies section)
- Nursing Care Checklist: Laparoscopy (Box 33-3)
- Laboratory Tests (Table 33-1)

Suggestions for Classroom Activities

1. Using visual aids, identify the major structures and functions of the male reproductive system.
2. Assign the students to define and discuss the key terms related to the female reproductive system.
3. Identify the major structures of the female reproductive system and discuss their functions.
4. Identify and describe the functions of female sex hormones.
5. Describe normal age-related changes in female reproductive system structure and function.
6. Identify the laboratory and diagnostic tests related to the male reproductive system. Discuss the nursing implications for each test.

Suggestions for Clinical Activities

In the clinical lab setting have students demonstrate:
- Preparation of patient for a pelvic examination
- Pap smear

© 2007 Pearson Education, Inc.

CHAPTER 34
CARING FOR MALE CLIENTS WITH REPRODUCTIVE SYSTEM DISORDERS

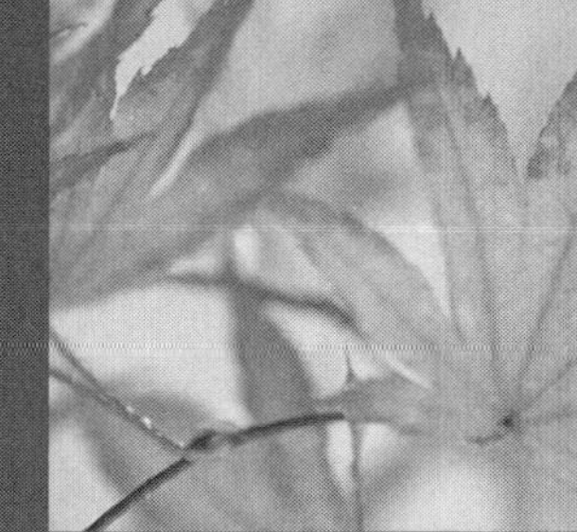

RESOURCE LIBRARY

IMAGE LIBRARY

Figure 34-1 Benign prostatic hyperplasia (BPH).
Figure 34-2 Transurethral resection of the prostate (TURP). A resectoscope inserted through the urethra is used to remove excess prostate tissue.
Figure 34-3 Operation of an artificial urinary sphincter.
Figure 34-4 Common scrotal masses.
Figure 34-5 Types of penile implants. (**A**) Semirigid rods implanted in the corpora cavernosa keep the penis in a constant state of semierection. (**B**) With an inflatable penile implant, the client compresses a pump in the scrotum to fill cylinders in the corpora cavernosa and achieve an erection. Pressing a release valve returns the fluid to a reservoir.

LEARNING OUTCOME 1

Describe the pathophysiology and manifestations of common disorders of the male reproductive system.

CONCEPTS FOR LECTURE

1. Prostate problems such as benign prostatic hyperplasia and prostate cancer are the most common problems affecting the male reproductive system, especially in older adults. Other disorders that will be discussed include prostatitis, structural and inflammatory disorders of the testes and scrotum, infertility, scrotal masses and trauma, testicular cancer, phimosis, priapism, cancer of the penis, erectile dysfunction, and ejaculatory dysfunction.

POWERPOINT LECTURE SLIDES

1 Benign prostatic hyperplasia (BPH)
- Pathophysiology
  - Testosterone produced in testes converted to DHT in prostate
  - DHT stimulates growth of prostate
  - Estrogen produced in small amounts in the male; ↑with aging
  - It is believed estrogen makes prostate more responsive to DHT, promoting growth
  - BPH develops as small nodules next to urethra, causing compression of urethra
- Manifestations (Box 34-1)

1a Prostate Cancer
- Pathophysiology
  - Usually adenocarcinoma originating in glandular epithelial cells
  - As tumor enlarges may compress urethra
  - Can spread locally to seminal vesicles or bladder, rarely to bowel
  - Metastasis is common
  - Pelvic lymph nodes most commonly involved
  - Can spread to liver and lungs; PSA significantly elevated
- Manifestations (Box 34-5)

1b Prostatitis
- Pathophysiology
  - Acute bacterial prostatitis associated with UTIs, usually *E. coli* infecting organism
  - Nonbacterial; may be caused by chlamydia, mycoplasmas, and viruses; exact cause unknown
  - May be a type of STD or autoimmune disorder
- Manifestations (Box 34-7)

PowerPoint Lecture Slides *continued*

Structural and Inflammatory Disorders of the Testes and Scrotum

- Testicular torsion
  - Pathophysiology
    - Twisting of the testes and spermatic cord
    - Elevated hormone levels and abnormal attachment of testes to scrotum contributing factor
    - Trauma to scrotum in predisposed individuals
    - Medical emergency
  - Manifestations
    - Sudden onset of scrotal pain
    - Nausea and vomiting
    - Cremasteric reflex depressed or absent
- Cryptoorchidism
  - Pathophysiology
    - Failure of one or both testes to descend through the inguinal ring into the scrotum
  - Manifestations
    - Primarily childhood problem
    - Problem in adolescence and adulthood; ↑ risk for testicular cancer and infertility
- Orchitis
  - Pathophysiology
    - Inflammation of testicle
    - Caused by:
      - Infection in other area of GU tract
      - Complication of mumps (adult men ↑ risk)
      - Trauma
      - Vasectomy
      - Scrotal surgeries
  - Manifestations
    - Severe testicular pain and swelling
    - Complications include hydrocele or abscess

1d Infertility

- Inability to conceive a child during a year or more of unprotected intercourse
- Sterility
  - Absolute inability to conceive
- Pathophysiology
  - Results from testicular disorders
  - Systemic disease
  - Hormonal disorder
  - Obstructed outflow of sperm from testes
- Manifestations
  - Sperm count below 20 million/mL

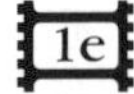
Scrotal Masses

- Hydrocele
  - Pathophysiology
    - Collection of fluid in the sac that encloses testes
    - Cause not always identified; may follow epididymitis, orchitis, injury, or tumor
    - Manifestations
      - Scrotal enlargement
      - Pain or tight sensation in scrotum

© 2007 Pearson Education, Inc.

PowerPoint Lecture Slides *continued*

1f Scrotal Trauma
- Pathophysiology
  - Minor injuries cause temporary hematomas from minor crushing or straddle-type injury
  - Severe crush injuries can rupture testicles
  - Scrotal skin or clothing trapped in machinery can cause avulsion injury
  - Penetrating injuries (gunshot or knife wounds)

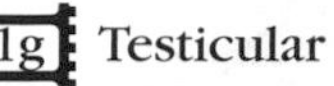

1g Testicular Cancer
- Most common cancer in men ages 15–35
- Most treatable cure rate 90%
- Pathophysiology
  - Unknown cause
  - Risk factors for testicular cancer include:
    - Age
    - Cryptorchidism
    - Family history
    - Race and ethnicity
  - Grows within one testicle; local spread limited
  - Can spread rapidly through lymph and blood vessels to other organs with metastasis to lungs, bone, or liver
- Manifestations
  - Painless hard nodule
  - Occasional dull ache in pelvis or scrotum

1h Phimosis
- Constriction of foreskin so that it cannot be pushed over the glans penis
- Pathophysiology
  - Can be congenital
  - Caused by infection or injury
- Manifestations
  - If foreskin forcibly retracted, can cause impaired circulation to glans penis

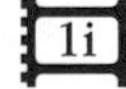

1i Priapism
- Sustained painful erection not associated with sexual arousal
- Pathophysiology
  - Caused by impaired blood flow in the corpora cavernosa of penis
  - Can be idiopathic or caused by certain drugs
- Manifestations
  - Sustained erection that is painful and harder than normal
  - Can cause tissue damage and impotence
  - Risk factors (Box 34-9)

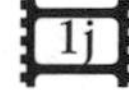

1j Cancer of the Penis
- Rare cause unknown
- Risk factors include phimosis, HPV, exposure to UV light, unprotected sex with multiple partners, cigarette smoking
- Pathophysiology
  - 95% squamous cell carcinoma
  - Nodular or wartlike growth or red velvety lesion on glans or foreskin

© 2007 Pearson Education, Inc.

POWERPOINT LECTURE SLIDES *continued*

- Manifestations
  - Mass or persistent sore or ulcer at distal end of penis involving the glans or foreskin
  - Lesions painless but may bleed or ulcerate
  - Purulent, foul-smelling discharge under foreskin

[1k] Erectile Dysfunction (Impotence)
- Inability to attain and maintain an erection
- Occurs in men over age 65
- Possible causes: diabetes, atherosclerosis, and many drugs
- Most caused by physiologic problem
- 10% to 20% psychologic
- Pathophysiology
  - Atherosclerosis interferes with blood supply to penis
  - Innervation can be disrupted by radical prostatectomy, diabetes, and multiple sclerosis
  - Antihypertensives, psychotropics, and hormones interfere with normal mechanisms
- Ejaculatory dysfunction types
  - **Premature ejaculation**—caused by psychologic factors or diabetes
  - **Delayed ejaculation**—related to aging or drugs
  - **Retrograde ejaculation**—semen discharged into bladder; related to treatment of prostate disorders or testicular cancer

LEARNING OUTCOME 2

Discuss nursing implications for medications used to treat disorders of the male reproductive system.

CONCEPTS FOR LECTURE

1. Several drugs may be used to shrink the enlarged prostate and reduce the manifestations of BPH. These drugs include Proscar and the $alpha_1$ blockers Hytrin, Cardura, and Flomax. Erectile dysfunction can be treated with drugs that work in a variety of ways. Viagra (Sidenafil) and related drugs do not directly cause an erection but enhance the natural response to sexual stimuli.

POWERPOINT LECTURE SLIDES

[1] Nursing Implications for Medications Used to Treat Disorders of the Male Reproductive System
- Proscar used for treatment of BPH inhibits conversion of testosterone to DHT in prostate; can cause impotence
- $Alpha_1$ blockers
- Hytrin, Cardura, Flomax relax smooth muscle in prostate, urethra, and bladder neck, reducing urethral obstruction and improving urinary flow and symptoms of BPH
- Hormone therapy for advanced prostate cancer
- Nursing implications for medications used to treat disorders of the male reproductive system
- Erectile dysfunction (Table 34-2)

LEARNING OUTCOME 3

Use the nursing process to provide care for clients with disorders of the male reproductive system.

CONCEPTS FOR LECTURE

1. The focus of nursing care for male clients with reproductive disorders is prevention by early detection and treatment. This can be accomplished through teaching

POWERPOINT LECTURE SLIDES

[1] Nursing Care: BPH
- Assess older men for:
  - Difficulty voiding, starting or stopping flow

© 2007 Pearson Education, Inc.

Concepts for Lecture *continued*

monthly testicular self-examination beginning at age 15. Additional nursing interventions for specific disorders are described in the slides.

PowerPoint Lecture Slides *continued*

- Size of urinary stream
- Symptoms of burning, frequency, urgency, nocturia
- Monitor output
- Check color, clarity, and odor of urine

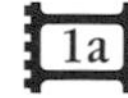

Nursing Care: Prostate Cancer

- Nursing Care Checklist: Transrectal Ultrasound-Guided Biopsy of the Prostate (Box 34-6)
- Nursing assessment of the client with prostate cancer done before admission to facility usually for radiation treatment or surgery (refer to Chapter 12 for data collection prior to radiation therapy)
- Client undergoing surgery—refer to Chapter 9 for preop and postop assessment
- Nursing priority for clients with prostate cancer are the effects on urinary elimination and sexual dysfunction
- Nursing diagnoses for client with prostate cancer
  - Impaired Urinary Elimination (Risk for Incontinence)
  - Sexual Dysfunction
  - Pain

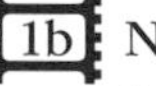

Nursing Care: Prostatitis

- Encourage client to ↑ fluids to 3 L/day
- Maintain regular bowel habits
- Use of local heat or sitz bath to relieve pain
- Stress importance of finishing antibiotic therapy
- Nonbacterial—frequent ejaculation will ↓ congestion of gland

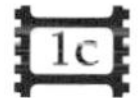

Nursing Care: Structural and Inflammatory Disorders of Testes and Scrotum

- Obtain data Hx of trauma, surgery swelling, or pain
- Ask about onset, duration, and severity of symptoms
- Inspect scrotum for swelling, redness, bruising, or discoloration
- Palpate testes and epididymis for tenderness warmth or masses
- Teach client about disorder and treatments
- If surgery planned, discuss fears about surgery, pain management postop, and measures to reduce bleeding
- Postop—report excessive swelling or discoloration

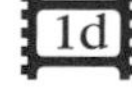

Nursing Care: Testicular Cancer

- Prevention—monthly testicular self-examination beginning at age 15 (Box 34-8)
- Identify testicular cancer early; ask client if any change in size of testicles
- Palpate scrotum and testicles, noting any difference in size
- Report immediately any testicle that is hard, irregular in shape, or fixed within scrotum

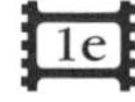

Client with Orchiectomy

- Focus is on teaching and psychologic support
- Nursing Diagnoses for postop orchiectomy:
  - Deficient Knowledge

© 2007 Pearson Education, Inc.

PowerPoint Lecture Slides *continued*

- – Discuss use of analgesics, ice bags, and scrotal support
- – Client should contact physician if complications arise such as gaps in incision or large amount of bleeding
- ○ Risk for Sexual Dysfunction
  - – Discuss concerns with client
  - – Assist to express concerns
  - – Reinforce teaching that sexual function is rarely affected by testicular cancer and treatment
- • Discuss follow-up care for testicular cancer including physical exams, chest x-rays, tumor markers, and CT scans for 5–10 years postorchiectomy

1f Nursing Care: Phimosis
- Teach client about importance of good hygiene to prevent infection and possible phimosis
- Teach client to perform self-examination for Ca of penis

1g Nursing Care: Priapism
- Initial Rx includes analgesics, sedation, fluids
- Ice packs to perineum
- Inspect penis for degree of erection
- Monitor urine output
- Report oliguria or signs of acute urinary retention
- Reassure client sexual function maintained after surgical shunting

1h Nursing Care: Cancer of the Penis
- Observe for visible lesions and report
- Postop—for localized lesion treated with laser or external radiation—monitor surgical site
- Penectomy with a urethrostomy done only when metastasized
- Intake and output; teach client perineal care
- Use sitz baths to relieve pain
- Teach client risks of unprotected sex and UV rays

1i Nursing Care: Erectile Dysfunction
- Assessment: ask about chronic diseases or medications that may be responsible
- Explore psychosocial stressors
- Ask specific questions about sexual function
- Provide information about treatment
- Refer client and partner for counseling

Learning Outcome 4

Contribute to the plan of care for male clients undergoing surgery for reproductive system disorders.

Concepts for Lecture

1. In both BPH and prostate cancer, surgery is often the treatment of choice. Minimally invasive procedures such as balloon dilation, laser prostatectomy, or transurethral incision of the prostate (TUIP) may be used to treat BPH. Prostate cancer, on the other hand, is treated with a prostatectomy.

PowerPoint Lecture Slides

1 Plan of Care For Male Patients Undergoing a Protestatectomy
- Transurethral resection of the prostate (TURP) checklist (Box 34-2)
- Approaches to protestatectomy (Table 34-1)

© 2007 Pearson Education, Inc.

Suggestions for Classroom Activities

1. Describe the pathophysiology and clinical manifestations of common disorders of the male reproductive system.
2. Using transparencies, identify the laboratory and diagnostic tests related to the male reproductive system.
3. Divide the class into three groups to discuss the disorders of the penis. Assign one group to develop a poster presentation of preventive measures for phimosis; another to develop a nursing care plan for priapism; and the third to develop a postoperative care plan for a client experiencing cancer of the penis.
4. Assign students to study the key terms for the chapter and to be prepared to define and discuss them.
5. Identify the laboratory and diagnostic tests related to the male reproductive system. Discuss the nursing implications for each test.
6. Discuss the use of the nursing process to provide care for clients with disorders of the male reproductive system.
7. Divide the class into small groups. Assign each group to one of the following scenarios. Ask them to use the nursing process to present a case study or a teaching plan for their scenario.

   Scenario A: A 26-year-old male with nonbacterial prostatitis

   Scenario B: A 62-year-old male postoperative suprapubic prostatectomy

   Scenario C: A 14-year-old male with testicular torsion

   Scenario D: A 35-year-old male who is thinking about having a vasectomy

   Scenario E: A 30-year-old male who is experiencing testicular cancer

Suggestions for Clinical Activities

Assign students to care for clients experiencing disorders of the male reproductive system. Have them discuss their observations in postconference. Ask the students to list nursing diagnoses and outcomes for the client, and have an open discussion on the nursing interventions needed to meet them.

© 2007 Pearson Education, Inc.

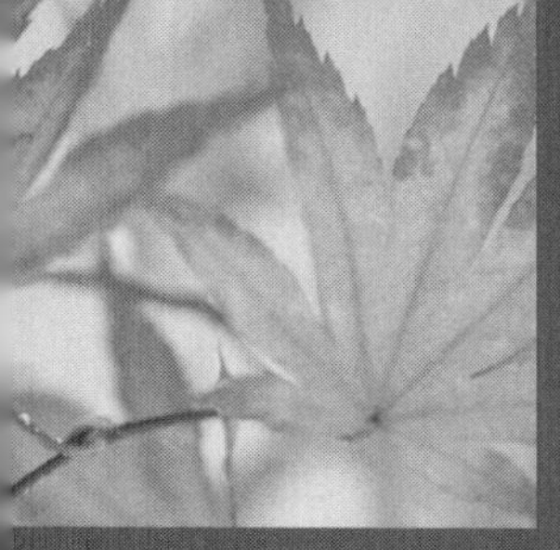

CHAPTER 35
CARING FOR FEMALE CLIENTS WITH REPRODUCTIVE SYSTEM DISORDERS

RESOURCE LIBRARY

IMAGE LIBRARY

LEARNING OUTCOME 1

Discuss the physiologic changes that occur during the perimenopausal period and the interdisciplinary care of clients during menopause.

CONCEPTS FOR LECTURE

1. Perimenopausal period includes 4–5 years surrounding menopause where estrogen production declines and menses permanently ceases.
2. Interdisciplinary care is focused on managing symptoms, teaching about menopause, and discussing postmenopausal health risks.

POWERPOINT LECTURE SLIDES

1 Menopause (Climacteric)

- Natural biologic end of reproduction
- Perimenopause—4–5 years surrounding menopause
- Estrogen production declines
- Menses ceases due to loss of ovarian function
- Normal physiologic process
- Hormonal changes lead to unpleasant side effects
- Occurs age 45–55
- Surgical menopause

PowerPoint Lecture Slides *continued*

- Physiology and manifestations
  - Ovarian follicles decline significantly
  - Ovarian estrogen production ceases
  - Loss of breast tissue, body hair, subcutaneous fat
  - Ovaries and uterus shrink in size
  - Skin less elastic
  - Vaginal and perineal tissue atrophy
  - Vaginal lubrication decreases
  - Imbalance of estrogen and FSH causes vasomotor instability (hot flashes, night sweats, palpitations, and headaches)
  - Vaginitis and dyspareunia
  - Irregular menstrual cycle

2 Interdisciplinary Care
- Focus on managing symptoms
- Hormone replacement therapy
- Complimentary therapy
- Nursing care
  - Deficient Knowledge: Menopause
  - Sexual Dysfunction
  - Risk for Situational Low Self-Esteem
  - Teaching

Suggestions for Classroom Activities

1. Discuss stereotypical attitudes about menopause.
2. Ask students to debate the benefits/risks of hormone replacement therapy.

Suggestions for Clinical Activities

Present case study of client experiencing surgical menopause after a hysterectomy.

Learning Outcome 2

Discuss the physiologic changes and the interdisciplinary care of clients with disorders of menstruation and abnormal uterine bleeding.

Concepts for Lecture

1. Monthly menstruation is often accompanied by minor discomforts and occasionally by episodes of abnormal uterine bleeding.
2. Interdisciplinary care is focused on managing symptoms during menstruation, and identifying and treating underlying causes of menstrual disorders and abnormal bleeding.

PowerPoint Lecture Slides

1 Disorders of Menstruation
- Monthly discomfort includes:
  - Breast tenderness
  - Feeling of heaviness and congestion in the pelvic region
  - Cramping
  - Backache
  - Other symptoms
- Premenstrual syndrome
  - Irritability
  - Depression
  - Edema
  - Breast tenderness
  - Cause unknown
  - Pathophysiology and manifestations
    - Hormonal changes
    - Increased aldosterone levels cause salt and water retention
    - Role of neurotransmitters
    - 7–10 days prior to onset of menstrual flow

PowerPoint Lecture Slides *continued*

- Dysmenorrhea
  - Pain with menstruation
  - Occurs in 75% of women
  - Pathophysiology and manifestations
    - Primary dysmenorrhea
      - Prostaglandin stimulations
      - Cramping and restriction of blood flow causing ischemia and pain
      - Lasts 12–24 hours
    - Secondary dysmenorrhea
      - Underlying disorder causing scarring or injury to reproductive organs

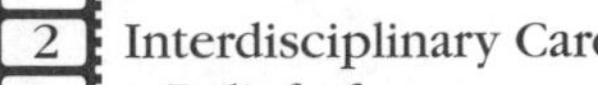

Interdisciplinary Care

- Relief of symptoms
- Diet, exercise, relaxation
- Reduce salt intake
- Restrict caffeine
- Vitamins
- Medications
  - NSAIDs
- Nursing care
  - Effective Therapeutic Regimen Management

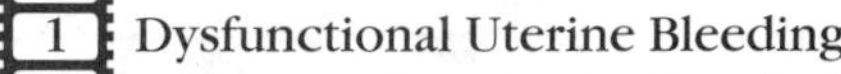

Dysfunctional Uterine Bleeding

- Abnormal amounts of vaginal bleeding
- Hormone imbalance or pelvic tumors
- Pathophysiology and manifestations
  - Hormone imbalance of progesterone deficiency
  - Anovulation—absence of ovulation
  - Amenorrhea—absence of menstruation
  - Oligomenorrhea—scant menses
  - Metrorrhagia—bleeding between menstrual periods
  - Postmenopausal bleeding

2 Interdisciplinary Care

- Focus on treating underlying disease
- H&P
- Abdominal and pelvic exam
- Diagnostic studies—hormone levels
- Pelvic ultrasound
- Laparoscopy
- Medications
  - Oral contraceptives
  - Iron preparations
- Surgery
  - D&C
  - Endometrial ablation
  - Uterine balloon heat therapy
  - Hysterectomy
    - Abdominal or vaginal
- Nursing care
  - Ineffective Coping
  - Sexual Dysfunction
  - Support and teaching

© 2007 Pearson Education, Inc.

Suggestions for Classroom Activities

1. Review anatomy of reproductive system and normal hormonal changes.
2. Discuss female stereotyping around menstrual discomforts.

Suggestions for Clinical Activities

Arrange for students to assist with pelvic exams in physician's office or emergency department.

Learning Outcome 3

Discuss the physiologic changes and the interdisciplinary care of clients with disorders of female reproductive tissue.

Concepts for Lecture

1. Disorders of female reproductive tissue include growths of female reproductive tissue that are benign in nature.
2. Interdisciplinary care is focused on identifying and correcting the disorder and on management of symptoms.

PowerPoint Lecture Slides

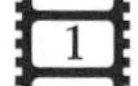

Disorders of Female Reproductive Tissue

- Endometriosis
  - Endometrial tissue outside of uterus
  - Found on ovaries, pelvic organs
  - Pathophysiology
    - Unknown
    - Backflow of menstrual blood carrying endometrial cells through fallopian tubes into the pelvis
    - Ectopic endometrial tissue responds to ovarian cycle and bleeding during menses
    - Cysts, scarring, inflammation, and adhesions
    - Infertility or bowel obstruction
  - Manifestations
    - Dysmenorrheal
    - Dyspareunia
    - Infertility
- Ovarian cysts
  - Fluid-filled sac on vulva, endometrium, ovaries
  - Follicular or corpus luteum cysts
  - May be asymptomatic or rupture, causing pain confused with pain of appendicitis
  - Polycystic ovary syndrome
- Uterine fibroids
  - Benign tumors of the uterus or cervix
  - Common among women of childbearing age
  - Primary cause for a hysterectomy
  - Three to nine times more common in African American women
  - Cause unclear—related to estrogen secretion
  - Classification (Figure 35-2)

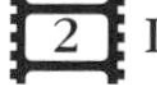

Interdisciplinary Care

- Diagnostic tests and evaluation
  - H&P
  - Pelvic exam
  - LH, FSH, and serum testosterone levels
  - GTT
  - Laparoscopy
- Medications
  - NSAIDs
  - Oral contraceptives
  - Analgesics
- Surgery

POWERPOINT LECTURE SLIDES *continued*

- Nursing care
  - Assessment of pain
  - Nursing diagnoses
    - Pain
    - Anxiety
  - Teaching
    - Disorder and treatment
    - Pain control

SUGGESTIONS FOR CLASSROOM ACTIVITIES

Compare and contrast symptoms of a ruptured ovarian cyst versus appendicitis.

SUGGESTIONS FOR CLINICAL ACTIVITIES

Assign students clients having hysterectomies for treatment of uterine fibroids.

LEARNING OUTCOME 4

Discuss the physiologic changes and the interdisciplinary care of clients with infections of the female reproductive system.

CONCEPTS FOR LECTURE

1. Common local infections of the reproductive system are in the vagina and are often caused by sexually transmitted diseases.
2. The interdisciplinary care for local infections is focused on the diagnosis and treatment of the underlying infection and supportive care to relieve symptoms.
3. Infections that involve the pelvic organs are systemic in nature and a result of an inflammatory process, toxic shock, or HIV/AIDS.
4. The interdisciplinary care for systemic infections of the reproductive organs is focused on the diagnosis and treatment of the underlying infection, care to manage the systemic effects, and supportive care to relieve symptoms.

POWERPOINT LECTURE SLIDES

1 Localized Infections of the Reproductive Organs

- Vaginitis
  - Inflammation or infection of the vagina
  - Causes
    - Fungal
    - Protozoan
    - Bacterial
  - Risk factors
    - Unprotected sexual activity
    - Multiple partners
    - Antiobiotics
    - Obesity
    - Diabetes
    - Pregnancy
    - Poor personal hygiene
  - Pathophysiology
    - Change in normal vaginal flora
    - Change in pH of vaginal secretions
    - Estrogen levels
    - Most cause vaginal discharge, itching and burning, and dysuria

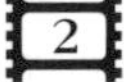

Interdisciplinary Care of Localized Infections of the Reproductive Organs

- Diagnosis by pelvic exam
- Vaginal cultures
  - Wet mount
  - Clue cells
- GTT
- Pregnancy test
- Medications
- Nursing care
  - Assessment
  - Diagnosis
    - Deficient Knowledge: Prevention of Vaginitis
    - Pain

© 2007 Pearson Education, Inc.

PowerPoint Lecture Slides *continued*

- Teaching
  - Sexual activity
  - Use of vaginal creams and lubricants
  - Medication administration

3 Systemic Infections of the Reproductive Organs

- Pelvic inflammatory disorder (PID)
  - Fallopian tubes, ovaries, uterus, and cervix
  - Cause—*Neisseria gonorrhoeae* and/or *Chlamydia trachomatis*
  - Major cause of female infertility
  - Pathophysiology
    - Infectious organ enters the vagina and travels to the uterus during intercourse or sexual activity
    - Can enter during childbirth, abortion, reproductive tract surgery
    - Spreads to surrounding pelvic organs
    - Enters lymphatic system and bloodstream, leading to systemic infection
  - Manifestations
    - Fever
    - Vaginal discharge
    - Severe lower abdominal pain
    - Scarring of fallopian tubes can lead to infertility
    - Pain during intercourse
- Toxic shock syndrome (TSS)
  - Rare
  - Caused by *Staphylococcus aureus* infection
  - Related to use of tampons during menstruation
  - Vaginal barrier contraceptives
  - Pathophysiology
    - Virulent strain of *S. aureus* enters bloodstream
    - Septic reaction of toxins causing shocklike syndrome

4 Interdisciplinary Care of Systemic Infections of the Reproductive Organs

- Diagnosis and treatment
  - Endocervical secretion cultures
  - Laparoscopy
  - Surgery
  - Medications
    - Treat infection
    - Restore stability to cardiovascular system and other body systems in TSS
  - Surgery
  - Nursing care
    - Assessment
    - Nursing diagnoses
      - Risk for Injury
      - Deficient Knowledge: STD Prevention
      - Ineffective Tissue Perfusion: TSS
      - Decreased Cardiac Output: TSS
    - Teaching directed to preventing future infections

© 2007 Pearson Education, Inc.

Suggestions for Classroom Activities

1. Create a crossword puzzle for students to identify common organisms that cause infections of the reproductive organs.
2. Discuss statistics and risks of unprotected sexual activity and incidence of infections of the reproductive organs.
3. Go to the Centers for Disease Control and Prevention website to find statistics on incidence of sexually transmitted diseases.

Suggestions for Clinical Activities

Arrange for clinical experience in outpatient clinic for the treatment of sexually transmitted diseases.

Learning Outcome 5

Discuss the physiologic changes and the interdisciplinary care of clients with malignant tumors of the female reproductive system.

Concepts for Lecture

1. Malignant tumors are located in the cervix, uterus and uterine lining, ovaries, and vulva. The most common is cervical cancer.
2. Diagnosis and screening procedures are essential in the early diagnosis of cancers of the female reproductive system.
3. Interdisciplinary care is directed at removal of the tumor, management of symptoms, and controlling the risk of metastasis.

PowerPoint Lecture Slides

1 Malignant Tumors of the Female Reproductive Organs

- Cervical cancer
  - Common
  - Early detection and intervention lead to decreased incidence and death
  - Related to infection of the cervix with HPV
  - Pathophysiology and manifestations
    - Changes in squamous cells of the cervix
      - Cervical intraepithelial neoplasia
      - Cells become abnormal over time
    - No symptoms in early stage
    - Bleeding and leukorrhea
- Endometrial cancer
  - Common
  - Older women, ages 50–70
  - Risk factors
  - Early diagnosis and treatment yields 90% survival
  - Pathophysiology and manifestations
    - Slow growing
    - Associated with estrogen excess
    - Tumor begins in the fundus of the uterus and spreads through the female reproductive tract
    - Metastasis occurs via the lymph and bloodstream
    - Abnormal uterine bleeding—painless
- Ovarian cancer
  - Most lethal, often asymptomatic
  - Spread beyond the ovaries at the time of diagnosis
  - European and American women
  - Risk factors
  - Pathophysiology
    - Different tissue types lead to different types of ovarian cancers
    - Grow and spread at different rates
    - Spread by shedding cancer cells into the peritoneal cavity by direct invasion of the bowel and bladder
    - Spread through lymph and blood

© 2007 Pearson Education, Inc.

POWERPOINT LECTURE SLIDES *continued*

- Cancer of the vulva
  - Older women, ages 60–70
  - Younger women associated with sexually transmitted disease, HPV
  - Pathophysiology and manifestations
    - Primary site—labia majora
    - Spreads by direct extension into surrounding tissue
    - May cause no symptoms
    - Puritis and irritation of the vulva are the most common symptoms

2 Interdisciplinary Care of Malignant Tumors of the Reproductive Organs

- Diagnosis
  - H&P
  - Pap smear—cervical cancer
  - Colposcopy
  - Biopsy
    - Cervix
    - Uterine tissue
  - CA125 tumor marker for ovarian cancer
  - Transvaginal ultrasound
  - Laparoscopy
- Treatment
  - Laser
  - Conization
  - Radioactive implants
  - Hysterectomy
  - Salpingo-oophrectomy
  - Pelvic lymph node removal
  - Pelvic exenteration (removal of all pelvic contents)
  - Chemotherapy
  - Vulvectomy
- Nursing care
  - Nursing diagnoses
    - Impaired Tissue Integrity
    - Fear
    - Disturbed Body Image
    - Pain
  - Teaching
    - Disease and treatment
    - Skin care
    - Symptom control during chemotherapy
    - Pain control

SUGGESTIONS FOR CLASSROOM ACTIVITIES

1. Discuss cancer screening procedures and lead debate on benefits.
2. Present a case study discussion on uterine cancer.

SUGGESTIONS FOR CLINICAL ACTIVITIES

1. Assign students to clinical experience in physician's office or clinic so that they can assist with Pap tests and vaginal exams.
2. Arrange for observational experience in OR to see hysterectomy surgery.

© 2007 Pearson Education, Inc.

Learning Outcome 6

Discuss the physiologic changes and the interdisciplinary care of clients with structural disorders of the female reproductive system.

Concepts for Lecture

1. Structural disorders occur that are either congenital or acquired or result from relaxation or weakening of the pelvic floor muscles.
2. Interdisciplinary care is directed toward symptom management and normal bowel and bladder function.
3. Abnormal openings may occur between the vagina and urinary bladder or rectum.

PowerPoint Lecture Slides

1 Structural Disorders of the Female Reproductive System

- Uterine displacement
  - Anteverted
  - Retroverted
  - Anteflexed
  - Retroflexed
- Pelvic organ prolapse
  - Cystocele—prolapse of the urinary bladder into the vagina
  - Rectocele—protrusion of the anterior rectal wall into the vagina
  - Uterine prolapse—prolapse of the uterus into the vagina

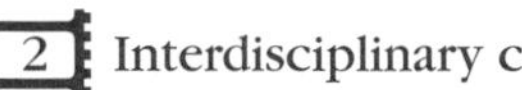

2 Interdisciplinary care

- Diagnosis made by physical exam
- H&P
- Surgical repair
- Nursing care
  - Kegel exercises
  - Stress incontinence
- Teaching
  - Anatomy of female reproductive system
  - Awareness of symptoms and management of incontinence

Suggestions for Classroom Activities

1. Discuss value of Kegel exercises.
2. Have students research articles on incontinence problems in women with structural disorders of the female reproductive tract.

Suggestions for Clinical Activities

Arrange for OR observation experience for surgical repairs of structural disorders.

Learning Outcome 7

Discuss the physiologic changes and the interdisciplinary care of clients with disorders of the breast tissue.

Concepts for Lecture

1. Noncancerous breast disorders include fibrocystic changes, inflammatory mastitis, and disorders related to breast augmentation.
2. Interdisciplinary care of noncancerous breast disorders encompasses diagnosis of underlying causes and symptom management.
3. Cancer of the breast is one of the leading causes of death among women, although its incidence is declining.
4. The pathophysiology, diagnosis, staging, and treatment of breast cancer encompass a multidisciplinary approach.

PowerPoint Lecture Slides

1 Noncancerous Breast Disorders

- Fibrocystic breast changes
  - Benign breast tissue changes
  - Swelling, pain, tenderness, and lumpiness
  - Excessive response to cyclic hormone changes
  - Common in women ages 30–50
  - Pathophysiology and manifestations
    - Nonproliferative
    - Proliferative
    - Bilateral or unilateral

© 2007 Pearson Education, Inc.

CONCEPTS FOR LECTURE *continued*

5. Nursing care of the client with breast cancer is comprehensive in nature and focuses on early detection, support through the diagnosis and treatment processes, and assisting the client to maintain a health body image.

POWERPOINT LECTURE SLIDES *continued*

- Mastitis
  - Inflammation of breast tissue
  - Tenderness, swelling, and redness
  - Lactating women
  - Caused by organisms from infant's nose and throat
  - Treated with antibiotics
- Disorders related to breast augmentation
  - Scarring
  - Implant rupture
  - Affect early detection of breast cancer

2 Interdisciplinary Care
- Diagnosis may be through biopsy
- Supportive care for symptom management
- Teaching
  - Self breast exam
  - Well-fitting bra
  - Medications and pain control

3 Breast Cancer
- Incidence is second only to lung cancer for cancer-related deaths in women
- Also strikes men but rare
- Incidence is stable and mortality is decreasing
- Lower in African American women but mortality higher

4 Multidisciplinary Approach to Care of Breast Cancer
- Pathophysiology
  - Unregulated growth of abnormal breast cells
  - Hormone dependent
  - Occur in ductal areas
  - Noninvasive (*in situ*)
    - Malignant cells proliferate within the ducts
    - Do not invade surrounding tissue
    - Nipple and subareolar region
    - Mass is seen on mammography
    - Increases the risk for invasive breast cancer
  - Invasive
    - Arise from the intermediate ducts
    - Differentiated by cell type
    - Prognosis and treatment depend on stage
    - Spread to surrounding tissue
    - Metastasize through regional lymph and blood
    - Common sites are bone, brain, lung, liver, and skin
  - Atypical types
    - Inflammatory carcinoma
      - Most malignant form
      - Metastasis develops early and widely
      - Poor prognosis
    - Paget's disease
      - Rare
- Manifestations
  - Small hard and painless lump or mass
  - Upper outer quadrant

PowerPoint Lecture Slides *continued*

- ○ Skin changes (Figure 35-8)
- ○ Metastasis to bone and lung
  - – Pathologic fractures
  - – Respiratory difficulties
- Breast Cancer Screening
  - ○ Self breast exam (Figure 35-9)
  - ○ Clinical breast exam
  - ○ Mammography
- Diagnostic tests
  - ○ Diagnostic mammography
  - ○ Ultrasonography
  - ○ CT, MRI, PET
  - ○ Cytologic exam
  - ○ Tissue biopsy
    - – Fine needle aspiration
    - – Core needle biopsy
    - – Excisional biopsy
- Staging
  - ○ Tumor size
  - ○ Lymph node involvement
  - ○ Metastasis
- Treatment
  - ○ Medications
    - – Systemic therapy
      - ▪ Tamoxifen
      - ▪ Chemotherapy
      - ▪ Biologic
  - ○ Radiation therapy
  - ○ Surgery
    - – Breast conserving
    - – Mastectomy
    - – Breast reconstruction
  - ○ Metastatic breast cancer treatment
    - – Palliation
    - – Extending life
    - – Ensuring comfort

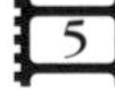

Nursing Care

- Assessing
  - ○ Risk factors for breast cancer
  - ○ Self breast exam
- Diagnosis, planning, and implementation
  - ○ Decisional Conflict: Treatment Options
  - ○ Anticipatory Grieving
  - ○ Risk for Infection
  - ○ Risk for Injury
  - ○ Risk for Disturbed Body Image
- Continued care
  - ○ Postoperative exercises
  - ○ Healing of surgical site
  - ○ Emotional support
  - ○ Balanced diet
  - ○ Prosthesis

© 2007 Pearson Education, Inc.

Suggestions for Classroom Activities

1. Discuss breast augmentation surgery and have students bring in articles about the risks of this type of surgery.
2. Review procedure for teaching self breast exam.
3. Invite representative from the American Cancer Society to discuss breast cancer research, support groups, and services for breast cancer patients.
4. Invite breast cancer survivors to share their personal experiences with breast cancer.
5. Invite prosthesis representative to bring in prosthetic devices that are used by women.

Suggestions for Clinical Activities

1. Ask students to prepare a teaching presentation on self breast exam.
2. Assign students to clients being treated for breast cancer.
3. Arrange for student experience in an outpatient setting where clients receive chemotherapy or radiation for the treatment of breast cancer.
4. Present a case study of a client with breast cancer during a postclinical conference.
5. Arrange for students to observe mastectomy procedures and breast reconstruction procedures in the operating room.

© 2007 Pearson Education, Inc.

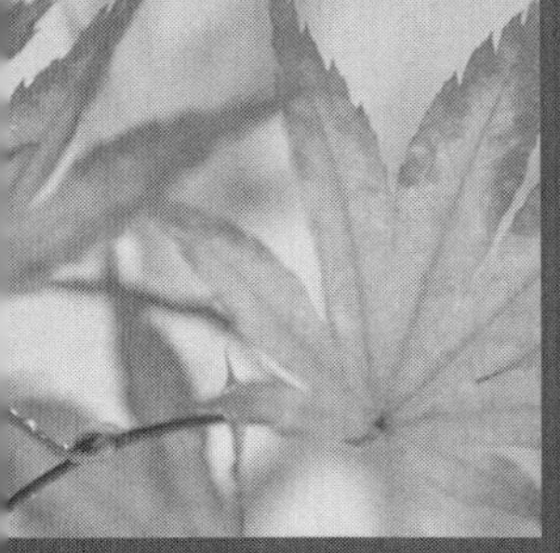

CHAPTER 36
CARING FOR CLIENTS WITH SEXUALLY TRANSMITTED INFECTIONS

RESOURCE LIBRARY

IMAGE LIBRARY

Figure 36-1 Genital herpes blisters as they appear on the penis.
Figure 36-2 Genital warts (condyloma acuminatum) on the penis.
Figure 36-3 Chancre of primary syphilis on the penis.
Figure 36-4 Palmar rash of secondary syphilis.

LEARNING OUTCOME 1

Describe the pathophysiology of the most common sexually transmitted infections (STIs).

CONCEPTS FOR LECTURE

1. Any infection transmitted by sexual contact, including vaginal, oral, and anal intercourse, is referred to as a sexually transmitted infection (STI).

POWERPOINT LECTURE SLIDES

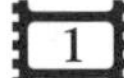
1 Chlamydial Infection
- Most common STI in U.S.
- Pathophysiology
  - Caused by a bacteria (*Chlamydia trachomatis*) that acts like a virus (only reproduces in host cell)
  - Spread by any sexual contact or to neonate by passage through birth canal
  - Incubation period 1 to 3 weeks
  - Invades the cervix in women
  - Invades the urethra in men
- Causes trachoma chronic contagious conjuntivitis

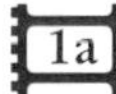
1a Genital Herpes
- Pathophysiology
  - Chronic asymptomatic STI
  - 45 million infected in U.S.
  - Caused by herpes simplex virus type 2 (HSV-2)
  - HSV-2 closely related to HSV-1, which causes cold sores
  - HSV-1 can also infect genitalia
  - Spread by vaginal, anal, or oral genital contact
  - Incubation period 3 to 7 days
  - Within a week develop painful red papules
  - Small painful blisters form after papules appear
  - Blisters break, shed virus, and create painful ulcers
  - First outbreak of herpes lesions called first episode infection
  - Subsequent episodes are recurrent and usually less severe
  - Period between episodes called latency
  - Still infected even during latency

- Prodromal symptoms (warning signals or clues) include burning, itching, tingling, or throbbing at sites where lesions commonly appear; sexual contact should be avoided during this time

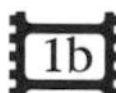
Genital Warts (*Condyloma acuminatum*)

- Pathophysiology
  - Caused by human papillomavirus (HPV)
  - Most common STI in U.S.
  - HPV transmitted by all types of sexual contact
  - Incubation period about 3 months
  - Different types of HPV cause chronic genital infections
  - Most people who carry HPV have no symptoms
  - Others develop single or multiple cauliflower-like growths on the vulvovaginal area, perineum, penis, urethra, or anus
  - In women growths may appear on the cervix
- Some subtypes of HPV are associated with cervical dysplasia and ↑ risk of cervical cancer
- Infants infected can develop papillomatosis chronic respiratory condition

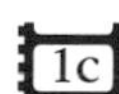
Gonnorhea

- Pathophysiology
  - Most common reportable communicable disease
  - Caused by *Neisseria gonorrhoeae* gram-negative diplococcus
  - Incubation period 2 to 8 days
  - Transmitted by direct sexual contact
  - Targets cervix and male urethra
  - Without treatment can spread to other organs
- In men causes acute painful inflammation of prostate, epididymis, and periurethral glands; can cause sterility
- In females can cause PID, endometritis, salpingitis, and pelvic peritonitis

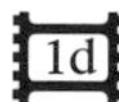
Syphilis

- Pathophysiology
  - Complex STI can infect almost any body tissue or organ
  - Caused by a spirochete (*Treponema pallidum*)
  - Transmitted through open lesions during any sexual contact
  - May also be transmitted through infected blood and body fluids such as saliva
  - Incubation period 20 to 30 days
  - Once in the system, spreads through blood and lymphatic system
- Has three clinical stages: primary, secondary, tertiary

© 2007 Pearson Education, Inc.

LEARNING OUTCOME 2

Identify laboratory and diagnostic tests used for STIs.

CONCEPTS FOR LECTURE

1. Early diagnosis and treatment of STIs can prevent complications and transmission of infection.

POWERPOINT LECTURE SLIDES

1 Laboratory and Diagnostic Tests Used for STIs

- Chlamydia
  - Culture of infected tissue
  - Detection of antigens, nucleic acid, or antibodies in blood or secretions
- Gonorrhea
  - Smear of urethral discharge in males
  - Cultures done if Gram stains of smears are negative despite clinical symptoms of gonorrhea
  - In women, cultures of cervical discharge necessary to confirm diagnosis
  - Individuals with gonorrhea are often infected with other STIs so are also tested for syphilis, chlamydia, and HIV
- Syphilis
  - VDRL and RPR are positive 4 to 6 weeks after infection
  - Tests nonspecific if positive further tests are done
  - FTA-ABS is specific for *T. pallidum* used to confirm VDRL and RPR findings
  - Immunofluorescent staining or darkfield microscopy can be used on specimen obtained from a chancre or lymph node

LEARNING OUTCOME 3

Identify general measures to prevent and treat common STIs.

CONCEPTS FOR LECTURE

1. Education of the general populace, especially high-risk groups, is essential in preventing transmission of STIs. Clients who are infected with STIs need to be encouraged to follow the plan of treatment to prevent reinfection and complications. All states require reporting of syphilis, gonorrhea, and AIDs to state and federal agencies. Chlamydia is reportable in some states. The CDC recommends screening asymptomatic women who are at high risk for chlamydia.

POWERPOINT LECTURE SLIDES

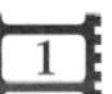

General Measures to Prevent and Treat STIs

- STIs directly related to lifestyle
- Teach all clients to use safer sex practices such as abstinence, mutual monogamy with uninfected partner, and barrier protection during sexual relations
- Syphilis, chlamydia, gonorrhea, can be treated effectively with single-dose antibiotic therapy
- Genital herpes and genital warts cannot be cured but can be treated
- Vaginal spermicides can help reduce risk for gonorrhea and chlamydia
- If an individual suspects exposure, seek medical attention and encourage partner to seek treatment
- Take all medication as prescribed
- Go back for follow-up exam annually; Pap smears recommended for females infected with HBV
- Do not have sex until you and partner completely cured

© 2007 Pearson Education, Inc.

Learning Outcome 4

List the signs and symptoms of the most common STIs.

Concepts for Lecture

1. The signs and symptoms of STIs vary. They can be localized to one area or manifested systemically.

PowerPoint Lecture Slides

1 Signs and Symptoms of Most Common STIs
- Selected sexually transmitted infections (Table 36-1)

Learning Outcome 5

Discuss nursing implications for medications prescribed for clients with STIs.

Concepts for Lecture

1. Medications to treat STIs vary. Chlamydia, syphilis, and gonorrhea can be cured with single-dose antibiotics. Genital herpes and genital warts can be managed but not cured.

PowerPoint Lecture Slides

1 Nursing Implications for Medications Prescribed for Clients with STIs
- Refer to Table 36-1 for specific medications to treat STIs
- Stress the importance of completing treatment plan and returning for follow-up visits
- Incomplete treatment may result in continued infection and organisms that are resistant to antibiotic therapy

Learning Outcome 6

Use the nursing process to provide individualized care for clients with STIs.

Concepts for Lecture

1. Teaching about the infection, its treatment, and potential effects on the reproductive health of the client and his or her partners is a priority for nursing care.

PowerPoint Lecture Slides

1 Utilizing Nursing Process for Clients with STIs
- Nursing care of the client with STIs focuses on:
  - Identifying the infection
  - Eradication
  - Prevention of future infections
  - Managing complications
- Assessing clients with an STI (Box 36-3)
- Nursing diagnoses and interventions related to STIs
  - Ineffective Health Maintenance
    - Interventions: Teach about infection, treatment, and potential effects on reproductive health of client and partners
    - Impaired Skin Integrity
      - Interventions: Teach client to keep perineal area clean and dry
    - Risk for Injury
      - Interventions: Stress importance of taking prescribed medication
    - Anxiety
      - Interventions: Emphasize most STIs can be effectively treated to prevent complication and transmission to infant
    - Situational Low Self-Esteem
      - Intervention: Create environment where client feels respected and safe to discuss concerns

© 2007 Pearson Education, Inc.

PowerPoint Lecture Slides *continued*

- Sexual Dysfunction
  - Interventions: Provide support for discussion of future sexual relationships
- Impaired Social Interaction
  - Intervention: Assist client to understand STI is consequence of sexual behavior not a punishment
- Pain
  - Interventions: Keep herpes blisters clean and dry
  - Teaching for discharge (Box 36-4)

Suggestions for Classroom Activities

1. Describe the pathophysiology of the most common sexually transmitted infections (STIs).
2. Divide the class into small groups. Have each group research the incidence of STIs and the populations at risk for each type of STI.
3. Identify and discuss the nursing implications for laboratory and diagnostic tests used for STIs.
4. Initiate a discussion on general measures to prevent and treat STIs.
5. Divide the class into small groups. Using Table 34-1, have each group present to the class manifestations, treatment, and complications for each STI. Presentations can be poster, demonstration, role-playing, or one of their own design with instructor approval.
6. Using transparencies, list the signs and symptoms of the most common STIs. Have the students list nursing interventions for each sign and symptom.
7. Discuss the nursing implications of the medications prescribed for clients with STIs.
8. Use the nursing process case studies and critical care thinking maps to provide individualized care for clients with STIs.
9. Ask students to volunteer to play the roles of a community health nurse and a client. Have them present a skit of the client asking questions regarding a particular STI and the nurse providing client teaching. The skit should include preventive measures, methods of transmission, and medications.

Suggestions for Clinical Activities

1. Invite a public health nurse to talk about the current statistics on STIs and public awareness information that is available.
2. Assign students to community health centers where STIs are treated. Have students share their thoughts and feelings on their experiences at the clinics.

© 2007 Pearson Education, Inc.

CHAPTER 37
THE NERVOUS SYSTEM AND ASSESSMENT

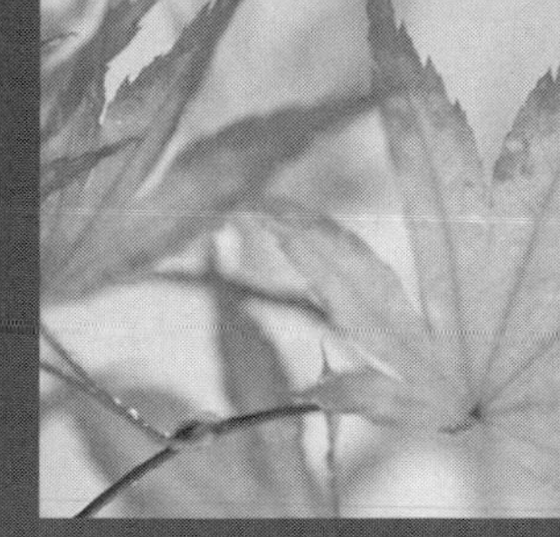

RESOURCE LIBRARY

IMAGE LIBRARY

Figure 37-1 A neuron.
Figure 37-2 The four major regions of the brain with an illustration of the meninges.
Figure 37-3 Cerebral lobes with their functions. The *frontal lobe* controls voluntary motor control on the opposite side of the body and determines emotions, motivation, complex thinking, judgment, and personality. Broca's area promotes speaking ability. The *parietal lobe* interprets sensations and determines right from left and where the body is in relation to the environment. The *temporal lobe* processes taste, smell, and hearing stimuli; it is also important in long-term memory. Wernicke's area promotes understanding of the spoken and written word. The *occipital lobe* processes visual stimuli.
Figure 37-4 Distribution of spinal nerves.
Figure 37-5 A typical reflex arc of the spinal nerve. The stimulus is transferred from the sensory neuron directly to the motor neuron at the point of synapse in the spinal cord.
Figure 37-6 Autonomic nervous system and the organs it affects. The right side shows the actions of the sympathetic nervous system. The left side shows the actions of the parasympathetic nervous system.
Figure 37-7 The external and accessory structures of the eye.
Figure 37-8 The internal structures of the eye.
Figure 37-9 The visual fields of the eyes and the optic pathways.
Figure 37-10 Structures of the external, middle, and inner ear.
Figure 37-11 Testing vision using a Rossenbaum eye chart.
Figure 37-12 Ptosis.

LEARNING OUTCOME 1

Describe the structure and functions of the central and peripheral nervous systems.

CONCEPTS FOR LECTURE

1. The functions of the various structures of the nervous system are interconnected, facilitating the maintenance of homeostasis of the internal environment and communication with and response to the external environment.
2. The neuron is the working cell of the nervous system.
3. There are two major divisions of the nervous system, each comprised of specific structures.

POWERPOINT LECTURE SLIDES

1 Nervous System
- Controls and integrates sensory, motor, and autonomic functions
- Maintains internal homeostasis
- Enables connection and response to external environment

2 Neuron (Figure 37-1)
- Working cell of the nervous system
- Carries impulses
  - Sensory (afferent)
  - Motor (efferent)
- Neurotransmitters (chemicals)
  - Facilitate or hinder impulse transmission across synapse

3 CNS
- Brain
- Spinal cord

3a PNS
- Cranial nerves
- Spinal nerves

PowerPoint Lecture Slides *continued*

- Somatic nervous system
- Autonomic nervous system
  - Sympathetic
  - Parasympathetic

CNS: Brain (Figure 37-2)
- Control center of the nervous system
- Cerebrum; sensation, movement
  - Left hemisphere; speech, problem solving, reasoning, calculations
  - Right hemisphere; visual, spatial

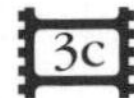

CNS: Brain
- Diencephalon
  - Thalamus; sensory relay
  - Hypothalamus; regulatory center
- Brainstem: vital centers
- Cerebellum
  - Involuntary muscle activity; fine motor
  - Balance and posture

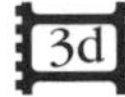

CNS: Spinal Cord
- Spinal tracts
  - Sensory and motor messages
  - White matter and gray matter

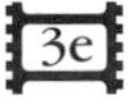

PNS
- Link between CNS and the body
- Spinal nerves
  - 31 pairs
  - Sensory and motor fibers
  - Involved in reflexes/reflex arc

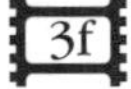

PNS: Cranial Nerves
- Cell bodies in brain/brainstem
- Sensory function, motor function, or both
- Mainly control head and neck functions

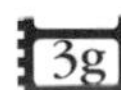

PNS: Autonomic Nervous System
- Maintains internal homeostasis
- Two divisions
  - Sympathetic: "flight or fight"
  - Parasympathetic: "rest and digest"

Suggestions for Classroom Activities

1. Instruct students to complete a simple task while remaining seated. For example, put pens down; raise their hands; cross their legs. Have students identify what components of the nervous system were used for the activity. Discuss the conscious and unconscious pieces to the activity.
2. Project a transparency depicting the four major regions of the brain onto a white board. Prepare a set number of brain functions prior to class. Have students volunteer to mark on the white board the region of the brain that corresponds to the function given. (If no white board is available, draw a brain on poster board.)

Suggestions for Clinical Activities

Pair this activity with assessment activity listed for Learning Outcome 3. When neurologic deficits are identified, have the student indicate the structures of the nervous system that correspond to the deficit.

© 2007 Pearson Education, Inc.

3. Prior to class, divide students into 12 groups. Preassign each group a cranial nerve. Instruct students to prepare a 2-minute presentation on the function of their assigned nerve, as well as deficits that might be seen indicating impairment.
4. Illustrate anatomy using medical models; charts; transparencies.

Learning Outcome 2

Identify the major structures and functions of the eye and the ear.

Concepts for Lecture

1. The eye is a sensory organ whose structures enable the brain to receive and interpret environmental input in the form of patterns of light.
2. Structures that enable vision include the eye itself, as well as accessory structures.
3. The ear is a sensory organ whose structures enable collection and transmission of sound waves to the brain for interpretation.
4. The structures of the ear enable hearing and help us maintain balance.

PowerPoint Lecture Slides

1 The Eye
- Sensory organ
- Converts patterns of light to nerve impulses sent to brain
- Brain interprets impulses, makes meaning of visual input

2 Accessory Structures of the Eye (Figure 37-7)

2a Eyeball
- Three layers
  - Outer: sclera, cornea
  - Middle: iris, ciliary body, choroids
    - Pupil, lens
  - Inner: retina
    - Rods, cones, optic disk (optic nerve)

2b Eyeball
- Two interior cavities
  - Posterior
    - Vitreous body
  - Anterior
    - Anterior chamber
      - Aqueous humor; canal of Schlemm
    - Posterior chamber

3 The Ear (Figure 37-10)
- Sensory organ
- Converts sound to vibrations then impulses
- Brain interprets impulses as sound
- Participates in maintaining balance, equilibrium, coordination of body movements

4 External Ear
- Pinna
- Auditory canal
- Eardrum

4a Middle Ear
- Auditory ossicles (bones)
  - Malleus, incus, stapes
- Eustachian tube

4b Inner Ear
- Labyrinth
  - Vestibule

PowerPoint Lecture Slides *continued*

- Semicircular canals
- Cochlea
  - Organ of Corti

Suggestions for Classroom Activities

1. Expand anatomy discussion by using medical models of the eye and ear.
2. Discuss the functions of each part of the eye as designated on PowerPoint slide.
3. Discuss the functions of each part of the ear as designated on PowerPoint slide.

Suggestions for Clinical Activities

Pair this activity with assessment activity listed for Learning Outcome 3. If vision or hearing deficits are identified during physical assessment, have students indicate the anatomic structure responsible for the deficit.

Learning Outcome 3

Identify subjective and objective assessment data to collect for clients with neurologic or sensory disorders.

Concepts for Lecture

1. The client's level of consciousness will determine the extent to which he or she can relay accurate information and participate in the neurologic exam.
2. Both subjective and objective data should be obtained when completing a focused assessment of the client with a neurologic disorder.
3. Data gathered during a neurologic assessment can reflect deficits in motor, sensory, or cognitive functioning.
4. Neurologic assessment should include data from the special senses of vision and hearing.

PowerPoint Lecture Slides

1 Beginning the neurologic assessment
- LOC always assessed first
  - Altered LOC → inaccuracies
- Determine alternate sources of information
  - Family, caregivers, health care professionals

2 Subjective Data: Health History
- Past medical history
  - Actual neurologic disorders/family history
- Medication use
- Symptom history; include pain assessment
- Social/environmental data

3 Subjective Data: Motor, Sensory, and Cognitive Functioning
- Motor: loss of movement; altered balance, coordination
- Sensory: numbness, tingling, sight, touch
- Cognitive: memory, speech, intellect, mood

4 Subjective Data: Special Senses
- Eye
  - PMH/family history related to the vision
  - Changes in vision; use of corrective lenses; irritation
- Ear
  - PMH/family history related to hearing
  - Changes in hearing; tinnitus drainage
  - Use of hearing aids

2 Objective Data
- General survey
  - Appearance, gait, balance, posture
- Vital signs
- Cranial nerve assessment

3 Objective Data
- Cognitive functioning
  - LOC, mental status, mood
- Sensory functioning
  - Sight, sounds, touch

© 2007 Pearson Education, Inc.

PowerPoint Lecture Slides *continued*

3a Objective Data
- Motor functioning
  - Muscle strength, tone symmetry
- Reflexes

4 Objective Data: Special Senses
- Eye
  - Snellen, Rossenbaum charts
  - Inspection
- Ear
  - Rinne, Webber, whisper tests
  - Inspection

Suggestions for Classroom Activities

1. Discuss the implications of an altered LOC on the validity of a neurologic exam.
2. Discuss in further detail the various techniques/exams used when assessing sensory, motor, eye, and ear functioning (Rhomberg, shoulder shrug, etc.).
3. Have students give examples of disease processes that might be present when various alterations in the neurologic exam are found.
4. Divide students into small workgroups. Have students practice a neurologic assessment in total or in part on a partner.
5. Show samples of Snellen and Rossenbaum charts.

Suggestions for Clinical Activities

1. Using a student volunteer, demonstrate a focused neurologic exam.
2. Assign students to clients having neurologic deficits/diseases. Have students perform a focused neurologic exam.
3. Have students share in postconference the differences in practicing a neurologic exam on a well classmate in lab versus completing an actual neurologic exam on a client.
4. Instruct students to identify a priority nursing diagnosis for any deficits found during assessment and develop an appropriate plan for care.

Learning Outcome 4

Describe changes in neurologic function, vision, and hearing that occur with aging.

Concepts for Lecture

1. Some changes in neurologic function can be expected as a result of aging.
2. It is imperative that health care professionals not make the assumption that neurologic deficits found in the elderly are expected, normal signs of aging. They often indicate neurologic or chronic physiologic problems that may be treatable.

PowerPoint Lecture Slides

1 Expected Neurologic Alterations Related to Aging
- Slower movement and reflexes
- Forgetfulness
- Changes in sleep patterns
- Changes in motor skills

1a Expected Alterations in the Special Senses
- Ptosis
- Presbyopia
- Decreased tear production
- Changes in eyelids
- Hearing difficulties
- Increased production of cerumen

2 Unexpected Neurologic Alterations Related to Aging
- *Significant* changes in
  - Long/short-term memory
  - Mental status
  - Coordination/motor skills
  - Speech
  - Pain perception
  - Sleep
  - Orientation
  - Psychologic status

© 2007 Pearson Education, Inc.

Suggestions for Classroom Activities

1. Have students share personal or clinical experiences with the elderly. Facilitate discussion related to normal and abnormal changes related to aging.
2. Encourage students to discuss their personal feelings and expectations related to aging.
3. Elaborate on the physiologic causes of neurologic changes such as confusion. Discuss the consequences of making assumptions about neurologic changes in the elderly in terms of poor client outcomes.
4. Invite a panel of "Well Elders" to speak with students. The panel should consist of three or four persons aged 75 or above who are living independently and caring for themselves. Invite the panel to share the experiences/factors in their lives that have enabled them to "age well."

Suggestions for Clinical Activities

1. Assign students to elderly clients experiencing neurologic changes related to physiologic alterations (medication toxicities, electrolyte imbalances, etc.).
2. Have students identify lab tests/other diagnostics that help differentiate between a treatable physiologic problem and a true neurologic problem.
3. Have students discuss their plan of care in relationship to client safety.

Learning Outcome 5

Identify nursing responsibilities for common diagnostic tests and monitors for clients with neurologic or sensory disorders.

Concepts for Lecture

1. It is important to complete diagnostics that will identify or rule out physiologic/metabolic causes of neurologic dysfunctions.
2. Imaging techniques and electrographic studies are done to identify actual neurologic pathologies.
3. Nurses have a role in preparing clients for neurologic diagnostic testing as well as caring for clients postprocedure.
4. Specific diagnostic tests are used to evaluate vision and hearing.
5. Nurses have a role in preparing clients for diagnostic exams of the special senses.

PowerPoint Lecture Slides

1 Diagnostics: Lab Tests
- Electrolytes
- Complete blood count
- Liver function tests
- Renal panel
- Arterial blood gases
- Cultures
- Urinalysis

2,3 Imaging Studies—Nursing Implications
- All radiographic studies
  - Allergy assessment—shellfish/iodine
  - Hydration, renal function
  - Pregnancy concerns
  - Client teaching re: procedure

2, 3a Imaging Studies—Nursing Implications
- Skull/spine x-rays
  - Client teaching/explanation
- MRI
  - Assess for implanted metal
  - Client teaching: enclosed space; noise

2, 3b Imaging Studies—Nursing Implications
- CT scan
  - ID shellfish/iodine allergy
  - Assess disorientation
  - Medicate for agitation
  - Teach: warm sensation with contrast

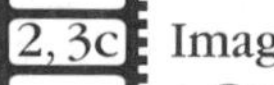
2, 3c Imaging Studies—Nursing Implications
- Cerebral angiography
  - NPO prior
  - Flushing with contrast media
  - Close neurologic/VS monitoring post

© 2007 Pearson Education, Inc.

PowerPoint Lecture Slides *continued*

- Pressure dressing/ice
- Report bleeding/swelling at site STAT

Imaging Studies—Nursing Implications

- Myelography
  - Post: elevate HOB, bed rest
  - Close neurologic/VS monitoring
  - Report leakage/bleeding at site STAT

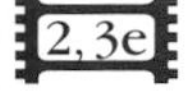

Imaging Studies—Nursing Implications

- PET
  - NPO 4 hours prior
  - IV start
  - Post: hydration
- Carotid duplex

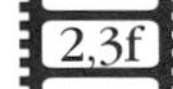

Electrographic Studies—Nursing Implications

- EEG, evoked potentials
  - Wash hair prior
- EMG
  - Discomfort with needle insertion

Vision Tests—Nursing Implications

- Fluorescein stain
  - Potential stinging; staining not permanent
- Visual fields
  - Tiring
- Facial x-rays/CT scan
  - Explain procedure
- Ultrasound
  - Cornea anesthetized

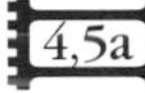

Hearing Tests—Nursing Implications

- Audiometry
  - Explain procedure
- X-ray/CT scan
  - Explain procedure
- Electronystagmography
  - Post assessment; vomiting
    - Aspiration precautions

Suggestions for Classroom Activities

1. Discuss in further detail the purposes of each diagnostic test and what neurologic disease would be identified by its use.
2. Discuss the importance of client teaching to alleviate client fears about diagnostics.
3. Discuss the challenges nurses face in preparing a client with neurologic impairments for certain diagnostic tests. Elicit from students strategies to facilitate the completion of testing for these clients.

Suggestions for Clinical Activities

1. Assign students to clients who are due to have any of the neurologic diagnostic tests completed during the clinical day. Have the student accompany the client to the testing area. Have students participate in both pre- and post-procedure care.
2. Assign students to develop patient teaching brochures for designated neurologic diagnostic tests.
3. If permitted, assign individual students to observe in diagnostic areas such as radiology for 2- to 4-hour blocks. Have students share observations in postconference.
4. Invite personnel from various neurologic diagnostic areas to speak with students at postconference.

© 2007 Pearson Education, Inc.

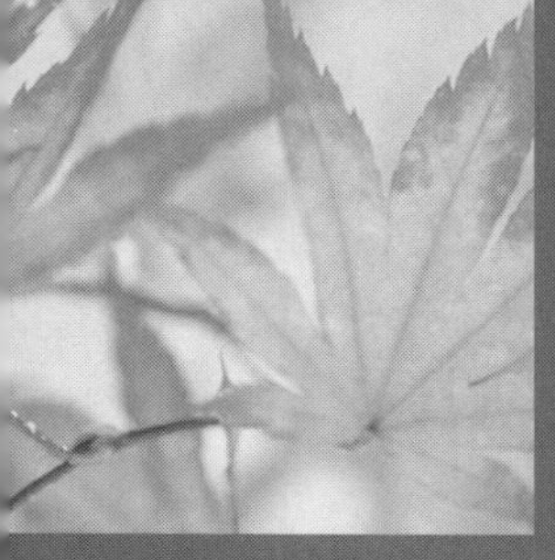

Chapter 38
Caring for Clients with Intracranial Disorders

Resource Library

IMAGE LIBRARY

Figure 38-1 Coup–contrecoup head injury. Following the initial injury (coup), the brain rebounds within the skull and sustains additional injury (contrecoup) in the opposite part of the brain.

Figure 38-2 Three types of hematomas: epidural, subdural, and intracerebral.

Figure 38-3 Burr holes are made in the skull to create a bone flap or to remove a blood clot or evaluate a hematoma.

Figure 38-4 Ommaya reservoir for medication administration.

Figure 38-5 In a craniotomy, a portion of the skull is surgically opened to allow access to the brain.

Figure 38-6 Types of paralysis. (**A**) Hemiplegia is paralysis of one-half of the body. (**B**) Paraplegia is paralysis of the lower part of the body.

Figure 38-7 Homonymous hemianopia. Loss of vision in the nasal field of the right eye and temporal field of the left eye.

Figure 38-8 Carotid endarterectomy. (**A**) The occluded area is clamped off and an incision is made in the artery. (**B**) Plaque is removed from the inner layer of the artery. (**C**) To restore blood flow through the artery, the artery is sutured or a graft is inserted.

Figure 38-9 Positioning the client with hemiplegia is important to prevent deformity of the affected extremities. (**A**) With the client in a supine position, place a pillow in the axilla (to prevent adduction) and under the hand and arm, with the hand higher than the elbow (to prevent flexion and edema). (**B**) When the client is lying supine, use a pillow from the iliac crest to the middle of the thigh to prevent external rotation of the hip. (**C**) When the client is in the prone position, place a pillow under the pelvis to promote hip hyperextension.

Figure 38-10 Types of aneurysms. (**A**) A berry aneurysm is a small sac on a stem or stalk. (**B**) A saccular aneurysm is formed from a distended small portion of the vessel wall. (**C**) A fusiform aneurysm is an enlarged area of the entire blood vessel. (**D**) A dissecting aneurysm is formed when blood fills the area between the tunica media and the tunica intima.

Figure 38-11 Tonic-clonic contractions in generalized seizures. (**A**) Tonic phase. (**B**) Clonic phase.

Learning Outcome 1

Identify the manifestations, neurologic effects, related laboratory/diagnostic tests, interdisciplinary interventions, and nursing implications for medications ordered for the client experiencing increased intracranial pressure. Use the nursing process to provide individualized nursing care.

Concepts for Lecture

1. Increased intracranial pressure (IICP) is a common manifestation and complication of several intracranial disorders.
2. Many manifestations and neurologic effects are associated with IICP that affect different functions of the brain.
3. Diagnostic tests for intracranial disorders include general diagnostics such as x-rays as well as diagnostic tests specific to the identification of neurologic disorders.
4. Altered level of consciousness is a common manifestation of many neurologic disorders, including IICP. Laboratory studies are done to identify the etiology of the altered LOC.
5. The client receiving pharmacotherapy for increased intracranial pressure should be closely monitored by

PowerPoint Lecture Slides

1 Intracranial Disorders
- Increased intracranial pressure
- Head injuries
- Brain tumors
- Cerebrovascular accidents
- Seizures
- Intracranial infections

2 Increased Intracranial Pressure
- Components of cranium
  - Brain
  - Blood in cerebral vessels
  - Cerebrospinal fluid

2a Common Causes of IICP
- Traumatic brain injury
- Cerebral edema

CONCEPTS FOR LECTURE *continued*

the nurse. The nurse is responsible for assessing the therapeutic effects of medications as well as monitoring for untoward effects.

6. The nursing process can be used to provide individualized nursing care for the client with increased intracranial pressure.
7. IICP is a complex syndrome that affects multiple systems. Interdisciplinary interventions are almost always needed.

POWERPOINT LECTURE SLIDES *continued*

- Brain tumor
- Cerebral hematoma
- Cerebrovascular accident
- Brain infections

Manifestations of IICP

- Change in LOC
  - Earliest sign; can progress to coma
- Pupils
  - Sluggish to fixed and dilated
- Vision
  - Blurry; diplopia

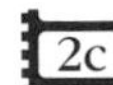

Manifestations of IICP

- Motor functioning
  - Hemiparesis; hemiplegia
  - Posturing
    - Decorticate
    - Decerebrate
- Difficulty speaking

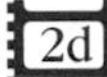

Manifestations of IICP

- Altered vital signs
  - Cushing's triad (Cushing's response)
    - Widening pulse pressure
    - Slow bounding bradycardic pulse
    - Alteration in respiratory pattern
- Other: change in body temperature; headache; projectile vomiting

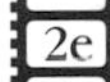

Fatal Complications of IICP

- Brain herniation
  - Shifting of brain
  - Compression of brain/brainstem
- Brain death
  - Cessation of cerebral blood flow/vital functions

Diagnostics: IICP

- Assessing for IICP
  - Cerebral monitoring
- Determining the cause
  - CT scan or MRI
  - Cerebral angiography
  - Lumbar puncture

Diagnostics: Altered LOC

- Laboratory tests
  - Blood glucose
  - Arterial blood gases
  - Toxicology screening
  - Serum creatinine/BUN
  - Liver function
  - Complete blood count

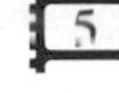

Medications Used in Managing IICP

- Osmotic diuretics/loop diuretics
  - Monitor client for fluid and electrolyte imbalances
  - Monitor client for dehydration

POWERPOINT LECTURE SLIDES *continued*

- Corticosteroids
  - Assess for GI irritation/ulcers
  - Administer H_2 blockers and/or antacids concurrently

5 Medications Used in Managing IICP
- Anticonvulsants
  - Monitor for signs of seizure activity
  - Document cessation of signs of seizure activity
- Barbiturate therapy for severe TBI, IICP
  - Artificial coma requiring ICU monitoring

6 Nursing Process: Assessing
- LOC/vital signs
- Altered cognitive functioning; headache, vomiting
- Sensory alterations: vision/hearing
- Numbness or tingling in extremities
- History; medication/alcohol use
- Reflexes; posturing

6a Nursing Process: Nursing Diagnoses
- Ineffective Tissue Perfusion
- Ineffective Breathing Pattern
- Risk for Imbalanced Nutrition
- Risk for Impaired Skin Integrity
- Impaired Physical Mobility
- Risk for Infection

6b Nursing Process: Evaluation
- LOC
- Grips, gait
- Absence of deficits

7 IICP: Interdisciplinary Care
- Pharmacotherapy
- Respiratory support
- Nutritional support
- Surgery
- Discharge planning

SUGGESTIONS FOR CLASSROOM ACTIVITIES

1. Discuss the concept of the cranium as a closed space. Use transparencies that depict the percentage of the cranium occupied by the three main components.
2. Obtain a preserved human brain (usually contained in a clear plastic container in fluid) from the science department. Use this as a method to further illustrate the concept of a closed space.
3. Link the discussion of increased intracranial pressure to the first two suggested activities.
4. Discuss the definition and pathophysiology of IICP. Use transparencies to illustrate the various methods used to measure intracranial pressure.
5. Point out to students how IICP is a common manifestation/complication of many intracranial disorders.
6. Assign students various vocabulary words related to the neurologic manifestations of IICP: hemiparesis,

SUGGESTIONS FOR CLINICAL ACTIVITIES

1. Assign students to clients in the clinical setting who have been hospitalized with IICP.
2. Assist students to refine their assessment skills when completing a neurologic assessment.
3. Assign students to clients who have altered levels of consciousness. Assist the student to assess LOC using the Glasgow Coma Scale on different clients. Have students describe what they observed during postconference.
4. Collaborate with the intensive care unit and determine if a client with IICP is being cared for there. Seek permission for one student per clinical day to observe that level of care.
5. Invite other members of the health care team to discuss their role postconference in the care of the client with IICP.

© 2007 Pearson Education, Inc.

hemiplegia, diplopia, etc. Have them share the definitions when the deficit is discussed in lecture.
7. Use clinical examples of alteration in lab results that would indicate a metabolic cause of altered LOC.
8. Divide students into small groups. Assign students to research the four main categories of medications used in the management of IICP. Have students report findings during lecture.
9. Using each nursing diagnosis, discuss in detail the nursing care that would be provided for the client with IICP. Include in the discussion ways to measure effectiveness of care.

LEARNING OUTCOME 2

Identify manifestations, neurologic effects, related diagnostic tests, and special client discharge teaching topics for the client who has sustained a head injury.

CONCEPTS FOR LECTURE

1. There are many types of head injuries that have both specific as well as overlapping signs and symptoms and neurologic effects.
2. Diagnostics for head injuries will identify disruptions in the continuity of the skull bones as well as swelling and/or bleeding into underlying brain tissue.
3. Care of the client who has sustained a head injury often focuses on assessing, monitoring, and implementing medical and nursing measures for the client with IICP.
4. Clients and their families will need individualized discharge teaching based on the severity of the head injury sustained and the chronicity of the postinjury neurologic deficits.

POWERPOINT LECTURE SLIDES

1 Head Injuries: Skull Fractures
- Linear: simple clean break in skull
- Comminuted: skull in fragmented pieces
- Depressed: skull bone fragments pushed into brain
- Basilar: at base of skull, may extend to temporal bone
  - Leakage of blood or CSF from nose/ears
  - Battle's sign
  - "Raccoon" eyes

1a Head Injuries: Open Head Injury
- Opening through skull and dura
  - Severe blunt trauma
  - Penetrating injuries
- Brain exposed to external environment
- Risk of meningitis; brain damage

1b Head Injuries: Closed Head injury
- Coup-contrecoup phenomenon
- Bruising of brain at two points
- Brain damage
  - Focal symptoms related to area of brain injured
  - Possible IICP

1c Head Injuries: Closed Head Injury
- Concussion r/t shaking of brain
  - Immediate loss of consciousness for < 5 min
  - Drowsiness, confusion
  - Headache, blurred/double vision

1d Head Injuries: Closed Head Injury
- Contusion: bruising/swelling of brain tissue
  - Initial loss of consciousness
  - Motionless, pale, clammy
  - Hypotensive, weak pulse, shallow respirations
  - Altered motor response

© 2007 Pearson Education, Inc.

PowerPoint Lecture Slides *continued*

1e Head Injuries: Epidural Hematoma
- Arterial bleed between skull and dura
- Can be caused by skull fracture/contusion
- Brief loss of consciousness → short period of alertness → rapid progression to coma with:
  - Posturing, pupil changes, seizures; IICP

1f Head Injuries: Subdural Hematoma
- Venous bleed between dura and subarachnoid layer
  - Acute: rapid progression to coma, pupil dilation, contralateral hemiparesis
  - Subacute: symptoms 48 hrs to 2 wks; alert period then slow progression to coma
  - Chronic: symptoms weeks to months later; impaired thinking, confusion; drowsiness; pupil changes; motor deficits

1g Head Injuries: Intracerebral Hematoma
- Bleeding into brain tissue
  - Decreasing LOC
  - Pupil changes
  - Motor deficits

2 Diagnostics: Head Injuries
- Skull series: x-ray
- CT scan

3 IICP in Head Injuries
- IICP results from:
  - Direct trauma to the brain tissue
  - Cerebral edema
  - Hematomas

4 Discharge Teaching Topics
- Symptoms of IICP
- Frequent monitoring at home
- Postconcussion syndrome
- Necessity for rehabilitation
- Necessity for long-term care

Suggestions for Classroom Activities

1. Discuss the incidence and causes of traumatic brain injury in the U.S.
2. Initiate a discussion about what health teaching could be done in the community to decrease the incidence of brain injuries.
3. Compare and contrast brain contusion and concussion.
4. Compare and contrast the three different types of hematomas.
5. Use transparencies to illustrate where the bleeding occurs in the three different types of hematomas.

Suggestions for Clinical Activities

1. Have students develop a teaching brochure featuring head injury prevention information for a community group.
2. Assign students to clients who have sustained a head injury. Assist the students in their assessment for IICP.
3. Assign one student each day to the emergency room to observe. Have the students report on the number of head injury victims admitted to the ER during the observation period.
4. Access a support group for head injury victims with chronic neurologic impairment. Invite a member to speak with students about the challenges faced by persons with chronic brain injuries.

© 2007 Pearson Education, Inc.

LEARNING OUTCOME 3

Identify the manifestations, neurologic effects, related laboratory/diagnostic tests, and nursing implications for medications ordered for the client having a brain tumor. Use the nursing process to provide individualized nursing care.

CONCEPTS FOR LECTURE

1. The extent of tumor growth and the area of the brain in which the tumor is located will determine which neurologic effects manifest.
2. Laboratory and diagnostic tests for brain tumors will identify the location of the tumor, sufficiency of cerebral blood flow, and type of tumor present.
3. The nurse needs to understand drug action related to chemotherapy when caring for a client receiving pharmacotherapy for brain cancer.
4. The nursing process can be used to create an individualized plan of care for the client with a brain tumor.

POWERPOINT LECTURE SLIDES

1 Brain Tumors
- Abnormal growths within the cranium
- Categorized as:
  - Benign or malignant
  - Primary: arising from brain cells/structures
  - Secondary: metastasis from other primary site of cancer

1a Brain Tumors: Types
- Glioma
  - Astrocytoma
  - Glioblastoma
- Meningioma
- Acoustic neuroma
- Metastatic brain tumors

1b Brain Tumors: Manifestations (Box 38-5)

2 Diagnostics: Brain Tumors
- CT scan or MRI
- EEG
- Cerebral angiogram
- Stereotactic needle biopsy
  - For certain tumors to identify type

3 Medications Used in Treating Brain Tumors
- Chemotherapy via:
  - Ommaya reservoir
  - Wafers in tumor cavity
- Assess for bone marrow suppression

4 Nursing Process: Assessing
- Cognitive changes
- Pain
- Sensory changes: vision, hearing
- Paresthesias
- Vital signs, LOC
- Strength, movement
- Gait, coordination

4a Nursing Process: Diagnoses
- Risk for Infection r/t chemotherapy
- Anxiety
- Disturbed Body image
- Deficient Knowledge r/t cranial surgery

4b Nursing Process: Evaluation
- Effectiveness of interventions: postop craniotomy
  - Absence of neurologic deficits
  - No signs of infection
- Knowledge re: follow-up care at home

© 2007 Pearson Education, Inc.

Suggestions for Classroom Activities

1. Discuss the potential harm/neurologic problems that can occur due to the presence of a benign brain tumor.
2. Discuss various survival rates for malignant brain tumors.
3. Divide students into small groups. Assign each group a different lobe of the brain. Have students report on the neurologic functions of each lobe.
4. Pair this lecture with the related topic of caring for the client following a craniotomy.
5. Ask students to identify commonalities when assessing a client with a brain tumor and other intracranial disorders.
6. Discuss the effect chemotherapy has on cells of the bone marrow.

Suggestions for Clinical Activities

1. Assign students to clients who have been either diagnosed with or treated for brain tumors. Assist the student to complete a focused neurologic exam.
2. If specialty departments exist in the clinical facility, have students observe stereotatic biopsy, gamma knife surgery, chemotherapy administration via the Ommaya reservoir, or craniotomy during a surgical rotation.
3. Invite a nurse from an oncology unit to speak with the students about caring for a client with a brain tumor.

Learning Outcome 4

Identify the manifestations, neurologic effects, related laboratory/diagnostic tests, and nursing implications for medications ordered for the client having a cerebrovascular accident. Use the nursing process to provide individualized nursing care.

Concepts for Lecture

1. Mortality and morbidity statistics for stroke illustrate how this pervasive neurologic disorder impacts the health of our nation.
2. There are both modifiable and nonmodifiable risk factors for stroke.
3. A transient ischemic attack can be a warning sign of an impending stroke. An impending stroke may be averted through surgical intervention.
4. Diagnostic tests for stroke will help to identify the area of the brain affected, the status of the cerebral vessels, and the presence or absence of RBCs in the CSF.
5. Manifestations of a stroke can be categorized according to the brain hemisphere that is affected as well as the brain function that is impaired.
6. The nurse participates in the interdisciplinary plan of care for the stroke client by administering medications that are ordered and monitoring for therapeutic effects.
7. The nursing process can be used to develop an individualized plan of care for the client who has experienced a stroke.

PowerPoint Lecture Slides

1 Cerebral Vascular Accident
- Terms preferred by National Stroke Association:
  - Stroke or brain attack
- Affects 700,000 people in the U.S. per year
- Third leading cause of death in the U.S.
- Most frequent cause of chronic neurologic disability

2 Risk Factors for Stroke/Brain Attack
- Race: African American
- Hypertension
- Obesity
- Diabetes mellitus
- Atrial fibrillation
- Atherosclerosis

2a Other Risk Factors: Lifestyle Choices
- Smoking
- High cholesterol
- Excessive use of alcohol, cocaine, and heroin
- Oral contraceptive use by women

3 TIA: Transient Ischemic Attack
- Temporary reduction in cerebral blood flow
- Reversible neurologic deficits
  - Several minutes to 24 hours
- Warning sign of an impending or future stroke
- Carotid endarterectomy

3a Manifestations
- Dizziness
- Loss of vision in one eye
- Numbness, weakness
  - One arm, hand, leg
- Aphasia

© 2007 Pearson Education, Inc.

PowerPoint Lecture Slides *continued*

4 Diagnostics: Stroke
- CT scan/MRI
- Cerebral arteriogram
- Doppler ultrasound
- PET scan
- Lumbar puncture

5 Stroke/Brain Attack
- Sudden loss of neurologic function due to decreased blood supply to a local area of the brain
- Ischemic
  - Thrombus
  - Emboli
- Hemorrhagic

5a Manifestations Right Hemisphere
- Left hemiplegia; visual field deficits
- Spatial-perceptual deficits
- Poor judgment; easily distracted
- Impulsive

5b Manifestations Left Hemisphere
- Right hemiplegia; visual field deficits
- Aphasia
- Impaired intellect
- Slow/cautious; high frustration

5c Motor Deficits
- Contralateral
- Hemiparesis
- Hemiplegia
  - Flaccidity moving to spacticity
- Problems associated with immobility

5d Speech Deficits
- Expressive aphasia
- Receptive aphasia
- Global aphasia
- Dysarthria

5e Visual Deficits
- Due to parietal and/or temporal lobe damage
- Diplopia
- Homonymous hemianopia

5f Sensory-Perceptual Deficits
- Agnosia
- Apraxia
- Unilateral neglect
- Alterations in perception
  - Temperature; vibration; pain; pressure; proprioception
- Increased risk for injury

5g Cognitive/Behavioral Changes
- Memory loss; decreased attention span
- Poor judgment; inability to solve problems
- Emotionally labile/loss of self-control
- Depression; stress manifesting as anger

© 2007 Pearson Education, Inc.

PowerPoint Lecture Slides *continued*

5h Urinary/Gastrointestinal Problems
- Urinary frequency, urgency, incontinence
- Constipation
- Dysphagia
  - Choking, drooling, aspiration

6 Medications Used in the Treatment of Stroke
- Preventive post TIA
  - Antiplatelets
- Thrombolytics
  - Only in ischemic stroke
  - Time frame critical
- Major nursing responsibility
  - Assess for bleeding

6a Medications Used in the Treatment of Stroke
- Anticoagulants (thrombotic stroke)
  - Assess for bleeding
- Antihypertensives
  - Assess BP
- Osmotic diuretics for IICP
  - Monitor I&O
- Anticonvulsants
  - Watch for seizure activity

7 Nursing Process: Assessing
- Cognitive changes
- Sensory changes
- Change in motor function
- Headache

7a Nursing Process: Assessing
- History of:
  - HTN, TIA, diabetes, cardiac dysrhythmias
  - Alcohol abuse, smoking
  - Use of anticoagulants
- Vital signs
- Focused neurologic exam

7b Nursing Process: Diagnoses
- Ineffective Tissue Perfusion: Cerebral
- Risk for Ineffective Airway Clearance
- Impaired Physical Mobility
- Impaired Verbal Communication

7c Nursing Process: Diagnoses
- Disturbed Sensory Perception
- Impaired Urinary Elimination/Constipation
- Impaired Swallowing
- Self-Care Deficit

7d Nursing Process: Evaluation
- Airway
- Self-care
- Communication
- Coping
- Knowledge of medications

© 2007 Pearson Education, Inc.

Suggestions for Classroom Activities

1. Instruct students to visit the National Stroke Association website prior to this lecture (*www.stroke.org*). Discuss the rationale behind the change in verbiage associated with cerebrovascular accident.
2. Compare and contrast modifiable and nonmodifiable risk factors for stroke.
3. Divide students into small groups. Assign each group a category of deficits seen following a stroke. Have students discuss in detail the pathologies and share with the class.
4. Discuss how the various neurologic deficits that occur with a stroke can affect the nurse's plan of care in terms of meeting the client's safety needs.
5. Compare and contrast TIA and stroke.
6. Divide students into small groups. Assign each group a different class of drug, used in the treatment of stroke. Have students share the nursing responsibilities associated with each drug.
7. Using previously discussed intracranial disorders, review the assessment data that is similar to and that which is different from stroke.
8. Discuss in detail the nursing interventions associated with each nursing diagnosis applicable to the client who has had a stroke.

Suggestions for Clinical Activities

1. Invite a member of the local Stroke Association to speak with the students about stroke prevention.
2. If a rehabilitation unit is accessible at the clinical facility, assign students to that unit. Have students report to their peers their observations related to rehabilitative care of the stroke client.
3. Assign students in the clinical area to clients with the diagnosis of TIA or stroke.
4. As with other intracranial disorders, assist students to complete a focused neurologic exam.
5. Invite other members of the interdisciplinary team such as the dietician or speech therapist to speak to the students about their role in the care of a client who has had a stroke.

Learning Outcome 5

Identify the manifestations, neurologic effects, related laboratory/diagnostic tests, and nursing implications for medications ordered for the client having a seizure disorder. Use the nursing process to provide individualized nursing care.

Concepts for Lecture

1. Seizure disorders involve the conduction of impulses in the brain. There can be anatomic as well as metabolic causes of seizures.
2. The diagnostic tests used to identify the presence of a seizure disorder identify changes in brain anatomy and brain electrical activity as well as metabolic changes that precipitate seizure activity.
3. The manifestations of seizures can include sensory alterations, changes in the level of consciousness, and alterations in motor functioning.
4. Continuous seizure activity can impair vital functions such as respiratory effort.
5. Nursing responsibilities related to medications used to control seizures are focused on client education and drug level monitoring.
6. The nursing process can be used to create an individualized plan of care for the client with seizure disorders. The plan should include emergency management.

PowerPoint Lecture Slides

1 Seizure Disorders
- Abnormal electrical activity in brain cells
- Involving all or part of brain
- Can be isolated event
- Chronic pattern → epilepsy

1a Seizures: Causes
- Most unknown
- In adults:
  - Brain infection
  - Stroke
  - Brain tumor
  - Hypoglycemia, high fever, hypoxia

2 Diagnostics: Seizures
- Radiologic
  - Skull x-rays; CT; MRI
- EEG
- CBC, electrolytes, BUN, glucose
- Testing for syphilis

3 Manifestations of Seizures: Partial
- Simple
  - Jacksonian march

© 2007 Pearson Education, Inc.

POWERPOINT LECTURE SLIDES *continued*

- Flashing lights; tingling sensation; hallucinations
- < 20–30 secs; no loss of consciousness

• Complex
- Automatisms
- Altered LOC
- Aura

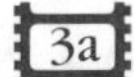 Manifestations of Seizures: Generalized

• Absence
- Brief change in consciousness
- Motor activity halts

• Tonic-clonic
- Aura
- Tonic contractions—rigidity
- Clonic contractions—muscle jerking; eyes roll; frothing at mouth; incontinence
- Postictal period

 Manifestations of Seizures: Status Epilepticus

• Life-threatening emergency
• Continuous tonic-clonic activity and loss of consciousness
• Can deprive brain of oxygen/glucose
• Causes physical exhaustion/respiratory distress
• Can cause permanent brain damage

 Medications Used in the Treatment of Seizures

• Halting status epilepticus
- Valium
- Ativan
- Phenobarbital

• Long-term seizure control
- Anticonvulsants

• Assess for effectiveness: monitor drug levels

 Nursing Process: Assessing

• Data r/t seizure experience
- Onset, duration, aura, postictal period

• History of intracranial disorders
• Observation
- Physical symptoms before, during, and after seizure

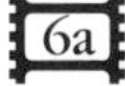 Nursing Process: Diagnoses

• Risk for Ineffective Airway Clearance
• Risk for Injury
• Anxiety

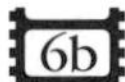 Nursing Process: Evaluation

• Seizure control
• Safety
• Knowledge of medications

SUGGESTIONS FOR CLASSROOM ACTIVITIES

1. Initiate a discussion with students about the stigma attached to seizure disorders.
2. Expand the discussion of extracranial factors that can precipitate a seizure.

SUGGESTIONS FOR CLINICAL ACTIVITIES

1. Devise a practice session wherein students must respond to a client having a seizure. Discuss emergency care, what is to be noted, how to keep the client safe.

© 2007 Pearson Education, Inc.

3. Compare and contrast partial and generalized seizures.
4. Discuss the physiology of status epilepticus in terms of being a potentially fatal problem.
5. Discuss the medications used in the emergency treatment of status epilepticus. Differentiate between the role of the registered nurse and the practical nurse in relationship to intravenous emergency drugs.
6. Using the nursing diagnoses listed on the PowerPoint slide, discuss in depth the nursing interventions associated with each when caring for the client with seizures.

2. Assign students to observe the performance of an EEG on a patient with seizure disorders.

Learning Outcome 6

Identify the manifestations, neurologic effects, related laboratory/diagnostic tests, and nursing implications for medications ordered for the client diagnosed with a brain infection. Use the nursing process to provide individualized nursing care.

Concepts for Lecture

1. Brain infections can affect either the meninges or brain tissue and be caused by either bacteria or viruses.
2. Brain infections have both specific as well as overlapping signs and symptoms and neurologic effects.
3. Diagnostic testing for clients with brain infections identifies the presence of microorganisms in the brain and CSF, as well as microorganisms originating in the blood, urine, ear, and nose that may have migrated to the brain and CSF.
4. The nurse is responsible for administering the medications ordered to treat brain infections as well as those ordered to relieve symptoms and prevent associated complications.
5. The nursing process can be used to develop an individualized plan of care for the client who is being treated for a brain infection.

PowerPoint Lecture Slides

1 Brain Infections: Meningitis
- Inflammation of the meninges: brain and spinal cord
  - Bacterial
  - Viral
- Viral meningitis: less severe, shorter course

2 Manifestations
- + Brudzinski's sign
- + Kernig's sign
- Headache, photophobia
- High fever, nausea, vomiting
- Restlessness, confusion, seizures
- Altered LOC
- Signs of IICP
- Altered vital signs

1,2 Brain Infections: Encephalitis
- Acute inflammation of white and gray matter: brain and spinal cord
- Damage of nerve cells
  - Cerebral edema, necrosis, localized hemorrhage
- Manifestations similar to meningitis

1,2a Brain Infections: Brain Abscess
- Collection of purulent material within the brain
- Caused by/often follow:
  - Middle ear/sinus infection
  - Head injury/intracranial surgery
  - Bacterial infections in hear, bone, lung
- Manifestations similar to meningitis

3 Diagnostics: Brain infections
- Lumbar puncture
- Culture, sensitivity and Gram stain of CSF
- Blood, urine, throat, and nasal cultures
- CT, MRI, skull x-rays

© 2007 Pearson Education, Inc.

PowerPoint Lecture Slides *continued*

4 Medications Used in the Treatment of Brain Infections
- Antibiotics: teaching related to completion
- Antivirals: teaching related to completion
- Anticonvulsants: monitor for seizures
- Antipyretics/analgesics: monitor temp
- Osmotic diuretics/corticosteroids: assess for signs of IICP
- Antiemetics: assess for nausea

5 Nursing Process: Assessment
- Nausea, vomiting
- Photophobia; stiff neck
- Confusion; headache
- History of:
  - Head injury; brain surgery; infections

5a Nursing Process: Assessment
- Vital signs/LOC
- Changes in vision/hearing
- Brudzinski's and Kernig's signs
- Seizures
- Petechial rash

5b Nursing Process: Diagnoses
- Risk for Ineffective Tissue Perfusion: Cerebral
- Hyperthermia
- Acute Pain

5c Nursing Process: Evaluation
- Afebrile
- Absence of headache/signs of IICP
- Knowledge r/t anti-infective therapy

Suggestions for Classroom Activities

1. Discuss the various pathologies that can lead to a brain infection.
2. Compare and contrast the course of disease for viral and bacterial meningitis and the populations they each affect.
3. Discuss the commonalities between the manifestations of brain infections and other intracranial disorders.
4. Demonstrate the technique for assessing Brudzinski's and Kernig's sign.
5. Using the nursing diagnoses listed on the PowerPoint slide, discuss in detail the nursing actions associated with each diagnosis.

Suggestions for Clinical Activities

Have students read the clinical agency policy regarding isolation for the client with meningitis. For example, for which type of meningitis would isolation be required?

Learning Outcome 7

Identify the preoperative and postoperative care for clients undergoing a craniotomy.

Concepts for Lecture

1. A craniotomy is a surgical procedure performed to treat a variety of different intracranial disorders.
2. Preoperative care for the client undergoing a craniotomy includes routine preoperative care as well as preoperative care specific to that particular procedure.

PowerPoint Lecture Slides

1 Craniotomy
- Surgical opening into the cranial cavity
- Purposes:
  - Elevate a depressed skull fracture
  - Remove foreign body

© 2007 Pearson Education, Inc.

CONCEPTS FOR LECTURE *continued*

3. Postoperative care for the client having a craniotomy includes routine postoperative care as well as postoperative care specific to that particular procedure such as positioning and assessing for IICP and CSF leakage.

POWERPOINT LECTURE SLIDES *continued*

    - Evacuate hematoma
    - Debulk/remove tumor

2 Preoperative Care
- Routine preoperative care/teaching
- Assess understanding of procedure
- Assess anxiety level
- Postoperative appearance

3 Postoperative Care
- Monitoring
    - Vital signs, respiratory status oxygenation status
    - IICP; CSF leak; manifestations of meningitis; seizures
- Pain control; antibiotic therapy
- Positioning
- Care of the wound/incision

SUGGESTIONS FOR CLASSROOM ACTIVITIES

1. Discuss the purposes for a craniotomy.
2. Describe the elements of preoperative teaching. Ask students to share their ideas on what precipitates anxiety in the preoperative craniotomy client.
3. Discuss each item to be monitored postoperatively. Expand on each topic, giving examples of abnormal findings for each.
4. Review signs and symptoms of IICP, meningitis seizures.
5. Discuss wound care related to craniotomy. Review wound/incision abnormalities the LPN would report to the RN.

SUGGESTIONS FOR CLINICAL ACTIVITIES

1. Assign students to an OR rotation. Have them observe a craniotomy should that surgery be available for student observation.
2. Assigns students to clients who have had a craniotomy. Assist the students to develop their neurologic assessment skills.
3. Have students perform dressing changes prn.
4. Invite an ICU nurse to speak with students about caring for a client who is status post-craniotomy in the ICU.

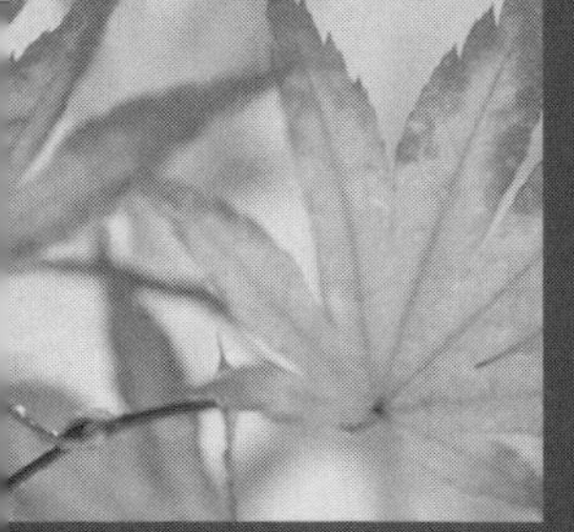

CHAPTER 39
CARING FOR CLIENTS WITH DEGENERATIVE NEUROLOGIC AND SPINAL CORD DISORDERS

RESOURCE LIBRARY

IMAGE LIBRARY

Figure 39-1 Neuron with neurofibrillary tangles seen in Alzheimer's disease.
Figure 39-2 Multisystem effects of multiple sclerosis.
Figure 39-3 In Parkinson's disease, the client's face lacks expression.
Figure 39-4 Sensory and motor branches of the trigeminal nerve. There are three sensory branches: ophthalmic, maxillary, and mandibular.
Figure 39-5 The client with Bell's palsy shows the typical drooping of one side of the face.
Figure 39-6 Spinal cord injury mechanisms. **(A)** Hyperflexion. **(B)** Hyperextension. **(C)** Cord compression.
Figure 39-7 Types of paralysis. **(A)** Tetraplegia. **(B)** Paraplegia.
Figure 39-8 Cervical traction with Gardner-Wells tongs.
Figure 39-9 Halo vest.
Figure 39-10 A herniated intervertebral disk. The herniated nucleus pulposus is applying pressure against the nerve root.

LEARNING OUTCOME 1

Describe the pathophysiology, etiology, manifestations, medical treatments, nursing implications, and the nursing plan of care for the client with Alzheimer's disease.

CONCEPTS FOR LECTURE

1. Alzheimer's disease is a degenerative neurologic disorder affecting millions of people in the U.S.
2. The pathophysiology of Alzheimer's involves changes in the anatomic structure of the brain and nerve cells.
3. The manifestations of Alzheimer's disease can be categorized by stages, which reflect increasing deterioration of neurologic function.
4. The goals of pharmacotherapy for Alzheimer's include slowing the decline of cognition, treating depression, and controlling behavior. Complementary therapy has also been used.
5. The nurse can use the nursing process to develop an individualized plan of care for the client with Alzheimer's.
6. The nursing care plan includes client/family teaching.

POWERPOINT LECTURE SLIDES

1 Alzheimer's Disease
- Brain deterioration
  - Progressive; irreversible
  - Gradual loss; intellectual functioning
- 4 million adults affected
- Most common type of dementia

2 Pathophysiology of Alzheimer's
- Loss of nerve cells
- Reduced brain size
- Neurofibrillary tangles
- Neuritic plaques

2a Consequences of Pathologic Changes
- Altered nerve impulse transmission
- Loss of memory
- Loss of cognition

3 Manifestations of Alzheimer's: Stage 1
- Short-term memory loss; forgets location and names of objects
- Attempts to cover up memory loss
- Has difficulty learning new information or making decisions
- Decreased attention span
- Can be angry or depressed

3a Manifestations of Alzheimer's: Stage 2
- Unable to remember family members' names
- Easily agitated and irritable

POWERPOINT LECTURE SLIDES *continued*

- Difficulty ready, writing, speaking
- Poor personal hygiene
- Unable to make decisions

3b Manifestations of Alzheimer's: Stage 3
- Cannot recognize self or others
- Inability to communicate
- Delusions and hallucinations
- Incontinence: bowel and bladder

4 Medications Used in the Treatment of Alzheimer's
- Cholinesterase inhibitor
- Glutamate inhibitor
- Antidepressant
- Antipsychotic

4a Complementary Therapy
- Gingko biloba
- Antioxidants
- Chinese medicine
- Massage; art and music therapy

5 Nursing Process: Assessment
- Cognitive changes
  - Memory; orientation; decisions; language
- Alterations in sleep
- Past medical history
- Appearance

5a Nursing Process: Diagnoses
- Disturbed Thought Processes
- Self-Care Deficit
- Caregiver Role Strain

5b Nursing Process: Evaluation
- Level of thought process/self-care
- Caregiver's ability to care for client
- Support systems
- Safety

6 Client/Patient Teaching
- Communication techniques
- Safety
- Support group contact
- Care for caregiver

SUGGESTIONS FOR CLASSROOM ACTIVITIES

1. Use transparency of Figure 39-1. Discuss the neurofibrillary tangles and their relevance to the diagnosis of Alzheimer's disease.
2. Compare and contrast Alzheimer's and other disease of dementia.
3. Give examples of manifestations in terms of actual thoughts and behaviors.
4. Bring attention to the devastating effect the disease has on the client/family group in terms of family process and loss of functioning as a family member.
5. Discuss the concept of "who cares for the caretaker."

SUGGESTIONS FOR CLINICAL ACTIVITIES

These clinical activities would be applicable in a long-term care facility or in a home health clinical rotation.

1. Assign students to a client with Alzheimer's disease. Have them complete a neurologic exam, focusing on cognitive functioning.
2. Have students practice correlating assessment findings with the stages of Alzheimer's.
3. Assign students to develop an art or music therapy program for the client with Alzheimer's and to implement that program in the clinical or home setting.

6. Using the nursing diagnoses listed, discuss in depth the nursing actions related to each diagnosis.
7. Discuss care of the client receiving antidepressant and antipsychotic medications.
8. Divide students into three groups. Assign each group to a stage of Alzheimer's. Have students discuss the different care needs of each group.
9. Discuss the safety needs for the client with Alzheimer's.

4. Have students interview a family member, gathering data related to the challenges of caring for a client with Alzheimer's in the home.
5. Have students attend a support group for families of clients with Alzheimer's.

Learning Outcome 2

Describe the pathophysiology, etiology, manifestations, medical treatments, nursing implications, and the nursing plan of care for the client with multiple sclerosis.

Concepts for Lecture

1. There are specific populations and geographic locations in which MS occurs more frequently.
2. The pathology of MS involves destruction of the myelin sheath in the CNS.
3. Patchy demyelination in the CNS causes manifestations to vary from client to client. The course of the disease includes periods of exacerbation and remission.
4. The goals of medications used in the treatment of MS include slowing the progression of the disease, altering the immune response, increasing periods of remissions, and treating accompanying symptoms.
5. There are other therapies for MS that are intended to improve the client's quality of life.
6. The nurse can use the nursing process to develop an individualized plan of care for the client with MS.
7. The nursing care plan includes client/family teaching.

PowerPoint Lecture Slides

1 Multiple Sclerosis
- Caucasian females
- Ages: 20–40
- Family history
- Northern U.S.

2 Pathophysiology of MS
- Autoimmune response with viral trigger
- Demyelination
  - Spinal cord
  - Brain
  - Nerves of the CNS
- Myelin replaced with plaque
- Impulse transmission interrupted/ halted

3 Manifestations of MS
- Exacerbations and remissions
  - Progression → longer exacerbations
- Triggers for exacerbations
  - Heat, sun, infections, stress

3a Manifestations of MS
- Figure 39-2

3b Long-Term Consequences
- Urinary tract infections
- Pressure ulcers/joint contractures
- Falls
- Pneumonia
- Depression

4 Medications for MS
- Immunomodulators
- Monoclonal antibody
- Steroids
- Antispasmotics
- Urinary agents
- Pharmacotherapy for fatigue

5 Other Therapies
- Physical therapy
- Surgical intervention
  - Neurectomy; rhizotomy
- Plasmapheresis
- Nutritional support

© 2007 Pearson Education, Inc.

POWERPOINT LECTURE SLIDES *continued*

6 Nursing Process: Assessment
- Motor assessment
  - Muscle strength; chewing/swallowing
- Sensory changes
  - Tingling; vision changes
- Mood changes
- Urinary elimination patterns
- Past medical/family history

6a Nursing Process: Assessment
- Respiratory effort
- ADLs
- Appearance

6b Nursing Process: Diagnoses
- Fatigue
- Self-Care Deficit
- Ineffective Coping
- Impaired Mobility
- Risk for Injury

6c Nursing Process: Evaluation
- ADLs
- Coping
- Knowledge level
  - Medications; diet; complications

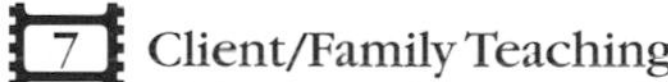

7 Client/Family Teaching
- Triggers for exacerbations/stressors
- Medications/side effects
- Coping with deficits
- Counseling/support groups

SUGGESTIONS FOR CLASSROOM ACTIVITIES

1. Discuss the statistics related to the prevalence of MS.
2. Review the concept of autoimmune disease processes.
3. Briefly discuss the four types of MS.
4. Discuss the concepts of exacerbations and remissions.
5. Divide students into small workgroups. Assign each group a class of drugs used in the treatment of MS. Have students report to the class on drug actions, interactions, expected effects, and side effects.
6. Discuss the nursing implications related to caring for a client receiving steroid and immunomodulating pharmacotherapy.
7. Assign students to visit the website for the National Multiple Sclerosis Society at *www.nmss.org* prior to class. Have students report on the information available at this site.
8. Using the nursing diagnoses on the PowerPoint slide, discuss in detail the nursing interventions to be used in caring for the client with MS.

SUGGESTIONS FOR CLINICAL ACTIVITIES

1. Assign students to a client with MS. If this is during a med/surg acute care rotation, have students explore how the condition for which the client was admitted is affecting the underlying MS.
2. In a postconference setting, have students share how nursing care changes when the client has an underlying diagnosis of MS.
3. Assign students to research the four different types of MS. Assist students to read history and physical information in patient charts to determine what kind of MS their client has.
4. If more than one student is caring for a client with MS, have them compare and contrast the varying manifestations experienced by the clients.
5. Have students design a client/family teaching brochure covering one of the teaching topics mentioned in lecture.
6. Invite a member from a local MS support organization to speak to the students in a postconference about community resources for the client/family.

© 2007 Pearson Education, Inc.

Learning Outcome 3

Describe the pathophysiology, etiology, manifestations, medical treatments, nursing implications, and the nursing plan of care for the client with Parkinson's disease.

Concepts for Lecture

1. Statistics related to Parkinson's disease illustrate how degenerative neurologic disorders affect differing populations in the U.S.
2. The pathophysiology of Parkinson's disease involves imbalances in critical neurotransmitters necessary for motor functioning.
3. Manifestations of Parkinson's disease appear as alterations in motor functioning and coordination.
4. The medications used to treat Parkinson's have therapeutic effects that control symptoms rather than cure.
5. Surgery, electrical stimulation, and complementary therapies may improve the quality of life for clients with Parkinson's disease.
6. The nurse can use the nursing process to create an individualized plan of care for the client with Parkinson's. This plan will include client/family teaching.

PowerPoint Lecture Slides

1 Parkinson's Disease: Statistics
- Most common neurologic disorder in the U.S.
- 1.5 million affected
- Most common > over 40 y/o
- Caucasian men vs. women

2 Pathophysiology of Parkinson's
- Deficiency of dopamine
  - Atrophy of cerebral cortex neurons
  - Decreased dopamine receptors
- Loss of inhibition of acetylcholine
  - Constant excitement of motor neurons

3 Manifestations of Parkinson's
- Cardinal signs
  - Tremor
  - Rigidity
  - Bradykinesia

3a Other Manifestations
- Tremor
- Rigidity of neck, shoulders, and trunk
- Bradykinesia
- Drooling

4 Medications Used in Parkinson's Disease
- Dopaminergics
- Dopamine agonists
- Anticholinergics
- MAOIs

5 Other Therapies for Parkinson's
- Surgery
  - Pallidotomy
  - Stereotactic thalamotomy
- Deep brain electrical stimulation
- Complementary therapy
  - Yoga, t'ai chi, massage, acupuncture

6 Nursing Process: Assessment
- Cognition, mood
- Motor functioning
  - Falls; stiffness; jerking movements
  - "Pill-rolling"
  - Facial muscle effects
- Weight loss; chewing/swallowing

6a Nursing Process: Diagnoses
- Impaired Physical Mobility
- Impaired Verbal Communication
- Imbalanced Nutrition: Less than Body Requirements
- Self-Care Deficit
- Ineffective Coping

© 2007 Pearson Education, Inc.

PowerPoint Lecture Slides *continued*

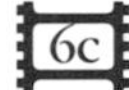

Nursing Process: Evaluation
- Ability to:
  - Ambulate
  - Chew and swallow
  - Communicate
- Complications
- Knowledge level related to disease process

6c Client/Family Teaching
- Assistive devices
- Communication techniques
- Decreasing aspiration risk
- Safety
- Diet
- Exercise

Suggestions for Classroom Activities

1. Compare and contrast Parkinson's disease with other degenerative neurologic disorders in this chapter. Include statistics on populations affected as well as pathophysiology.
2. Ask students to share experiences with family or friends with Parkinson's disease.
3. Divide students into small workgroups. Assign each group a classification of medication used in the treatment of Parkinson's. Have students report on the effects and side effects of the medications.
4. Discuss the concept of neurotransmitters.
5. Discuss other symptoms of Parkinson's from Box 39-5. Use transparency if available.
6. Explain how surgical treatments help to relieve symptoms

Suggestions for Clinical Activities

As with other degenerative neurologic diseases, these activities are better implemented in a skilled care or home care setting.

1. Assign students to clients with Parkinson's disease requiring long-term skilled nursing care. Have students complete a neurologic assessment. Discuss how the assessment finding for a client with Parkinson's differs from that of a client with MS or Alzheimer's.
2. Have students evaluate the nutritional status of their assigned clients.
3. In the home setting, have students assess the home environment for safety issues. If safety concerns arise, have the students complete client/family teaching on the topic.
4. Instruct students to create a one-day meal plan for a client with late-stage Parkinson's.
5. Assign students to the physical therapy department for one clinical day. Have students report in postconference the types of therapy and/or exercise that is used for the client with Parkinson's.
6. Invite a member of a local support group to speak with the clinical group.

Learning Outcome 4

Describe the pathophysiology, etiology, manifestations, medical treatments, nursing implications, and the nursing plan of care for the client with myasthenia gravis.

Concepts for Lecture

1. There are both similarities and differences in the pathophysiology of myasthenia compared to other degenerative neurologic disorders.
2. Myasthenia is a disease that affects the neuromuscular junction and the neurotransmitter involved is acetylcholine.
3. Clinical manifestations are seen in the facial muscles, as well as those used for speech and chewing. There are two life-threatening manifestations associated with myasthenia.

PowerPoint Lecture Slides

1 Myasthenia Gravis
- Women ages 20–30
- Exacerbations and remissions
- Triggers for exacerbations

2 Pathophysiology of Myasthenia
- Auto-antibodies from thymus gland
  - Block acetylcholine receptors
  - Decrease number of receptors

CONCEPTS FOR LECTURE *continued*

4. The goal of pharmacotherapy related to myasthenia is to reduce the breakdown of acetylcholine and/or decrease the number of circulating receptor antibodies.
5. There are two short-term treatments for myasthenia gravis.
6. The nursing process can be used to create an individualized plan of care for the client with myasthenia gravis. This plan includes client/family teaching.

POWERPOINT LECTURE SLIDES *continued*

- Blockage of nerve impulses to:
  - Face, lips, tongue, neck, and throat
- Can affect fine motor skills
- Can affect respiratory muscles

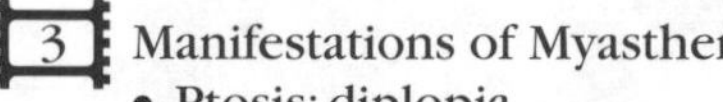

3 Manifestations of Myasthenia
- Ptosis; diplopia
- Slurred speech
- Difficulty chewing and swallowing
- Respiratory insufficiency
- Fatigue
- Altered facial expressions
- Difficulty writing

3a Life-Threatening Complications of Myasthenia
- Cholinergic crisis
  - Severe muscle weakness, nausea, vomiting
  - Salivation, sweating, bradycardia
- Myasthenia crisis
  - Muscle weakness
  - Inability to swallow; respiratory distress

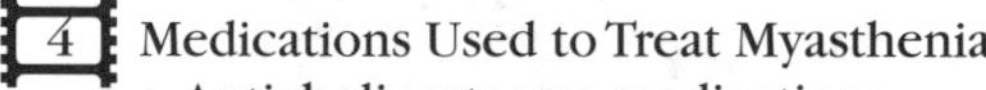

4 Medications Used to Treat Myasthenia
- Anticholinesterase medications
- Steroids
- Cytotoxic agents

5 Short-Term Treatments
- Thymectomy
  - Removal of the thymus
  - Decreased auto-antibody production
- Plasmapheresis
  - Removes auto-antibodies

6 Nursing Process: Assessment
- Muscle weakness
- Respiratory effort
- Ability to swallow
- Speech
- Vision

6a Client/Family Teaching
- Medication regimen
  - Strict time schedule
  - Effects; side effects
- CPR: airway management
- Symptoms of myasthenia and cholinergic crisis

SUGGESTIONS FOR CLASSROOM ACTIVITIES

1. Compare and contrast myasthenia gravis and other degenerative neurologic disorders. Include pathophysiology and manifestations.
2. Discuss the impact of the manifestations on client's ability to complete ADLs.
3. Discuss the impact of chewing and swallowing on the client's nutritional status.
4. Discuss the difference between early manifestations and late; e.g., diplopia versus respiratory involvement.

SUGGESTIONS FOR CLINICAL ACTIVITIES

1. Have students discuss the impact of hospitalization on a client with myasthenia gravis.
2. Assign students to a client with myasthenia. Have students complete a neurologic exam, identifying the manifestations of the disease.
3. If the experience is available, have students observe plasmapheresis.
4. Have a member of a community support group for clients with myasthenia gravis speak to the students.

© 2007 Pearson Education, Inc.

5. Compare and contrast myasthenia and cholinergic crises.
6. Have students research the two short-term treatments of thymectomy and plasmapheresis. Ask students to explain the procedures during lecture.

5. Have students develop a client/family teaching brochure for anticholinesterase medications, including the concepts of myasthenia and cholinergic crisis.

LEARNING OUTCOME 5

Describe the basic pathophysiology and common manifestations of less common degenerative neurologic diseases including amyotrophic lateral sclerosis, Guillain-Barré syndrome, trigeminal neuralgia, and Bell's palsy.

CONCEPTS FOR LECTURE

1. Degenerative neurologic disorders have varying pathologies that affect motor neurons, the peripheral nervous system and specific cranial nerves.
2. Each degenerative neurologic disorder has manifestations that are particular to that disorder.

POWERPOINT LECTURE SLIDES

1 Amyotrophic Lateral Sclerosis
- Rapidly progressively fatal
- Loss of motor neurons
  - Spinal cord and brain
- Loss of impulses to voluntary muscles
  - Decreased strength; atrophy
- Cognitive ability/intellect intact

2 Manifestations of ALS
- Muscle weakness; fasciculations
- Muscle wasting: arms, legs, trunk
- Speech/swallowing difficulties
- Compromised respiratory effort
  - Respiratory failure
  - Death

1 Guillain-Barré Syndrome
- Inflammation of PNS
  - Acute, progressive
  - Most clients recover; no residual deficits
- Follows respiratory/GI infection, viral vaccination, surgery
- Myelin sheath destroyed
  - Cell-mediated reaction
  - Poor impulse conduction

2 Manifestations of Guillain-Barré
- Progressive weakness/numbness/tingling
  - Ascending; legs to arms
- Respiratory muscles
- Eventual paralysis
- Cranial nerve involvement
  - Chewing, swallowing, talking
- Potential respiratory failure

1 Trigeminal Neuralgia
- Two sensory branches of the trigeminal nerve
- Pain along branches
- No known cause: could be related to:
  - Dental procedure/surgery; facial trauma, infection, tumor

2 Manifestations of Trigeminal Neuralgia
- Severe one-sided facial pain
- Stabbing/burning: forehead, nose, lips, cheek
- Exacerbations and remissions
- Simple actions can trigger symptoms

POWERPOINT LECTURE SLIDES *continued*

1 Bell's Palsy
- Herpes virus: associated organism
- Inflammation
  - Edema/pressure on facial nerve
  - Necrosis of nerve
- Sudden one-sided facial paralysis
- Can recover; can have residual deficits

2 Manifestations of Bell's Palsy
- Distorted facial features
  - Ptosis, tearing
  - Mouth droop; can't smile
  - Drooling/difficulty chewing

SUGGESTIONS FOR CLASSROOM ACTIVITIES

1. Discuss each less common degenerative neurologic disorder, comparing and contrasting the various pathophysiologic changes that occur.
2. Divide students into small workgroups. Using all the less common disorders in the chapter, assign each student group to a disorder and have them create a nursing plan of care for each. Have the students share their care plans in class.
3. Discuss the impact even "less common" degenerative disorders have on clients and their families in terms of family processes, e.g., jobs, family role, residual deficits.
4. Discuss diagnostics, treatment, and nursing care as time permits.

SUGGESTIONS FOR CLINICAL ACTIVITIES

1. Either in the acute care or home care setting, assign students to clients with the various less common degenerative neurologic disorders listed in the text.
2. Have students compare and contrast the various disorders in terms of disease course and manifestations.
3. Have members of the interdisciplinary team speak to students about their role in the care of clients with the disorders covered in the text.
4. Invite a nurse from a critical care area to speak to the students about the use of ventilators in supporting the respiratory effort of clients with degenerative neurologic disorders.

LEARNING OUTCOME 6

Describe the causes, pathophysiology, and manifestations of spinal cord injuries.

CONCEPTS FOR LECTURE

1. Many types of traumatic injuries result in spinal cord injury. Certain populations are more prone to SCIs.
2. The pathophysiology of spinal cord injury involves initial injury, injury caused by the resulting edema and hypoxia, and deficits resulting from the inability of the cord to regenerate.
3. Manifestations of spinal cord injury can be classified in two ways.
4. Complications of spinal cord injury manifest in all body systems. Two complications are specific to spinal cord injuries.

POWERPOINT LECTURE SLIDES

1 Spinal Cord Injuries: Common Causes
- Affect adolescent and adult males
- Motor vehicle accidents
- Falls
- Violent acts
  - Shootings
- Sports injuries

2 Pathophysiology of SCI
- Bruising or compression of cord via injury
- Bleeding into gray matter
- Inflammatory response
  - Edema
  - Hypoxia
  - Ischemia
- No regeneration

3 Classifications of SCI Manifestations
- Level of injury
  - Cervical—tetraplegia
  - Thoracic—paraplegia
  - Sacral

 © 2007 Pearson Education, Inc.

PowerPoint Lecture Slides *continued*

- Amount of cord damage
  - Complete
  - Incomplete

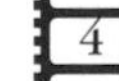
Complications of Spinal Cord Injury
- *Integument:* Decubitus (pressure) ulcers
- *Neurologic:* Pain, hypotonia, autonomic dysreflexia
- *Cardiovascular and peripheral vascular:* Spinal shock, orthostatic hypotension, bradycardia, deep vein thrombosis
- *Respiratory:* Limited chest expansion, pneumonia

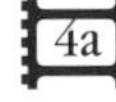
Complication of Spinal Cord Injury
- *Gastrointestinal:* Stress ulcers, paralytic ileus, stool impaction, stool incontinence
- *Genitourinary:* Urinary retention, urinary incontinence, neurogenic bladder, urinary tract infections, impotence, decreased vaginal lubrication
- *Musculoskeletal:* Joint contractures, muscle spasms, muscle atrophy, pathologic fractures, hypercalcemia

Special Complications
- Spinal shock: 30–60 minutes postinjury
  - Loss of reflex activity below injury
  - Bradycardia and hypotension
  - Loss of sweating and temp control
  - Bowel and bladder dysfunction
  - Flaccid paralysis

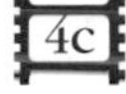
Special Complications
- Autonomic dysreflexia
  - Exaggerated sympathetic response
  - SCIs T6 or above
- Involves triggers/stimuli
- Medical emergency

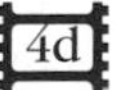
Manifestations of Autonomic Dysreflexia
- Hypertensive crisis
- Pounding headache
- Flushed diaphoretic above lesion
- Cold, pale, dry below lesion
- Goosebumps; anxiety
- Possible CVA/death

Suggestions for Classroom Activities

1. Ask students to list commonly known public personalities who have experienced SCI, e.g., Christopher Reeves. Discuss the common causes of SCI.
2. Use transparency of Figure 39-6 to illustrate cord compression.
3. Divide students into small workgroups. Assign each group a "section" of the spinal column. Have students research the functions carried out by the different nerves in the assigned region.

Suggestions for Clinical Activities

1. Assign students to clients who have experienced a spinal cord injury. Assist students to complete a neurologic exam focusing on functional ability.
2. Invite a nurse from the ICU area to speak with the students about immediate emergent care of the client with a SCI.
3. Invite a member of a rehab team to speak with students about the latest in rehabilitation strategies for the client with an SCI.

© 2007 Pearson Education, Inc.

4. Compare and contrast spinal shock and autonomic dysreflexia. Discuss the "triggers" for autonomic dysreflexia.
5. Discuss the complications of spinal cord injury according to body systems affected.

Learning Outcome 7

Describe the client's functional ability according to the level of damage to the spinal cord.

Concepts for Lecture

1. Manifestations of spinal cord injury are dependent on the level at which the injury occurred to the cord. These manifestations are often discussed in terms of the client's functional level.

PowerPoint Lecture Slides

1 Cervical Spinal Cord Injuries
- C1, C2, C3: No movement or sensation below the neck; ventilator-dependent
- C4: Movement and sensation of head and neck; some partial function of the diaphragm
- C5: Controls head, neck, and shoulders; flexes elbows
- C6: Uses shoulder, extends wrist.
- C7–C8: Extends elbow, flexes wrist, some use of fingers

1a Thoracic and Sacral Spinal Cord Injuries
- T1–T5: Has full hand and finger control, full use of thoracic muscles
- T6–T10: Controls abdominal muscles, has good balance
- T11–L5: Flexes and abducts the hips; flexes and extends the knees
- S1–S5: Full control of legs; progressive bowel, bladder, and sexual function

Suggestions for Classroom Activities

1. Using a medical model of a skeleton, review the three different regions of the "spinal cord" by referring to the associated vertebrae.
2. Discuss in detail the functions that remain following injury according to the level of injury.
3. Begin discussion of how the amount of nursing care provided will correspond to the degree of function that is lost.
4. Compare and contrast tetraplegia with paraplegia.

Suggestions for Clinical Activities

1. If possible, assign students to clients who have experienced differing levels of spinal cord injury. Have students share their assessment findings in terms of functional ability.
2. Have students discuss how the nursing plan for care changes depending on the client's functional ability.
3. Assign students to a rehab department. Have them participate in the rehab plan of care for the client with an SCI.

Learning Outcome 8

Describe the interdisciplinary care required for clients with tetraplegia and other spinal cord disorders.

Concepts for Lecture

1. Interdisciplinary care for the client who has experienced a spinal cord injury involves emergent care to preserve life.
2. Diagnostic testing following a spinal cord injury helps to detect the level and extent of injury to the cord.
3. Pharmacotherapy following a spinal cord injury is aimed at decreasing and controlling cord edema.

PowerPoint Lecture Slides

1 Spinal Cord Injury: Emergent Care
- Airway, breathing circulation
- Pain; sensation
- Immobilization: neck, spine
- Oxygenation needs
- Intravenous fluids

© 2007 Pearson Education, Inc.

CONCEPTS FOR LECTURE *continued*

Other medications control spasms and prevent stress ulcers, thrombophlebitis, and constipation.

4. Several devices are used to stabilize and immobilize the spinal cord following an injury.
5. Surgery can be used to remove bone fragments or hematomas and to stabilize and support the spine.

POWERPOINT LECTURE SLIDES *continued*

2 Diagnostic Testing
- Cervical spine x-rays
- CT scan
- MRI

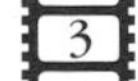

Pharmacotherapy
- Corticosteroids
- Histamine blockers
- Anticoagulants
- Stool softeners

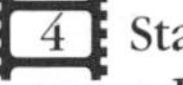

Stabilization/Immobilization
- Braces
- Body casts
- Cervical tongs/traction
- Halo vest

Surgical Interventions in SCI
- Spinal fusion
- Decompression laminectomy
- Insertion of rods

SUGGESTIONS FOR CLASSROOM ACTIVITIES

1. Discuss specific examples of emergent care of the client with spinal cord injury.
2. Invite a member of a paramedic rescue team to speak to the students about emergency care of the SCI victim.
3. If possible, obtain x-ray films from a local clinical agency (observing HIPAA regulations) featuring views of anatomic damage from SCIs.
4. Divide students into small workgroups. Assign each workgroup a class of drugs used in the treatment of spinal cord injury. Have students report on the nursing responsibilities for each class of drug.
5. Using transparencies or other photos, discuss the various devices used to stabilize the spinal cord.

SUGGESTIONS FOR CLINICAL ACTIVITIES

1. Assign students on a clinical day to the radiology department for a desired block of time. Have students observe for clients having radiologic exams for spinal cord injury. Ask students to share their experiences in postconference.
2. Ask a member from an "Air-Life" or other helicopter rescue team to discuss the emergent care in the field for the client with spinal cord injury.

LEARNING OUTCOME 9

Use the nursing process to assess, plan, and implement individualized care for the client with spinal cord disorders.

CONCEPTS FOR LECTURE

1. The nursing plan of care will be prioritized. Promoting respiratory function is a priority intervention.
2. The plan of care will be based on the nurse's assessment of the client's level of functioning.
3. The plan of care includes addressing the client's psychologic needs related to changes in social and personal roles.

POWERPOINT LECTURE SLIDES

Nursing Process: Assessment
- Respiratory
  - Rate, depth, effort
  - Breath sounds
- Sensory level
- Elimination
- History of the trauma

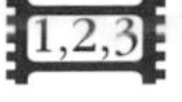

Nursing Process: Diagnoses
- Ineffective Breathing Pattern
- Impaired Physical Mobility
- Impaired Urinary Elimination/Constipation
- Situational Low Self-Esteem

POWERPOINT LECTURE SLIDES *continued*

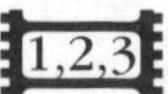 Nursing Process: Evaluation

- Gas exchange/respiratory functioning
- Ability to manage ADLs
- Bowel and bladder function
- Skin integrity
- Absence of system based complications

SUGGESTIONS FOR CLASSROOM ACTIVITIES

1. Discuss assessment findings that would alert the nurse to the client's need for ventilatory assistance.
2. Discuss the assessment techniques used to assess sensation.
3. Review the technique of palpating for bladder fullness.
4. Using each nursing diagnosis listed in the text, describe in full the nursing interventions associated with each.

SUGGESTIONS FOR CLINICAL ACTIVITIES

1. Assign students to clients with spinal cord injuries of varying degrees. Assist students to complete head-to-toe assessments, focusing on level of functioning. Have students compare assessment findings in post conference.
2. Have students develop a nursing plan of care for their assigned clients.
3. Invite a client who has sustained a spinal cord injury (and is now living independently) to speak to the students about his or her experience.

 © 2007 Pearson Education, Inc.

CHAPTER 40
CARING FOR CLIENTS WITH EYE AND EAR DISORDERS

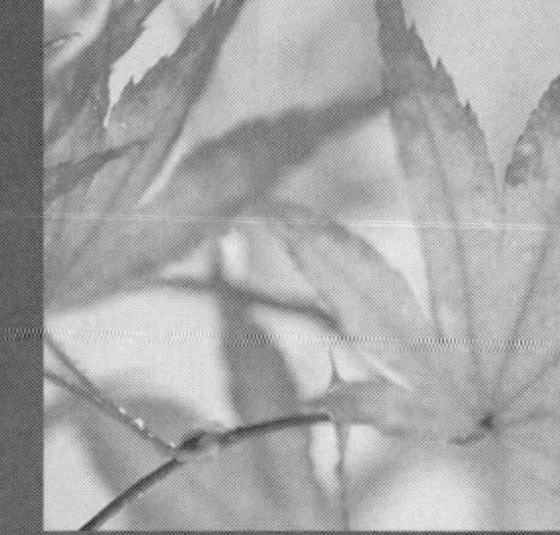

RESOURCE LIBRARY

IMAGE LIBRARY

Figure 40-1 (**A**) Hordeolum (sty); (**B**) Chalazion.
Figure 40-2 An eye with acute conjunctivitis.
Figure 40-3 Corneal ulcers.
Figure 40-4 LASIK surgery corrects refractive error by flattening the cornea of the eye.
Figure 40-5 Blurring of near and distant vision with a cataract.
Figure 40-6 Cataract removal with intraocular lens implant. (**A**) The lens and anterior capsule are removed. (**B**) The intraocular lens is implanted within the posterior capsule behind the pupil.
Figure 40-7 Types of glaucoma. (**A**) Chronic open-angle glaucoma. Drainage of aqueous humor through the trabecular meshwork is impaired. (**B**) Angle-closure glaucoma. The angle between the cornea and iris closes, completely blocking aqueous humor drainage.
Figure 40-8 Narrowing of the visual field with glaucoma.
Figure 40-9 The Schiötz tonometer for measuring intraocular pressure.
Figure 40-10 Detached retina.
Figure 40-11 Blurred central vision occurs in age-related macular degeneration.
Figure 40-12 A red, bulging tympanic membrane of otitis media.
Figure 40-13 Types of hearing aids. (**A**) An in-ear hearing aid. (**B**) A behind-the-ear hearing aid.

LEARNING OUTCOME 1

Describe the pathophysiology, manifestations, and the nurse's role in the care of the client with infectious/inflammatory eye disorders including the nursing implications for medications ordered.

CONCEPTS FOR LECTURE

1. Inflammatory and infectious disorders can affect many different anatomic structures of the eye.
2. Bacteria as well as viruses can cause infectious processes of the eye.
3. The manifestations of inflammatory and infectious eye disorders can range from discomfort to blindness.
4. The goals of pharmacotherapy for infectious and inflammatory eye disorders include eradicating the infectious organism and decreasing inflammation and irritation.
5. The nursing process can be used to develop an individualized nursing plan of care for the client with problems that affect vision.

POWERPOINT LECTURE SLIDES

1 Inflammatory/Infectious Eye Disorders
- Blepharitis; eyelid inflammation
  - Infection/dermatitis
  - Irritation; itchy
- Hordeolum (sty)
  - Eyelid infection; Staphylococcus aureus
  - Red; painful

1a Inflammatory/Infectious Eye Disorders
- Conjuctivitis ("pink eye")
  - Bacterial or viral; direct contact
  - Redness, itching, tearing, discharge
  - Trachoma-corneal damage, blindness

1b Inflammatory/Infectious Eye Disorders
- Keratitis: corneal inflammation
  - Infection; lack of tears, trauma
  - Tearing, discharge, photophobia
  - Blepharospasm

POWERPOINT LECTURE SLIDES *continued*

2 Inflammatory/Infectious Eye Disorders
- Corneal ulcer
  - Infection, trauma, contact lens
  - Herpes virus
  - Scarring, clouding
  - Perforation; vision loss

3 Inflammatory/Infectious Eye Disorders
- Uveitis: inflammation of vascular layer
- Iritis: inflammation of iris
- For both:
  - Severe eye pain; photophobia
  - Blurred vision
  - Constricted pupil; red limbus

4 Medications for Inflammatory/Infectious Eye Disorders
- Topical anti-infectives
- Antihistamines
- Corticosteroids
- Mydriatics

5 Nursing Process: Assessment
- Symptoms: local, systemic
- Structures of the eye
- Vision/corrective lens use
  - Snellen chart
  - Rosenbaum chart
- Injury; exposure

5a Nursing Process: Diagnoses
- Risk for Disturbed Sensory Perception: Visual
- Pain
- Risk for Injury

6 Nursing Process: Evaluation
- Eye appearance/vision
- Client's psychomotor skills related to:
  - Eyedrops
  - Contact lens care
  - Eye cleansing

SUGGESTIONS FOR CLASSROOM ACTIVITIES

1. Using a medical model, review the anatomic structures of the eye.
2. Discuss the concept that inflammation can occur as a manifestation of an infection.
3. Compare and contrast the structures of the eye that are affected by both inflammatory and infectious processes.
4. Discuss the four different categories of medications used for the infectious and inflammatory eye disorders and the nursing responsibilities for each.
5. Review with students the correct technique for drop instillation and ointment application.
6. Using the nursing diagnoses given on the PowerPoint slide, discuss in detail the correlating nursing interventions for each.

SUGGESTIONS FOR CLINICAL ACTIVITIES

These activities would be most appropriate in an outpatient/clinic setting.

1. Assign students to assist with eye exams. Include physical inspection of external structures as well as obtaining subjective data from the client.
2. If the experience is available, have students assist in assessing vision using the Snellen and Rossenbaum charts.
3. Have students teach clients the proper technique for instilling eyedrops as well as applying eye ointment.

© 2007 Pearson Education, Inc.

LEARNING OUTCOME 2

Describe the etiology, manifestations, interdisciplinary, and nursing care for the client who has sustained trauma to the eye.

CONCEPTS FOR LECTURE

1. Eye trauma can affect the internal structures of the eye as well as those parts exposed to the external environment.
2. Eye trauma includes the presence of foreign bodies, abrasions, and lacerations as well as blunt trauma.
3. The manifestations of a traumatic injury to the eye can range from pain and burning to loss of eye contents.
4. Interdisciplinary care for traumatic injuries to the eye includes diagnostic testing.
5. The nursing process can be used to develop an individualized plan of care for the client who has sustained a traumatic injury to the eye.

POWERPOINT LECTURE SLIDES

1 Eye Trauma: Corneal Abrasion
- Scratch of the cornea
  - Contact lenses, eyelashes
  - Small foreign bodies, fingernails
- Pain, photophobia, tearing

2 Eye Trauma: Burns
- Chemical/thermal
  - Ammonia, drain cleaner/UV lights
- Pain, vision changes
- Swollen eyelids; red edematous conjunctiva
- Cornea: cloudy/hazy

2a Eye Trauma: Perforation
- Metal flakes; glass shards
- Weapons
  - Guns, knives, arrows
- Pain; partial or complete loss of vision
- Possible bleeding, loss of eye contents

3 Eye Trauma: Blunt Trauma
- Sports injuries
- Lid ecchymosis, subconjunctival hemorrhage
- Hyphema; fractured orbit
- Diplopia, reddish tint
- Pain; enophthalomos

4 Eye Trauma: Interdisciplinary Care
- Eye inspection/examination
- Fluorescein staining
- Opthalmoscopic examination
- Facial x-rays/CT scan
- Eye irrigations
- Surgery

5 Nursing Process: Assessment
- Type of trauma
- Vision
- Pain

5a Nursing Process: Diagnoses
- Impaired Tissue Integrity: Ocular
- Pain
- Anxiety

5b Nursing Process: Evaluation
- Vision
- Client and/or family are able to verbalize:
  - Prevention
  - Irrigation procedure
  - Medications
  - Patches
  - Intraocular pressure

© 2007 Pearson Education, Inc.

Suggestions for Classroom Activities

1. Divide students into small workgroups. Assign the various categories of eye trauma to individual groups. Have students find alternative causes for each (not found in the text) and share with the class during lecture.
2. Discuss the connection between the risk for eye trauma and certain occupations.
3. Discuss in greater detail the various diagnostic tests used to identify damage caused by each traumatic injury.
4. Using the diagnoses given on the PowerPoint slide, discuss in detail the nursing interventions for the client with eye trauma.

Suggestions for Clinical Activities

1. Assign students to clients who have sustained one of the types of eye trauma discussed in lecture. Have students determine the degree of vision loss experienced by the client.
2. Discuss with students how the even minimal loss of vision affects the client's ability to complete ADLs. Encourage students to discuss with clients their perception of how the loss of vision affects their life.
3. Have students develop a teaching brochure about preventing eye trauma related to sports injuries.

Learning Outcome 3

Describe the pathophysiology, manifestations, and the nursing care for the client undergoing surgery for cataracts.

Concepts for Lecture

1. Cataracts are a common eye disorder that affects older clients, the pathology of which results in impairment of vision.
2. Interdisciplinary care for cataracts involves diagnosis and surgery.
3. The nursing plan of care for the client having surgery for cataracts reflects general principles of care that are applicable to clients having eye surgery for other eye disorders.

PowerPoint Lecture Slides

1 Cataracts
- Affect most people over 65
- Clouding of the lens
  - Immature/mature
- Impairment of vision
  - Glare; dark/light adjustment problems

1a Risk Factors for Cataracts
- Exposure to sunlight
- Cigarette smoking
- Heavy alcohol use
- Congenital conditions
- Medications

2 Interdisciplinary Care
- Ophthalmoscopic exam
  - Lens changes; loss of red reflex
- Elective surgery
  - Lens removal
  - Intraocular lens implant

3 Nursing Care: Eye Surgery
- Preoperative care
  - Routine preop care
  - Assessing vision
  - Reinforcement of postop restrictions

3a Nursing Care: Eye Surgery
- Postoperative care
  - Vital signs, pain control
  - Dressings/patch/shield
  - Positioning
  - Prevent increase in intraocular pressure
  - Report sudden eye pain

© 2007 Pearson Education, Inc.

POWERPOINT LECTURE SLIDES *continued*

3b Nursing Care: Eye Surgery
- Client/family teaching
  - Medication administration techniques
  - Patch/shield application
  - Preventing eye injury
  - Preventing increased intraocular pressure
  - Symptoms to report

SUGGESTIONS FOR CLASSROOM ACTIVITIES

1. Discuss the impact of cataracts on the elderly. Include a discussion of other chronic illnesses that may exacerbate or compound the deficits created by cataracts.
2. Describe each of the risk factors for cataracts related to the concept of preventive health.
3. Use a transparency or printed copy of Box 40-2 to discuss in detail the preoperative and postoperative responsibilities of the nurse when caring for the client having eye surgery.
4. Describe the activities that will increase intraocular pressure postoperatively.
5. Have students cover one eye with a removable gauze dressing. Invite students to complete a common task (i.e., writing, walking around the classroom) then share their experience in terms of having vision in only one eye.

SUGGESTIONS FOR CLINICAL ACTIVITIES

1. Assign students to clients who have had eye surgery. Have students participate in both the preoperative and postoperative care.
2. Have students observe/participate in client/family postoperative teaching.

LEARNING OUTCOME 4

Describe the pathophysiology, manifestations, pharmacotherapy, nursing implications, and nursing care for the client with glaucoma.

CONCEPTS FOR LECTURE

1. The basic etiology of glaucoma is an imbalance between the production and drainage of aqueous humor. There are two types of glaucoma.
2. The manifestations of glaucoma are type specific.
3. Pharmacotherapy for glaucoma is aimed at reducing intraocular pressure and preserving vision.
4. The nursing process can be used to develop an individualized plan of care for the client with glaucoma.
5. Interdisciplinary care for the client with glaucoma includes early detection and potential surgery.

POWERPOINT LECTURE SLIDES

1 Glaucoma
- Aqueous humor
  - Produced by ciliary body
    - Space between lens and cornea
    - Anterior chamber
    - Canal of Schlemm
- Production/drainage disrupted

1a Types of Glaucoma
- Open-angle
  - Obstruction of flow through canal
  - Slow onset
- Angle-closure
  - Cornea/iris angle closure
  - Rapid onset

1b Types of Glaucoma
- Figure 40-7

2 Manifestations: Open-Angle Glaucoma
- Painless
- Gradual loss of peripheral vision
- Blurred vision
- Halos around lights
- Difficulty focusing on near objects

PowerPoint Lecture Slides *continued*

2a Manifestations: Angle-Closure Glaucoma
- Acute severe eye pain
- Blurred or cloudy vision
- Halos around lights
- Affected eye red, cornea clouded
- Nonreactive pupil

3 Medications for Glaucoma
- Miotics
- Sympathomimetics
- Beta blockers
- Prostaglandin analogs
- Carbonic anhydrase inhibitors

4 Nursing Process: Assessment
- Identify clients at risk
- Changes in vision
- Family history of glaucoma
- Inspection of eye structures
- Visual fields

4a Nursing Process: Diagnoses
- Ineffective Health Maintenance
- Risk for Injury
- Anxiety

4b Nursing Process: Evaluation
- Client's knowledge of medications
  - Instillation technique for drops
- Safety issues with vision loss
- Ability to perform ADLs

5 Interdisciplinary Care
- Diagnostics for detection
  - Tonometry
  - Gonioscopy
- Surgery
  - Laser trabeculoplasty
  - Cyclocryotherapy
  - Laser iridotomy

Suggestions for Classroom Activities

1. Review the production, flow, and drainage of aqueous humor.
2. Compare and contrast open-angle and angle-closure glaucoma. Use Fig. 40-7.
3. Discuss the populations affected by glaucoma. Include a brief review of other disorders that also may impair vision (e.g., diabetes).
4. Divide students into small workgroups. Assign each group a class of drugs used in the treatment of glaucoma. Have students list the nursing responsibilities for each drug used.
5. Using the nursing diagnoses provided on the PowerPoint slides, discuss in detail the nursing interventions for the client with glaucoma.

Suggestions for Clinical Activities

1. Have students observe diagnostic testing for glaucoma. When applicable, have students participate in the testing.
2. Assign students to a nurse preceptor in the clinic setting. Have students observe and/or assist with gathering assessment data related to glaucoma.
3. If in an applicable clinical area, have students observe the various surgical interventions for glaucoma.
4. Ask students to develop a teaching brochure for clients with visual impairments, giving the client and family information on how to reduce the risk for injury in the home.

© 2007 Pearson Education, Inc.

LEARNING OUTCOME 5

Describe the pathophysiology, manifestations, and nursing plan of care for the client experiencing a detached retina.

CONCEPTS FOR LECTURE

1. A detached retina can occur slowly over time or spontaneously as a result of trauma.
2. The pathophysiology of a detached retina involves the separation of the retina from the choroid.
3. The retina contains neurons integral to the sense of vision; therefore, the classic symptoms of a detached retina manifest as changes in vision.
4. Interdisciplinary care for a detached retina includes proper positioning and procedures to reconnect the retina and the choroid.
5. The nursing process can be used to develop an individualized plan of care for the client with a detached retina, which focuses on early identification and treatment.

POWERPOINT LECTURE SLIDES

1 Detached retina
- Etiologies
  - Shrinking of the vitreous humor with age
  - Trauma
    - Hole/tear in retina
  - Certain disease processes

2 Detached retina: Pathophysiology
- Retina separates from choroid
  - Intact but separate
  - Folds back on self
- Hole/tear
  - Fluid seeps between layers

3 Manifestations of Detached Retina
- Painless
- Curtain/veil across vision
- Floaters
- Flashes of light

4 Interdisciplinary Care
- Positioning
- Air into vitreous cavity
- Laser or cryotherapy
- Scleral buckling

5 Nursing Process: Assessment
- Sudden change in vision
- Client knowledge level
- Treatment planned
  - Assessments r/t the client having eye surgery

5a Nursing Process: Diagnoses
- Ineffective Tissue Perfusion: Retinal
- Anxiety
- Deficient Knowledge r/t surgery

5b Nursing Process: Evaluation
- Anxiety level
- Client knowledge of:
  - Importance of positioning
  - Future detachments
  - Safety
  - Follow-up treatment

SUGGESTIONS FOR CLASSROOM ACTIVITIES

1. Use Figure 40-10 to illustrate further the pathophysiology of a detached retina. Use a medical model if necessary to show the layers of the inner eye.
2. Describe the manifestations of a detached retina, stressing that these are classic symptoms for this disorder.

SUGGESTIONS FOR CLINICAL ACTIVITIES

1. Assign students to participate in the assessment of the client with a detached retina. Have the students share which classic signs and symptoms have manifested in varying clients.
2. Have students observe the various procedures used to treat a detached retina.

© 2007 Pearson Education, Inc.

3. Compare and contrast the various treatments for a detached retina. Clarify for students that these are most often carried out in the outpatient or clinic area.
4. Using the nursing diagnoses provided, discuss in detail the nursing interventions for the client with a detached retina.

3. In postconference, have students devise a discharge teaching instruction sheet for clients having treatment for a detached retina.
4. Invite a member of the eye clinic/ophthalmologist's office to speak with the students about the care and treatment of a client with retinal detachment.

LEARNING OUTCOME 6

Describe the pathophysiology, manifestations, interdisciplinary care, and nurse's role in the care of client with otitis media, including the nursing implications for medications ordered.

CONCEPTS FOR LECTURE

1. Otitis media most often occurs as a result of changes in the patency of the eustachian tube.
2. There are two different classifications of otitis media, each having specific pathophysiologic processes and manifestations.
3. Ineffective treatment of otitis media can lead to complications.
4. Interdisciplinary care for otitis media includes pharmacotherapy and surgery.
5. The nursing plan of care for the client having surgery for otitis media reflects general principles of care that are applicable to clients having ear surgery for other ear disorders.
6. The nursing process can be used to develop an individualized plan of care for the client with otitis media.

POWERPOINT LECTURE SLIDES

1 Otitis Media
- Inflammation/infection of the middle ear
- Eustachian tube
  - Connects middle ear to nasopharynx
  - Involved in development of otitis media

2 Pathophysiology and Manifestations
- Serous otitis media
  - Obstruction of eustachian tube
  - Negative pressure draws fluid
- "Snapping," "popping"
- Retracted/bulging ear drum
- Acute pain/bleeding in middle ear/ruptured drum

2a Pathophysiology and Manifestations
- Acute otitis media
  - Follows URI; impaired tube drainage
  - Collection of fluid and mucous/bacterial growth
- Pus; increased pressure/rupture
- Severe pain, fever
- Hearing loss, vertigo, tinnitus
- Possible purulent drainage

3 Complications of Otitis Media
- Acute mastoiditis
  - Destroys air cells
  - Recurrent earaches/hearing loss
- Chronic otitis media
  - Permanent eardrum perforation
  - Recurrent ear infections
  - Conductive hearing loss

4 Pharmacotherapy: Otitis Media
- Decongestants
- Antibiotics
- Analgesics

4a Surgical Interventions
- Tympanocentesis
- Myringotomy
- Tympanostomy (tubes)
- Mastoidectomy

5 Nursing Care: Ear Surgery
- Preoperative care
  - Routine preop care

© 2007 Pearson Education, Inc.

POWERPOINT LECTURE SLIDES *continued*

- Assess hearing
- Plan communication strategies
- Explain postop restrictions

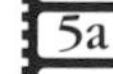

Nursing Care: Ear Surgery
- Postoperative care
  - Assess:
    - Bleeding/drainage/hearing
  - Control nausea
  - Positioning
  - Safety r/t vertigo
- Home care instructions

Nursing Process: Assessment
- Symptoms: onset, duration
- URI history
- Pain; exacerbating/alleviating factors
- Hearing
- Visual inspection: otoscope

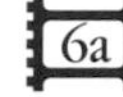

Nursing Process: Diagnoses
- Pain
- Deficient Knowledge: Antibiotic Therapy
- Impaired Tissue Integrity

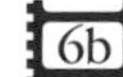

Nursing Process: Evaluation
- Client's knowledge of:
  - Treatment plan
  - Antibiotic regimen compliance
  - Symptoms to report
  - Hearing

SUGGESTIONS FOR CLASSROOM ACTIVITIES

1. Using a transparency or medical model, review the structures of the ear, focusing on the middle ear.
2. Discuss the populations usually affected by otitis media.
3. Compare and contrast the two types of otitis media and their associated manifestations.
4. Divide students into small workgroups. Assign each group a class of drugs used in the treatment of otitis media. Have students present the nursing responsibilities associated with each class.
5. Review routine preoperative care for any surgical procedure. Discuss the various types of surgical interventions.
6. Describe the activities to be avoided postoperatively that may increase inner ear pressure.
7. Using Box 40-8, discuss the discharge instructions for home care for the client having ear surgery.
8. Using the nursing diagnoses given in the text, describe in full detail the nursing interventions for the client having otitis media/ear surgery.

SUGGESTIONS FOR CLINICAL ACTIVITIES

1. If possible, assign students to the day-surgery area to observe the various surgical interventions for otitis media.
2. Obtain an otoscope. Allow students to practice visualization of the eardrum on peers. Have students describe their observations.
3. Assist students to practice techniques used to assess hearing.
4. Have students participate in both preoperative and postoperative client teaching.

Learning Outcome 7

Describe the pathophysiology, manifestations, and nursing care for the client with inner ear disorders.

Concepts for Lecture

1. Labyrinthitis and Ménière's disease are two inner ear disorders.
2. There are commonalities in the pathophysiology and manifestations of both inner ear disorders.
3. Interdisciplinary care for the client with labyrinthitis or Ménière's disease can include diagnostic testing, pharmacotherapy, symptom management, or surgery.
4. The nursing process can be used to develop an individualized plan of care for the client with an inner ear disorder. The plan focuses on symptom management and prevention of permanent hearing loss.

PowerPoint Lecture Slides

1 Labyrinthitis
- Inner ear inflammation
- Severe vertigo; nausea, vomiting
- Hearing loss
- Nystagmus
- Risk for falls

2 Ménière's Disease
- Chronic: excess fluid and pressure
- Recurring vertigo; abrupt, unpredictable
- Tinnitus
- Gradual hearing loss

3 Interdisciplinary Care
- Diagnostic testing
  - Electronystagmography
  - X-rays/CT scan
  - Glycerol test
- Pharmacotherapy
  - Antivert, Compazine, Vistaril

3a Interdisciplinary Care
- Symptom management
  - Control environmental stimuli
  - Bed rest; decreased movement
  - Dietary changes; tobacco, alcohol, caffeine
- Surgery

4 Nursing Process: Assessment
- Balance/safety
- Hearing
- Nystagmus
- Nutritional status
- Sleep/rest/activity

4a Nursing Process: Diagnoses
- Risk for Trauma
- Disturbed Sleep Pattern

4b Nursing Process: Evaluation
- Client's knowledge of:
  - Safety measures
  - Disease process
  - Measures to decrease reoccurrence
  - Disease management

Suggestions for Classroom Activities

1. Using a medical model, describe the structures of the inner ear and their involvement in both hearing and balance.
2. Compare the similarities between labyrinthitis and Ménière's disease.
3. Discuss the nursing implications for the three classes of drugs used to treat symptoms of inner ear disorders.

Suggestions for Clinical Activities

1. Assign students to clients who have inner ear disorders. Have students describe how their plan for care incorporates addressing safety concerns related to vertigo.
2. Have students assess the effects of disease manifestations on the client's quality of life.

 © 2007 Pearson Education, Inc.

4. Using the nursing diagnoses given in the text, describe in detail the nursing interventions for the client with inner ear disorders.

3. Have student assess the effects of disease manifestations on the client's nutrition, activity, safety, sleep patterns, etc.

Learning Outcome 8

Describe the pathophysiology, interdisciplinary care, and nursing care for the client with hearing loss.

Concepts for Lecture

1. There are two different classifications of hearing loss, each having specific pathophysiologic processes.
2. Interdisciplinary care for the client with hearing loss includes diagnostic testing, sound amplification, and possible surgical intervention.
3. The nursing process can be used to develop an individualized plan of care for the client with a hearing loss. The plan is dependent on the type and extent of the hearing loss.

PowerPoint Lecture Slides

1 Conductive Hearing Loss
- Sound transmission affected
  - Obstruction of the ear canal
  - Perforated eardrum
  - Damage to ossicles
  - Fluid/scarring/tumors

1a Sensorineural Hearing Loss
- Inner ear/auditory pathway affected
  - Trauma/infection
  - Ménière's disease
  - Ototoxic medications
  - Noise exposure: major cause

2 Interdisciplinary Care
- Diagnostic testing
  - Rinne test; Weber test
  - Audiometry
- Amplification
  - Hearing aid; pocket talkers
- Surgery
  - Cochlear implant

3 Nursing Process: Assessment
- Voice volume
- Body language
  - Cupping ear, turning head
- Changes in social participation
- Visual inspection
- Hearing tests

3a Nursing Process: Diagnoses
- Impaired Verbal Communication
- Disturbed Sensory Perception: Auditory
- Social Isolation

3b Nursing Process: Evaluation
- Observation of:
  - Social behavior, anxiety and stress level
  - Absence of coping behaviors
- Client's knowledge of:
  - Hearing aide use
  - Community resources

© 2007 Pearson Education, Inc.

SUGGESTIONS FOR CLASSROOM ACTIVITIES

1. Using a transparency or medical model, describe the structures of the ear involved in hearing loss.
2. Compare and contrast sensorineural and conductive hearing loss.
3. Divide students into small workgroups. Assign each group a common environmental noise, including items such as construction noise, traffic, different types of music. Have each group research the decibel level for each type of noise. Have students share their findings during lecture.
4. Using Box 40-9, describe the techniques used for the Rinne and Weber hearing tests.
5. Using the nursing diagnoses given in the text, discuss in detail the nursing interventions for the client with a hearing loss.
6. Discuss the nursing responsibilities in terms of caring for amplification devices.

SUGGESTIONS FOR CLINICAL ACTIVITIES

1. Assign students to observe diagnostic testing for hearing loss at an outpatient clinic. Have students participate in the testing as appropriate.
2. Have students place a clean cotton ball in the outermost aspect of the ear canal. Have students describe the impact on their hearing.
3. With hearing "impaired" by a cotton ball, encourage students to speak to each other in low tones or a whispered voice. Have students share the impact of hearing loss on social interactions.
4. Collaborate with a local school district. Have students participate in hearing screenings for elementary students.
5. Have a representative from a hearing aid company speak with students about amplification products available to clients with a hearing loss.

 © 2007 Pearson Education, Inc.

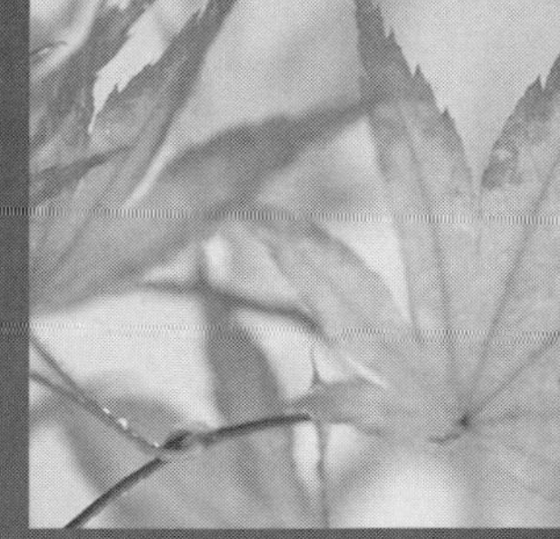

CHAPTER 41
THE MUSCULOSKELETAL SYSTEM AND ASSESSMENT

RESOURCE LIBRARY

IMAGE LIBRARY

Figure 41-1 Bones of the human skeleton.
Figure 41-2 Classification of bones by shape.
Figure 41-3 (**A**) Muscles of the anterior body. (**B**) Muscles of the posterior body.
Figure 41-4 Checking for the bulge sign.
Figure 41-5 Checking for ballottement.

LEARNING OUTCOME 1

Describe the structure and function of bones, joints, muscles, ligaments, and tendons.

CONCEPTS FOR LECTURE

1. The musculoskeletal system includes bones and joints of the skeleton, connective tissues such as tendons and ligaments, and the skeletal muscles. The musculoskeletal system allows us to remain upright and to move and protect our vital organs.

POWERPOINT LECTURE SLIDES

1 Structure and Function of Bones
- Human skeleton has 206 bones
- Functions
  - Provide structure and support for soft tissue
  - Protect vital organs
- Bones classified according to shape
  - Long bones
  - Short bones
  - Flat bones
  - Irregular bones

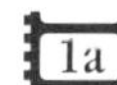

1a Types of Bone
- Compact bone—smooth and dense; forms shaft of long bones and outside layer of other bones
- Spongy bone—contains spaces; spongy sections contain bone marrow
- Two types of marrow
  - Red bone marrow—found in flat bones of sternum, ribs, and ileum; produces blood cells and hemoglobin
  - Yellow bone marrow—found in shaft of long bones; contains fat and connective tissue

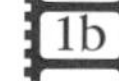

1b Joints (Articulations)
- Area where two or more bones meet
- Function
  - Holds skeleton together while allowing body to move
- Three types of joints
  - Synarthrosis—immovable (e.g., skull)
  - Amphiarthrosis—slightly movable (e.g., vertebral joints)
  - Diarthrosis or synovial—freely movable (e.g., shoulders, hips)
- Synovial joints found at all limb articulations
- Surface covered with cartilage

POWERPOINT LECTURE SLIDES *continued*

- Joint cavity covered with tough fibrous capsule
- Cavity lined with synovial membrane and filled with synovial fluid

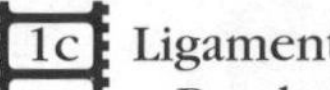
1c Ligaments

- Bands of connective tissue that connect bone to bone
- Function
  - Either limit or enhance movement
  - Provide joint stability
  - Enhance joint strength

1d Tendons

- Fibrous connective tissue bands that connect bone to muscles
- Function:
  - Enable bones to move when muscles contract

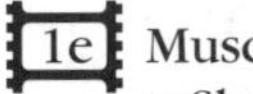
1e Muscles

- Skeletal muscle (voluntary muscle)—allows voluntary movement
  - Structure: 600 skeletal muscles
  - Made up of thick bundles of parallel fibers
  - Each muscle fiber made up of smaller structure myofibrils
  - Myofibrils are strands of repeating units called sarcomeres
  - Skeletal muscle contracts with the release of acetylcholine
  - The more fibers that contract, the stronger the muscle contraction
- Smooth muscle—involuntary muscle movement controlled by internal mechanism (e.g., muscles in bladder wall and GI system)
- Cardiac muscle (involuntary muscle)—found in heart

LEARNING OUTCOME 2

Identify age-related changes in the musculoskeletal system.

CONCEPTS FOR LECTURE

1. Aging commonly affects the musculoskeletal system. Although some musculoskeletal changes appear to relate to the aging process itself, others result from decreased activity, lifestyle factors, or pathophysiologic processes.

POWERPOINT LECTURE SLIDES

1 Changes in Older Adult

- Musculoskeletal changes can be due to:
  - Aging process
  - Decreased activity
  - Lifestyle factors

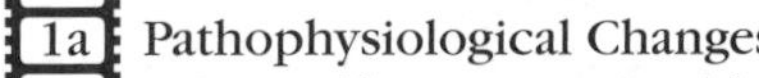
1a Pathophysiological Changes

- Loss of bone mass in older women
- Joint and disk cartilage dehydrates causing loss of flexibility contributes to degenerative joint disease (osteoarthritis); joints stiffen, lose range of motion
- Cause stooped posture, changing center of gravity
- Elderly at greater risk for falls
- Endocrine changes cause skeletal muscle atrophy
- Muscle tone decreases

© 2007 Pearson Education, Inc.

LEARNING OUTCOME 3

Collect appropriate subjective and objective assessment data related to the musculoskeletal system and its function.

CONCEPTS FOR LECTURE

1. The data may be collected as part of the total health assessment of the client or it may be collected from a client with a complaint or disorder related to the musculoskeletal system. Pain and limited mobility are the primary manifestations of musculoskeletal trauma and disorders. The assessment should include subjective data from the health history as well as well as objective data from the physical examination.

POWERPOINT LECTURE SLIDES

1 Assessment of Musculoskeletal System
- Health history
- Chief complaint
- Onset of problem
- Effect on ADLs
- Precipitating events, e.g., trauma
- Examine complaints of pain for location, duration, radiation character (sharp dull), aggravating, or alleviating factors
- Inquire about fever, fatigue, weight changes, rash, or swelling

1a Physical Exam—Assess:
- Posture
- Gait
- Ability to walk with or without assistive devices
- Ability to feed, toliet, and dress self
- Muscle mass and symmetry
- Muscle strength on scale of 0–5, 5 full ROM against resistance (Tables 41-2 and 41-3)
- Inspect and palpate bone, joints for visible deformities, tenderness or pain, swelling, warmth, and ROM
- Assess and compare corresponding joints
- Palpate joints knees and shoulder for crepitus (grating sound during ROM)
- Clinical alert: Never attempt to move a joint past normal ROM or past point where patient experiences pain
- Bulge sign and ballottment sign used to assess for fluid in the knee joint
- Thomas test performed when hip flexion contracture suspected

LEARNING OUTCOME 4

Provide nursing care for clients undergoing diagnostic tests for musculoskeletal system disorders.

CONCEPTS FOR LECTURE

1. The diagnostic tests used to diagnose a musculoskeletal disorder are the arthrocentesis, arthroscopy, and bone scan.

POWERPOINT LECTURE SLIDES

1 Arthrocentesis
- Procedure to obtain fluid from joint
- Nursing Care Checklist (Box 41-2)

1a Bone scan
- Nuclear medicine procedure in which amount of radioactive isotope taken up by bones is evaluated
- Abnormal bone scans show hot spots due to malignancies or infection
- Cold spot uptakes show areas of bone that are ischemic
- Nursing Care Checklist (Box 41-3)

© 2007 Pearson Education, Inc.

PowerPoint Lecture Slides *continued*

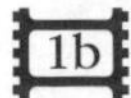
Arthroscopy
- Flexible fiberoptic endoscope used to view joint structures and tissues
- Used to identify torn tendon and ligaments, injured meniscus, inflammatory joint changes, and damaged cartilage
- Nursing Care Checklist (Box 41-4)

Suggestions for Classroom Activities

1. Review the structures of the musculoskeletal system, using an anatomic model that illustrates bones, joints, and attachment of muscles, ligaments, and tendons.
2. Differentiate between musculoskeletal problems caused by deconditioning and those related to normal effects of aging.
3. Describe the physical examination of the musculoskeletal system and demonstrate measurements of limbs and joint motion.
4. Discuss common diagnostic studies of the musculoskeletal system, emphasizing the nurse's responsibility in arthroscopy and arthrocentesis.

Suggestions for Clinical Activities

Have student perform a physical assessment of a client who has a musculoskeletal disorder.

© 2007 Pearson Education, Inc.

CHAPTER 42
CARING FOR CLIENTS WITH MUSCULOSKELETAL TRAUMA

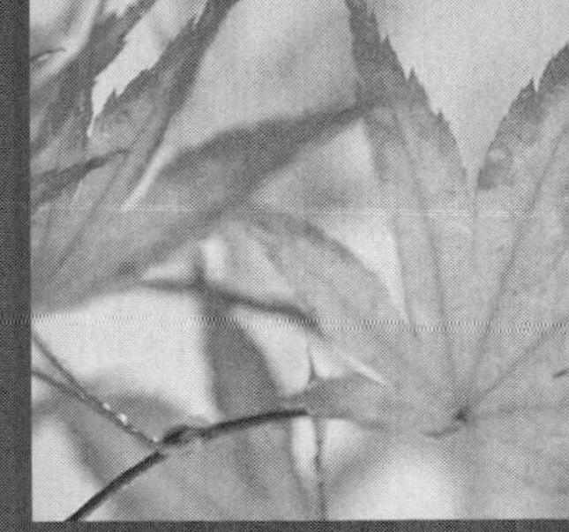

RESOURCE LIBRARY

IMAGE LIBRARY

Figure 42-1 Fracture healing.
Figure 42-2 Common types of casts.
Figure 42-3 Bivalving a cast.
Figure 42-4 Examples of traction. **(A)** Buck's traction, a straight, skin traction. **(B)** Balanced suspension traction for a femur fracture. **(C)** Skeletal traction to stabilize a fractured humerus.
Figure 42-5 An external fixator device used to stabilize a fractured tibia and fibula.
Figure 42-6 Internal fixation devices. **(A)** A plate and screws used to stabilize an oblique fracture. **(B)** Screws inserted through the fracture. **(C)** A medullary nail inserted into the bone to stabilize a segmental fracture.
Figure 42-7 A clavicular strap to immobilize a fractured clavicle.
Figure 42-8 The *head* of the femur fits into the socket of the pelvis. The *neck* is the narrower area below the head. The *trochanteric* region is below the neck.
Figure 42-9 **(A)** A surgical nail or screw is used to stabilize an intertrochanteric hip fracture. **(B)** A hip prosthesis is used if the femoral head is damaged.
Figure 42-10 Phalen's test. The wrist is flexed 90 degrees with the fingers extended. Finger numbness during the test may indicate carpal tunnel syndrome.
Figure 42-11 Common sites of amputation. **(A)** The upper extremities and **(B)** the lower extremities.
Figure 42-12 With an above-knee amputation, a figure-8 bandage is wrapped around the waist, then brought down over the stump and back up around the hips.

LEARNING OUTCOME 1

Discuss risk factors for and mechanisms of musculoskeletal trauma.

CONCEPTS FOR LECTURE

1. Trauma occurs when tissue is subject to more force than it can absorb with the severity dependent on the amount and location.
2. Education is the key to prevention.
3. Older clients are at higher risk.

POWERPOINT LECTURE SLIDES

1 Mechanisms of Musculoskeletal Trauma
- Tissue is subjected to more force than it can absorb
- Severity depends on:
  - Amount of force
  - Location of impact
- Musculoskeletal trauma
  - Mild to severe
  - Soft tissue
  - Fractures
    - Affect function of muscle, tendons, and ligaments
  - Complete amputation

2 Education
- Teach importance of using safety equipment
  - Seat belts
  - Bicycle helmets
  - Football pads
  - Proper footwear
  - Protective eyewear
  - Hard hats

PowerPoint Lecture Slides *continued*

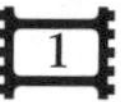

Older Clients Are at Highest Risk
- Falls
- Safety in the home
  - Lighting
  - Handrails
  - Throw rugs
  - Bath mats and grab bars
  - Shoes with good treads

Suggestions for Classroom Activities

1. Have students research state laws on seat belts, helmets, and other protective equipment.
2. Have students do an assessment of their home and the safety risks for injury.

Suggestions for Clinical Activities

1. Discuss risks of the elderly for musculoskeletal trauma in a postclinical conference.
2. Have students prepare a teaching plan for their elderly clients on home safety to prevent musculoskeletal trauma.

Learning Outcome 2

Describe the pathophysiology, interdisciplinary care, and nursing care of clients with soft tissue trauma.

Concepts for Lecture

1. Common injuries result from bleeding into soft tissue and stretching and tears of tissue and ligaments.
2. Interdisciplinary care is focused on decreasing swelling, alleviating pain, and restoring function of the affected tissue.

PowerPoint Lecture Slides

1 Soft Tissue Injuries Are Common
- Contusion
  - Bleeding into soft tissue
    - Significant bleeding can cause a hematoma
    - Swelling and discoloration (bruise)
- Sprain
  - Ligament injury
    - Twisting motion
    - Overstretching or tear
      - Grade I—mild bleeding and inflammation
      - Grade II—severe stretching and some tearing and inflammation and hematoma
      - Grade III—complete tearing of ligament
      - Grade IV—bony attachment of ligament broken away
- Strain
  - Microscopic tear in the muscle
    - May cause bleeding
    - "Pulled muscle"
    - Inappropriate lifting or sudden acceleration-deceleration

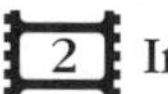

Interdisciplinary Care
- Diagnosis
  - X-ray to rule out fracture
  - MRI
- Measures to decrease swelling, decrease pain, and encourage rest
  - Ice for first 48 hours
  - Splint to support extremities and limit movement
  - Compression dressing
  - Elevation to increase venous return and decrease swelling
  - Nonsteroidal anti-inflammatory drugs (NSAIDs)

© 2007 Pearson Education, Inc.

POWERPOINT LECTURE SLIDES *continued*

- Nursing care
  - Assessment
    - Mechanism of injury
    - Protective devices
    - Pain assessment
    - Inspection for redness, swelling, deformity
    - Range of motion
    - Palpation for warmth, tenderness, crepitus
  - Diagnosing, planning, and implementing
    - Teaching measures
      - Promote comfort
      - Prevent further injury
      - Allow healing
    - Pain control
      - RICE acronym:
        - Rest
        - Ice
        - Compression
        - Elevation
      - Heat after several days
      - NSAIDs
    - Impaired physical mobility

SUGGESTIONS FOR CLASSROOM ACTIVITIES

Ask students to share their personal experiences with soft tissue injuries.

SUGGESTIONS FOR CLINICAL ACTIVITIES

Arrange for clinical experience in emergency department rapid treatment section to observe clients who come in with soft tissue trauma.

LEARNING OUTCOME 3

Describe the pathophysiology, interdisciplinary care, and nursing care of clients with fractures.

CONCEPTS FOR LECTURE

1. Fractures are breaks in the continuity of the bone and vary in severity according to their location and type.
2. The process of fracture healing is affected by age, physical condition, and type of fracture and involves the repair of bone, tissue, and blood vessels.
3. Manifestations of fractures are similar to what is seen in soft tissue injuries.
4. Major complications can occur from infection, blood loss resulting in shock, and excess pressure that restricts blood flow to nerves, fat globules leaving the bone marrow and entering the bloodstream, and from delayed union of the bone.
5. Interdisciplinary care comprises the emergency treatment and diagnosis to restore alignment and accomplish proper immobilization.
6. Other aspects of care includes the use of casting, traction, surgery, and medications.
7. The nursing process is utilized to provide individualized care to the client with fractures.
8. Older adults are at high risk for hip fractures that require comprehensive interdisciplinary and nursing care.

POWERPOINT LECTURE SLIDES

1 Fractures

- Break in the continuity of bone
  - Direct blow
  - Crushing force (compression)
  - Sudden twisting motions (torsion)
  - Severe muscle contraction
  - Disease (pathologic fracture)
- Types
  - Closed or simple
  - Open or compound
  - Complete or incomplete
  - Stable or unstable
  - Direction of the fracture line
    - Oblique
    - Spiral
    - Lengthwise plane (greenstick)

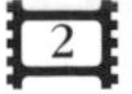
Fracture Healing

- Affected by age, physical condition, and type of fracture
- Damage occurs to blood vessels forming a hematoma
- Local inflammatory response

POWERPOINT LECTURE SLIDES *continued*

- Healing process starts within 48 hours
  - Fibroblasts and new capillaries form granulation tissue
  - Bone cells form osteoblasts build a collagen web
  - Chondroblasts lay down patches of cartilage
  - Fibrocartilaginous callus connect bone fragments splinting the fracture
  - Mineralization with calcium and mineral salts
  - Osteoclasts repair site
  - Excess callus is removed and new bone is laid along the fracture
  - Healing time varies
    - 6–8 weeks to 12–16 weeks for a fractured hip

3 Common Manifestations of Fractures

- Deformity
- Swelling, ecchymosis
- Pain
- Tenderness
- Numbness
- Crepitus
- Muscle spasms

4 Complications

- Infection
  - Risk with open fractures
- Shock
  - Pelvic and femur fractures
- Compartment syndrome
  - Compartment—space enclosed by a fibrous membrane or fascia
  - Within the limbs, fascia enclose and support bones
  - Compartment syndrome
    - Excess pressure restricts blood vessels and nerves within a compartment
    - Bleeding or edema
    - External compression of the limb
    - Nerve damage occurs within 30 minutes
    - Impaired tissue perfusion and necrosis
    - "5 Ps" (Box 42-3)
- Fat embolism
  - Fat globules lodge in a pulmonary vessel or peripheral circulation
    - Fat globules leave the bone marrow and enter the bloodstream after a fracture
    - Combine with platelets
    - Travel to the brain, lungs, kidney, and other organs, causing ischemia
    - Femur (long bone) is at high risk
    - Occurs within few hours to a week after injury
    - See symptoms of altered cerebral perfusion of respiratory distress depending on location of the emboli
- Delayed union
  - Prolonged healing
    - Delayed fracture reduction
    - Inadequate immobilization

© 2007 Pearson Education, Inc.

- Infection
- Age

5 Interdisciplinary Care

- Goal is to reduce (restore normal alignment) and immobilize
- Emergency care and diagnosis
  - Immobilize before moving client
  - Joint above and below
  - Check pulse, color, movement, sensation before splinting
  - Sterile dressing for open wounds
- Fracture reduction
  - Closed—external manipulation
  - Open—surgery

6 Casts, Traction, Surgery, and Medications

- Casts
  - Rigid device to immobilize bones and promote healing
  - Plaster or fiberglass
  - Joints above and below fracture
  - Avoid pressure until cast is dry
  - Type of cast depends on type of fracture
  - Cast care (Box 42-4)
  - Observe for swelling, blood flow, and nerve damage
  - Bivalve casts
- Traction
  - Used to straighten or pull force to decrease muscle spasms and restore proper alignment
    - Types
      - Manual
      - Skin
      - Skeletal
      - Straight
      - Balanced suspension
    - Nursing care checklist of clients with traction (Box 42-5)
- Surgery
  - Align and stabilize fractured bone
    - External fixator
    - Internal fixation
      - ORIF (open reduction and internal fixation)
    - Nursing care check for ORIF (Box 42-6)
- Medications and other interventions
  - Analgesics
  - NSAIDs
  - Parenteral pain medications
  - Stool softners
  - Antiulcer drugs
  - Electrical bone stimulation

7 Nursing Process

- Assessment
  - Pain
  - Pulses
  - Sensation

© 2007 Pearson Education, Inc.

PowerPoint Lecture Slides *continued*

- Skin color
- Temperature
- Motion

- Diagnosis, planning, and implementation
  - Manage pain
  - Impaired Mobility
  - Risk for Ineffective Tissue Perfusion
  - Evaluate effectiveness
    - Pain control
    - Safety and mobility
    - Tissue perfusion
  - Documentation
  - Teaching
    - Care at home
    - Risk for falls

Focus on Older Adults

- Decreasing fractures
  - Fall prevention
  - High risk for hip fractures
    - Decreased bone mass and muscle strength
    - Slowed reflexes
    - Medications affecting cognition and balance
    - Osteoporosis
  - Hip fractures
    - Break in the femur at the head, neck, or trochanter regions
      - Intracapsular
      - Extracapsular
    - Pain, shortening, and external rotation of the affected lower extremity
    - Interdisciplinary care includes:
      - Diagnosis
      - Buck's traction
      - ORIF
        - Arthroplasty
        - Total hip replacement
    - Nursing care
      - Assessment
      - Diagnosis, planning, and implementation
        - Pain
        - Impaired Physical Mobility
        - Impaired Skin Integrity
      - Evaluation
      - Documentation
      - Continuity of care
        - Plan for discharge
        - Inclusion of family
        - Teaching

Suggestions for Classroom Activities

1. Have students match picture of fracture types with terms.
2. Present a case study that discusses compartment syndrome, emphasizing assessment by the nurse.

Suggestions for Clinical Activities

1. Assign students care of hip fracture patients.Ask students to present client at a postclinical conference.
2. Assign students to observe at an orthopedic physician's office or clinic where they will see clients at all stages of injury and care.

© 2007 Pearson Education, Inc.

3. Invite physical therapist to demonstrate use of casts and traction.	3. Arrange for students to observe an ORIF procedure in the operating room.

LEARNING OUTCOME 4

Describe the pathophysiology, interdisciplinary care, and nursing care of clients with joint trauma and injury.

CONCEPTS FOR LECTURE

1. Injury and trauma to joints result in the separation of the joint either partially (subluxation) or fully (dislocation) and are manifested by pain and deformity
2. Interdisciplinary care is required to diagnose, treat, control pain and discomfort, and restore the usual relationship of the bones.
3. Repetitive use of joints also results in joint trauma that results in pain and disability.
4. Interdisciplinary care is required to diagnose, treat, control pain and discomfort, and maintain function of the joints and bones.

POWERPOINT LECTURE SLIDES

1 Joint Trauma

- Dislocation
  - Separation of contact between two bones of a joint
  - Trauma or spontaneous
- Subluxation
  - Partial separation
- Manifestations
  - Pain
  - Change in shape of joint
  - Change in length of extremity
  - Immobility
  - Change in the axis of the bone

2 Interdisciplinary Care of Dislocations and Subluxations

- Manual traction to reduce dislocation
- Narcotics, muscle relaxants, conscious sedation to control pain
- Nursing care
  - Assessment of pain, neurovascular status
  - Traction to maintain alignment
  - Implement care to prevent complications of immobility
  - Teaching to include:
    - Immobilization recommendations
    - Skin care
    - Pain control
    - Rehabilitation exercises

3 Repetitive Use Injuries

- Results from repeated twisting and turning of joint
  - Types
    - Carpal tunnel syndrome
      - Most common work-related injury
      - More common in women than men
      - Tunnel narrows, compressing median nerve
      - Numbness and tingling of thumb, index finger, and middle finger
      - Weakness of affected hand
    - Bursitis
      - Inflammation of the bursa (fluid-filled sac)
      - Shoulder, hip, leg, elbow
      - Pain
    - Epicondylitis
      - Inflammation of a tendon
      - Tennis elbow, golfer's elbow
      - Repeated trauma causes tears, bleeding, and inflammation

© 2007 Pearson Education, Inc.

PowerPoint Lecture Slides *continued*

4 Interdisciplinary Care of Repetitive Use Injuries

- Diagnosis related to cause
- Phalen's test for carpel tunnel
- Initial treatment is rest and immobilization of joint
- NSAIDs
- Surgery for carpel tunnel to enlarge tunnel and relieve pressure on nerve
- Nursing care
  - Pain control
  - Impaired physical mobility
  - Teaching focused on cause and prevention

Suggestions for Classroom Activities

1. Discuss conscious sedation used for pain control during reduction of dislocation.
2. Present case study example of carpel tunnel syndrome.

Suggestions for Clinical Activities

Arrange clinical experience in the OR for surgery for treatment of carpel tunnel syndrome.

Learning Outcome 5

Describe the pathophysiology, interdisciplinary care, and nursing care of clients with amputations.

Concepts for Lecture

1. Amputations are partial or total removal of a body part and may be done to treat disease or chronic conditions or may occur as a result of trauma with the primary pathophysiology a result of impaired blood flow or infection.
2. Complications of amputations include infections, delayed healing, and contractures.
3. Interdisciplinary care focuses on care of the wound, control of pain, prevention of infection, grieving, disturbance of body image, and restoring thc clicnt's function of the lost extremity.

PowerPoint Lecture Slides

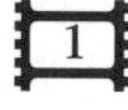
1 Amputation

- Partial or total removal of body part
- Treat cancer
- Chronic condition [peripheral vascular disease (PVD) or diabetes]
- Trauma

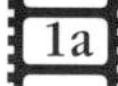
1a Pathophysiology

- Impaired blood flow
- Untreated infection
- Gangrene (tissue death)
- PVD
  - Impaired circulation
  - Edema and tissue damage
- Level determined by extent of tissue damage

2 Complications

- Infection
- Delayed healing
- Contractures
  - Prevention of contractures (Box 42-9)
- Phantom pain
  - Felt along nerves of body part
  - Management is challenging

3 Interdisciplinary Care of the Client with an Amputation

- Open wound (guillotine)
  - Done when infection is present
  - Stump is left open to drain
  - Wound closed when infection is cleared

© 2007 Pearson Education, Inc.

PowerPoint Lecture Slides *continued*

- Closed (flap)
  - Skin is formed to cover end of wound
  - Rigid plaster shell or soft compression dressing applied
- May have a temporary prosthesis
- Once the stump is healed, client is fitted for a prosthesis to aid in restoring function of extremity
- Nursing care
  - Assessment
  - Diagnosis, planning, and evaluation
    - Relieve pain, promote healing, and prevent complications
      - Pain
      - Risk for Infection
      - Risk for Dysfunctional Grieving
      - Disturbed Body Image
      - Impaired Physical Mobility
    - Teaching
      - Knowledge to care for needs
      - Home management

Suggestions for Classroom Activities

Invite representative from prosthetic device company to demonstrate prosthesis fitting and equipment.

Suggestions for Clinical Activities

Assign students to rehabilitation unit to care for clients after their amputation surgery.

© 2007 Pearson Education, Inc.

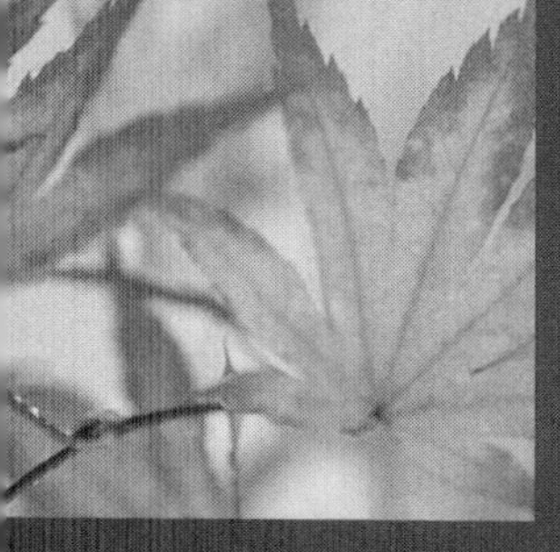

CHAPTER 43
CARING FOR CLIENTS WITH MUSCULOSKELETAL DISORDERS

RESOURCE LIBRARY

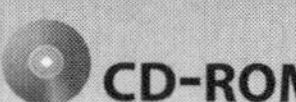

CD-ROM

Video: Osteoporosis
Video: Using a Walker
Video: Using a Cane
Video: Arthritis
Video: MD
Video: Muscle Atrophy

IMAGE LIBRARY

Figure 43-1 (A) Scoliosis, a lateral curvature of the spine. (B) Kyphosis, exaggerated posterior curvature of the thoracic spine.
Figure 43-2 Changes in height, posture, and spinal curves caused by osteoporosis.
Figure 43-3 Osteomyelitis. (A) Bacteria enter and multiply in the bone. (B) The infection spreads to other parts of the bone. If the infection reaches the outer part of the bone, the periosteum separates from the surface of the bone.
Figure 43-4 (A) Hallux valgus (bunion). (B) Hammertoe.
Figure 43-5 (A) Total hip replacement. (B) Total knee replacement.
Figure 43-6 Joint inflammation and destruction in rheumatoid arthritis.
Figure 43-7 Typical hand deformities associated with rheumatoid arthritis. (*Source:* Custom Medical Stock Photos, Inc.)
Figure 43-8 The butterfly rash of systemic lupus erythematosus. (*Source:* Photo Researchers, Inc.)
Figure 43-9 The multisystem effects of systemic lupus erythematosus.

LEARNING OUTCOME 1

Describe the pathophysiology, interdisciplinary care, and nursing care of clients with structural disorders of the spine.

CONCEPTS FOR LECTURE

1. The two most common disorders are scoliosis and kyphosis, which are manifested by structural changes in the spine.
2. Interdisciplinary care is directed toward the identification of the disorder, the determination of risk for injury and impairment of normal activity, and the prevention of skin irritation from braces and devices used to stabilize the spine.

POWERPOINT LECTURE SLIDES

1 Scoliosis
- Diagnosed in adolescence
- More common in girls
- Idiopathic
- Lateral curve
  - Thoracic
  - Lumbar
  - Thoracolumbar
- X-rays show lateral curvature and rotation of the spine
- Severe scoliosis results in:
  - Back pain
  - Dyspnea
  - Anorexia
  - Crowding of internal organs

1a Kyphosis
- Structural changes from multiple causes
- Increased curvature of thoracic spine, "hunchback"
- Results in impaired mobility and potential respiratory problems if severe

2 Interdisciplinary Care
- Diagnosis by x-rays
- Physical exam
  - Symmetry of shoulders, scapulae, waist creases, length of arms

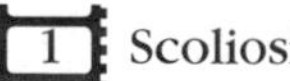

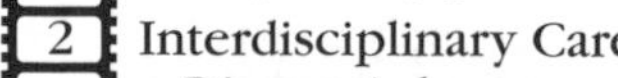

POWERPOINT LECTURE SLIDES *continued*

- Prominence of scapula or hip when bending over
- Thoracic rounding or lumbar swayback
- Nursing care
  - Risk for Injury
  - Potential for skin breakdown from braces

SUGGESTIONS FOR CLASSROOM ACTIVITIES

1. Show pictures of deformities.
2. Demonstrate screening exam for scoliosis and kyphosis.

SUGGESTIONS FOR CLINICAL ACTIVITIES

Assign students to pediatric orthopedic clinic that specializes in treatment of scoliosis.

LEARNING OUTCOME 2

Describe the pathophysiology, interdisciplinary care, and nursing care of clients with bone disorders.

CONCEPTS FOR LECTURE

1. Osteoporosis is a bone disorder that results from loss of bone mass. This leads to fragile brittle bones that are at risk for fractures.
2. Inadequate mineralization of the bone occurs in two conditions that are a result of inadequate intake of minerals or excessive breakdown of the bone minerals.
3. Infections of the bone occur at any age with an increased risk in the elderly. Infections may be difficult to treat and resolve.
4. Bone tumors can be benign or malignant but are more commonly malignant.
5. The common foot disorders cause pain and difficulty walking.

POWERPOINT LECTURE SLIDE

1 Osteoporosis—"Porous Bones"

- Fragile bones with risk of fractures
- 80% are women over the age of 60
- Cause unclear
- Risk factors (Box 43-1)
- Pathophysiology
  - Reduced bone mass
  - Imbalance of bone growth and maintenance
  - Peak bone mass at age 35
  - Formation does not keep pace with resorption, resulting in loss of bone mass
  - Type I osteoporosis
    - Postmenopausal women ages 51–75
    - Caused by estrogen deficiency
  - Type II osteoporosis
    - Men and women over age 70
    - Slow development
    - Calcium deficiency
- Interdisciplinary care
  - Focus is on stopping or slowing process
  - Relieving symptoms
  - Preventing complications
  - Bond density measurement
  - Calcium
    - Vital in prevention
    - Adequate intake may slow process
    - Calcium needs change over lifetime
    - NIH calcium intake recommendations (Table 43-1)
  - Medications
    - Calcium supplements
    - Hormone replacement
    - Other drugs
  - Nursing care
    - Risk for Injury
    - Imbalanced Nutrition: Less than Body Requirements
    - Pain

© 2007 Pearson Education, Inc.

- Health teaching
  - Prevention
  - Calcium intake in diet
  - Physical activity
  - Hormone replacement therapy
  - Smoking
  - Fall prevention

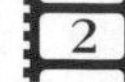

Osteomalacia and Paget's Disease

- Osteomalacia—adult rickets
  - Inadequate mineralization of bone
  - Insufficient amounts of calcium or phosphate result in no mineralization of the bone matrix
  - Bone is unable to bear weight
  - Results in deformities and pathologic fractures
  - Cause is lack of vitamin D
- Paget's disease
  - Increase of osteoclasts
  - Osteoblasts are stimulated but produce soft and poorly mineralized bone
  - Prone to fracture
  - Cause unknown
- Collaborative care
  - Replace vitamin D
  - Calcium and phosphate supplements
  - Biphosphonates and calcitonin drugs

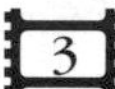

Osteomyelitis

- Infection in the bone
  - *Staphylococcus aureus*
  - Any age
  - Older adults at risk
  - Pathogens enter the bone from an open wound
  - Spread to the bone from local tissue
  - Lodge and multiply, causing an inflammatory and immune system response
  - Phagocytes attempt to contain the infection, but release enzymes that destroy bone tissue
  - Canals in the marrow cavity of the bone allow the infection to spread
  - Spreads along the surface
  - Disruption of blood supply leads to necrosis
- Interdisciplinary care
  - Early diagnosis and antibiotic therapy
    - WBC
    - Blood and tissue cultures
    - MRI
    - Bone scan
  - Medications intravenously
  - Surgery
    - Cultures
    - Debridement
  - Nursing care
    - Assessing
    - Diagnosis, planning, and implementation
      - Pain
      - Hyperthermia
      - Impaired Physical Mobility

© 2007 Pearson Education, Inc.

POWERPOINT LECTURE SLIDES *continued*

- Teaching
  - Medications and wound management
  - Rest and limited weight bearing
  - Good nutrition

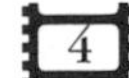

Bone Tumors

- Definitions
  - Benign or malignant
  - Primary or secondary
    - Primary
      - Adolescents
    - Metastatic
      - Adults
      - Originates from tumors of the prostate, breast, kidney, thyroid, and lung
- Pathophysiology and manifestations
  - Classification
    - Bone—osteogenic
    - Cartilage—chondrogenic
    - Collagen—collagenic
    - Bone marrow—myelogenic
  - Primary tumors cause bone breakdown
  - Malignant tumors invade and destroy adjacent bone tissue
  - Benign tumors have a symmetric controlled growth, weakening bone structure and causing risk for fractures
- Interdisciplinary care
  - Diagnosis
    - X-rays
    - CT scan and MRI
    - Biopsy
    - Serum alkaline phosphatase, RBC, serum calcium
  - Treatment
    - Chemotherapy
    - Radiation therapy
    - Surgery
  - Nursing care
    - Pain
    - Impaired Physical Mobility
    - Disturbed Body Image
    - Anticipatory Grieving
  - Teaching
    - Disease
    - Potential consequences
    - Treatment options
    - Home environment needs
    - Wound care
    - Activity and weight restrictions
    - Resources

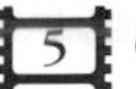

Common Foot Disorders

- Hallux valgus
  - Bunion—enlargement and lateral displacement of great toe
  - Due to chronic pressure against the great toe
  - Heredity

© 2007 Pearson Education, Inc.

PowerPoint Lecture Slides *continued*

- Pointed-toe shoes or high heels
- Metatarsophalangeal (MTP) joint enlarged
- Callus develops

- Hammertoe
  - Flexion of the proximal interphalangeal joint with hyperextension of the MTP and distal interphalangeal joints
  - Affects any toe
  - Causes painful corns to develop
- Interdisciplinary care
  - Corrective shoes and orthotic devices
  - Analgesics and corticosteroids
  - Surgery
- Nursing Care
  - Pain
  - Risk for infection

Suggestions for Classroom Activities

1. Arrange for bone density testing of students.
2. Conduct a brainstorming exercise or game to help students identify sources of calcium.
3. Discuss famous people who were diagnosed with bone cancer.

Suggestions for Clinical Activities

1. Assign student on orthopedic unit to care for patients with hip fractures who have osteoporosis.
2. Develop a case study to discuss in a postclinical conference on the treatment of osteomyelitis.

Learning Outcome 3

Describe the pathophysiology, interdisciplinary care, and nursing care of clients with joint disorders.

Concepts for Lecture

1. Disorders that cause pain and stiffness of a joint are the result of an inflammatory process called arthritis.
2. Osteoarthritis is limited to the joint and surrounding tissue and results in a progressive degeneration of the joint cartilage.
3. The goal of interdisciplinary care of osteoarthritis is directed to relief of pain and restoration of joint function.

PowerPoint Lecture Slide

1 Arthritis
- Inflammation of a joint
- Localized
  - Osteoarthritis
- Systemic (connective tissue disorders)
  - Rheumatoid arthritis
  - Systemic lupus erythematosus

2 Osteoarthritis
- Degenerative joint disease with progressive loss of joint cartilage
  - Most common type
  - Leading cause of disability in older adults
  - Equal in men and women
  - Risk factors
    - Age
    - Repetitive joint use and trauma
    - Heredity
    - Obesity
    - Congenital and acquired defects
- Pathophysiology
  - Entire joint affected
  - Cartilage loses strength and elasticity and erodes and ulcerates
  - Underlying bone exposed
  - Cartilage-coated osteophytes (bony outgrowths)

© 2007 Pearson Education, Inc.

POWERPOINT LECTURE SLIDES *continued*

- Manifestations and complications
  - Inflammation in the joint
  - Pain (arthralgia)
  - Decrease in joint range of motion
  - Enlarged joints
  - Herniated disk

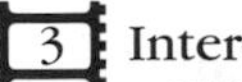

Interdisciplinary Care

- H&P, x-ray examination
- Weight reduction and exercise
- Heat for local pain relief
- Medications
- Surgery
- Arthroscopy
- Arthroplasty—reconstruction or replacement of the joint
  - Total joint replacement—hip, knee, shoulder, elbow, ankle, wrist, joints of finger and toes
  - Total hip replacement (Figure 43-5A)
  - Total knee replacement (Figure 43-5B)
  - Infection is a major complication of total joint replacement
- Nursing Care
  - Assessment focuses on effects of the disease and ADLs
  - Nursing diagnosis
    - Chronic Pain
    - Impaired Physical Mobility
    - Self-Care Deficit
  - Teaching
    - Environmental safety
    - Use of assistive devices to maintain independence
    - Medications
    - Activity and weight bearing
    - Signs and symptoms of infection

SUGGESTIONS FOR CLASSROOM ACTIVITIES

1. Invite prosthesis representative to discuss joint replacement and demonstrate how devices are made.
2. Have students do a web search of the Arthritis Foundation and ask them to identify what research support and patient services the foundation provides.

SUGGESTIONS FOR CLINICAL ACTIVITIES

1. Assign students observation of joint replacement surgery.
2. Assign students to joint replacement unit to care for patients postoperatively.
3. Arrange for clinical experience in rehabilitation department.

LEARNING OUTCOME 4

Describe the pathophysiology, interdisciplinary care, and nursing care of clients with connective tissue disorders.

CONCEPTS FOR LECTURE

1. Rheumatoid arthritis is a systemic inflammatory disorder of the joints resulting in chronic pain and disability.
2. Systemic lupus erythematosus is a systemic inflammatory disorder affecting multiple body systems.

POWERPOINT LECTURE SLIDE

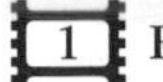

Rheumatoid Arthritis

- Chronic systemic inflammatory disorder of the joints
- More women than men
- Ages 30–50
- Multiple joints

CONCEPTS FOR LECTURE *continued*

3. Other connective tissue disorders of various types and causes include gout, Lyme disease, ankylosing spondylitis, fibromyalgia, and low back pain.
4. Muscular dystrophy is a genetic disorder of progressive muscle degeneration and wasting.
5. The goal of interdisciplinary care is early diagnosis and treatment to preserve bone, muscles, and joint function, to reduce pain and discomfort, and to maintain the highest level of independent functioning.

POWERPOINT LECTURE SLIDES *continued*

- Remission and exacerbations
- Pathophysiology
  - Autoimmune response
  - Autoantibodies (rheumatoid factors) bind with IgG to form immune complexes
  - Complement activated and WBCs attracted to the area
  - Cells phagocytize immune complexes and also destroy the joint
- Manifestations
  - Red, swollen, and painful joints
  - Pannus erodes cartilage and joints (Figure 43-6)
  - Systemic symptoms
    - Fatigue
    - Anorexia
    - Weight loss
    - Aching and stiffness
  - Destruction of joints and immobility

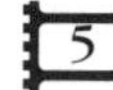 Interdisciplinary Care

- Diagnosis
  - H&P
  - Rheumatoid factors
  - Erythrocyte sedimentation rate
  - Synovial fluid aspirate
  - X-rays
- Rest and exercise
- Medications
  - Aspirin and NSAIDs
  - Steroids
  - Drugs to modify the autoimmune response
- Surgery
  - Relieve pain and repair or replace joints
  - Arthrodesis (joint fusion)
- Other therapies
  - Plasmapheresis
  - Total lympoid radiation
- Nursing care
  - Assessment focuses on progress of disease and effect on functional abilities
  - Nursing diagnoses
    - Pain
    - Fatigue
    - Ineffective Role Performance
    - Disturbed Body Image
  - Teaching
    - Disease and systemic effects
    - Rest and exercise
    - Medications
    - Assistive devices
    - Safety

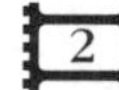 Systemic Lupus Erythematosus

- Chronic inflammatory connective tissue disorder affecting multiple systems
  - Mild to severe, even fatal
  - More women than men

© 2007 Pearson Education, Inc.

- Common and severe in African ancestry
- Cause unknown

- Pathophysiology
  - Autoantibodies target normal cells, depositing immune complexes in the connective tissue of
    - Blood vessels
    - Lymphatic vessels
    - Kidneys
    - Musculoskeletal system
    - Brain
    - Heart
    - Lung
    - GI tract
    - Skin
    - Peritoneum
  - Manifestations
    - Mimic rheumatoid arthritis
    - Fever
    - Skin manifestations (butterfly rash)
    - Photosensitivity
    - Course is mild and chronic
    - Remissions and exacerbations
    - Risk for infections

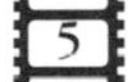

Interdisciplinary Care

- Diagnosis
  - H&P
  - Antinuclear antibodies
  - Anti-DNA
  - C-reactive protein
  - ESR
  - Urinalysis
  - Renal function tests
- Medications
  - Aspirin and NSAIDs
  - Antimalarial drugs
  - Corticosteorids
- Other therapies
  - Sunscreen
  - End-stage renal disease treatment
- Nursing care
  - Similar to arthritis patients
  - Nursing diagnoses
    - Impaired Skin Integrity
    - Ineffective Protection
  - Teaching
    - Disease
    - Psychosocial issues
    - Skin care
    - Exposure to infection
    - Treatment plan

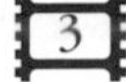

Other Connective Tissue Disorders

- Gout—metabolic disorder
  - Accumulation of urate crystals in joints
  - Men more than women
  - Primary gout—genetic disorder
  - Secondary gout—other causes or drugs

© 2007 Pearson Education, Inc.

- Pathophysiology
  - Imbalance of uric acid
  - Joints become red, hot, swollen, and painful
  - Frequent site is great toe
- Treatment focus
  - NSAIDs
  - Indocin
  - Aspirin
- Nursing care
  - Acute pain
- Teaching
  - Disease signs and symptoms
  - Medications

- Lyme disease
  - Inflammatory disorder caused by spirochete *Borrelia burgdorferi*
  - Spread by ticks
  - Seen in children
  - More common in northeast, upper Midwest, and Pacific Coast
  - Pathophysiology
    - Enters skin at site of tick bite
    - Incubation 30 days
    - Lesion—erythema migrans
    - Spread through lymph or blood to other sites
    - Flat, slightly raised red lesion
  - Systemic symptoms
    - Fatigue
    - Malaise
    - Fever
    - Muscle pain
    - Secondary skin lesions and musculoskeletal symptoms
    - Other chronic manifestations
  - Treatment
    - NSAIDs and aspirin
  - Nursing care
    - Educational to prevent infection
- Ankylosing spondylitis
  - Chronic inflammatory arthritis of the spine
    - Pain and progressive stiffening
  - Pathophysiology and manifestations
    - Insidious
    - Pain worse at night with morning stiffness
    - Intermittent or persistent bouts of low back pain
  - Treatement
    - NSAIDs to relieve pain and stiffness
    - Supportive care and education
- Fibromyalgia
  - Fibrositis
  - Common rheumatic syndrome of musculoskeletal pain, stiffness, and tenderness
  - Women over the age of 50
  - Cause unknown
  - Chronic achy muscle pain and tenderness at trigger points
  - Systemic effects

© 2007 Pearson Education, Inc.

POWERPOINT LECTURE SLIDES *continued*

- May resolve spontaneously or become chronic and recurrent
- Supportive treatment and care

- Low back pain
  - Acute or chronic low back pain due to strains in muscles and tendons of the back
  - Lumbar or lumbosacral or sacroiliac areas
  - Degenerative disk disease or herniated vertebral disks
  - Five types of pain
    - Local
    - Referred
    - Pain of spinal origin
    - Radicular
    - Muscle spasm
  - Diagnosis
    - H&P
    - X-rays, CT scan, MRI
  - Treatment
    - Rest
    - Ice packs
    - Exercise
    - Diathermy
    - TENS
    - NSAIDs and analgesics
  - Nursing care
    - Ineffective Health Maintenance
    - Pain
  - Teaching
    - Safe lifting, bending, and turning
    - Body mechanics, posture, sleeping on a firm mattress, chairs with good support

Muscular Dystrophy

- Inherited muscle disease of progressive degeneration and wasting
  - Most common form—Duchenne's muscular dystrophy
  - Inherited sex-linked recessive disorder
    - Mother to male children
    - One out of 3,500 live male births
  - Muscle fiber atrophy, necrosis, regeneration, and fibrosis lead to progressive weakness of voluntary muscle
  - No cure
  - Care focused on preserving and promoting mobility

SUGGESTIONS FOR CLASSROOM ACTIVITIES

1. Create a matching practice quiz with types of arthritic disorders and cause/manifestation.
2. Have students conduct a web search for information from the Arthritis Foundation.

SUGGESTIONS FOR CLINICAL ACTIVITIES

1. Arrange for clinical experience in the rehabilitation services department (physical therapy, occupational therapy).
2. Assign students to case studies of clients with arthritic disorders.
3. Visit pediatric centers or Shriner's centers to observe children with arthritic and muscle disorders.

© 2007 Pearson Education, Inc.

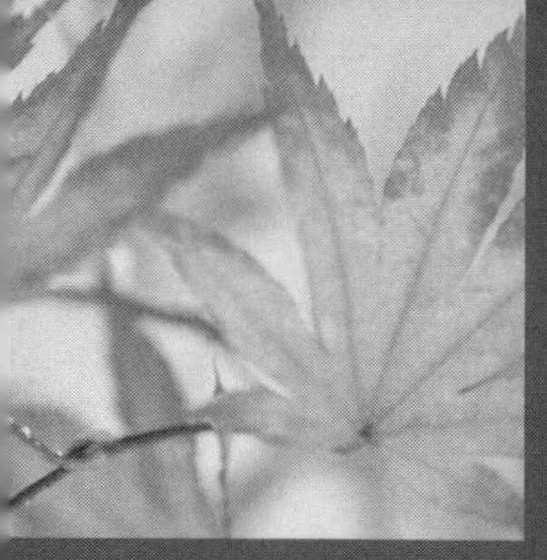

Chapter 44
The Integumentary System and Assessment

Resource Library

IMAGE LIBRARY

Figure 44-1 Anatomy of the skin.

Figure 44-2 Tenting in an elderly client.

Learning Outcome 1

Identify the structure and functions of the skin and its appendages.

Concepts for Lecture

1. The skin, glands, hair, and nails make up the integumentary system. The skin provides an external covering for the body, separating organs and tissues from the external environment. The skin contains receptors for touch and sensation, helps regulate body temperature, and assists in fluid and electrolyte balance.

PowerPoint Lecture Slides

1 Structures and Functions of the Skin and Its Appendages
- Table 44-1

Learning Outcome 2

Describe factors that influence skin color.

Concepts for Lecture

1. The color of skin is the result of varying levels of pigmentation. Skin color can also be affected by emotions, disease, and injuries.

PowerPoint Lecture Slides

1 Factors that Influence Skin Color
- Skin color is result of varying levels of pigmentation
- Melanin—yellow to brown pigment produced in greater amounts in persons with dark skin
- Exposure to sun causes a buildup in melanin, causing light skin to tan
- Carotene (yellow to orange pigment) found in greater abundance in persons of Asian ancestry
- Caucasian skin has very little melanin; color of red blood cells shows through, giving skin pinkish tone
- Skin color influenced by emotions or illnesses
- Erythema—reddening of skin caused by blushing, fever, inflammation, hypertension
- Cyanosis—bluish discoloration of skin and mucous membranes results from poor oxygenation of hemoglobin, lack of adequate RBCs or hemoglobin
- Pallor—paleness of skin caused by shock, fear, anemia, anger, or hypoxia
- Jaundice—yellow to orange color visible in skin and mucous membranes usually results from a liver disorder

Learning Outcome 3

Describe skin changes in the older adult.

Concepts for Lecture

1. A variety of normal skin changes are seen in the older adult.

PowerPoint Lecture Slides

1 Skin Changes in the Older Adult
- Loss of subcutaneous tissue
- Dermal thinning
- Decreased elasticity causes wrinkles and sagging
- Turgor decreased
- Inability to respond to heat and cold quickly, which ↑ the risk for heat stroke and hypothermia
- Loss of oil and sweat gland causes dry itchy skin
- Localized hyperpigmentation caused by localized proliferation of melanocytes causes senile lentigines (liver spots), flat brown macules on hands and arms
- Keratosis caused by hyperpigmentation
- Seborrheic keratosis—dark raised lesions
- Actinic keratosis—reddish raised plaques on areas of high sun exposure can become malignant
- Skin tags (small flaps excessive skin) normal with aging
- Hair and nail growth decreases
- Postmenopausal may develop facial hair over and under chin
- Hair grays due to reduction of melanocytes
- Nails may thicken, yellow, and peel

Learning Outcome 4

Identify subjective and objective assessment data to collect for clients with integumentary disorders.

Concepts for Lecture

1. Subjective and objective data are collected through the health history and the physical exam. The health history may be part of a health screening, total health assessment, or focused on the client's chief complaint such as a rash or itching. The physical examination should be conducted in a warm, private room. The client removes all clothing and puts on a gown that allows access to skin areas.

PowerPoint Lecture Slides

1 Subjective and Objective Assessment Data to Collect
- Health History
  - Changes in health, skin color, dryness, or oiliness
  - Growth or changes in warts or moles
  - Presence of lesions
  - Delayed wound healing
  - Determine whether client takes hormones, vitamins, or antibiotics that cause skin side effects
  - If client complains about itching, ask client to describe and identify any precipitating causes such as medications, soaps,
  - Inquire about excessive hair loss
  - For nail problems ask about nail splitting, breakage, discoloration, infection, diet, exposure to chemicals
  - Obtain past medical Hx, previous problems with allergies, surgeries, or lesions
  - Skin problems can indicate other health disorders such as cardiovascular, hematologic, diabetes mellitus, thyroid, and liver problems

© 2007 Pearson Education, Inc.

PowerPoint Lecture Slides *continued*

- ○ Family Hx of skin cancer, light-colored hair and eyes, excessive exposure to sun, and skin trauma
- ○ Explore risk factors for malignant melanoma—large moles, family history of melanomas, freckling and sun burning
- Physical exam:
  - ○ Inspect skin for:
    - Pallor, cyanosis rashes, inflammations lesions bruising
    - Table 44-2
  - ○ Assess for:
    - Vitiligo (abnormal patchy loss of melanin over face, hands, and groin
    - Petechiae—small reddish purple pinpoint spots over abdomen and buttocks
  - ○ Inspect
  - ○ Palpate
  - ○ Check skin temperature, texture, moisture, and turgor
  - ○ Inspect skin for tenting or edema
  - ○ Hair distribution—hirsutism (excessive hair) or alopecia
  - ○ Inspect scalp for lesions, pustules, and nits
  - ○ Inspect nails for clubbing, nail beds for red splinter hemorrhages

Learning Outcome 5

Identify nursing responsibilities for common diagnostic tests and monitors for clients with integumentary disorders.

Concepts for Lecture

1. Biopsy, cutaneous immunofluorescence biopsy, potassium hydroxide, culture and sensitivity, Tzanck test, skin scrapings, patch test, and Wood's light examination are common diagnostic tests done for integumentary disorders.

PowerPoint Lecture Slides

1 Nursing Responsibilities for Common Diagnostic Tests

- Table 44-3

Suggestions for Classroom Activities

1. Differentiate among the various skin cancers as to risk factors, rate of growth and spread, clinical manifestations, and treatment.
2. Identify the most common benign skin disorders.
3. Discuss the importance of history in the diagnosis of skin problems.

© 2007 Pearson Education, Inc.

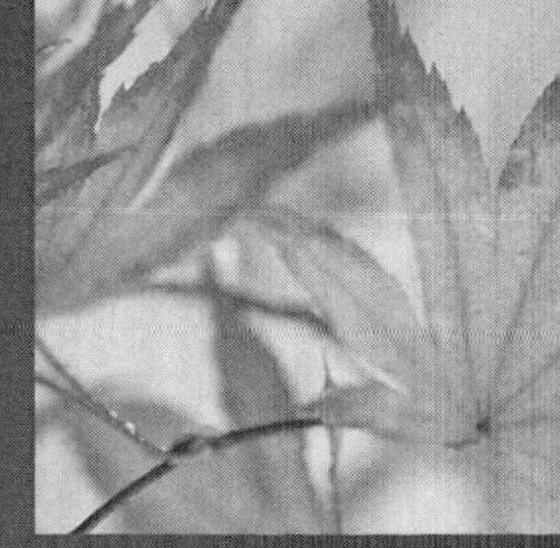

CHAPTER 45
CARING FOR CLIENTS WITH SKIN DISORDERS

RESOURCE LIBRARY

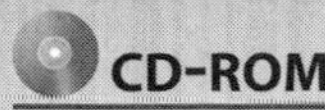

Video: Eczema
Pressure Ulcers

IMAGE LIBRARY

Figure 45-1 The characteristic lesions of psoriasis are raised, red, round plaques covered with thick, silvery scales.
Figure 45-2 Atopic dermatitis or eczema.
Figure 45-3 Inflammatory acne lesions include comedones, erythematous pustules, and cysts. These lesions often leave scars when they heal.
Figure 45-4 Cellulitis is a bacterial infection localized in the dermis and subcutaneous tissue. The involved area is red, swollen, and painful.
Figure 45-5 As a squamous cell cancer grows, it tends to invade surrounding tissue. It also ulcerates, may bleed, and is painful.
Figure 45-6 Malignant melanoma is a serious skin cancer that arises from melanocytes.

LEARNING OUTCOME 1

Relate skin changes in the older adult to an increased risk for dry skin, pruritus, skin cancer, and pressure ulcers.

CONCEPTS FOR LECTURE

1. Dry skin is the most common skin disorder seen in the elderly due to the decreased activity of sebaceous and sweat glands. The primary manifestation of dry skin is pruritus.
2. The incidence of skin cancers occurs most frequently in adults between the ages of 30 and 60 years. The incidence increases with excess exposure to the sun.
3. Pressure ulcers are a risk for the older adult because of the high incidence of limited mobility, incidence of paralysis, and incidence of clients with critical illnesses and other conditions that affect mobility.
4. Incontinence, poor nutrition, and chronic illness create an increased risk for skin breakdown in the older adult.

POWERPOINT LECTURE SLIDES

1 Dry Skin and Pruritis
- Occurs at any age
- Increased in the elderly
  - Decreased activity of sebaceous glands and sweat glands
  - Exposure to sunlight
  - Decreased fluid intake
  - Pruritis is the primary manifestation of dry skin

2 Skin Cancer
- Adults between age of 30 and 60 years
- Factors that influence incidence
  - Exposure to ultraviolet radiation
  - Exposure to chemicals
  - Skin pigmentation

3 Pressure Ulcers
- High risk for the older adult due to:
  - Limited mobility with aging
  - Conditions that alter mobility of the elderly
    - Arthritis
    - Osteoporosis and fractures
    - Chronic illness and debility
    - Critical illness
  - Illnesses that result in paralysis
    - Stroke
    - Spinal injury and disease

4 Skin Breakdown
- Conditions that contribute to skin breakdown
  - Altered nutrition less than body requirements
  - Incontinence
  - Chronic illness

Suggestions for Classroom Activities

1. Discuss the risks of ultraviolet light exposure at a young age and how this can affect the skin as the individual gets older.
2. Ask students to identify skin problems they see in their parents, grandparents, and elderly friends.
3. Have students read an article on the incidence of pressure ulcers in the older adult.

Suggestions for Clinical Activities

Have students identify elderly patients on the clinical unit that are at risk for common skin disorders. Include the reason why the client is at risk.

Learning Outcome 2

Compare and contrast the pathophysiology, manifestations, and interdisciplinary care of clients with common skin disorders, infections and infestations of the skin, malignant skin disorders, and pressure ulcers.

Concepts for Lecture

1. Common skin disorders are changes in the skin of a minor nature. Included in this category are pruritis, dry skin, psoriasis, dermatitis, and acne.
2. Infections and infestations occur when a break in the skin surface allows a virulent agent to invade or when a compromised immune system results in decreased resistance. Included in this category are bacterial, viral, fungal, and parasitic agents.
3. The most common of all cancers, skin cancer is a result of malignant changes of the cellular structure and function of the skin. They fall into two categories: the nonmelamona (basal cell and squamous cell carcinomas) and the melanoma type cancers.
4. Ischemic lesions of the skin and underlying tissue caused by external pressure that impairs flow of blood and lymph are termed pressure ulcers. If left untreated, they will lead to tissue necrosis and ulceration.

PowerPoint Lecture Slides

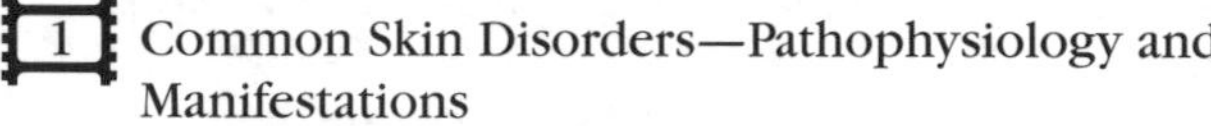

1 Common Skin Disorders—Pathophysiology and Manifestations

- Pruritis
  - Itching sensation producing the urge to scratch
  - Small or widespread with or without a rash
  - Triggered by heat and prostaglandins
  - Increased by release of histamine and chemical mediators
  - Caused by anything in the internal or external environment
  - Stimulation or irritation of receptors in the junction between the epidermis and dermis
    - Itch-scratch-itch cycle
- Dry skin
  - Decreased activity of sebaceous and sweat glands reducing skin lubrication
  - More common in older adults
  - Exposure to environmental heat and low humidity, sunlight, excessive bathing, and decreased intake of liquids
  - Pruritis and flaking of skin
- Psoriasis
  - Chronic, noninfectious skin disorder
  - Raised, reddened, round circumscribed plaques covered by silvery white scales
  - Appear anywhere in the body
  - Plaques shed gray scales
  - Cause unknown but may be an autoimmune disorder
  - Sunlight, stress, hormone fluctuations, steroid withdrawal, seasonal changes, and drugs may make condition worse
  - Family history
  - Pruritis, pain, discoloration of nails
- Dermatitis
  - Acute or chronic inflammation of the skin
  - Erythema and pain or pruritis
  - Vesicles, scales, and pruritis initially
  - Progresses to edema, serous discharge, and crusting
  - Types

© 2007 Pearson Education, Inc.

- Contact
- Atopic—eczema
- Seborrheic
- Exfoliative

- Acne
  - Disorder of the sebaceous glands
  - Sebum is produced in response to hormonal stimulation by:
    - Testicular androgens in men
    - Adrenal and ovarian androgens in women
  - Sebaceous glands are on the face, scalp, and scrotum
  - Lesions are called comedones
  - Types
    - Acne vulgaris
      - Adolescents and young to middle-aged adults
    - Acne rosacea
      - Chronic facial acne in middle and older adults

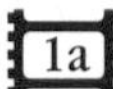

Common Skin Disorders—Interdisciplinary Care

- Most treated by self-care at home
- Focus of treatment is identifying, modifying, or eliminating precipitating factors
- Diagnosis
  - Culture
  - Skin scrapings
  - Biopsy
  - Ultrasound tests
- Medications and treatments—pruritis
  - Antihistamines
  - Tranquilizers—stress related to pruritis
  - Antibiotics
  - Topical steroids
  - Therapeutic baths
- Medications and treatments—psorisis
  - Topical corticosteroids
  - Tar preparations
  - Retinoids to decrease inflammation
  - Photochemotherapy
  - Ultraviolet-B
- Medications and treatments—acne
  - Based on type and severity of lesions
  - Retinoic acid, Retin-A
  - Benzoyl peroxide
  - Azelaic acid
  - OTC medications
  - Accutane
  - Surgery—dermabrasion
- Complimentary therapy
  - Aloe

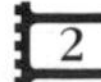

Infections and Infestations—Pathophysiology and Manifestations

- Bacterial infections
  - Arise from the hair follicle where bacteria accumulate and grow

© 2007 Pearson Education, Inc.

POWERPOINT LECTURE SLIDES *continued*

            - Localized infection
            - Systemic if invade into deeper tissue
            - Types
                - Foliculitis
                    - *Staphylococcus aureus*
                    - Skin surface and extends into hair follicle
                    - Inflammation sets in
                    - Scalp and extremities, face of bearded men, legs of women who shave, eyelids (stye)
                    - Poor hygiene, nutrition, prolonged moisture, trauma
                - Furuncle
                    - Infection of the hair follicle
                    - Carbuncle—group of infected hair follicles
                    - *Staphylococcus aureus*
                    - Deep red nodule that gets larger and cystic
                    - May cause fever, chills, or malaise
                - Cellulitis
                    - Localized infection of the dermis and subcutaneous layers
                    - Spreads as a result of spreading factor hyaluronidase
                    - Breakdown of fibrin network and other barriers
                    - Red swollen, painful
                    - Fever, chills, malaise, headache, swollen lymph glands
        - Fungal infections
            - Plantlike organisms that live in soil, on animals, on humans
            - Dermatotypes live on stratum corneum, hair, and nails
            - Superficial infections—ringworm or tinea
            - Mycoses
            - Types
                - Dermatophyte (tinea) infections
                    - Tinea pedis
                    - Tinea curis
                - Candidiasis infections
                    - *Candida albicans*—yeastlike infections on skin, vagina, gastrointestinal tact
        - Viral infections
            - RNA or DNA core surrounded by a protein coat
            - Depend on live cells for reproduction
            - Increase cell growth or cause cellular death
            - Types
                - Warts
                    - Human papillomavirus
                    - Skin and mucous membranes
                    - Nongenital warts are benign lesions
                    - Genital warts are precancerous
                    - Transmitted through skin contact
                    - Types
                        - □ Common
                        - □ Plantar
                        - □ Condylomata acuminate (venereal warts)

 © 2007 Pearson Education, Inc.

POWERPOINT LECTURE SLIDES *continued*

- Herpes simplex
  - Herpesvirus I and II
  - Fever blister or cold sore
    - HSV I—lips, face, and mouth
    - HSV I or II—genital herpes, sexually transmitted
  - Begins with a tingling sensation followed by erythema, vesicle formation, and pain
  - Lasts 10–14 days
- Herpes zoster
  - Varicella zoster
  - Reactivation of dormant virus
  - Painful vesicles on the face, trunk, and thorax
  - Prevalent in people who are immunocompromised
  - Recovery 4–6 weeks
  - Postherpetic neuralgia

- Parasitic infestations
  - Skin invaded by parasites or insects
  - Most common parasites are mites and lice
    - Pediculosis
      - Infestation of lice
      - First stage is an unhatched egg (nit)
      - Three types live on humans
        - *Pediculosis corporis*—body lice
        - *Pediculosis capitus*—head lice
        - *Pediculosis pubis*—pubic lice (crabs)
    - Scabies
      - Female mite
      - Infestation between fingers and inner surfaces of wrist, elbow, axillae, nipple, penis, belt line, and gluteal crease
      - Occur up to 4 weeks after contact
      - Small red mite burrows into skin

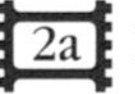

Infections and Infestations—Interdisciplinary Care

- Treatment focused on identifying causative agent
- Administer medication to kill bacteria or eradicate the organism
- Prevent secondary infection
- Environmental surveillance and control
- Diagnosis
  - Culture and sensitivity
  - Scrapings and microscopic examination
  - Ultraviolet light inspection
  - Lab studies
- Medications and treatment
  - Bacterial infections
    - Antiobiotics—topically or systemically
  - Fungal infections
    - Antifungal agents—topically or systemically
  - Viral infections
    - Antiviral agents
    - Medications to relieve pain and pruritis
  - Parasitic infestations
    - Topical agents to kill the parasite
      - Single or multiple treatment

© 2007 Pearson Education, Inc.

- Complementary therapy
  - Tea tree oil

3 Skin Cancer—Pathophysiology and Manifestations

- Most common of all cancers
- Result of long-term exposure to the sun or environment
- Exposure to chemicals, ultraviolet light
- Skin pigmentation—the more melanin, the more you are protected
- Types
  - Nonmelanoma skin cancer
    - Basal cell
      - Epidermis
      - Sun-exposed areas of the head and neck
      - Slow growing and rarely metastasize
    - Squamous cell carcinoma
      - Squamous epithelium of the skin or mucous membranes
      - UV ray exposure
      - Forehead, helix of ear, top of nose, lower lip, back of hands
      - Firm flesh-colored or erythematous papule
      - Can be recurring and invasive increasing risk of metastasis
  - Melanoma
    - Cutaneous or malignant melanoma
    - Arises from the melanocytes that produce melanin
    - Lesions can be benign until they infiltrate the dermis and mingle with blood and lymph
    - Increases the risk of metastasis
    - Precursor lesion is a dysplastic nevi (mole)
    - Change in the color or size of a nevus occurs in 70% of people diagnosed with melanoma
    - ABCD rule of the American Cancer Society
      - A = asymmetry
      - B = border irregularity
      - C = color variation
      - D = diameter greater than 6 mm

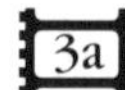

Skin Cancer—Interdisciplinary Care

- Treatment focuses on removal of malignant tissue
- Staging of malignant melanoma
- Treatment with chemotherapy, immunotherapy, radiation therapy, and biological therapies
- Diagnosis
  - Microscopic exam and tissue biopsies
  - Liver function tests
  - Chest x-rays
  - Microstaging
- Surgery
- Curretage and electrodesiccation or cryosurgery
- Radiation
- Immunotherapy

© 2007 Pearson Education, Inc.

PowerPoint Lecture Slides *continued*

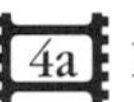
Ischemic Lesions—Pathophysiology and Manifestations

- Pressure develops over bony prominences
- Shearing forces, friction, external pressure cause damage
- Impairment of flow of blood and lymph causing ischemia from distortion of capillaries
- If pressure continues, platelets clump and form microthrombi
- Microthrombi impede blood flow, resulting in ischemia and hypoxia
- Cells and tissue die and become necrotic
- Injury can be
  - Superficial
    - Red or blister
  - Deep
    - Deeper structures where tissue becomes necrotic and dies
- Shearing forces
  - Result when one tissue layer slides over another
  - Stretching and bending of blood vessels
    - Head of bed elevated and torso slides down toward foot of bed
    - Pulling client up in bed
- Increased risk with immobility
- Pressure ulcer staging (Box 45-5)

4a Ischemic Lesions—Interdisciplinary Care

- Goal is prevention
- Laboratory tests to determine infection
- Topical and systemic antibiotics
- Surgical debridement
- Specialty dressings and beds

Suggestions for Classroom Activities

1. Prepare pictures of the different common skin disorders. Ask students to match the name of the disorder with the picture.
2. Prepare a matching quiz for students to identify whether the infection/infestation is bacterial, viral, fungal, or parasitic.
3. Ask students do an online search for articles that discuss risks of skin cancer.
4. Ask students to read an article on pressure ulcers that discusses prevention and intervention techniques.

Suggestions for Clinical Activities

1. Arrange for clinical experience in a dermatology clinic or dermatologist's office.
2. Arrange for clinical experience in the rapid treatment section of the emergency department where they see patients with minor illnesses.
3. Find a client in the clinical area who has stage III and/or stage IV pressure ulcers. Use this as a case study presentation in a postclinical conference.

Learning Outcome 3

Use the nursing process to collect data and provide interventions for clients with common skin disorders, infections and infestations of the skin, malignant skin disorders, and pressure ulcers.

Concepts for Lecture

1. Data collected include subjective and objective data related to history and description of skin condition and factors relevant to exposure to causative agents.

PowerPoint Lecture Slides

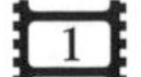
Common Skin Disorders—Assessment

- Present health status
- Past medical history
- Inspection of the entire skin for color and lesions

© 2007 Pearson Education, Inc.

CONCEPTS FOR LECTURE *continued*

2. The focus of nursing care centers on promoting comfort and decreasing risk of spread of infection, promoting healing, and preventing disfiguration, deformity, and loss of function.

POWERPOINT LECTURE SLIDES *continued*

- Palpate skin for temperature, texture, moisture, and turgor

1a Infections and Infestations—Assessment

- Subjective data
  - History of contact
  - Living conditions
  - Chronic illnesses
- Objective data
  - Inspect skin, hair, mucous membranes
  - Note location, appearance, and size of lesions

1b Skin Cancers—Assessment

- Subjective data
  - Present health status
    - Change in mole, wart, birthmark, scar
    - Exposure
    - Other
  - Past medical history
    - Skin cancer or family history
    - Geographic residence
    - Serious sunburn
- Objective data
  - Inspection and palpation of skin lesions
  - Measure and document location
  - Monitor report results

1c Pressure Ulcers—Assessment

- Identify patients at risk
- Describe appearance
- Measure size and depth

2 Common Skin Disorders—Nursing Diagnosis, Planning, and Implementation

- Impaired Skin Integrity
  - Strategies to relieve itching
  - Therapeutic baths
- Disturbed Body Image
  - Trusting relationship
  - Self-perception
  - Involvement of family
- Deficient Knowledge

2a Infections and Infestations—Nursing Diagnosis, Planning, and Implementation

- Acute pain
- Disturbed sleep pattern
- Risk for infection

2b Skin Cancer—Nursing Diagnosis, Planning, and Implementation

- Anxiety
- Impaired Skin Integrity
- Hopelessness

2c Pressure Ulcers—Nursing Diagnosis, Planning, and Implementation

- Risk for Impaired Skin Integrity and Impaired Skin Integrity
  - Minimize risk
  - Conduct systematic inspection

© 2007 Pearson Education, Inc.

POWERPOINT LECTURE SLIDES *continued*

- Keep skin clean and manage incontinence
- Minimize environmental factors
- Minimize friction and shearing forces
- Maintain adequate nutritional intake
- Maintain activity level
- Teach client to shift weight
- Use positioning devices, pillows
- Keep head of bed at lowest position
- Use specialty devices

SUGGESTIONS FOR CLASSROOM ACTIVITIES

1. Invite a wound care nursing specialist to discuss nursing care of pressure ulcers.
2. Contact skin care product representatives. Invite them to speak to the class about skin care and use of various products, beds, and supportive devices to treat skin conditions.
3. Invite school nurse to discuss processes for preventing spread of parasitic infections in schoolchildren.

SUGGESTIONS FOR CLINICAL ACTIVITIES

1. Have students conduct a prevalence study of the occurrence of pressure ulcers in the clinical agency.
2. Have students spend a day with the wound/ostomy/skin care nursing specialist.
3. Arrange for clinical experience in a wound clinic.

LEARNING OUTCOME 4

Provide client and family teaching appropriate for prevention and self-care of disorders of the skin.

CONCEPTS FOR LECTURE

1. The focus of client family teaching relates to eliminating factors that contribute to skin conditions and teaching proper medication administration, skin and wound care, environmental control to reduce spread of infection and infestation, and recognition and prevention of the risks of skin cancer.

POWERPOINT LECTURE SLIDES

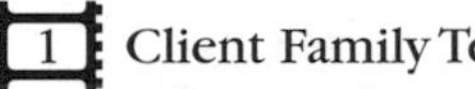

Client Family Teaching

- Supportive role
- Report complications of treatments
- Proper medication administration
- Care to facilitate healing and eliminate spread of infection
- Dressing changes and direct care of skin lesions
  - Cleansing skinfolds
  - Bathing
- Nutrition
- Environmental control
  - Washing of clothing, linens
  - Bathing
  - Clothing
  - Treatment of partner
  - Home environment
  - Sexual practices
- Early detection and care of skin cancers
- Prevention of skin cancer
- Prevention of pressure ulcers in clients cared for at home
  - Inspection of skin
  - Daily skin care
  - Reporting problems
  - Eliminating pressure, friction, and shearing forces

© 2007 Pearson Education, Inc.

Suggestions for Classroom Activities

1. Have students prepare and present a teaching plan to parents on the treatment of head lice.
2. Discuss the various OTC skin products that people use and the recommended value of those products. Ask students to reflect on how they would incorporate this information when teaching clients and their families.

Suggestions for Clinical Activities

In a postconference discuss how families can be involved in the care of the clients they cared for that day in the clinical area.

© 2007 Pearson Education, Inc.

CHAPTER 46
CARING FOR CLIENTS WITH BURNS

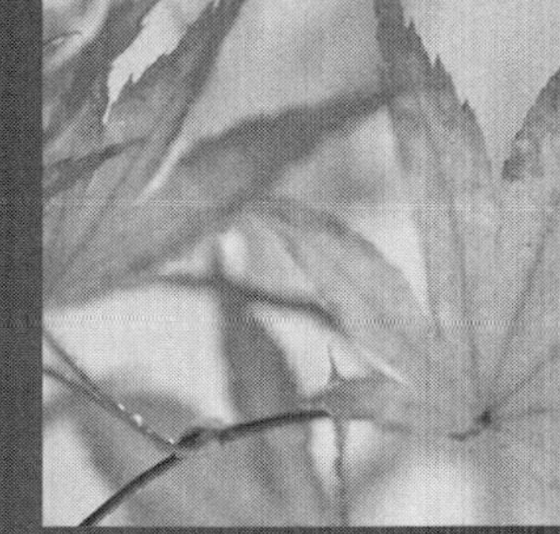

RESOURCE LIBRARY

CD-ROM

Burn
Electrical Burn
Partial Burn

IMAGE LIBRARY

Figure 46-1 Burn injury classification according to the depth of the burn.
Figure 46-2 Partial-thickness burn injury.
Figure 46-3 Full-thickness burn injury.
Figure 46-4 The "rule of nines" is a way to estimate the percentage of TBSA affected by a burn injury. This quick method is useful in emergency situations, but it is not accurate for adults who are short, obese, or very thin.
Figure 46-5 Skin graft for burn injury (autograft).

LEARNING OUTCOME 1

Discuss types, classification, extent estimation, and stages of treatment for burns.

CONCEPTS FOR LECTURE

1. Burns are discussed by the type of heat source that affects the tissue in different ways.
2. Classification of burns is determined by the extent and depth of the burn measured by percentage of body surface area affected and layers of skin and tissue involved.
3. Stages of treatment are divided in three overlapping stages: immediate or emergent care, ongoing care in the acute care setting, and restorative or rehabilitative treatment months to years after the initial injury.

POWERPOINT LECTURE SLIDES

1 Types of Heat Sources
- Thermal
  - Dry heat—flame
  - Moist heat—steam or hot liquid
- Chemical—acid or alkaline agents
- Electrical—current or voltage
- Radiation—sunburn or radiation treatment of cancer

2 Classification of Burns
- Superficial—first degree
  - Epidermal layer only (examples: sunburn, UV light, minor flash injury)
- Partial-thickness burn—second degree
  - Superficial—dermis
    - Surface appears red, moist with blister formation
  - Deep—dermis plus hair follicles
    - Surface appears pale, waxy, and moist or dry
    - Large, easily ruptured blisters
- Full-thickness burn—third degree
  - All layers of skin
    - Extend to subcutaneous fat, connective tissue, muscle, and bone
    - Appears pale, waxy, yellow, brown, mottled, charred, or nonblanching red
    - Pain and touch receptors destroyed

3 Stages of Burn Injury Care
- Emergent or resuscitative stage—onset of injury through successful fluid resuscitation
  - Immediate care to prevent shock and respiratory distress
  - Fluid resuscitation is important in severe burns

PowerPoint Lecture Slides *continued*

- Acute stage—start of diuresis; ends with closure of burn wound
  - Hydrotherapy
  - Excision and grafting
  - Nutritional support
  - Topical and systemic antimicrobial agents
  - Narcotic for pain control
  - Physical therapy
- Rehabilitative stage—wound closure to highest level of health
  - Biophysical adjustment
  - Prevention of contractures and scars
  - Resumption of work; return to family and social roles

Suggestions for Classroom Activities

1. Create a matching quiz or crossword puzzle to help students identify the definitions of the types, classifications, and stages of burn treatment.
2. Have students research an article in a journal or newspaper that discusses burn safety issues and risks of the type of burn injury.

Suggestions for Clinical Activities

1. Arrange for a visit to a regional burn center if burn patients are not treated in your clinical agencies.
2. If possible, have students assigned to burn patients at the various stages of treatment. Have the students present these cases for group discussion in a post-clinical conference format.

Learning Outcome 2

Describe the pathophysiology of a major burn.

Concepts for Lecture

1. Burns affect all body systems.
2. Within minutes of the burn, the cell wall is damaged causing movement of fluid in the cardiovascular system. This can lead to profound hypovolemic shock called burn shock.
3. The destruction of the skin and burn shock lead to an impairment of immune function and high risk for infection.
4. Inhalation injury can lead to respiratory failure.
5. The GI system is affected by the risk of ulcers and paralytic ileus.
6. Fluid losses can alter renal function and lead to renal failure.
7. Metabolism is affected in two distinct phases, which include an ebb phase in the early stage and a flow phase or hypermetabolic state.

PowerPoint Lecture Slides

1 Pathophysiology and Manifestations of Major Burns
- Burns affect all body systems

2 Cardiovascular
- Loss of cell wall integrity at the injury site and capillary bed
- Massive fluid shift from the intracellular space to the interstitial space
- Fluid leads from the capillaries at the burn wound site
- All lead to decrease in intravascular volume and hypovolemic shock called burn shock

2a Further Changes of the Cardiovascular System
- Vasoconstriction
- Platelet aggregation
- Ischemia and thrombosis
- Hemolysis of RBCs
- Elevated RBCs (hemoconcentration) and WBCs
- Edema
- Potassium loss and dysrhythmias

3 Immune System
- Impairs active components of cell-mediated and humoral immunity
- Decrease in serum immunoglobulins

 © 2007 Pearson Education, Inc.

PowerPoint Lecture Slides *continued*

- Decrease in serum protein
- Acquired immunodeficiency and risk for infection

3a Integumentary System
- Microcirculation
  - If intact, cools and protects deeper layers
  - If lost, continues to burn even if heat source removed
  - Thickness of the dermis and epidermis varies from one area to another in the body

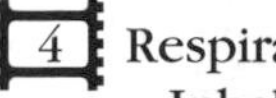

4 Respiratory System
- Inhalation injury
  - Respiratory inflammation
  - Pulmonary failure
- Carbon monoxide and smoke inhalation
  - Carbon monoxide displaces oxygen
  - Smoke inhalation results in toxic gases and soot deposited on pulmonary mucosa and causes inflammation
  - Interstitial pulmonary edema secondary to movement of fluid in pulmonary blood vessels
  - Inactivation of surfactant and alveolar collapse
  - Upper airway thermal injury and edema

5 Gastrointestinal System
- Curling's ulcer
- Paralytic ileus

6 Urinary System
- Massive fluid loss leads to dehydration, hemoconcentration, and decreased urinary output
- Hemoglobinuria
- Renal failure

7 Metabolism
- Ebb phase
  - Decreased metabolic state
  - First 3 days of injury
- Flow phase
  - Hypermetabolic state
  - Increased BMR—twice normal rate
  - Body weight and heat decrease
  - Persists after wound closure and may reappear

Suggestions for Classroom Activities

1. Discuss the normal function of each system and then illustrate what happens when major burns occur.
2. Discuss each system affected using a concept map to show the interrelationship of the effect of skin disruption and fluid loss.

Suggestions for Clinical Activities

Have students look at lab values for burn patients identifying electrolyte changes, CBC counts, protein levels, and blood gases. Ask students to discuss which body system is affected by the lab value.

Learning Outcome 3

Identify the interdisciplinary care necessary for the client with a major burn, including diagnostic tests; medications; fluid resuscitation; respiratory management; nutritional support; wound management; surgery; biologic and biosynthetic dressings; scar, keloid, and contracture prevention; and wound dressings.

Concepts for Lecture

1. Interdisciplinary care is required immediately from the stabilization in the emergency room through to the transfer to the critical care unit or specialized burn center.
2. Diagnostic studies include a comprehensive analysis of blood counts, chemistries, protein and albumin levels, blood gas levels, pulse oximetry, chest x-ray, urinalysis, and electrocardiogram studies. Cultures of sputum, blood, urine, and wound tissue are done due to risk of infection.
3. Medications are used to provide pain relief and to eliminate infection. Narcotics are used for pain control, and systemic and topical antimicrobial agents are used.
4. Fluid resuscitation is a major focus to prevent and treat burn shock and is calculated based on total body surface area (TBSA) and is warranted when burns involve 20% or more of the TBSA.
5. Two large-bore peripheral and central access lines are used along with invasive hemodynamic monitoring to evaluate intravascular volume and cardiac output with the goal of maintaining urine output at 30–50 mL/hr. Fluids used include colloids, crystalloids, blood, and blood products.
6. Goal of respiratory management is to maintain the airway and ensure oxygenation. Mechanical ventilation may be required.
7. Nutrition is essential for metabolism and wound healing. Caloric needs will increase to 4,000–6,000 kcal/day. Enteral or parenteral nutrition is often needed. Feeding tubes and monitoring for ulcer or ileus formation are required.
8. Wound management is a major initiative in the interdisciplinary care of a burn patient to promote healing, prevent infection, and decrease the incidence of scarring and deformity.

PowerPoint Lecture Slides

1 Interdisciplinary Care
- Stabilization in the Emergency Department
- Transfer to critical care or specialized burn center

2 Diagnostic Tests
- Cultures
- Urinalysis
- Complete blood count
- Serum electrolytes
- Total protein and albumin
- Arterial blood gases
- Pulse oximetry
- Chest x-ray and flexible bronchoscopy
- Electrocardiogram

3 Medications
- Narcotics for pain control
- Antimicrobials
  - Systemic
  - Topical
    - Sulfamylon
    - Silver sulfadiazine (silvadene)
  - Other

4, 5 Fluid Resusitation
- Necessary in all burn wounds that involve >20% TBSA
- Rule of Nines for calculating TBSA
- Colloids, crystalloids, blood, and blood products
- Goal 30–50 mL/hr urine output
- Invasive monitoring, two large-bore IVs

6 Respiratory Management
- Elevate head of bed 30 degrees
- Monitor for airway obstruction
- Mechanical ventilation

7 Nutrition
- Caloric needs increase to 4,000–6,000 kcal/day
- Enteral and parenteral feedings may be needed
- Monitor for Curling's ulcer, bowel obstruction, and ileus

8 Wound Management
- Major initiative in the care of a burn patient
- Debridement is the process of removing dead tissue
  - Cleansing with an antimicrobial soap
    - Chlorhexidine gluconate
    - Dial soap or Shurclens for the face
  - Mechanical debridement
    - Performed during hydrotherapy
    - Removal of eschar and blistered skin
  - Enzymatic debridement

© 2007 Pearson Education, Inc.

POWERPOINT LECTURE SLIDES *continued*

- Surgery
  - Debridement
  - Escharotomy
  - Autografting
  - Cultured epithelial autographing
- Biologic and biosynthetic dressings
  - Temporary material
  - Prepares the burn wound for permanent autograft coverage
  - Bibrane, Dermagraft, Integra, Alloderm, TransCyte
- Scar, keloid, and contractures
  - When burns extend to dermal layer, the skin is repaired through scar formation
  - Hypertrophic scar
    - Overgrowth of dermal tissue within the boundaries of the wound
  - Keloid scar
    - Extends beyond the boundaries of the original wound
  - People with dark skin are at greater risk for scars
  - Burn scars shrink and become fixed and inelastic, leading to contractures
- Wound dressings
  - Open
    - Open to air and covered with the topical antimicrobial agent
  - Closed
    - Topical antimicrobial agent
    - Gauze or nonadherent dressing
    - Wet-to-dry dressings
  - Splints used to prevent contractures
  - Uniform pressure garments
    - Reduces hypertrophic scarring
    - May be required to wear for 6 months to 1 year postgraft
  - Complementary therapy
    - Aloe gel for minor burns

SUGGESTIONS FOR CLASSROOM ACTIVITIES

1. Discuss the diagnostic workup of a burn client. Correlate the evaluation with the systems affected as discussed with the pathophysiology material.
2. Ask students to label a picture of the human body to illustrate the Rule of Nines to calculate TBSA.
3. Invite wound care specialist as a guest speaker to discuss wound management of burn clients.

SUGGESTIONS FOR CLINICAL ACTIVITIES

1. Using a case study approach, discuss pain control of a burn client who undergoes debridement of burn wounds.
2. Ask students to calculate caloric needs of their clients with burns and ask them to discuss in conference what is being done to meet these needs.
3. Demonstrate wound care for selected clients in the clinical area.

LEARNING OUTCOME 4

Use the nursing process to collect data and provide interventions for clients with major burns.

CONCEPTS FOR LECTURE

1. All elements of the nursing process are utilized in the care of clients with burns.
2. Assessment and collection of data involve history of the incident and the evaluation of all body systems that may be affected by the burn injury.
3. The major nursing diagnoses for planning and implementing care of a client with a burn injury include focus in the injury to the skin, the risk of infection, fluid resuscitation, monitoring for respiratory failure, nutritional support, pain control, wound management, and wound healing.
4. Clients with major burns require extensive care through the rehabilitative phase that can last for several months to years.

POWERPOINT LECTURE SLIDES

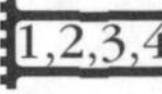
1,2,3,4 Nursing Process for a Client with a Burn Injury

- Assessment
  - Refer to Box 46-1—Initial Focused Assessment of the Client with a Major Burn
  - Assessment of body systems
  - Total body surface area (TBSA) affected
    - Rule of Nines
- Diagnosis, planning, and implementation
  - Priority nursing diagnoses
    - Impaired Skin Integrity
    - Deficient Fluid Volume
    - Risk for Infection
    - Impaired Physical Mobility
    - Imbalanced Nutrition: Less than Body Requirements
    - Acute Pain
    - Powerlessness
- Evaluation
  - Wound healing
  - Fluid status
  - Absence of infection
  - Adequate nutrition
  - Pain relief
  - Client perceptions of control of outcomes, treatment, and care
  - Effectiveness of exercises and prevention of contractures

SUGGESTIONS FOR CLASSROOM ACTIVITIES

1. Discuss the role of the nurse in each of the stages of care of a client with a major burn. Illustrate how the nursing process is used in the emergency department and critical care unit, through the rehabilitative stages.
2. Prepare a list of potential client problems that may occur in a client with a major burn. Ask students to work in groups of two to three students. Give each group a problem. Ask the students in the group to identify what additional data they could collect about the problem, what care would be appropriate to resolve the problem, and how would they evaluate the effectiveness of the care.

SUGGESTIONS FOR CLINICAL ACTIVITIES

1. Have students care for clients with burns in the clinical setting. Assign students to create a client problem list along with nursing care interventions.
2. Have students present an actual case study of a burn client that illustrates the powerlessness that a burn client may experience. Ask students to express how they would feel in the same circumstances.

LEARNING OUTCOME 5

Provide client and family teaching for care of the burn after discharge.

CONCEPTS FOR LECTURE

1. Clients with major burns need care through an integrated approach over a long period of time.

POWERPOINT LECTURE SLIDES

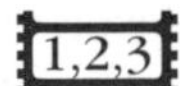
1,2,3 Continuity of Care

- Client teaching in all phases
- Include family
- Establish short-term and long-term goals

© 2007 Pearson Education, Inc.

Concepts for Lecture *continued*

2. Ensuring continuity of care requires a comprehensive plan for the client and the family and includes teaching as a major component.
3. Rehabilitative therapies play an integral role in partnership with nursing in helping the client with a major burn return to the highest level of health and functioning possible.

PowerPoint Lecture Slides *continued*

- Areas on which to focus
  - Prevention of infection and deformity
  - Fluid resuscitation
  - Nutrition
  - Wound healing
  - Pain control
  - Role of therapies
- Emotional support
  - Powerlessness
  - Fears and concerns

Suggestions for Classroom Activities

1. Discuss the long-term care of a burn client to include discussion of community agencies and web searches for support groups and burn recovery sites.
2. If possible, invite representatives of a burn recovery or burn support group to share their personal experiences in dealing with clients with burn injuries.

Suggestions for Clinical Activities

Ask students to develop a teaching plan for their burn patients in the clinical area.

© 2007 Pearson Education, Inc.

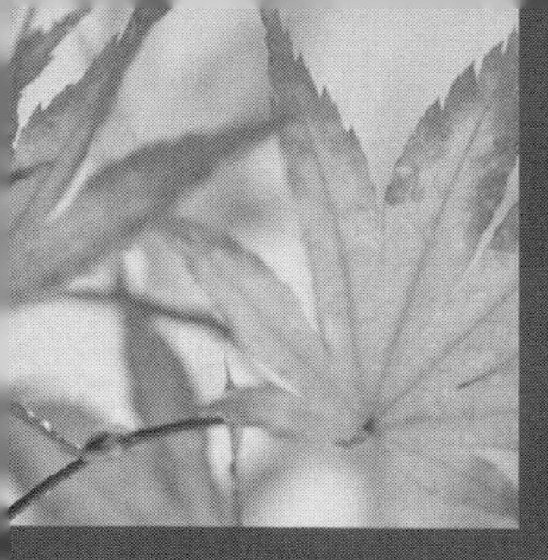

CHAPTER 47
MENTAL HEALTH AND ASSESSMENT

RESOURCE LIBRARY

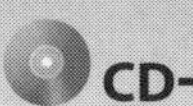 **CD-ROM**

Brain/Brainstem
Neurosynapse
Video: English as Second Language

IMAGE LIBRARY

Figure 47-1 Dimensions of a person. All are included in holistic nursing care.
Figure 47-2 Risk factors for mental illness and factors that promote mental health.
Figure 47-3 Brain anatomy.
Figure 47-4 Neurotransmission. First inset shows axon-dendrite interface. Second inset illustrates step-by-step neurotransmission.

LEARNING OUTCOME 1

Compare and contrast mental health and mental illness.

CONCEPTS FOR LECTURE

1. Mentally healthy persons are able to live full, productive lives filled with satisfying social relationships. They have a realistic self-concept, adapt well to change, and have the ability to control instinctive behavior.
2. Mental illness is a point on a continuum wherein the aspects associated with mental health are impaired, resulting in symptoms related to thinking, feeling, and behaving.
3. It is critical for nurses to examine their own beliefs and prejudices about mental illnesses in order to see beyond the stigma commonly associated with them and provide competent, evidence-based nursing care.

POWERPOINT LECTURE SLIDES

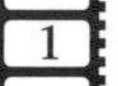 1 Mental Health
- An integral part of the whole person; body, mind, spirit
  - An important part of overall health
- A relative state
  - Minimally healthy mental behavior does not equate to a mental disorder

1a Attributes of a Mentally Healthy Person
- Ability to assess reality accurately
- Healthy self-concept/insight
- Ability to relate to others
- Achievement of a sense of meaning in life
- Ability to contribute to the world; creative/productive
- Control over own behavior
- Adaptability

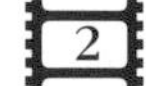 2 Mental Illness
- Interferes with a person's ability to think, feel, or behave

 3 Carries a Stigma:
- Based on stereotypes/fear
- Inability to "see" disease physically
- Not valued illnesses
- Shame

Suggestions for Classroom Activities

1. Based on the premise that mental illness would be an alteration in or absence of the attributes of mental health, elicit from students characteristics of a client with a mental illness.
2. Discuss terms other than those listed in the text that students have heard used to describe persons with mental illnesses.
3. Discuss the number of aspects of mental health that might be altered before mental illness would be diagnosed. Include the concept of mental health on a continuum.
4. Have students share their own personal beliefs, prejudices, and biases about mental illness. Ask students to share their thoughts about mental health being part of overall wellness.
5. Discuss the prevalence and impact of mental illness on society. Include a discussion of the underdiagnosing of mental illnesses.

Suggestions for Clinical Activities

1. Invite a nurse who works in the mental health clinical area to speak with students about the challenges faced when caring for a client with a mental illness.
2. In postconference, have students identify what aspects of mental health seemed to be impaired in the client assigned to them. What aspects of mental health were intact?

Learning Outcome 2

Identify risk factors for mental illness.

Concepts for Lecture

1. Certain factors will place clients at risk for mental illness.

PowerPoint Lecture Slides

1 Risk Factors for Mental Illness
- Figure 47-2

Suggestions for Classroom Activities

1. Relate the risk factors from Figure 47-2 to the aspects of mental health. Ask students to identify any relationship between the two.
2. Review the concept of mental health as being on a continuum. Discuss the risk factors in terms of how many need be present for mental illness to occur.
3. Ask students if they can identify other risk factors for mental illness not listed in the text.

Suggestions for Clinical Activities

Have students review patient histories in the mental health clinical setting. Ask them to share in postconference what risk factors the client had for mental illness according to the text.

Learning Outcome 3

Identify factors that prevent mental illness.

Concepts for Lecture

1. Certain factors are associated with the prevention of mental illness.

PowerPoint Lecture Slides

1 Factors That Promote Mental Health
- Healthy self-concept
- Positive attitude
- Flexibility
- Adequate rest
- Conflict management skills
- Sense of meaning in life
- Control over one's own behavior
- Satisfying interpersonal relationships

© 2007 Pearson Education, Inc.

Suggestions for Classroom Activities

1. Discuss the general concept of preventive health. Ask students to share their beliefs about preventive health.
2. Compare and contrast risk factors for mental illness with factors associated with the prevention of them.

Suggestions for Clinical Activities

1. Instruct students to investigate varying treatment modalities for clients with mental disorders. Have students determine if any treatments incorporate the concept of prevention.
2. Have students create a patient education brochure, identifying strategies to prevent mental illness.

Learning Outcome 4

Describe neurotransmission in the brain.

Concepts for Lecture

1. Successful physiologic functioning of the brain is dependent on the transmission of neurologic impulses between neurons (communication between neurons).
2. Chemicals known as neurotransmitters, working at receptors in neural synapses, are responsible for either facilitating or halting the transmission of impulses.
3. Either an abundance of or deficit in particular neurotransmitters is associated with the development of certain mental disorders.

PowerPoint Lecture Slides

1 Neurotransmitters
- Chemical messengers manufactured in neurons
- Released into synapse
- Work at receptor site
- Alter electrical environment; electrical charge
- Facilitate passage of impulses between neurons

2 Neurotransmission
- Figure 47-4

3 Neurotransmitters and Mental Disorders
- Acetylcholine
  - Alzheimer's; Parkinson's
- Dopamine
  - Schizophrenia, mania
  - Parkinson's; depression

3a Neurotransmitters and Mental Disorders
- Norepinephrine
  - Depression
  - Schizophrenia, mania, anxiety
- Serotonin
  - Schizophrenia
  - Depression, anxiety, OCD

Suggestions for Classroom Activities

1. Develop a skit wherein students line up and act out the process of neurotransmission. Assign students to play the role of the neurons, the impulses, and the neurotransmitters.
2. Using illustrations from the text or other transparencies, review the concept of receptors in the body.
3. Invite students to begin thinking about the relationship between neurotransmitter abnormalities and pharmacotherapy for mental disorders.

Suggestions for Clinical Activities

1. Invite a pharmacist to speak with the students about drug therapy for mental disorders, focusing on pharmacotherapy related to neurotransmitter abnormalities.
2. Have students identify medical conditions that are "caused" or exacerbated by chemical imbalances.

Learning Outcome 5

Explain why psychosocial assessment is important.

Concepts for Lecture

1. Human beings are comprised of physical, mental, and spiritual aspects, each being an integral part of the

PowerPoint Lecture Slides

1 The Whole Person
- Figure 47-1

© 2007 Pearson Education, Inc.

Concepts for Lecture *continued*

"whole" person. Due to the interconnectedness of the three aspects, a change in one will affect not only the other two aspects, but the client's total health as well.

2. In completing a psychosocial assessment, the nurse identifies factors that may affect both psychologic and social functioning.
3. The psychosocial assessment should be included in the initial assessment of a client being admitted to any health care facility.

PowerPoint Lecture Slides *continued*

2 The Psychosocial Assessment
- Psychologic functions include:
  - Thinking
  - Feelings
  - Behavior
  - Responses to current stressors

3 The Psychosocial Assessment
- Social functions include:
  - Relationships with self and others
  - Community support

Suggestions for Classroom Activities

1. Discuss the concept of delivering health care using a holistic approach. Have students give examples from their own experiences of health care delivered using solely a medical model.
2. Using Figure 47-1, discuss how the mind, body, and spirit are interconnected. Encourage students to share their beliefs about this idea.
3. Use examples from clinical practice to illustrate how mental and spiritual distress can cause or exacerbate physical illnesses and vice versa.

Suggestions for Clinical Activities

1. Invite a chaplain or other spiritual adviser to speak with students about tending to the client's spiritual needs.
2. Obtain an admission assessment form from a clinical agency where students are currently assigned. Have students identify where the psychosocial assessment is documented on the form.

Learning Outcome 6

Identify subjective and objective psychosocial assessment data.

Concepts for Lecture

1. As with the physical assessment of a body system, the psychosocial assessment includes gathering both subjective and objective data.
2. Psychosocial assessment of the client also includes completing a mental status assessment.

PowerPoint Lecture Slides

1 Psychosocial Subjective Data
- Culture and information about family
- Patient's perception of reason for admission
- Current medical problems

1a Psychosocial Subjective Data
- Use of alcohol or drugs
- Social support systems
- Self-concept
- Coping skills

1b Psychosocial Objective Data
- Appearance
- Motor activity
- Quality of speech
- Affect

2 Mental Status Assessment
- Appearance
- Motor activity

PowerPoint Lecture Slides *continued*

- Characteristics of speech and content
- Interpersonal behavior
- Mood
- Affect
- Thought processes
- Cognition
- Judgment
- Abstract thinking

Suggestions for Classroom Activities

1. Discuss differences and similarities between a psychosocial assessment and a physical assessment. Ask students to identify data that are common to both.
2. Discuss in further detail using examples: How does each piece of subjective/objective data give a clue to the presence of a mental disorder?
3. Have students problem solve whether the mental status assessment should be completed at the beginning or the end of the assessment process.
4. Using the mental assessment form found in Box 47-4, have students practice a mental status assessment on a peer partner.
5. Discuss the challenges of getting accurate data from a client with a mental disorder during the psychosocial exam.

Suggestions for Clinical Activities

1. Have the students participate in or complete the psychosocial assessment on an assigned client.
2. In a postconference, encourage students to share their experiences when obtaining data for the psychosocial assessment. Ask them to identify the major differences between the head-to-toe physical exam and the psychosocial exam.

© 2007 Pearson Education, Inc.

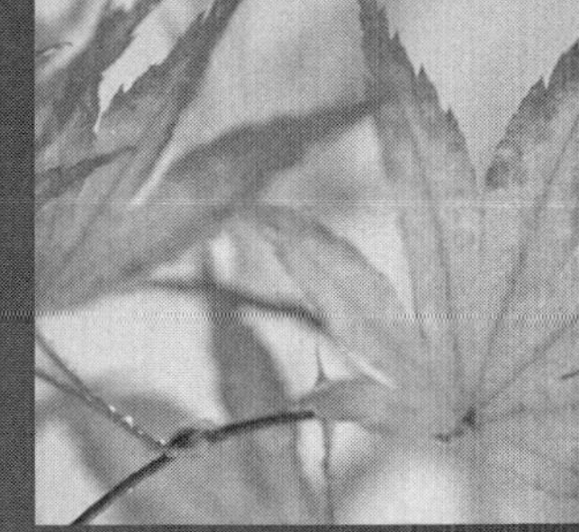

Chapter 48
Caring for Clients with Psychotic Disorders

Resource Library

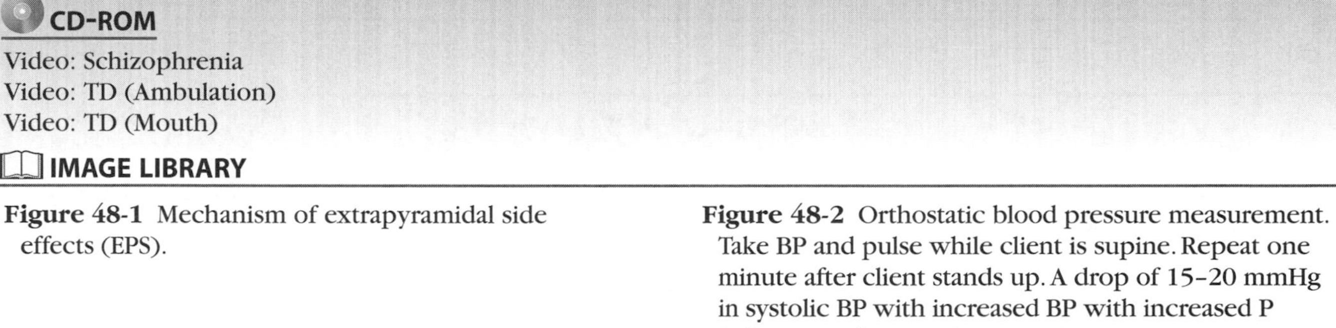

CD-ROM

Video: Schizophrenia
Video: TD (Ambulation)
Video: TD (Mouth)

IMAGE LIBRARY

Figure 48-1 Mechanism of extrapyramidal side effects (EPS).

Figure 48-2 Orthostatic blood pressure measurement. Take BP and pulse while client is supine. Repeat one minute after client stands up. A drop of 15–20 mmHg in systolic BP with increased BP with increased P indicates orthostatic hypotension.

Learning Outcome 1

Explain the role of brain neurotransmitters in causing schizophrenia.

Concepts for Lecture

1. Schizophrenia is a thought disorder that affects a person's ability to perceive reality accurately, thereby disrupting normal social functioning.
2. In schizophrenia, there is an imbalance in brain neurotransmitters that normally mediate thought, mood and behavior.

PowerPoint Lecture Slides

1 Manifestations of Schizophrenia
- Psychosis
- Disorganized personality
- Impaired ability to interpret reality
- Cannot relate to self and others

2 Neurotransmitters Involved in Schizophrenia
- Dopamine (increased)
  - Cognition/motivation
  - Pleasure/emotional response
- Norepinephrine (increased)
  - Affects attention, learning, memory
  - Regulates mood, sleep, and wakefulness

2a Neurotransmitters Involved in Schizophrenia
- Serotonin (increased)
  - Sleep, wakefulness
  - Mood, thought processes
- Gamma-aminobutyric acid (GABA)
  - Modulates other neurotransmitters

Suggestions for Classroom Activities

1. Discuss the term *psychosis* and processes that can cause it.
2. Compare and contrast the symptoms of psychosis: delusions and hallucinations.
3. Describe the statistics of and populations affected by schizophrenia.

Suggestions for Clinical Activities

1. Assign students to care for a client with schizophrenia. Assist them to assess (through observation) the degree to which the disease is impairing the client's ability to carry out the functions mediated by the various neurotransmitters.
2. Have students work in small groups. Assign to each group one of the neurotransmitters involved in the

SUGGESTIONS FOR CLASSROOM ACTIVITIES *continued*

4. Discuss the other contributing factors to the development of schizophrenia besides neurochemical imbalances.
5. Give examples of the manifestations of schizophrenia.
6. Review brain chemistry in terms of neurotransmitters. Include a discussion of the physiology of receptors.
7. Give examples of the functions of daily living that are mediated by brain neurotransmitters.

SUGGESTIONS FOR CLINICAL ACTIVITIES *continued*

development of schizophrenia. Have students research the functions of each neurotransmitter and have them present their findings to the group.

LEARNING OUTCOME 2

Describe the actions and side effects of antipsychotic drugs.

CONCEPTS FOR LECTURE

1. It is critical for nurses to know and understand the actions and side effects of antipsychotic drugs due to the many issues surrounding pharmacotherapy for schizophrenia.
2. There are three categories of antipsychotic agents. Their actions alter brain chemistry; therefore, they can have both desired and untoward effects.

POWERPOINT LECTURE SLIDES

1 Antipsychotic Agents: Issues
- Manifestations of schizophrenia are client specific
- Acknowledgment of illness
- Side effects contribute to noncompliance
- Onset of therapeutic action

2 Antipsychotic Agents
- Typical: first generation
- Atypical: second generation
- New generation

2a Typical: First-Generation Antipsychotics
- Box 48-3

2b Typical Antipsychotics
- Action
  - Target dopamine-2 receptors
  - Mesolimbic area of brain
  - Act as antagonists

2c Typical Antipsychotics
- Side Effects
  - Extrapyramidal effects
    - Dystonia
    - Dyskinesia
    - Akathisia
    - Tardive dyskinesia

2d Typical Antipsychotics
- Other side effects
  - Neuroleptic malignant syndrome
  - Endocrine
  - Anticholinergic
  - Weight gain

2e Typical Antipsychotics
- Other side effects
  - Orthostatic hypotension
  - Cardiac
  - Seizures
  - Photosensitivity

© 2007 Pearson Education, Inc.

PowerPoint Lecture Slides *continued*

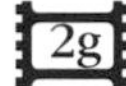 Atypical Antipsychotics
- Action
  - Wider variety of dopamine receptors
  - Serotonin receptors
  - Muscarinic receptors
  - Alpha receptors
  - Histamine receptors

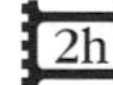 Atypical Antipsychotics
- Side effects
  - EPS
  - Diabetes
  - Agranulocytosis

2h New-Generation Antipsychotics
- Action
  - Stabilize/modulate dopamine
  - Reduce high levels
  - Preserves dopamine transmission when it is low

Suggestions for Classroom Activities

1. Discuss in detail issues connected with pharmacotherapy for the client with schizophrenia. Include length of time needed to see therapeutic effects; client's lack of perception of own health status; correlation between side effects and compliance issues.
2. Describe the importance of client/family teaching in relationship to medication compliance for the client with schizophrenia.
3. Divide students into small workgroups. Assign each group a particular antipsychotic medication. Have students research prior to class all potential untoward side effects of their assigned drug. Have groups present the information to the class detailing why the effects would increase noncompliance with therapy.

Suggestions for Clinical Activities

1. Assign students to care for a client with schizophrenia. Following HIPAA regulations, have students share in postconference the medication regimen for their assigned clients.
2. Assist students to assess clients with schizophrenia (through observation) for side effects of antipsychotic medication therapy. Have students share their findings in postconference.
3. Invite a pharmacist to speak with students about the actions and side effects of antipsychotic therapy.
4. Invite a registered nurse to speak with the students about the challenges faced by the medical team in terms of patient compliance with drug therapy for schizophrenia.

Learning Outcome 3

Identify subjective and objective data to collect for the client with schizophrenia.

Concepts for Lecture

1. Subjective information may be difficult to obtain from the client with schizophrenia due to alterations in cognition and inability to interpret reality.
2. Subjective information will be gathered by listening to the client and by completing a mental status assessment.
3. Due to the client's altered perception of reality, the nurse must limit his or her physical assessment to priority concerns.
4. Certain objective data for the client with schizophrenia can be gathered through observation.

PowerPoint Lecture Slides

 Subjective Assessment Data
- Past medical history/family history
- Speech: rate, content
- Interpersonal skills
- Mood/affect
- Thought process:
  - Hallucinations, judgment, memory

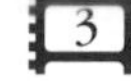 Objective Assessment Data
- Limit data gathering due to clients:
  - Hallucinations: alter perception of reality
  - Delusional thinking
  - Touching: misperceived

© 2007 Pearson Education, Inc.

PowerPoint Lecture Slides *continued*

4 Objective Assessment Data
- Pertinent illnesses
- Drug response
- Violent behaviors:
  - Clenched fists
  - Loud; yelling
  - Increased motor activity
  - Hitting inanimate objects

Suggestions for Classroom Activities

1. As the course instructor, perform a short skit for the students in which behaviors of the client with schizophrenia are demonstrated. Have students "assess" for subjective and objective data.
2. Review how an altered perception of reality in the client with schizophrenia will skew assessment findings. Give examples.
3. Discuss the various misperceptions about physical touching that occur in the client with schizophrenia.
4. Ask students to share their perceptions of what constitutes a "priority" physical assessment.

Suggestions for Clinical Activities

1. Assign students to care for a client with schizophrenia. Assist the students to obtain subjective and objective assessment data.
2. Obtain assessment forms from the clinical agency. Review the form with students, discussing how to obtain the data required.

Learning Outcome 4

Identify the nursing responsibilities and nursing interventions for clients experiencing schizophrenia.

Concepts for Lecture

1. Schizophrenia is considered the prototype disorder for all nursing care provided for clients with psychoses.
2. The primary responsibility of the nurse caring for the client with schizophrenia is assessing the client for risk for violence and creating a safe environment based on assessment findings.
3. Four priority nursing diagnoses can be used to create an individualized plan of care for the client with schizophrenia.

PowerPoint Lecture Slides

1 Nursing Diagnosis: Risk for Violence
- Avoid touching
- Use calm approach
- Interventions
  - Start with least restrictive
- Decrease environmental stimuli

1a Nursing Diagnosis: Disturbed Thought Processes
- Drug therapy
- Reinforce reality
- Avoid arguing
- Active listening

2 Nursing Diagnosis: Ineffective Individual Coping
- Trusting relationship
- Continuity of care
- Establish expectations
- Role model acceptable social behavior

3 Nursing Diagnosis: Impaired Social Interaction
- Accepting attitude
  - Honesty, sincerity
- Positive reinforcement
- Group activities

© 2007 Pearson Education, Inc.

Suggested Classroom Activities

1. Review other conditions/disorders in which clients may exhibit psychosis. Describe how the plan of care for the client with schizophrenia may be applicable in these instances as well.
2. Discuss in detail the assessment data that would indicate a client is experiencing paranoia or command hallucinations.
3. Using each nursing diagnosis given, describe in full detail the nursing interventions for each. Give clinical examples of each intervention.
4. Have students give examples for interventions used in the text such as "low stimulation environment," "trusting relationship," "calm approach." Give students feedback about the accuracy of their interpretation of these terms.

Suggestions for Clinical Activities

1. Have students observe the psychiatric clinical environment. Instruct students to note how the environment is constructed/arranged to promote client safety.
2. Demonstrate for students the skill of modeling acceptable social behavior for clients. Have students practice in postconference with a partner.
3. Invite a registered nurse from the psychiatric clinical agency to speak with students regarding promoting safety for the client experiencing paranoia or command hallucinations.
4. If allowed, have students observe in a group therapy session. Have students discuss the social behavior of their assigned client in that setting.

© 2007 Pearson Education, Inc.

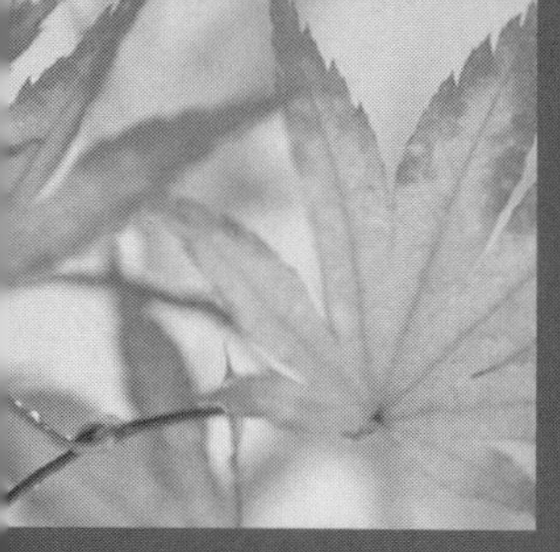

CHAPTER 49
CARING FOR CLIENTS WITH MOOD DISORDERS

RESOURCE LIBRARY

CD-ROM

Video: Bipolar Disorder

IMAGE LIBRARY

Figure 49-1 Characteristics of a major depressive episode.
Figure 49-2 Neurotransmission and antidepressant drug action.
Figure 49-3 Comparison of mood disorders.
Figure 49-4 Characteristics of a manic episode.
Figure 49-5 Desired outcomes for clients with mood disorders.

LEARNING OUTCOME 1

Explain the pathophysiology of mood disorders in relation to brain neurotransmitters.

CONCEPTS FOR LECTURE

1. Mood disorders alter the intensity of emotions that clients experience in their daily lives.
2. Two disorders serve as prototypes for the conditions known as mood disorders.
3. Several factors play a part in the pathophysiology of mood disorders including a disturbance in brain neurotransmitter balance.
4. Several brain neurotransmitters are involved in the development of mood disorders.

POWERPOINT LECTURE SLIDES

1 Mood Disorders
- Emotions beyond normal intensity

2 Prototypes
- Major Depressive Disorder
- Bipolar Disorder

3 Neurotransmitters Involved in Major Depressive Disorder
- Decreased levels of:
  - Serotonin
  - Norepinephrine
  - Dopamine
  - Acetylcholine
  - GABA

4 Neurotransmitters Involved in Bipolar Disorder
- Manic episodes: increased
  - Norepinephrine
  - Dopamine
- Depressive episodes
  - Same neurotransmitters, decreased levels

SUGGESTIONS FOR CLASSROOM ACTIVITIES

1. Discuss mood disorders. Define the two prototypes, including signs and symptoms of depression and those for the manic aspect of bipolar disorder.
2. Assign the following terms to the students: *mood, affect, dysphoric, euthymic*. Have students define the terms and share the definitions in class.
3. Compare and contrast normal "highs and lows" in terms of emotional responses and the intensity of mood alterations found in mood disorders.

SUGGESTIONS FOR CLINICAL ACTIVITIES

1. Assign students to care for clients with mood disorders. Have students observe for the abnormal intensity of responses that occur. Have them share their observations with their peers.
2. Invite a registered nurse from the psychiatric setting to speak with the students about the differences between schizophrenia and mood disorders.

Suggestions for Classroom Activities *continued*

4. Describe the other mood disorders that are listed in the chapter besides the two prototypes.
5. Using Figure 49-1, discuss the characteristics of a major depressive episode.
6. Review the brain neurotransmitters involved in mood disorders.
7. Compare and contrast the alterations in brain neurotransmitters between schizophrenia, major depressive disorders, and bipolar disorders.

Learning Outcome 2

Identify subjective and objective data to collect related to a client's mood.

Concepts for Lecture

1. Client observation, mental status assessment, and specific screening tools are all methods the nurse can use to assess for both subjective and objective data related to mood disorders.

PowerPoint Lecture Slides

1 Assessing Mood: Objective Data
- Appearance
- Motor activity
- Speech
- Anxiety
- Affect

1a Assessing Mood: Subjective Data
- Mental status exam
    - Client's rating of mood
    - Memory/judgment/thinking
- Geriatric Depression Scale
- Beck Depression Inventory
- Culture

Suggestions for Classroom Activities

1. Review the components of the mental status exam. Describe how alterations in each section can be a reflection of a mood disorder.
2. Discuss what behavior a client with major depression or bipolar disorder might exhibit.
3. Use transparencies of the Geriatric Depression Scale and Beck Depression Inventory to enhance student understanding of the components of each assessment tool.
4. Have students practice using the assessment tools mentioned in Activity 3 on a peer.
5. Discuss how cultural behavior might influence assessment findings.
6. Show a clip from a current popular movie that illustrates a mood disorder. Have students identify assessment data that supports the diagnosis.

Suggestions for Clinical Activities

1. Assign students to an admission area in a psychiatric clinical facility. If allowed/appropriate, have students participate in obtaining subjective information related to mood disorders using screening assessment tools.
2. Assign students to care for a client with a mood disorder. Assist the student to identify subjective and objective data that support the diagnosis. Have students share their observations in a postconference.

© 2007 Pearson Education, Inc.

Learning Outcome 3

Assess clients for suicidal thinking.

Concepts for Lecture

1. Certain client populations are at higher risk for suicide than others.
2. Assessing for suicide is critical to promoting client safety as well as the safety of others.
3. The process of assessing for suicidal ideation consists of questions designed to determine if the client has a solid, lethal plan for suicide with the means to carry it out.

PowerPoint Lecture Slides

1 The Elderly: Risk Factors for Suicide
- Prior attempt, family history
- Mental disorders
- Hopelessness, isolation
- Losses, isolation
- Unwillingness to seek help, stigma

2 Assessing for Suicide
- Will not "suggest" the idea
- Promotes prevention
- Allows verbalization
- Promotes problem clarification

3 Process of Assessing for Suicide
- Determine if client has:
  - Suicidal thoughts
  - An organized plan
  - Access to means
- Lethality of plan
- Inform health care team

Suggestions for Classroom Activities

1. Use a transparency of Box 49-3 to discuss risk factors for suicide.
2. Discuss the factors that relate to the elderly client with a chronic illness. Ask students to give example of chronic illnesses that lead to depression and, thus, potential for thoughts of suicide.
3. Compare and contrast general statements made by the client and statements that are a clear indication of suicidal ideation.
4. Explain how active listening enables the client to verbalize thoughts.
5. Expand on the questions listed in the text that are part of the assessment for suicidal ideation.
6. Discuss the nurse's responsibility in reporting a client who has clear thoughts, intention, a plan, and means to commit suicide to the treatment team.

Suggestions for Clinical Activities

1. Have students work in pairs. Assign them to "issues" that might be faced by a client with depression and have the students practice active listening.
2. Have students share their fears and insecurities about assessing a client for suicide. Role model what a client might say during the assessment process.
3. Ask students to share their thoughts about the concept of "having a plan" for suicide.
4. Invite members of the treatment team to speak with students about how their individual roles as team members ensure the safety of the client with a plan for committing suicide

Learning Outcome 4

Safely and effectively administer antidepressant and mood stabilizing medications.

Concepts for Lecture

1. The safe and effective administration of antidepressants and mood stabilizing medications requires knowledge of pharmacodynamic facts related to overall drug therapy.
2. The safe and effective administration of antidepressants and mood stabilizing medications is also dependent on the nurse's knowledge of expected drug action.

PowerPoint Lecture Slides

1 General Pharmacodynamic Concepts
- Effectiveness is client specific
- 2–6 weeks → full therapeutic effect
- Side effects affect compliance
- Combination therapy common
- Act on major brain neurotransmitters

 © 2007 Pearson Education, Inc.

CONCEPTS FOR LECTURE *continued*

3. Antidepressant and mood stabilizing medications can have serious and potentially fatal side effects. The nurse must understand these effects in order to administer these medications safely.

POWERPOINT LECTURE SLIDES *continued*

2 Antidepressants: SSRIs
- Action
  - Inhibit serotonin reuptake
- Side effects
  - Some anticholinergic, cardiac, sedation
  - Sexual
  - GI: nausea, weight loss
  - Headache, anxiety, insomnia

2a Antidepressants: Tricyclics
- Action
  - Block reuptake: serotonin, norepinephrine
- Side effects
  - Anticholinergic
    - Glaucoma alert
  - Overdose → fatal
  - Cardiac

2b Antidepressants: MAOIs
- Action
  - Inhibit breakdown of monoamines
- Side effects
  - Hypertensive crisis: tyramine
  - Potentially fatal drug interactions

3 Novel Antidepressants
- NDRI
- SNRI
- NaSSAs
- SARIs
- NRIs

3a Mood Stabilizers: Lithium
- Action
  - Affects neurotransmitter function
- Common side effects
  - Fine hand tremors
  - Polyuria
  - Weight gain
  - GI discomfort, mild nausea
  - Subjective feeling of mental dullness
  - Thyroid dysfunction
- Lithium toxicities
  - Coarse hand tremor
  - Slurred speech, mental confusion
  - Muscle weakness → irritability
  - Seizures
  - Kidney and cardiac dysfunction
  - Coma and death

3b Mood Stabilizers: Anticonvulsants
- Action
  - Exact action unknown
  - GABA increase
  - Reduced calcium influx
- Side effects
  - GI
  - Thrombocytopenia
  - Fetal anomalies
  - Skin reactions

© 2007 Pearson Education, Inc.

Suggestions for Classroom Activities

1. Discuss the principles of pharmacologic management of mood disorders in terms of matching therapy to specific client symptoms; potential for no effect; length of time for therapeutic effect; use of combination therapies.
2. Divide students into small workgroups. Assign each group a specific medication used to treat mood disorders. Have students identify the one side effect that would most likely lead to noncompliance with therapy.
3. Review brain neurotransmitters and their functions (see Chapter 47).
4. Discuss the three categories of side effects associated with lithium.

Suggestions for Clinical Activities

1. Assign students to care for clients with mood disorders. Have students choose one medication from the clients' prescribed regimen. Have students develop a client teaching brochure related to the medication.
2. Invite a clinical pharmacist to speak to the students about common medication combinations/regimens used to treat mood disorders.

Learning Outcome 5

Apply the nursing process to clients with mood disorders.

Concepts for Lecture

1. The nursing process can be used to develop an individualized plan of care for the client with a mood disorder.
2. The plan of care focuses on attending to the client's risk for violence, social interactions, nutrition, and thought processes.

PowerPoint Lecture Slides

1 Nursing Process: Assessment
- Mood
- Risk for suicide
- Appearance and affect
- Psychomotor activity
- Thought processes
- Reactions to medication therapy

2 Nursing Process: Diagnoses
- Risk for Violence
  - Self-directed/directed at others
- Impaired Social Interaction
- Imbalanced Nutrition
- Hopelessness

2a Nursing Process: Evaluation
- Cognition
- Mood
- Behavior
- Physical findings

Suggestions for Classroom Activities

1. Review the mental status assessment form found in Chapter 47 with the students.
2. Using the nursing diagnoses given in the chapter, elicit from students the nursing interventions they believe will address them.
3. Discuss how a nurse develops a trusting relationship with a client who has a mood disorder.

Suggestions for Clinical Activities

1. Assign students to care for patients with major depressive disorder and bipolar disorder in the manic phase. Have students compare and contrast the plans of care for these clients.
2. Assist students to understand the critical elements of the plan of care for a client exhibiting violent behavior.

© 2007 Pearson Education, Inc.

CHAPTER 50
CARING FOR CLIENTS WITH ANXIETY DISORDERS

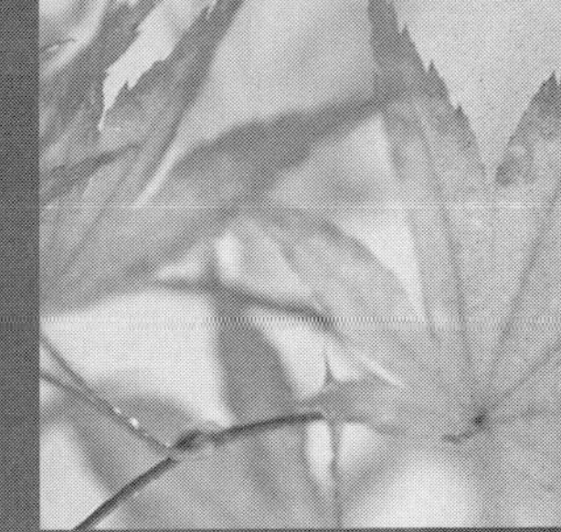

RESOURCE LIBRARY

CD-ROM
Video: Panic Attacks
Video: OCD

IMAGE LIBRARY

Figure 50-1 The limbic system is surrounded by the cerebral cortex. It plays a role in motivation, emotion, and memory. It is composed of the thalamus, amygdala, hippocampus, and hypothalamus.

LEARNING OUTCOME 1

Collect subjective and objective data about clients' anxiety.

CONCEPTS FOR LECTURE

1. In collecting assessment data, the nurse must be able to differentiate between "normal" feelings of uneasiness in response to a stressor and overwhelming feelings of anxiety that are incapacitating.
2. Anxiety is a manifestation that is common to many anxiety-related disorders.
3. There is both general subjective and objective assessment data that indicate the presence of anxiety as well as data that are specific to the degree of anxiety experienced by the client.

POWERPOINT LECTURE SLIDES

1 Concepts Related to Anxiety
- Anxiety
  - Feeling of uneasiness
  - Response to vague threat
  - Normal response to stress
- Anxiety disorder
  - Anxiety overwhelming
  - Impaired functioning

2 Anxiety-Related Disorders
- Generalized Anxiety Disorder
- Panic Disorder
- Agoraphobia
- OCD
- Acute Stress Disorder
- PTSD

3 Subjective Assessment Data
- Box 50-2

3a Subjective Assessment Data
- Perception of threat
- Feelings
- Use of alcohol/drugs
- Medication use
- Usual coping methods
- Verbalization of any objective manifestation

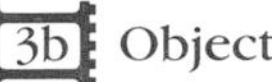

3b Objective Assessment Data
- Vital signs
- Physical symptoms
  - Trembling/shaking
  - Sweating
  - Chest pain

PowerPoint Lecture Slides *continued*

- Vertigo
- Increased arousal
- GI distress

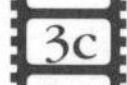
Objective Assessment Data
- Cognitive changes
  - Difficulty concentrating
  - Irritability
  - Irrational fears

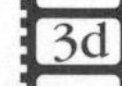
Data Related to Mild Anxiety
- Widened perceptual field
- Alert/heightened perceptions
- Motivated

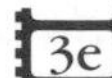
Data Related to Moderate Anxiety
- Narrow perceptual field
- Direction changes attention
- Speech faster
- Increased vital signs
- Expresses anxiety

Data Related to Severe Anxiety
- More reduced perceptual field
- Unable to redirect focus
- Erroneous assumptions
- Unaware of anxiety
- Uses coping measures

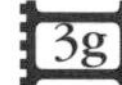
Data Related to Panic
- Distorted perception/single detail
- Flight of ideas
- Feels threatened/dread/terror
- Loss of control/pacing
- Potential violence
- Confused/altered reality

Suggestions for Classroom Activities

1. Compare and contrast normal anxiety and anxiety disorders.
2. Ask students to share examples of instances when they experienced "normal" anxiety.
3. Describe the anxiety-related disorders given in the text in further detail. Discuss the other manifestations of the disorders besides anxiety.
4. Discuss the changes in vital signs that would be seen in a client with an anxiety disorder. Describe the degree of elevation in vital signs that occurs as anxiety progresses from mild anxiety to panic.
5. Compare and contrast the subjective and objective data specific to the varying degrees of anxiety.

Suggestions for Clinical Activities

1. Assign students to care for clients with varying anxiety disorders. Have students observe their assigned clients for manifestations of anxiety. Ask students to compare their assessment findings.
2. In the general med/surg clinical setting, have students assess their assigned clients for anxiety. Ask students to determine if the client's anxiety is related to a general medical condition.

© 2007 Pearson Education, Inc.

Learning Outcome 2

Apply the nursing process to the care of clients with anxiety disorders.

Concepts for Lecture

1. The nursing process can be used to develop an individualized plan of care for the client with an anxiety disorder.

PowerPoint Lecture Slides

1 Nursing Process: Assessment
- Subjective data
- Objective data
- General medical conditions
- Assess own anxiety level

1a Nursing Process: Diagnoses
- Anxiety
- Ineffective Coping
- Post-Trauma Syndrome

1b Nursing Process: Evaluation
- Anxiety symptoms
- Client safety from self-harm
- Ability to cope with stress
- Coping methods used
- Medication regimen
  - Effects/side effects

Suggestions for Classroom Activities

1. Discuss the medical conditions found in Box 50-2, which may produce the symptoms of anxiety. Review how this type of anxiety is different from that which is found in anxiety disorders.
2. Review the subjective and objective data assessment data given on previous slides.
3. Describe how the anxiety level of the nurse may exacerbate feelings of anxiety in the client.
4. Using the nursing diagnoses listed in the text, explain in detail the nursing interventions for the client with anxiety.
5. Discuss the concept of "healthy" anxiety.

Suggestions for Clinical Activities

1. Generate a discussion with students about their own anxiety in the clinical setting. Have students identify strategies that they use to cope with or reduce their anxiety.
2. Have students create a plan of care for their assigned client.
3. Assist the students in assessing the client for risk of self-harm.
4. Ask students to assess the clinical setting for safety.
5. Role model for the students the concept of "therapeutic use of self" in relationship to developing a therapeutic relationship with clients.

Learning Outcome 3

Explain the role of coping mechanisms in the management of anxiety.

Concepts for Lecture

1. Coping behaviors are ways in which people act in order to manage and/or alleviate anxiety.
2. There are three basic categories of conscious coping behaviors. The behaviors in each category can be either healthy or unhealthy.
3. Another method of coping with anxiety is the unconscious use of defense mechanisms.

PowerPoint Lecture Slides

1 Conscious Coping Behaviors
- Used to control anxiety
- Become a pattern
- Adaptive/maladaptive
- Three main categories

2 Categories
- Taking action
- Avoidance or withdrawal
- Compromise

2a Taking Action
- Adaptive
  - Active problem solving
  - Considers others' rights

© 2007 Pearson Education, Inc.

PowerPoint Lecture Slides *continued*

- Maladaptive
  - Anger
  - Hostility
  - Aggression

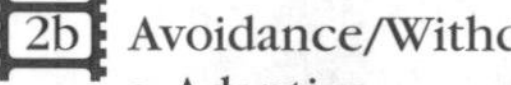

2b Avoidance/Withdrawal

- Adaptive
  - Removing self from harm
- Maladaptive
  - Avoiding resolution of an issue/problem

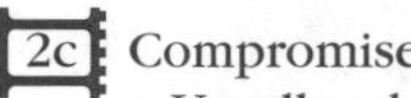

2c Compromise

- Usually adaptive
  - Changing behavior
  - Substituting goals
  - Giving up aspects of needs

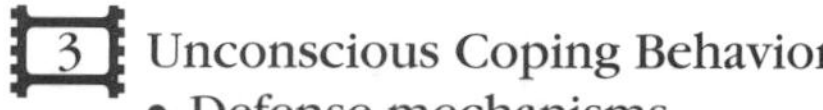

3 Unconscious Coping Behavior

- Defense mechanisms
- Table 50-4

Suggestions for Classroom Activities

1. Discuss the three categories of conscious coping behaviors.
2. Use examples, both clinical and from daily life, to illustrate each behavior fully. Examples should be different from those listed in the text.
3. Compare and contrast the concept of adaptive and maladaptive coping behaviors.
4. Ask students to list two coping strategies they have used in dealing with any anxiety experienced during nursing school. Have the students privately determine whether their behavior is adaptive or maladaptive. Ask for volunteers to share their findings.
5. Give examples of unconscious coping behaviors.

Suggestions for Clinical Activity

1. In any clinical setting, have students determine if their assigned client is anxious. Have students determine if the client is using any type of coping behavior.
2. Depending on the degree of rapport developed with the students, design a small but very difficult quiz or test to administer to the students after a full clinical day (a drug dose calculation test would work well). Tell the students that the grade for that day will include their score on the quiz. Several minutes into the test, instruct students to stop and examine their anxiety level. Generate a discussion about the coping mechanisms that may have been used during the exercise.

Learning Outcome 4

Plan nonpharmacologic nursing interventions to treat or prevent client anxiety.

Concepts for Lecture

1. Nonpharmacologic interventions are often used in conjunction with medications to treat anxiety disorders.
2. Cognitive behavioral therapy helps clients to identify the source of their anxiety as well as change their reaction to it.
3. Nurses can assist clients to develop resilience, a trait that is often linked to the ability to cope more effectively and function more fully in life.

PowerPoint Lecture Slides

1 Nonpharmacologic Interventions

- Cognitive behavioral therapy
- Promoting resilience

2 Cognitive Behavioral Therapy

- Goal
  - Relieve anxiety by eliminating supporting beliefs
- Dual focus
  - Cognitive
  - Behavioral

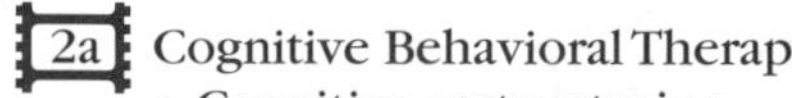

2a Cognitive Behavioral Therapy

- Cognitive restructuring
  - Identify negative thinking
  - See it as erroneous
  - Replace with supporting thinking

© 2007 Pearson Education, Inc.

PowerPoint Lecture Slides *continued*

2b Cognitive Behavioral Therapy
- Behavioral changes
- Relaxation techniques
- Exposure
  - Confronting fears
  - Gradual, increased exposure to fear
  - Supported by therapist

Resilience
- Hardy; stress resistant
- Adaptive coping
- Factors associated with resilience

Suggestions for Classroom Activities

1. Discuss the interrelationship between pharmacologic and nonpharmacologic therapies for clients with anxiety disorders.
2. Describe cognitive behavioral therapy: overall goal and dual aspects.
3. Ask students to share examples of negative thinking expressed either by a client during a clinical experience or by other persons associated with the student.
4. Describe how erroneous negative thinking can lead to avoidance. Include the concept of this becoming a self-perpetuating problem/issue.
5. Explain cognitive restructuring. Use student examples of negative thinking. Ask students what positive supportive statement might be used.
6. Explain the concept of exposure in behavioral therapy.
7. Discuss the concept of resilience.

Suggestions for Clinical Activities

1. In the psychiatric clinical experience, assign students to observe the use of cognitive behavioral therapy by a trained practitioner. Have students report their observations to their peers during a postconference.
2. Assign each student to a specific phobia, found in Table 50-3 in the text. Have the students discuss strategies for implementing "exposure" principles for a client with each specific phobia.
3. Invite an elder person or panel of elder persons who are "living well" in the community to speak with students. Invite them to share the life experiences they believe have enabled them to "live well," overcoming/surviving life's stressors. Have students compare what is shared to the list of resilience factors in the text.

Learning Outcome 5

Safely administer antianxiety and sedative hypnotic agents.

Concepts for Lecture

1. The safe administration of antianxiety and sedative hypnotic agents requires knowledge of drug names and categories, expected effects, and/or potential side effects.
2. There are different target symptoms for each class of drugs.

PowerPoint Lecture Slides

1 Antianxiety Agents: Benzodiazepines
- Effects
  - CNS depressant
  - Enhance GABA
  - Affects certain neurotransmitters

1a Benzodiazepines
- Side effects
  - Sedation, drowsiness
  - Dizziness/decreased coordination
  - Paradoxical response
- Physical dependence
- Tolerance

1b Antianxiety Agents: BuSpar
- Effects
  - Serotonin agonist
- No sedation
- No euphoria
- 6 wks for full effect

© 2007 Pearson Education, Inc.

PowerPoint Lecture Slides *continued*

1c Sedative Hypnotics: Nonbenzodiazepines

- Zaleplon
  - Benzodiazepine receptor agonist
  - Sedation; muscle relaxant
- Zolpidem
  - Benzodiazepine receptor agonist
  - Daytime drowsiness, dizziness, diarrhea

1d Sedative Hypnotics: Barbiturates

- Rarely used
  - Overdose/withdrawal potential high
  - Fatal interaction with alcohol/CNS depressants
- Secobarbital
- Pentobarbital

2 Target Symptoms: Antianxiety Agents

- Nervousness: sweating, tachycardia
- Phobias: dread, fearfulness
- Compulsiveness
- Nausea, vomiting, diarrhea
- Vertigo, irritability

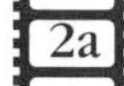

2a Target Symptoms: Sedative-Hypnotic Agents

- Insomnia: difficulty
  - Falling asleep
  - Staying asleep
  - Falling back to sleep
- Sleep disorders

Suggestions for Classroom Activities

1. Discuss the merits of pharmacotherapy for the client with an anxiety disorder.
2. Describe how pharmacotherapy aids in the implementation of other therapies.
3. Divide students into small workgroups. Assign each group a drug used to treat anxiety disorders. Have student investigate and share the expected effects as well as side effects for their assigned drug.
4. Compare and contrast antianxiety medications and sedative hypnotic agents.
5. Discuss the prototype medications for each classification. Describe the nursing responsibilities with each.

Suggestions for Clinical Activities

1. Invite a clinical pharmacist to speak with the students about the most current medications in each of the two classes of antianxiety medications discussed in class.
2. If possible, have student observe/assess clients who are prescribed any of the medications discussed in the chapter. Have students report any side effects of drug therapy noted.

© 2007 Pearson Education, Inc.

CHAPTER 51
CARING FOR CLIENTS WITH PERSONALITY DISORDERS

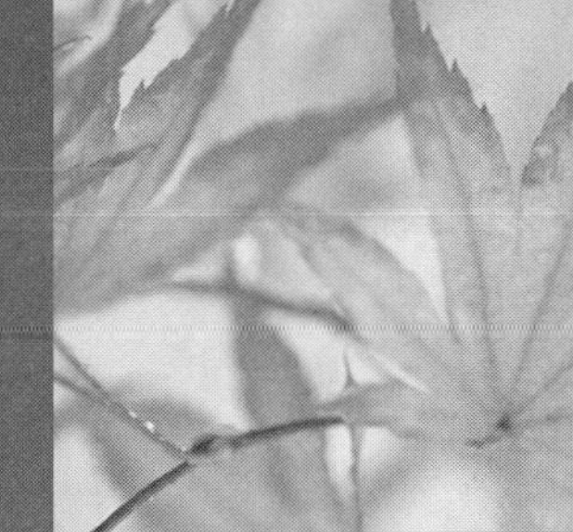

RESOURCE LIBRARY

CD-ROM

Video: Antisocial Behavior

IMAGE LIBRARY

Figure 51-1 Vicious cycle of personality disorders.
Figure 51-2 Self-injury is sometimes used as a coping mechanism by clients with Borderline Personality Disorder.

LEARNING OUTCOME 1

Perform basic client teaching about personality disorders.

CONCEPTS FOR LECTURE

1. Basic teaching about personality disorders should include defining the term *personality* as well as describing the patterns that characterize personality disorders.

POWERPOINT LECTURE SLIDES

1 Personality
- The way a person:
  - Thinks, feels, behaves
- Psychosocial traits/characteristics
- Affected by:
  - Genetic predisposition
  - Life experiences
- Unique to each person

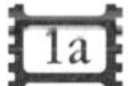

1a Characteristics of Personality Disorders
- Deviates from cultural expectations
- Pervasive/inflexible
- Starts in adolescence/young adulthood
- Stable over time
- Leads to distress/impaired functioning

SUGGESTIONS FOR CLASSROOM ACTIVITIES

1. Prior to class, ask students to define their own personality. In class, discuss the definition of personality. Have students share their definitions of themselves.
2. Have students examine the traits or characteristics given in peer definitions of their personalities. Have students list commonalities and differences in what their peers have listed.
3. Discuss cultural variations with respect to behavior and personality.
4. Give examples of the characteristics of personality disorders.
5. Compare and contrast true personality disorders with changes in personality that accompany medical conditions and substance abuse.
6. Compare and contrast personality disorders with other mental health disorders in terms of treatment options.

SUGGESTIONS FOR CLINICAL ACTIVITIES

1. During a postconference for any clinical experience, have students describe the personality of their assigned client. If students perceive the presence of abnormalities, assist students to differentiate between a personality disorder and personality changes/alterations caused by medical disorders or substance abuse.
2. In the psychiatric setting, assign students to a client with a diagnosed personality disorder. Assist students to identify the presence or absence of one of the general characteristics of personality disorders discussed in class.

Learning Outcome 2

Identify the major features and client-related behaviors of odd and eccentric personality disorders.

Concepts for Lecture

1. Personality disorders identified by the American Psychiatric Association are clustered into three groups having similar behaviors.
2. There are four main categories of features common to all personality disorders.
3. Each disorder in the odd and eccentric cluster has its own particular features.
4. Each odd and eccentric disorder is distinguished by specific client behavior.

PowerPoint Lecture Slides

1 Categories of Personality Disorders
- Odd and eccentric
- Dramatic and emotional
- Anxiety and fear based

2 General Manifestations
- Impaired self-identity
- Distorted thinking patterns
- Blunted/distorted emotions
- Impulsive/inflexible behavior

3,4 Features: Paranoid Personality Disorder
- Distrust
- Suspiciousness
- Assumption of intent without evidence
- Hidden/threatening messages

3,4a Behaviors: Paranoid Personality
- Hostile
- Defensive
- Attack without reason
- Hold grudges

3,4b Features: Schizoid Personality
- Pervasive detachment
- Restricted affect
- Prefer being alone

3,4c Behaviors: Schizoid
- No strong emotions shown
- Reduced/flattened affect
- Do not share confidences
- Choose isolation

3,4d Features: Schizotypal Personality
- Cannot form close relationships
- Cognitive/perceptual deficits
- Eccentric behavior

3,4e Behaviors: Schizotypal
- Superstitious
- Ideas of reference
- Inappropriate affect
- Odd thinking/speech
- Excessive social anxiety

Suggestions for Classroom Activities

1. Discuss the general manifestations of personality disorders.
2. List the three main clusters of personality disorders. Include the concept of those that do not meet the APA diagnostic criteria.
3. Describe the person with a paranoid personality disorder. Have students share their perceptions of the degrees to which a person might be paranoid.

Suggestions for Clinical Activities

1. Assign students to care for the client with odd and eccentric personality disorders.
2. Assist students to compare and contrast the client behaviors they observe for each disorder.
3. Generate a discussion about what necessitates an inpatient admission in relationship to manifestations of the disorder.

© 2007 Pearson Education, Inc.

4. Compare and contrast "normal" suspiciousness with that experienced by the person with paranoia.
5. Describe the features and client behaviors for schizoid and schizotypal personalities.
6. Give examples of behaviors listed on the PowerPoint slide.
7. Assign students to define the terms from this section in the text such as *affect, paranoia,* and *ideas of reference*. Have them share the definitions in their own words with the class.

LEARNING OUTCOME 3

Adapt the nurse-client relationship to the client who has an odd and eccentric personality disorder. Apply the nursing process.

CONCEPTS FOR LECTURE

1. The nurse must include several specific strategies in his or her relationship with the client who has an odd and eccentric personality in order for the interaction to be therapeutic.
2. The nurse can use the nursing process to guide the plan of care for the client with odd and eccentric personality disorders.

POWERPOINT LECTURE SLIDES

1 Effective Therapeutic Strategies
- Know yourself
  - Stressors
- Direct communication
- Clear expectations
- Clear and consistent limitations
- Remain objective

2 Nursing Process: Assessment
- Mental health assessment
- Verbal and nonverbal behavior
- Anxiety level
- Medication history

2a Nursing Process: Diagnoses
- Disturbed Thought Processes
- Impaired Social Interaction

2b Nursing Process: Evaluation
- Client interactions
- Verbal/nonverbal behavior
- Anxiety level

SUGGESTIONS FOR CLASSROOM ACTIVITIES

1. Ask students to reflect/think about what types of behaviors cause them stress. Review this idea in terms of working with clients with personality disorders.
2. Define and give examples of clear expectations and setting clear limitations.
3. Review the mental health assessment questions found in Chapter 47.
4. Discuss each phase of the nursing process in relationship to care of the client with a personality disorder. Using the nursing diagnoses from the text, identify appropriate nursing interventions for each.

SUGGESTIONS FOR CLINICAL ACTIVITIES

1. In the psychiatric clinical setting, assign students to read treatment plans for clients with odd and eccentric personality disorders. Have students identify what limits are being set for each client.
2. Assist the students to collect subjective and objective assessment data.
3. Have students create a plan of care for their assigned client.

© 2007 Pearson Education, Inc.

LEARNING OUTCOME 4

Identify the major features and client-related behaviors of dramatic and emotional personality disorders.

CONCEPTS FOR LECTURE

1. Each disorder in the dramatic and emotional personality disorder cluster has its own particular features.
2. Each dramatic and emotional personality disorder is distinguished by specific client behavior.

POWERPOINT LECTURE SLIDES

1 Features: Antisocial Personality Disorder
- Disregarding/violating others' rights
- Conduct disorder in childhood
- Disregard for societal expectations
- Impulsiveness/irresponsibility
- Show no remorse

2 Behaviors: Antisocial Personality Disorder
- Repeated illegal acts
- Deceitful
- Manipulative
- Repeated fights/assaults
- Irresponsible behaviors

1 Features: Borderline Personality Disorder
- Pattern of impulsiveness/instability
  - Interpersonal relationships
  - Self-image
  - Emotions
- Parasuicidal behavior
- Depersonalization

2 Behaviors: Borderline Personality Disorder
- Emotional vulnerability
- Self-invalidation
- Unrelenting crises
- Inhibited grieving
- Active passivity
- Apparent competence

1 Features: Histrionic Personality Disorder
- Excessive emotionality
- Excessive attention seeking

2 Behaviors: Histrionic Personality Disorder
- Inappropriately provocative sexually
- Impressionistic speech
- Strong opinions without foundation
- Exaggerated emotions
- Easily influenced by others

1 Features: Narcissistic Personality Disorder
- Pervasive grandiosity
- Need for admiration
- Lack of empathy for others
- Inflated self-importance
- Fantasy thinking

2 Behaviors: Narcissistic Personality Disorder
- Arrogant and conceited
- Exploit others
- Emotionally cold
- Quick to criticize
- Unable to take risks

© 2007 Pearson Education, Inc.

Suggestions for Classroom Activities

1. Divide the class into small workgroups. Assign each group a personality disorder from this category. Have students identify the main features and client behaviors for each disorder.
2. Compare and contrast the features and behaviors for each disorder. Give clinical examples for each behavior.
3. Distinguish between the commonly used phrase "he or she is antisocial" and the difference in that phrase when used in relationship to a true personality disorder.
4. Define histrionic. Contrast this term with the concept of someone who is "melodramatic."
5. Define narcissism. Contrast this term with the concept of someone who is merely self-absorbed.

Suggestions for Clinical Activities

1. Assign students to observe clients with dramatic and emotional personality disorders in a psychiatric clinical setting. Have students observe the clients for the behaviors associated with each disorder.
2. Ask students to predict which of the clients might need inpatient care and for what reason.
3. Help students to identify which client is at most risk for harming themselves. Others.

Learning Outcome 5

Adapt the nurse-client relationship to the client who has a dramatic and emotional personality disorder. Apply the nursing process.

Concepts for Lecture

1. The nurse must include several specific strategies in his or her relationship with the client who has a dramatic and emotional personality disorder in order for the interaction to be therapeutic.
2. The nurse can use the nursing process to guide the plan of care for the client with dramatic and emotional personality disorders.

PowerPoint Lecture Slides

1 Effective Therapeutic Strategies
- "No self-harm" contract
- Directing away from others
- No tolerance for verbal abuse
- Consistent application of rules

2 Nursing Process: Assessment
- Violence toward self
- Violence toward others
- Mental status
- Behavior

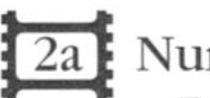

Nursing Process: Diagnoses
- Risk for Self-Directed Violence
- Risk for Other-Directed Violence

Suggestions for Classroom Activities

1. Expand on the concept of a "no self-harm" contract.
2. Discuss how disruptive clients with these types of personality disorders can become in a client care area. Review strategies in Box 51-4 to prevent this upset.
3. Review the nurse's responsibility in creating a therapeutic and safe environment for clients with any mental health disorder.
4. Describe the steps in the ACCEPTS mnemonic. Discuss when this is to be used.
5. Discuss how the five senses exercise listed in the text can assist a client who may be having thoughts of self-harm.
6. Using the nursing diagnoses given in the text, describe other nursing interventions that will assist the client to control violent behavior.

Suggestions for Clinical Activities

1. Have students develop a client teaching booklet using the ACCEPTS mnemonic. Have them participate in client teaching as applicable.
2. Instruct students to read any unit rules that are intended to prevent clients with personality disorders from disrupting the unit.
3. Invite a psychiatric nurse to speak with students about protecting themselves from clients who are potentially violent.

© 2007 Pearson Education, Inc.

Learning Outcome 6

Identify the major features and client-related behaviors of anxiety/fear-based personality disorders.

Concepts for Lecture

1. Each disorder in the anxiety/fear-based personality disorder cluster has its own particular features.
2. Each anxiety/fear-based personality disorder is distinguished by specific client behavior.

PowerPoint Lecture Slides

1 Features: Avoidant Personality Disorder
- Social shyness
- Feelings of inadequacy
- Hypersensitive to negative evaluations
- Negative self-view

2 Behaviors: Avoidant Personality Disorder
- Avoid:
  - Situation that may draw criticism
  - Making new friends
  - Social activities/new activities
- Fearful/tense manner

1 Features: Dependent Personality Disorder
- Need to be taken care of
- Fear separation/abandonment
- Poor decision maker

2 Behaviors: Dependent Personality Disorder
- Passivity
- Act incompetent
- Self-sacrificing
- Avoid decision making
- Warm and giving

1 Features: Obsessive-Compulsive Personality Disorder
- Preoccupation with
  - Orderliness
  - Perfectionism
  - Control
- Inflexible
- Overly conscientious

2 Behaviors: Obsessive-Compulsive Personality Disorder
- Abnormal attention to details, rules
- Meticulous with details
- Defer to authority
- Cannot delegate
- Miserly
- Rigid/indecisive/stubborn
- Controlled emotions

Suggestions for Classroom Activities

1. Compare and contrast the normal concept of being shy, and the shyness associated with avoidant personality disorder.
2. Give examples of the behaviors associated with avoidant personality disorders.
3. Discuss self-esteem. Ask students to share their ideas on how self-esteem is developed.
4. Compare and contrast the concepts of compromise and submissiveness.

Suggestions for Clinical Activities

1. Assign students to care for clients diagnosed with one of the anxiety/fear-based personality disorders. Have them discuss the manifestations observed.
2. Ask students to share known stereotypical behavior for clients with Obsessive-Compulsive Personality Disorder. Have them decide whether the manifestations are truly for OCD instead.

© 2007 Pearson Education, Inc.

5. Describe how a dependent personality disorder might affect a person's job performance.
6. Discuss how culture may play a part in "submissive" behavior. Have students share their thoughts about whether this constitutes a personality disorder.
7. Show clips from the movie *As Good As It Gets* to illustrate Obsessive-Compulsive Personality Disorder.
8. Compare and contrast Obsessive-Compulsive Personality Disorder and Obsessive-compulsive disorder.

3. Have students identify with which client with a disorder in this category it would be most difficult to develop a therapeutic relationship.

LEARNING OUTCOME 7

Adapt the nurse–client relationship to the client who has an anxiety/fear-based personality disorder. Apply the nursing process.

CONCEPTS FOR LECTURE

1. The nurse must include several specific strategies in his or her relationship with the client who has an anxiety/fear-based personality disorder in order for the interaction to be therapeutic.
2. The nurse can use the nursing process to guide the plan of care for the client with an anxiety/fear-based personality disorder.

POWERPOINT LECTURE SLIDES

1 Effective Therapeutic Strategies
- Use calm approach
- Give client choices regarding care
- Establish a trusting relationship

2 Nursing Process: Assessment
- Functional ability
- Mental status
- Interpersonal relationships

2a Nursing Process: Diagnosis/Evaluation
- Diagnosis
  - Anxiety

2b Nursing Process: Evaluation
- Adequate self-esteem
- Appropriate interactions with others
- Positive statements about self
- Taking initiative to solve problems

SUGGESTIONS FOR CLASSROOM ACTIVITIES

1. Discuss the strategies nurses can use to develop a calm approach to the client in a psychiatric care area.
2. Describe the types of choices about care that can be reasonably given to clients.
3. Ask students to share their ideas on how to assess a client for functional ability.
4. Review, if necessary, the mental status exam questions.
5. Using the nursing diagnosis of anxiety, describe specific nursing interventions that may help alleviate this problem.
6. Discuss how to evaluate a client's self-esteem.

SUGGESTIONS FOR CLINICAL ACTIVITIES

1. Assign students to care for a client with one of the anxiety/fear-based personality disorders. Have students discuss how they have tailored their nurse–client relationship based on the client diagnosis.
2. Assign students to a group therapy session. Have students report their observations of client reactions to suggested treatment.
3. Have students share their ideas about how Obsessive-Compulsive Personality disorder would disrupt a client's ability to function.

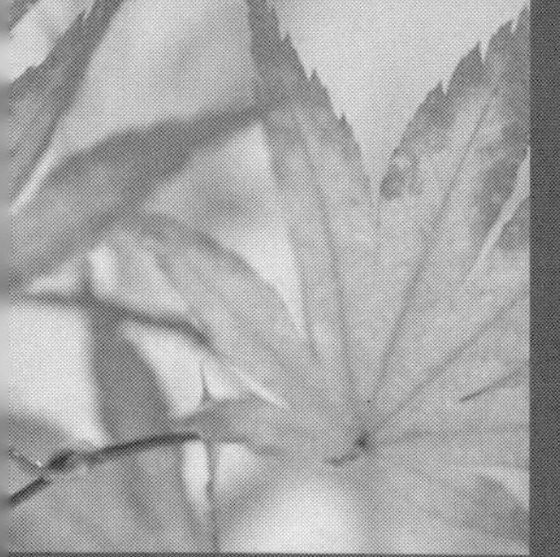

CHAPTER 52
CARING FOR CLIENTS WITH SUBSTANCE ABUSE OR DEPENDENCY

RESOURCE LIBRARY

IMAGE LIBRARY

Figure 52-1 Fatal events in which alcohol is a factor.
Figure 52-2 Physiologic effects of alcoholism.
Figure 52-3 Common sources of caffeine, with doses per serving.

LEARNING OUTCOME 1

Explain substance abuse, substance dependency, tolerance, and withdrawal.

CONCEPTS FOR LECTURE

1. The consequences of substance abuse are far reaching in terms of cost and effect on the overall health of the U.S. population.
2. Person's who abuse certain substances continue the behavior despite adverse outcomes that occur in social, physical, and legal aspects of their lives.
3. Dependency on certain substances significantly impairs daily functioning and physical health.
4. The pathophysiologic changes associated with tolerance are discussed in relationship to alcohol abuse and involve the interrelated concepts of increased CNS self-stimulation and CNS depression.
5. The symptoms of withdrawal (also discussed within the context of alcohol abuse) occur due to the overstimulation of the CNS in conjunction with the loss of the depressive effects of alcohol.

POWERPOINT LECTURE SLIDES

1 Substance Abuse
- Affects 20% of the U.S. population
- Network of interrelated social effects
- High financial cost

1a Substance Abuse
- Maladaptive behavior pattern
- Involves use of certain substances
- Continued despite bad outcomes

2 Manifestation of Substance Abuse
- Unable to fulfill role obligations
- Placing self in physical danger
- Legal issues
- Disruption in social/interpersonal relationships

2a Commonly Abused Substances
- Alcohol
- Opioids
- Sedatives, hypnotics, and anxiolytics
- Cocaine
- Amphetamines and similar drugs
- Hallucinogens
- Phencyclidine (PCP) and similar drugs
- Inhalants
- Cannabis
- Caffeine
- Nicotine

3 Substance Dependency
- More severe than abuse
- Significant impairment
  - Social
  - Physical
  - Legal

3a Manifestations of Dependency
- Tolerance/withdrawal syndrome
- High amounts/longer period
- Desire to control or stop

PowerPoint Lecture Slides *continued*

- Occupies time
- Affects social interactions
- Ignoring physical/psychologic problems

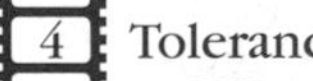

4 Tolerance

- CNS suppression
- Increased CNS activity to compensate
- Higher amount of substance
- *Must* use substance to avoid withdrawal symptoms

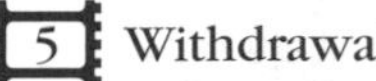

5 Withdrawal

- Overstimulated CNS
- Sudden cessation of alcohol use
- Loss of depressant effects
- Symptoms related to stimulated CNS

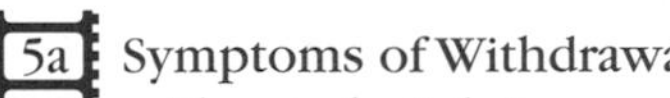

5a Symptoms of Withdrawal

- Elevated vital signs
- Anxiety
- Tremors/diaphoresis
- GI
- Ataxia/disorientation

5b Delirium tremens

- Severe alcohol withdrawal
  - Confusion
  - Delusions/hallucinations
- Medical emergency

Suggestions for Classroom Activities

1. Discuss the economic and other long-term effects of substance abuse. Include statistics related to morbidity and mortality.
2. Define substance abuse. Include a discussion of the abuse of illegal substances.
3. Describe in detail the manifestations of substance abuse, using clinical examples.
4. Ask students to list the most commonly abused substances. Compare students' beliefs with the DSM-IV list in the text.
5. Compare and contrast substance abuse and dependency.
6. Explain the relationship between tolerance and withdrawal.

Suggestions for Clinical Activities

1. Assign students to care for clients being treated for substance abuse. Have students identify the substance used and the client history related to the abuse.
2. Assist students to assess the client who has abused alcohol for the presence of long-term physical effects.
3. If the experience is available, assign students to observe a client being treated for delirium tremens in the intensive care unit. Have students report on their observations. Generate a discussion about the serious nature of this problem related to alcohol withdrawal.

Learning Outcome 2

Collect information from clients who are using commonly abused drugs.

Concepts for Lecture

1. Several principles guide the collection of subjective data by the nurse from clients with substance abuse problems.

PowerPoint Lecture Slides

1 Collecting Information: Substance Abuse

- Assess every client
- Use open-ended questions
- Answers skewed by guilt/denial
- Nonjudgmental/accepting

CONCEPTS FOR LECTURE *continued*

2. Subjective data related to substance abuse problems can be gathered through traditional admission nursing assessment as well as through the use of screening tools.
3. The objective data found in the client with a substance abuse problem could be symptoms reflective of the substance being abused or symptoms related to more serious consequences of that abuse.

POWERPOINT LECTURE SLIDES *continued*

2 Subjective Data: Substance Abuse
- Box 52-4

2a Subjective Data: Alcohol Abuse
- Acronym
  - CAGE
- Cut down
- Annoyed
- Guilty
- Eye-opener

3 Objective Data: Alcohol Abuse
- Intoxication
- Euphoria
- Decreased mental concentration
- Ataxia
- Emotional lability

3a Objective Data: Alcohol Abuse
- Long-term effects
  - Pancreatitis
  - Hepatitis
  - Cardiomyopathy
  - Korsakoff's syndrome
  - Wernicke's syndrome

3b Objective Data: Opiate Abuse
- Euphoria
- Loss of inhibition
- Reduced cognition/impaired judgment
- Decreased libido
- Nausea/constipation

3c Objective Data: Opioid Toxicity
- Pinpoint pupils
- Respiratory depression
- Seizures/coma
- Hypoxia/respiratory arrest

3d Objective Data: CNS Stimulant Abuse
- Euphoria/elation/energy
- Anorexia
- Weight loss
- Elevated vital signs
- Grandiosity

3e Objective Data: Steroid Abuse
- Severe acne
- Tremors
- Mood swings/paranoia
- Delusions/aggression
- Gender-related symptoms

SUGGESTIONS FOR CLASSROOM ACTIVITIES

1. Describe the techniques used by the nurse to obtain subjective assessment data from a client who is suspected of substance abuse. Give examples of open-ended versus "yes/no" questions.

SUGGESTIONS FOR CLINICAL ACTIVITIES

1. Assign students to care for the client with a substance abuse problem. Role model the techniques to be used when gathering subjective data. Have students practice open-ended questions with their peers.

© 2007 Pearson Education, Inc.

2. Generate a discussion about the societal judgments placed on persons who abuse certain substances.
3. Discuss in detail the items in the acronym "CAGE" as it applies to screening for alcohol abuse.
4. Divide students into small workgroups. Assign one commonly abused substance to each group. Have students report on the objective data that might be seen in the client with this particular problem. Include symptoms of abuse as well as symptoms of overdose/toxicity.
5. Compare and contrast the objective data associated with abuse versus those associated with severe abuse/toxicity/withdrawal.

2. If the experience is available, have students attend an Alcoholic's Anonymous meeting in either an outpatient or inpatient setting. Have students discuss any subjective "symptoms" of alcohol abuse shared by participants.
3. If students care for clients who abuse different substances, have them compare and contrast their assessment findings in terms of objective data.
4. In the traditional medical/surgical clinical rotation, assign students to care for clients who have long-term health issues related to alcohol abuse, for example, cirrhosis or cardiomyopathy.

LEARNING OUTCOME 3

Identify adverse effects caused by interactions between commonly abused substances and medications used in surgery or emergency care.

CONCEPTS FOR LECTURE

1. Medications that are commonly administered in the emergency and surgical areas can cause potentially harmful drug interactions in the client who has a substance abuse problem.
2. It is critical for the nurse to understand the concepts of additive effect and cross-tolerance.

POWERPOINT LECTURE SLIDES

1 Drug Interactions and Substance Abuse
- Area for concern
  - Emergency room
  - Surgery

2 Additive Effect: CNS Depression
- Polysubstance abuse
- Alcohol plus other CNS depressants
  - Narcotic analgesics
  - Sedatives/sleep agents
  - Benzodiazepines
  - Anesthetics

2a Cross-Tolerance in Substance Abuse
- Dependence leads to tolerance
  - Fewer CNS effects with higher doses
- Issues
  - Analgesia
  - Pain control

SUGGESTIONS FOR CLASSROOM ACTIVITIES

1. Describe the areas in which it is critical for the nurse to assess for substance abuse.
2. Discuss the role of the nurse in terms of assessing for substance abuse and promoting client safety.
3. Define the concept of "additive effect." Give examples of medications in different classes that will cause an additive effect.
4. Describe how cross-tolerance can lead to poor pain control in the client with a substance abuse problem.
5. Generate a discussion with students about common myths held by health care workers about using high doses of analgesics in order to control pain in the client with a substance abuse problem. Link this discussion to the concept of building tolerance.

SUGGESTIONS FOR CLINICAL ACTIVITIES

1. Assign students to care for the client with a substance abuse problem. This client is often admitted to the general medical/surgical unit for a condition unrelated to the abuse. Have students assess the client's medication list for potential drug/substance interactions.
2. Invite a health care member with expertise in the area of pain control to speak with the students about the myths associated with high-dose analgesia required by the client with a substance abuse problem.
3. Have students share what they have observed on the med/surg unit in terms of nursing attitudes toward clients with substance abuse problems and providing adequate analgesia. (listen for judgmental phrases such as "druggie" or "drug seeking") Generate a discussion about the theory of cross-tolerance and providing analgesia in a nonjudgmental manner.

© 2007 Pearson Education, Inc.

LEARNING OUTCOME 4

Provide appropriate nursing interventions for a client in drug or alcohol withdrawal.

CONCEPTS FOR LECTURE

1. Withdrawal from drug or alcohol use can lead to life-threatening symptoms.
2. Nursing interventions for the client experiencing withdrawal are aimed at supporting vital functions and promoting client safety.

POWERPOINT LECTURE SLIDES

Withdrawal: Nursing Interventions

- Supporting vital functions
  - Vital signs
- Assess for delirium tremens
  - Cognitive changes
- Promote client safety
- Provide symptom relief
- Pharmacotherapy

SUGGESTIONS FOR CLASSROOM ACTIVITIES

1. Describe the varying degrees of withdrawal a client may experience related to detoxification. Review the concept that the development of delirium tremens is considered to be a medical emergency.
2. Ask students to share their ideas on how the nurse keeps the patient in withdrawal safe. Discuss the use of restraints: physical and chemical.
3. Give a more detailed list of symptoms experienced by the client in withdrawal and the nursing interventions for each. For example, GI disturbances, anxiety, or ataxia.
4. Discuss pharmacologic management of the client in withdrawal.

SUGGESTIONS FOR CLINICAL ACTIVITIES

1. If available, assign students to the intensive care unit. Have them observe the care of the client experiencing detoxification. Ask students to share their observations with their peers in a postconference.
2. Generate a discussion with students about the stigma associated with the withdrawal process. Have students share what they have observed in terms of nursing attitudes.
3. Compare and contrast the care of the client experiencing a "mild" withdrawal versus a client experiencing delirium tremens.

LEARNING OUTCOME 5

Apply the nursing process to clients experiencing substance abuse or dependency. Include appropriate nursing interventions for the client experiencing withdrawal.

CONCEPTS FOR LECTURE

1. The nursing process can be used to develop an individualized plan of care for the client with a substance abuse or substance dependency problem.
2. The nursing interventions for the client with a substance abuse/dependency problem are aimed at ensuring client safety.

POWERPOINT LECTURE SLIDES

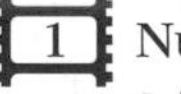

Nursing Process: Assessment

- Substance used
- Pattern of use
- Subjective data
- Objective data

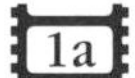

Nursing Process: Diagnoses

- Risk for Injury
- Deficient Knowledge
- Ineffective Coping
- Compromised/Disabled Family Coping
- Powerlessness
- Social Isolation

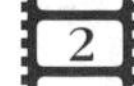

Nursing Process: Implementation

- Monitoring vital signs
- Promoting nutrition
- Decreasing environmental stimuli
- Client/family education
- Promoting safety r/t withdrawal

© 2007 Pearson Education, Inc.

PowerPoint Lecture Slides *continued*

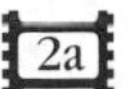 Nursing Process: Evaluation
- Alternative to substance use
- Effective coping mechanisms
- Identify resources/peer support
- Verbalize feelings

Suggestions for Classroom Activities

1. Review the subjective and objective data to be assessed by the nurse in the client with a substance abuse problem. Have students list the objective data indicative of acute withdrawal. Have students list what data might necessitate an inpatient admission.
2. Discuss other potential nursing diagnoses for the client who abuses certain substances found in the text and not on the PowerPoint slide. Ask students if any other diagnoses might apply.
3. Describe in detail how the various nursing interventions are to be carried out in both the acute-care and outpatient settings. Compare and contrast the two settings. For example, ask students how the nurse would decrease environmental stimuli in the hospital. In the home.

Suggestions for Clinical Activities

1. Using the nursing diagnoses suggested in the text, have students identify priorities in terms of developing a plan of care for the client with a substance abuse/dependency problem.
2. Have students share their thoughts about how difficult the intervention of "decreasing environmental stimuli" might be in the ICU setting. On the med/surg unit? In the home?
3. Assign students to develop a list of community resources for the client with substance abuse/dependency issues.
4. Seek permission for students to attend a meeting of a peer support group for persons with substance abuse problems.

© 2007 Pearson Education, Inc.

NCLEX-PN® Test Questions

The following questions are similar to those that may appear on the NCLEX-RN® exam. Some questions may have more than one correct response. During this review, you should select the one best response.

Chapter 1

1.1 A client is being discharged and needs instructions on wound care. When planning to teach the client, the nurse should: a. identify the client's learning needs and learning ability. b. identify the client's learning needs and advise him what to do. c. identify the client's problems and make the appropriate referral. d. provide pamphlets or videotapes for ongoing learning.	Answer: a Rationale: To provide the most appropriate teaching, the nurse first needs to identify what the client needs to know and determine the client's educational level and learning ability. Comprehension Implementation Health Promotion: Prevention and/or Early Detection of Health Problems
1.2 A client is requesting a second opinion. The nurse who supports and promotes the client's rights is acting as the client's: a. teacher. b. adviser. c. supporter. d. advocate.	Answer: d Rationale: The nurse's role as client advocate involves actively promoting clients' rights to make decisions and choices. Comprehension Assessment Safe, Effective Care Environment: Coordinated Care Health Promotion: Prevention and/or Early Detection of Health Problems
1.3 The client tells the nurse she has been smoking one pack of cigarettes a day for the past 20 years. The nurse recognizes this is what part of the nursing process? a. assessment b. planning c. implementation d. evaluation	Answer: a Rationale: Data collection occurs during the assessment phase; the information can be obtained during the initial assessment as well as during ongoing assessment. Knowledge Assessment Health Promotion: Prevention and/or Early Detection of Health Problems
1.4 During the assessment step of the nursing process, the nurse collects subjective and objective data. The nurse uses the information to identify: a. medical diagnoses. b. actual or potential problems. c. client's response to illness. d. need for community support groups.	Answer: b Rationale: Information obtained during the assessment step is used in planning and implementing nursing care, based on the problems identified from the assessment data. Analysis Planning Health Promotion: Prevention and/or Early Detection of Health Problem
1.5 The nurse performs daily, routine equipment checks to detect possible malfunction. This is part of the nurse's role in the: a. nursing process. b. quality assurance plan. c. care management. d. assessment plan.	Answer: b Rationale: Quality of care is evaluated through documentation reviews, interviews and surveys, observation and equipment checks. Application Implementation Health Promotion: Prevention and/or Early Detection of Health Problems
1.6 The nurse is developing a nursing diagnosis for a client who has pneumonia. The nurse recognizes the diagnosis describes an actual or potential problem that: a. the nurse can treat independently.	Answer: a Rationale: Nursing diagnoses reflect client problems that the nurse can treat independently. Application Planning Safe, Effective Care Environment: Coordinated Care

© 2007 Pearson Education, Inc.

b. the nurse can treat with a physician's order. c. requires physician's intervention. d. relates to the clients' primary diagnosis.	
1.7 After administering pain medication, the nurse returns to check the client's level of comfort. This stage of the nursing process is known as: a. assessment. b. planning. c. implementation. d. evaluation.	Answer: d Rationale: In the evaluation step the nurse determines if the interventions were effective. Analysis/Diagnosis Evaluation Safe, Effective Care Environment: Coordinated Care
1.8 A client has lost 10 pounds related to nausea and vomiting. The nurse identifies an appropriate expected outcome: The client will: a. gain weight. b. gain 2 pounds within 1 week. c. not lose weight. d. gain 10 pounds in 2 days.	Answer: b Rationale: Expected outcomes should reflect a goal that is client centered, realistic, and measurable. Answers a and c are not measurable; d is not realistic. Analysis/Diagnosis Planning Physiological Integrity: Physiological Adaptation
1.9 A problem-solving process that requires empathy, knowledge, divergent thinking, discipline, and creativity is known as: a. critical thinking. b. nursing process. c. framework for nurses. d. care management.	Answer: a Rationale: Critical thinking involves self-directed thinking, combining the nurse's cognitive skills as well as attitude, experience, empathy, and discipline. Comprehension Analysis/Diagnosis Safe, Effective Care Environment: Coordinated Care
1.10 At the end of the shift, the nurse is ready to leave but has not been relieved by the oncoming shift nurse. The nurse's responsibility to provide care for clients is part of the nurse's: a. Code of Ethics. b. nursing process. c. critical thinking. d. quality assurance.	Answer: a Rationale: The Code of Ethics guides the behavior of nurses. The nurse's primary commitment is to the client, ensuring he or she receives safe, competent, and continual care. Comprehension Implementation Safe, Effective Care Environment: Coordinated Care

CHAPTER 2

2.1 According to Havighurst, the developmental tasks that describe adults as learning to live with a mate, have children, and hold a job are found in which of the following stages? a. young adult (18–35 years of age) b. middle adult (36–60 years of age) c. older adult (over 60 years of age) d. productive adult (18–60 years of age)	Answer: a Rationale: These tasks occur predominantly in the young adult age group. Knowledge Assessment Health Promotion: Growth and Development
2.2 When caring for the middle age adult the nurse recognizes a major risk factor is: a. cigarette smoking. b. multiple sex partners. c. decreased physical activity. d. obesity.	Answer: c Rationale: Due to a decrease in basal metabolic rate and often activity level as well, the middle adult is at risk for weight gain and obesity. Comprehension Integrative process: Assessment Test plan: Health Promotion: Prevention and/or Early Detection of Health Problems

2.3 Because of the physiologic changes in the gastrointestinal system, the nurse should encourage the older adult to consume a diet high in: a. Na. b. fiber. c. carbohydrates. d. calories.	Answer: b Rationale: A decrease in peristalsis can lead to constipation; increasing fiber in the diet will help to combat this. Comprehension Planning Health Promotion: Growth and Development
2.4 Women in the middle adult age group are at risk for cancer of the breast and reproductive organs. The nurse can suggest the following in health promotion teaching: a. "You need to contact your physician about mammography." b. "If there is not a history of cancer in the women of your family, you need not be concerned." c. "An annual physical exam is important to detect early signs and symptoms of cancer." d. "Self-breast exam monthly and an annual Pap smear are necessary for early detection of cancer."	Answer: d Rationale: This option gives the most specific recommendations for tests that should be done to detect cancer. The other options provide more general information. Application Implementation Health Promotion: Prevention and/or Early Detection of Health Problems
2.5 When teaching the old-old adult (over age 85) who has been diagnosed with a new illness, the nurse recognizes this age group: a. needs client teaching at a slower pace, with visual aids and repetition. b. does not profit from patient teaching. c. learns at the same rate as young-old adults. d. is generally cognitively impaired and unable to learn new information.	Answer: a Rationale: Due to neurovascular and sensory losses, older adults need adjustment in teaching methods, although they still have the ability to learn. Application Planning Health Promotion: Growth and Development
2.6 When planning care for elderly clients in long-term care facilities, the nurse gives highest priority to: a. ensuring that they consume at least 1,200 calories a day. b. providing regular periods of exercise daily. c. maintaining a safe environment. d. providing opportunities for social interactions.	Answer: c Rationale: Although all the options are important, maintenance of a safe environment is always of highest priority. Application Implementation Safe, Effective Care Environment: Safety and Infection Control
2.7 The nurse visits an elderly client who lives alone, is not eating well, and has very little food available in the home. The nurse may also want to assess the client's: a. ability to do her own grocery shopping. b. access to local restaurants. c. number of visits by family. d. availability of local grocery stores.	Answer: a Rationale: Assessing the client's ability to obtain food would be essential to determine why the client isn't eating and has little food available. Analysis Assessment Health Promotion: Prevention and/or Early Detection of Health Problems

© 2007 Pearson Education, Inc.

2.8 A client is experiencing a significant change from his normal health. In the first stage of an acute illness, the nurse can expect the client to report having: a. bleeding. b. cough. c. fever. d. pain.	Answer: d Rationale: Pain is the most frequently reported manifestation of acute illnesses. Analysis Assessment Physiological Integrity: Physiological Adaptation
2.9 When caring for a client with a chronic illness, the nurse is aware the client will have: a. impaired function. b. persistent pain. c. reversible conditions. d. severe symptoms.	Answer: a Rationale: Chronic illness is characterized by impaired functioning of one or more body systems. Persistent pain and severity of symptoms vary with the client and condition. Chronic conditions are not reversible. Comprehension Assessment Physiological Integrity: Physiological Adaptation
2.10 The nurse is planning interventions beneficial to clients with chronic illness. The nurse should focus on: a. pain management. b. education to promote independent functioning. c. securing assistance from family members. d. assisting the client to accept her illness.	Answer: b Rationale: Nursing interventions should focus on promoting independence, reducing health care costs, and improving quality of life. Application Intervention Safe, Effective Care Environment: Coordinated Care

CHAPTER 3

3.1 The nurse is planning to teach an older client how to check her blood sugar. To promote short-term memory activity, the nurse should: a. have the client repeat the steps of the procedure back to the nurse. b. ensure environment is free of distracting stimuli. c. review the procedure with client on several occasions. d. limit teaching session to 5 to 10 minutes in length.	Answer: c Rationale: Repetitive presentations promote short memory retention. All of the other options are helpful to the learning process, but c is the best option. Application Planning Health Promotion and Maintenance; Growth and Development
3.2 When doing a physical assessment of an old-old client, the nurse could expect to see which of the following? a. dilated pupils b. thin and brittle nails c. an increase in tear production d. a decrease in pubic hair	Answer: d Rationale: Age-related physical changes include decreased scalp, axillary, and pubic hair. Pupils are smaller. Nails often become thick and brittle. Tear production decreases. Comprehension Assessment Health Promotion and Maintenance; Growth and Development
3.3 A client who was previously independent with bathing is hospitalized for a possible bowel obstruction. When the client asks the nurse for help with bathing the nurse recognizes the client's need to: a. revert to a more dependent stage of development. b. adjust for disease symptoms by restricting activity. c. use the physical ailment to solicit more attention for himself. d. have more physical contact with another human being.	Answer: b Rationale: Restriction of activity allows the elder client to adapt to an acute illness or change in routine. Restriction of activity may be misinterpreted as dependent or attention-seeking behavior. Application Evaluation Health Promotion and Maintenance; Growth and Development

3.4 An elder client is being prepared for transfer to a long-term care facility and expresses sorrow at not being able to return to his own home. The nurse can best help the client cope with this change by: a. explaining why it is necessary to move to the new facility. b. explaining why it would be unsafe to remain in his own home. c. showing him pictures of the new facility. d. asking him to tell you about significant events in his life.	Answer: d Rationale: Life review or reminiscence can be used therapeutically to facilitate coping with change and allows the older adult to maintain/achieve ego integrity. The other options can be used as the client moves into the adjustment phase. Application Planning Health Promotion and Maintenance: Growth and Development
3.5 An elderly client is seen in the clinic. When reviewing his health care maintenance, the nurse recommends that the client should have: a. a digital rectal examination for prostate enlargement every 3 months. b. a blood test for prostate specific antigen (PSA) yearly. c. a monthly screening for fecal occult blood. d. An eye examination every 2 years.	Answer: b Rationale: A digital rectal exam and PSA blood test should be done yearly in males over 65 years of age. Screening for fecal occult blood is indicated yearly. Application Implementation Health Promotion and Maintenance: Prevention and Early Detection of Health Problems
3.6 The nurse is teaching an elder client who is recovering from a prolonged illness about a new medication regimen. The most appropriate teaching aid would be: a. assist client with making a written list of medication times. b. instruct a family member on the times of the new medications. c. encourage the client to ask frequent questions. d. have the client repeat the instructions back to you.	Answer: a Rationale: Since short-term memory loss frequently occurs in the elderly, written lists and use of calendars is helpful in assisting elderly clients with recall of information. Instructing family members doesn't involve the client, although they should have a copy of the list as well. Options c and d are helpful techniques, but the client may still forget the instructions. Application Implementation Health Promotion and Maintenance: Prevention and Early Detection of Health Problems.
3.7 The nurse is assisting in a teaching program for clients in a senior citizen center. The nurse informs the clients that healthy behaviors in the older adult include: a. having a pneumonia immunization if over age 65. b. consuming at least 2000 mg of calcium daily. c. having a yearly tetanus immunization. d. engaging in 60 minutes of aerobic exercise daily.	Answer: a Rationale: It is recommended that people over age 65 or with chronic illness have a pneumonia vaccine. The recommended calcium intake is 1200 mg. Tetanus immunizations are recommended every 10 years. Thirty to 60 minutes of moderately strenuous, but aerobic activity is not necessarily recommended. Application Implementation Health Promotion and Maintenance: Prevention and Early Detection of Health Problems
3.8 A client is admitted with complaints of right upper quadrant pain, nausea, and vomiting. The nurse recognizes these symptoms correlate with which of the following physical changes in the elder adult? a. a greater risk to develop gallstones b. an increased gag reflex c. decreased sense of smell d. increased stomach emptying	Answer: a Rationale: Intestinal motility and liver function decrease, putting elderly at greater risk for gallstone formation. The gag reflex and stomach emptying decrease. Sense of smell is decreased, but would not contribute to the listed symptoms. Analysis Assessment Health Promotion and Maintenance: Growth and Development

© 2007 Pearson Education, Inc.

3.9 When developing a care plan for the older adult the nurse recognizes that age-related physical changes indicate: a. a need for greater analgesic since the pain threshold decreases. b. strong odors are more offensive since the sense of smell is increased. c. night lights should be available since night vision is decreased. d. bathing should be done daily since sebum production is increased.	Answer: c Rationale: Pupils are smaller, therefore reducing night vision. The pain threshold and sense of smell both increase. Sebaceous gland activity decreases, resulting in dry skin. Application Planning Health Promotion and Maintenance: Growth and Development
3.10 When caring for a client in a long-term care facility, the nurse facilitates reminiscing by: a. encouraging client to focus on her current situation. b. reminding client what her current strengths are. c. asking client to tell about her childhood. d. helping client to remember what activities she did in the past week.	Answer: c Rationale: Reminiscing involves recall of past events that are significant to the individual. Remembrance of recent activities would only involve recall of short-term memory. Application Implementation Health Promotion and Maintenance: Growth and Development

CHAPTER 4

4.1 A nurse is planning to recommend a community clinic to a client. The nurse will need to consider the: a. socioeconomic status of the client. b. ethnicity of the client. c. gender of the client. d. availability of transportation.	Answer: d Rationale: The nurse will need to determine if the client has access to the community clinic. The other options will not affect the client's use of the clinic. Analysis Assessment Safe, Effective Care Environment: Coordinated Care
4.2 The nurse is caring for an elderly person with a fractured hip who lives alone. The client may require which of the following types of care after discharge from the hospital? a. transitional care b. nursing home care c. intermediate care d. retirement center	Answer: a Rationale: Before returning to their home independently, clients often need a skilled nursing care facility while transitioning from the acute care setting to home. Comprehension Planning Safe, Effective Care Environment: Coordinated Care
4.3 The nurse understands that home health care is provided to clients who are: a. chronically ill, disabled, or recuperating. b. acutely ill. c. unable to afford hospitalization. d. not covered by medical insurance.	Answer: a Rationale: Home health care is provided to the chronically ill, those with disabilities, or clients recovering from an acute illness. Acutely ill clients need to be in an inpatient facility. Insurance and payment options may impact the type and/or length of care provided in the home. Knowledge Implementation Safe, Effective Care Environment: Coordinated Care
4.4 A client who is scheduled to have home health services asks the nurse who will come to see her in her home. The nurse explains home health care is provided by: a. registered nurses only. b. a multidisciplinary team of providers. c. home health aides. d. volunteers.	Answer: b Rationale: Home health care may involve a variety of services, including nursing, social services, therapists, and volunteers. Assessment Comprehension Safe, Effective Care Environment: Coordinated Care

4.5 A 75-year-old client expresses concern over not being eligible for home health visits. The nurse explains to the client that the elderly are entitled to home care under which of the following legislation? a. diagnosis-related groups (DRGs) b. Omnibus Reconciliation Act c. Medicaid Act d. Medicare Act	Answer: d Rationale: Medicare legislation entitles the elderly to home care services. DRGs and Medicaid have affected home health services, but came into effect after Medicare. Assessment Comprehension Safe, Effective Environment: Coordinated Care
4.6 The nurse is caring for a client in the acute care setting who will need home care. The client will initially need to have: a. physician's order and treatment plan. b. nursing orders and care plan. c. a referral source and recommendation. d. approval by Medicare for payment.	Answer: a Rationale: Home care cannot begin without physician orders and a physician-approved treatment plan. Options b and c become a part of the treatment plan. Home care reimbursement may include Medicare, Medicaid, private insurance, and self-pay. Comprehension Assessment Safe, Effective Care Environment: Coordinated Care
4.7 When providing care to a client in the home setting, the nurse understands reimbursement sources such as Medicare will approve payment only on: a. medications ordered by the physician. b. interventions provided by licensed nurses. c. interventions documented on the progress notes. d. interventions identified on the treatment plan.	Answer: d Rationale: The nurse must confirm that all interventions are included in the physician's treatment plan. Payment will not be made if the intervention is not part of the treatment plan. Assessment Comprehension Safe, Effective Care Environment: Coordinated Care
4.8 The nurse providing home care is a guest in the client's home and must: a. make home visits only when it is convenient for the client. b. respect boundaries and maintain confidentiality. c. obtain written consent from family members to make visits. d. take direction from the client for interventions.	Answer: b Rationale: Patient confidentiality and respect for property are part of a home health agency's bill of rights. Visit times are arranged between the nurse and the family. The client gives written consent and interventions are based on the physician's treatment plan. Application Implementation Safe, Effective Care Environment: Coordinated Care
4.9 Infection control can present a challenge to the home care nurse, especially with clients who have open wounds. Important client teaching by the nurse must include: a. avoiding contact with the open wound. b. prohibiting family members to change dressings. c. hand washing and proper disposal of waste. d. documentation of wound care procedures.	Answer: c Rationale: Effective hand washing and waste disposal are of paramount importance to infection control. Clients may have contact with their own wounds and family members are taught to do the dressing changes. Documentation is important, but a not a part of infection control Application Implementation Physiological Integrity: Reduction of Risk Potential

© 2007 Pearson Education, Inc.

4.10 The rehabilitation nurse performs a primary assessment in order to determine the client's: a. medical condition. b. insurance provider. c. level of function. d. nutritional status.	Answer: c Rationale: To develop an individualized plan of care, the nurse must first determine the client's level of physical function. The medical condition and insurance provider will already be documented. Nutritional assessment will be determined after the primary assessment. Analysis Assessment Physiological Integrity: Physiological Adaptation

CHAPTER 5

5.1 During the assessment the client tells the nurse he has pain in the left knee. This information is considered: a. objective data. b. subjective data. c. nonrelevant data. d. historical data.	Answer: b Rationale: Subjective data is information only the client can describe. Objective data is observable and measurable. A complaint of pain is also relevant and current data. Comprehension Assessment Physiological Integrity: Physiological Adaptation
5.2 When collecting assessment data on a client, the nurse can obtain data from a secondary source if: a. the client is under 21 years of age. b. the client is over 65 years of age. c. the client refuses care. d. the client is unable to speak English.	Answer: d Rationale: When the client does not speak the same language as the nurse, information may need to be obtained from another source; a translator may also assist. Comprehension Assessment Health Promotion: Prevention and/or Early Detection of Health Problems
5.3 During an assessment the client complains of back pain. It is important for the nurse to determine: a. the exact cause of the pain. b. the length of time the client has experienced the pain. c. the location on the back and severity of the pain. d. the client's exercise schedule.	Answer: c Rationale: The client's complaint of pain is general in nature and warrants further clarification. The other options can be explored when more specific information about the pain has been determined. Analysis Assessment Physiological Integrity: Physiological Adaptation
5.4 When assessing the client, the nurse uses percussion to determine: a. equal symmetry of chest expansion. b. heart sounds. c. presence of gas in the intestines. d. presence of fluid in the lungs.	Answer: c Rationale: Percussion is most often used to assess abdominal structures and check for tympany or dullness. Options b and d would be assessed through auscultation. Option a involves inspection. Comprehension Assessment Health Promotion: Prevention and/or Early Detection of Health Problems
5.5 In the general survey, the nurse can obtain an indication of the client's general health by inspecting the: a. general environment. b. respiration rate. c. skin, hair, and nails. d. range of motion of the extremities.	Answer: c Rationale: The integumentary system often provides a general indication of overall health. The general environment does not reflect the client's health. Respiration and range of motion are more specific to one body system. Comprehension Assessment Health Promotion: Prevention and/or Early Detection of Health Problems
5.6 The nurse observes the client has cyanosis, a blue or gray discoloration of the skin, and recognizes this is seen in clients with decreased: a. oxygen levels. b. activity. c. heart sounds. d. lung sounds.	Answer: a Rationale: Cyanosis is a result of decreased levels of oxygen in the blood. Comprehension Assessment Health Promotion: Prevention and/or Early Detection of Health Problems

5.7 On assessment the nurse observes small red spots caused by capillary bleeding and documents the client has: a. erythema. b. petechiae. c. lesions. d. rash.	Answer: b Rationale: The spots describe petechiae. Erythema is a redness of the skin. Lesions involve disruption of the skin surface and rashes occur secondary to irritation or allergic reactions. Comprehension Assessment Health Promotion: Prevention and/or Early Detection of Health Problems
5.8 The nurse determines a client's skin turgor is nonelastic and the skin folds remain elevated. The nurse recognizes a cause of this is: a. edema. b. cold temperature. c. dehydration. d. lesions.	Answer: c Rationale: A lack of water as seen with dehydration decreases the fullness and elasticity of the skin. Excess fluid would cause edema. Temperature and lesions usually do not affect skin turgor. Analysis Assessment Physiological Integrity: Physiological Adaptation
5.9 A client is able to breathe more easily in an upright position. The nurse reports the client is experiencing: a. apnea. b. orthopnea. c. dyspnea. d. eupnea.	Answer: b Rationale: Orthopnea is shortness of breath in a reclining position that is relieved by sitting upright. Apnea involves periods of no breathing. Dyspnea is difficulty breathing. Eupnea is normal breathing. Comprehension Assessment Health Promotion: Care and Comfort
5.10 A client's mental status is evaluated by the nurse by determining the client's: a. ability to communicate. b. awareness about their surroundings. c. orientation and level of consciousness. d. ability to remember recent and past events.	Answer: c Rationale: Mental status is determined by checking both level of awareness (orientation) and client's state of arousal, or level of consciousness. The other options only measure a portion of the client's mental status. Comprehension Assessment Health Promotion: Prevention and/or Early Detection of Health Problems

CHAPTER 6

6.1 The nurse brings A.M. medications to a client who has just eaten breakfast, noticing the client has just consumed 8 ounces of milk. Which of the following medications should the nurse hold? a. aspirin b. calcium channel blocker c. diuretic d. tetracycline antibiotic	Answer: d Rationale: The calcium in antacids and dairy products reduces the absorption of tetracyclines. Application Implementation Physiological Integrity: Pharmacological and Parenteral Therapies
6.2 A client is being discharged on warfarin (Coumadin), an anticoagulant. To avoid food-drug interactions, the nurse instructs the client to restrict which of the following foods? a. green leafy vegetables b. citrus foods c. dairy products d. whole grains	Answer: a Rationale: The vitamin K found in green leafy vegetables can interfere with the clotting cascade and prolong bleeding time, thereby enhancing the anticoagulant effect. Application Implementation Physiological Integrity: Pharmacological and Parenteral Therapies
6.3 The nurse administers a drug with a half-life of 12 hours. To maintain a steady state of the drug, the nurse recognizes the medication will need to be administered every: a. 4 hours. b. 6 hours. c. 12 hours. d. 24 hours.	Answer: c Rationale: After 12 hours 50% of the drug will have been metabolized and will need to be given again in order to maintain a steady blood level of drug. Comprehension Planning Physiological Integrity: Pharmacological and Parenteral Therapies

 © 2007 Pearson Education, Inc.

6.4 The nurse is caring for a client who has had a temperature of 38.8°C for the past 24 hours. When medicating the client for pain, the nurse is aware that: a. elimination of the drug may be prolonged. b. the analgesic should be given by a parenteral route. c. the analgesic effect may be shortened. d. absorption of the drug will be reduced.	Answer: c Rationale: Fever increases metabolism of drugs, resulting in a shorter duration of action and faster elimination. The analgesic does not need to be given by a parenteral route and absorption isn't affected by the fever. Analysis Planning Physiological Integrity: Pharmacological and Parenteral Therapies
6.5 A client is receiving an antihypertensive and a diuretic medication. Since these two medications will have a synergistic effect, the nurse can expect the client will have: a. a decrease in blood pressure. b. an increase in urinary output. c. a decrease in heart rate. d. signs of dehydration.	Answer: a Rationale: Synergism occurs when two drugs have a greater response than each drug given separately. The combined effect of both drugs will lower the blood pressure. Diuretic action alone will increase urinary output and may cause some dehydration. A decrease in heart rate may be seen with some types of antihypertensive agents. Analysis Evaluation Physiological Integrity: Pharmacological and Parenteral Therapies
6.6 A client with chronic renal failure informs the nurse he frequently uses over-the-counter medications to manage headaches. The nurse's best response would be: a. "As long as you don't exceed the recommended dose, it is okay." b. "It would be better to use herbal supplements than most over-the-counter analgesics." c. "The FDA ensures that all over-the-counter medications are safe to consume." d. "You should check with your primary care provider before using any over-the-counter medications."	Answer: d Rationale: Some over-the-counter medications are contraindicated in liver and renal disease, even when taken at recommended doses. Herbal supplement safety and effectiveness are not regulated and they may be contraindicated in certain disease states as well. Application Implementation Physiological Integrity: Pharmacological and Parenteral Therapies
6.7 A client becomes agitated and restless a few hours after being given a sleeping pill. The nurse recognizes the client is most likely experiencing: a. an idiosyncratic drug reaction. b. a toxic effect from the medication. c. an allergic reaction to a chemical in the medication. d. a side effect of the medication.	Answer: a Rationale: An idiosyncratic reaction is unusual or unexpected response to a medication, such as the opposite of the intended effect. Toxic effects are harmful, undesirable effects occurring at high drug doses. Allergic responses usually include rashes, hives, or itching. Side effects are anticipated and usually mild. Comprehension Assessment Physiological Integrity: Pharmacological and Parenteral Therapies.
6.8 A client informs the nurse she is allergic to a certain medication. To verify the allergic condition, the nurse should ask the client: a. "Can you explain what happens when you take the medication?" b. "Are you allergic to any other medications?" c. "How many times did you take the medication?" d. "Did you take the medication on an empty stomach?"	Answer: a Rationale: To distinguish an allergic reaction from side effects or toxic effects, it is best to clarify what occurred when the medication was taken. The other options will not elicit specific information as to the nature of the allergic response. Application Implementation Physiological Integrity: Pharmacological and Parenteral Therapies

6.9 A client has been started on an antihypertensive medication and is not exhibiting the expected response. Which of the following factors does the nurse recognize could contribute to the lack of drug effect? The client: a. has never taken an antihypertensive medication before. b. is of Asian descent. c. is African American. d. was not given a loading dose of the medication.	Answer: c Rationale: Ethnicity plays a role in drug response. Some antihypertensive medications are less effective in African Americans. Application Evaluation Physiological Integrity; Pharmacological and Pareteral Therapies
6.10 When administering medications the client states: "I've never taken this pill before. I really am not comfortable taking it." The best response of the nurse would be: a. "Let me check the physician's order and verify it is the correct medication." b. "It is probably a generic formulation of the drug and it doesn't look like the medication you are familiar with taking." c. "It is okay if you are not comfortable taking the medication. You have a right to refuse." d. "The physician probably added a new medication to your regimen."	Answer: a Rationale: To prevent med errors, the nurse should always recheck the medication administration record (MAR) and physician orders before assuming the medication is a generic formulation or that a new medication has been added. Clients have a right to refuse, but further exploration of the medication is the best response. Application Implementation Physiological Integrity: Pharmacological and Parenteral Therapies

CHAPTER 7

7.1 A client's extracellular fluid (ECF) exceeds 20% of his normal body weight. The nurse's findings on assessment may include: a. weight loss. b. edema and weight gain. c. increased output. d. decreased intake.	Answer: b Rationale: The excess fluid in the extracellular spaces contributes to edema and will be reflected as weight gain. The other options indicate a loss of fluid has occurred. Analysis Assessment Health Promotion: Prevention and/or Early Detection of Health Problems
7.2 When caring for the elderly population, the nurse recognizes they are at risk for dehydration related to: a. decline of the thirst mechanism in the hypothalamus. b. altered mobility. c. renal failure. d. excessive antidiuretic hormone (ADH) released by the posterior pituitary.	Answer: a Rationale: The primary regulator of water intake is thirst and this mechanism declines in the elderly. Comprehension Assessment Physiological Integrity: Reduction of Risk Potential
7.3 A dehydrated client experiences a drop in blood pressure. The nurse understands the body responds by: a. decreasing the antidiuretic hormone (ADH). b. decreasing the production of renin by the kidneys. c. suppressing the release of aldosterone by the adrenals. d. increasing ADH, renin, and aldosterone production.	Answer: d Rationale: An increase in ADH, renin, and aldosterone secretion is the body's compensatory mechanism to conserve water and reduce urine output, which is designed to maintain intravascular fluid volume. Comprehension Assessment Physiological Integrity: Reduction of Risk Potential

 © 2007 Pearson Education, Inc.

7.4 The nurse assesses the fluid balance in a client. Which of the following findings would support a fluid volume deficit? a. dry skin, decreased heart rate, and increased blood pressure b. increased heart rate, increased blood pressure, and cold clammy skin c. decreased heart rate, decreased blood pressure, and diaphoresis d. decreased blood pressure, increased heart rate, and dry skin	Answer: d Rationale: Fluid volume deficit is characterized by a decrease in extracellular fluid, which would manifest as a drop in blood pressure and dry skin. Heart rate increases to compensate for the reduction in blood volume. Analysis Assessment Physiological Integrity: Reduction of Risk Potential
7.5 The nurse is caring for a client who has been experiencing nausea and vomiting for several days. The client is at risk for developing which of these imbalances? a. respiratory alkalosis b. respiratory acidosis c. metabolic alkalosis d. metabolic acidosis	Answer: c Rationale: The vomiting causes loss of acidic fluids, resulting in alkalosis. The cause is metabolic, not respiratory, in origin. Analysis Assessment Physiological Integrity: Reduction of Risk Potential
7.6 Your client has returned from a parathyroidectomy and must be monitored for hypocalcemia. The nurse should assess for: a. muscle cramps, tingling, tetany. b. flaccid paralysis. c. bradycardia and weight loss. d. hypotension and headache.	Answer: a Rationale: These symptoms result when insufficient ionized calcium causes excitability of the neuromuscular tissues. Paralysis or muscle weakness would indicate hypercalcemia. Weight loss and headache are not necessarily seen with hypocalcemia. Analysis Assessment Physiological Integrity: Reduction of Risk Potential
7.7 The nurse observes a client to have a central venous pressure (CVP) reading of 9 cm of water. The nurse determines this to be: a. fluid volume deficit. b. fluid volume overload. c. homeostasis. d. dehydration.	Answer: b Rationale: A normal CVP reading is 2 to 8 cm of water. Elevated levels are indicative of fluid overload, heart failure, and some lung disorders. Analysis Assessment Physiological Integrity: Reduction of Risk Potential
7.8 The nurse suspects dehydration in an elderly client. The nurse assesses for skin turgor on the client's: a. abdomen. b. upper extremities. c. lower extremities. d. sternum.	Answer: d Rationale: Due to loss of skin elasticity with aging, the sternum or forehead provide the most reliable indication of skin turgor and hydration level. Application Assessment Health Promotion: Prevention and/or Early Detection of Health Problems
7.9 The nurse assesses for presence of edema in the bedridden client by checking the: a. sacral area. b. lower extremities. c. upper extremities. d. periorbital area.	Answer: a Rationale: Edematous fluid settles to dependent area, which is found above the sacrum in bedridden clients. Comprehension Assessment Physiological Integrity: Physiological Adaptation
7.10 A client is experiencing a fluid volume excess and dyspnea. The nurse positions the client: a. dorsal recumbent with legs elevated. b. prone, with head to one side. c. reverse Trendelenburg. d. high Fowler's.	Answer: d Rationale: This position allows for improved ventilation and lung expansion. The other positions would promote drainage of fluid toward the heart and lungs, thereby increasing dyspnea. Application Intervention Physiological Integrity: Basic Care and Comfort

© 2007 Pearson Education, Inc.

CHAPTER 8

8.1 Nurses can assist clients experiencing pain by stimulating large-diameter A-delta and A-beta fibers by using techniques such as: a. high-intensity exercise. b. relaxation and massage. c. electrical stimulation therapy. d. group therapy.	Answer: b Rationale: Stimulation of the alpha, or touch, fibers close the gait and blocks transmission of pain. Massage would stimulate these fibers. Application Implementation Physiological Integrity: Basic Care and Comfort
8.2 The nurse is caring for a postoperative client who is experiencing sweating, tachycardia, and increased blood pressure. The nurse recognizes these symptoms are due to: a. chronic pain. b. postoperative shock. c. acute pain. d. phantom pain.	Answer: c Rationale: The tissue injury caused from surgery produces acute pain and initiates the fight-or-flight response, resulting in physical responses of sweating, pallor, tachycardia, and blood pressure increase. Analysis Assessment Health Promotion: Prevention and/or Early Detection of Health Problems
8.3 A client who has just had a heart attack reports experiencing intense pain in the left shoulder. The nurse explains this type of pain is called: a. acute pain. b. chronic pain. c. phantom pain. d. referred pain.	Answer: d Rationale: Referred pain starts in one site but is perceived in another area, distant from the site of the stimuli. There are sometimes nerve tracts connecting the two sites. Analysis Assessment Health Promotion: Prevention and/or Early Detection of Health Problems
8.4 A client with a right lower extremity amputation complains of pain in the lost limb. The nurse plans care of the client based on the understanding that phantom limb pain should be: a. ignored, as it is not possible to have pain in the lost limb. b. referred to a grief counselor. c. given small doses of pain medication to prevent addiction. d. treated as any other client experiencing pain.	Answer: d Rationale: Phantom limb pain is experienced in the missing body part and is very real to the patient. Pain may be due to stimulation of severed nerves in the limb and should be treated as any other type of pain. Application Implementation Physiological Integrity: Basic Care and Comfort
8.5 The nurse should watch for which of the following side effects when clients are receiving NSAIDs, nonsteroidal anti-inflammatory drugs, for pain: a. diarrhea and vomiting. b. tarry black stools and epigastric pain. c. vertigo and syncope. d. confusion and memory loss.	Answer: b Rationale: NSAIDs block the action of protective prostaglandins in the stomach and cause GI irritation and bleeding. Analysis Evaluation Physiological Integrity: Pharmacological and Parenteral Therapies
8.6 A client in hospice care has received large doses of morphine but is still unable to sleep. The nurse should administer which of the following adjuvant drugs? a. amitriptyline (Elavil) b. lisinopril (Zestril) c. meperidine (Demerol) d. acetaminophen (Tylenol)	Answer: a Rationale: In cases of chronic pain and cancer, the use of antidepressants, such as Elavil, some anticonvulsants, corticosteroids, and psychostimulants have been found to provide analgesia. Application Implementation Physiological Integrity: Pharmacological and Parenteral Therapies

© 2007 Pearson Education, Inc.

8.7 The nurse evaluates the effectiveness of a client's intravenous injection of morphine sulfate, 15 mg, given for pain. How soon can the nurse expect the client to begin to get some relief? a. 1 to 5 minutes b. 10 to 15 minutes c. 20 to 30 minutes d. 1 to 2 hours	Answer: a Rationale: Medication given by the intravenous route should begin working within 1 to 5 minutes. Application Evaluation Physiological Integrity: Pharmacological and Parenteral Therapies
8.8 A client feels reluctant to ask for pain medication frequently to keep from bothering the nurse. The nurse recognizes an appropriate type of pain control for this client would be: a. narcotic tablets left at the bedside. b. relaxation exercises. c. transcutaneous electrical nerve stimulation (TENS) unit. d. patient-controlled analgesia (PCA) pump.	Answer: d Rationale: A PCA pump allows the client to self-administer pain medication as needed, within limits set for safe dosing. It would be unsafe to leave meds at the bedside. Relaxation and TENS units are often used as compensatory therapies to medication. Analysis Intervention Physiological Integrity: Pharmacological and Parenteral Therapies
8.9 A 5-year-old client was admitted with severe dog bites and was experiencing pain. The nurse can best evaluate level of pain intensity by: a. showing pictures of happy, sad, and crying faces and have the client point to the one like him. b. asking the parents about how much pain the client seems to be experiencing. c. recognizing the level of intensity cannot be evaluated at that early age. d. asking the child to rate the pain on a scale of 1 to 10.	Answer: a Rationale: The child can relate to pictures and help define degree of pain in that way. Information is always best obtained from the client. A child may not relate to a 1–10 pain scale as well as using pictures. Application Evaluation Physiological Integrity: Basic Care and Comfort
8.10 The nurse notes a client is crying and holding the operative site, yet continues to refuse pain medication. The nurse might initially explore the client's: a. religious beliefs. b. cultural beliefs. c. beliefs about the frequent use of narcotics. d. socioeconomic status.	Answer: c Rationale: Fears of developing addiction or being labeled an addict prompt clients to refuse pain meds. Religious and cultural beliefs often influence clients as well, often displayed by stoic behavior, but these options should be explored as well. Analysis Assessment Health Promotion: Prevention and/or Early Detection of Health Problems

CHAPTER 9

9.1 A client is being given 0.6 mg atropine (an anticholinergic) IM preoperatively and asks the nurse what the medication is for. The nurse explains the medication will prevent: a. anxiety. b. nausea. c. aspiration. d. pain.	Answer: c Rationale: Atropine, an anticholinergic, reduces oral and respiratory secretions in order to reduce risk of aspiration. Analgesics and benzodiazepines are given to decrease anxiety and pain. Antiemetics are given help to reduce nausea. Application Intervention Physiological Integrity: Pharmacological and Parenteral Therapies

9.2 During the preoperative assessment, the nurse learns that the client had gestational diabetes with her three pregnancies. The nurse will obtain an order for the following test: a. urinalysis. b. blood sugar. c. electrolytes. d. partial thromboplastin time (PTT).	Answer: b Rationale: Clients with a history of diabetes mellitus should have blood glucose levels monitored before, during, and after surgery. Urinalysis, electrolytes, and clotting studies may be ordered routinely for any patient preoperatively. Application Implementation Physiological Integrity: Prevention of Risk Potential
9.3 The preoperative client asks the nurse for some tea before surgery. The nurse explains that it is important to have nothing by mouth (NPO) prior to surgery to prevent: a. abdominal cramping. b. urine formation. c. hyperglycemia. d. aspiration.	Answer: d Rationale: Keeping a client NPO for at least 8 to 10 hours prior to surgery reduces the risk of aspirating stomach contents. Abdominal cramping would not be life threatening. It would not be desirable to prevent urine formation. Tea would not cause hyperglycemia. Application Implementation Physiological Integrity: Prevention of Risk Potential
9.4 The nurse is preparing to obtain a client's signature on an informed consent. It is the nurse's responsibility to: a. witness the signature. b. explain the procedure. c. describe surgical risks. d. determine the client's understanding about the procedure.	Answer: a Rationale: The nurse is only responsible for witnessing the signature. Options b, c, and d are the physician's responsibility. Comprehension Implementation Safe, Effective Care Environment: Coordinated Care
9.5 When providing preoperative teaching for a client scheduled to have abdominal surgery, the nurse should include: a. assisting with the bed bath. b. self-medication using a PCA pump. c. changing the dressings. d. turning, coughing, and deep breathing (TCDB).	Answer: d Rationale: Coughing and deep breathing is required of all postoperative patients in order to reduce the risk of complications. Clients may or may not be expected to assist with their baths and to have a PCA device. Clients do not change their own dressings. Application Implementation Physiological Integrity: Reduction of Risk Potential
9.6 After abdominal surgery a client has difficulty coughing, saying, "It hurts too much." The nurse teaches the client to: a. support the abdomen with a pillow during the coughing exercises. b. ask for pain medication if the pain is severe. c. cough without straining the abdomen. d. turn and deep breathe without coughing.	Answer: a Rationale: Teaching the client to splint the incision aids in decreasing discomfort. Premedicating client for pain may also help, but not waiting until pain is severe. Options c and d would not allow for proper coughing technique. Application Implementation Physiological Integrity: Basic Care and Comfort
9.7 When changing the client's sterile dressings on the second postoperative day, the nurse notes that the suture line is red and slightly inflamed. The nurse recognizes these findings are: a. abnormal and need to be reported to the charge nurse. b. signs of infection and need to be reported to the physician. c. normal signs of the inflammatory response. d. abnormal and need to be documented.	Answer: c Rationale: Slight redness and inflammation is a normal sign of the inflammatory process, caused by increased blood flow to site of tissue trauma. Analysis Assessment Physiological Integrity: Physiological Adaptation

 © 2007 Pearson Education, Inc.

9.8 After abdominal surgery, a client feels bloated and is unable to pass gas. Appropriate nursing interventions include: a. restrict foods to reduce gas production. b. encourage fluid intake of 3000 mL/day. c. assist with ambulation. d. press gently on the abdomen to promote expulsion of gas.	Answer: c Rationale: Ambulation stimulates peristalsis, which will promote gas expulsion. Restricting gas-forming foods prevents gas production, but wouldn't be the best intervention to promote gas expulsion. Fluid intake would also not promote gas expulsion. Pressing on the abdomen may be painful following abdominal surgery. Application Intervention Physiological Integrity: Physiological Adaptation
9.9 A postoperative client complains of dizziness when getting out of bed to ambulate. The nurse should: a. have the client use a walker. b. walk alongside the client. c. return the client to bed. d. administer medication for dizziness.	Answer: b Rationale: Walking alongside the client provides support and safety. Dizziness is a common occurrence postoperatively and does not usually require medication. Application Intervention Safe, Effective Care Environment: Safety and Infection Control
9.10 A nurse is preparing to discharge a client who has had outpatient surgery. It is important for the nurse to assess the client's: a. knowledge of sterile technique. b. food preferences. c. family support at home. d. understanding of the surgical procedure.	Answer: c Rationale: Since client will be discharged to home following outpatient surgery, it is necessary to know who will be available to assist with recovery. Analysis Assessment Safe, Effective Carc Environment: Coordinated Care

CHAPTER 10

10.1 The nurse is caring for an elderly client who does not exhibit an elevated temperature but is suspected of having a severe infection. The nurse should look for other signs and symptoms such as: a. Diarrhea. b. Nausea and vomiting. c. Hypertension. d. Change in mental function or delirium.	Answer: d Rationale: In the elderly confusion is a frequent atypical sign of infection, along with restlessness, fatigue, and behavioral changes. The other options would be indicative of GI and blood pressure problems. Analysis Assessment Physiological Integrity: Physiological Adaptation
10.2 Laboratory studies on a client with pneumonia reveal leukopenia. The nurse knows this may be indicative of a(n): a. viral infection. b. bacterial infection. c. fungal infection. d. absence of infection.	Answer: a Rationale: Leukopenia, a decrease in WBC, is seen in anemias, viral infections, and autoimmune disorders. Bacterial and fungal infections cause leukocystosis, or an elevated WBC. Analysis Assessment Physiological Integrity: Physiological Adaptation
10.3 The nurse obtains a specimen of wound drainage ordered for a client. The specimen is sent for a culture and sensitivity test to determine the: a. severity of the disease. b. most effective antibiotic. c. effectiveness of the client's immune system. d. type of pathogen.	Answer: b Rationale: The culture identifies the type of pathogen and defines which antibiotic it is sensitive and resistant to. Comprehesion Assessment Physiological Integrity: Reduction of Risk Potential

© 2007 Pearson Education, Inc.

10.4 The client is caring for a client who has been taking nonsteroidal anti-inflammatory drugs (NSAIDs). The nurse should monitor the client for: a. occult blood in the stool. b. acoustic toxicity. c. tinnitus. d. irregular heart rhythms.	Answer: a Rationale: Occult blood would be a sign of gastrointestinal bleeding, a common side effect of NSAIDs. Acoustic toxicity and tinnitus are seen with aspirin and some antibiotics. Irregular heart rhythms are a side effect of many different drugs. Analysis Assessment Physiological Integrity: Pharmacological and Parenteral Therapies
10.5 The nurse instructs the mother of a child with chickenpox to avoid giving aspirin because it may cause: a. meningitis. b. Reye's syndrome. c. acoustic toxicity. d. seizures.	Answer: b Rationale: Giving aspirin to children with chickenpox or influenza may precipitate Reye's syndrome. Application Planning Physiological Integrity: Reduction of Risk Potential
10.6 In corticosteroid therapy it is important for the nurse to teach the clients: a. to increase the dosage when symptoms appear. b. to watch for signs and symptoms of hypoglycemia. c. to take the medication on an empty stomach. d. to taper the doses gradually and never stop the medication abruptly.	Answer: d Rationale: Abruptly stopping corticosteroids can cause a client to go into an Addisonian crisis. Tapering the dose allows the adrenal gland to return to normal function. Clients should be monitored for hyperglycemia and the med should be taken with food. Application Implementation Physiological Integrity: Reduction of Risk Potential
10.7 To promote blood clotting and tissue healing, the nurse instructs the client recovering from multiple wounds to increase intake of foods high in: a. vitamins E and C. b. vitamins E and A. c. vitamins C and B. d. vitamins K and B.	Answer: d Rationale: B complex vitamins promote wound healing and vitamin K is essential for blood clotting. Vitamin C is necessary for collagen synthesis and vitamin A fosters capillary formation. Vitamin E is not indicated for wound healing. Application Planning Health Promotion: Prevention and/or Early Detection of Health Problems
10.8 Adequate fluid intake is essential to wound healing. If not contraindicated, the nurse should encourage the client to drink at least: a. 600 mL daily. b. 1200 mL daily. c. 1800 mL daily. d. 2500 mL daily.	Answer: d Rationale: Adequate hydration helps maintain blood flow and nutrition supply to tissues; 2500 mL provides an optimal amount. Application Implementation Physiological Integrity: Reduction of Risk Potential
10.9 The nurse notes that a client with a Foley catheter has developed a bladder infection. The nurse recognizes this is a type of: a. sterile infection. b. noninvasive infection. c. nosocomial infection. d. systemic infection.	Answer: c Rationale: Nosocomial infections are infections acquired in a health care setting, often secondary to the presence of indwelling urinary catheters. Analysis Assessment Physiological Integrity: Physiological Adaptation
10.10 The nurse admits a client with methicillin-resistant *Staphylococcus aureus* (MRSA). The nurse knows that this client: a. cannot be treated with any antibiotics. b. must be isolated using Contact Precautions. c. can be placed in a room with another client with an infection. d. can be treated with no restrictions.	Answer: b Rationale: Since MRSA is often transmitted on the hands of health care workers, contact isolation reduces the transmission of direct skin contact and skin to clothing. Clients should be isolated to prevent spread of the bacteria. MRSA is treated with antibiotics not yet resistant to it. Application Planning Safe, Effective Care Environment: Safety and Infection Control

 © 2007 Pearson Education, Inc.

CHAPTER 11

11.1 A client exposed to hepatitis A is given a human immune globulin vaccine. The nurse explains this will provide: a. natural immunity. b. active acquired immunity. c. natural acquired immunity. d. passive acquired immunity.	Answer: d Rationale: Passive immunity comes from injection of serum containing antibodies from other humans or animals. Natural immunity is a person's resistance to foreign substances. Active immunity can be naturally acquired by developing the disease. Naturally acquired immunity occurs when neonates receive antibodies from their mothers. Application Implementation Health Promotion: Prevention and/or Early Detection of Health Problems
11.2 A nurse has accepted a position working in a high-risk area such as an emergency room. It is recommended by the Occupational Safety and Health Administration (OSHA) that the nurse receive vaccinations against: a. hepatitis B. b. hepatitis C. c. tuberculosis. d. influenza.	Answer: a Rationale: Hepatitis B vaccine is recommended for anyone at high risk for exposure to blood and/or other body fluids. Comprehension Implementation Health Promotion: Safety and Infection Control
11.3 The nurse is preparing to administer influenza immunizations to a group of clients. The nurse should not administer the immunization to clients who are: a. elderly b. naturally immune. c. immunosuppressed. d. not exposed to the influenza virus.	Answer: c Rationale: Reactions to the vaccine may be enhanced in the immunocompromised client. The elderly are advised to have yearly influenza immunizations. Natural immunity doesn't occur because strains of influenza change yearly. The vaccine is given to stimulate antibody production in case the person is exposed to the virus. Application Planning Health Promotion: Prevention and/or Early Detection of Health Problems
11.4 The nurse administering a vaccination should have the patient stay for observation for at least: a. 2 hours. b. 20 to 30 minutes. c. 10 to 15 minutes. d. 45 to 60 minutes.	Answer: b Rationale: Allergic reactions usually occur within 20 to 30 minutes. Application Implementation Health Promotion: Prevention and/or Early Detection of Health Problems
11.5 The nurse suspects a client is hypersensitive to a vaccine just administered. Nursing management of an allergic response includes immediate assessment of the: a. dose of medication taken by the client. b. skin to check for urticaria. c. injection site for signs and symptoms of the inflammatory response. d. respirations to determine airway patency.	Answer: d Rationale: Allergic reactions may include anaphylaxis with laryngeal swelling and difficulty breathing. Airway assessment is the number one priority. Application Assessment Physiological Integrity: Reduction of Risk Potential
11.6 A client receiving intravenous therapy suddenly develops dyspnea. The nurse should immediately: a. call a code. b. administer oxygen. c. administer epinephrine. d. stop the intravenous flow.	Answer: d Rationale: This action prevents any further infusion of the antigen, the probable cause of the dyspneic response. Application Implementation Physiological Integrity: Reduction of Risk Potential

11.7 Discharge instructions given to a client who has had a severe allergic reaction should include: a. wear a Medic-Alert bracelet identifying the allergen. b. check with physician prior to the use of any new product. c. written instructions on intravenous administration of epinephrine. d. written directions to all local emergency rooms.	Answer: a Rationale: A Medic-Alert bracelet identifies the client's allergies and is valuable in emergency situations. Options b and d are not realistic. Client should be instructed on how to administer subcutaneous epinephrine. Application Implementation Health Promotion: Prevention and/or Early Detection of Health Problems
11.8 A client who received an allograft develops symptoms of vomiting, diarrhea, and a pruritic rash on the palms of the hands and soles of the feet. The nurse recognizes this is indicative of: a. an allergic response. b. graft-versus-host disease. c. chronic rejection. d. acute rejection.	Answer: b Rationale: Graft-versus-host disease begins with a maculopapular rash on the palms and soles of the feet, as well as gastrointestinal symptoms. Allergic responses usually involve urticaria, swelling, itching, and/or anaphylaxis. Acute and chronic rejections involve symptoms related to failure of the transplanted organ. Application Assessment Physiological Integrity: Physiological Adaptation
11.9 When caring for a client who is a recipient of a transplanted kidney, the nurse monitors for early indications of rejection, which include: a. an increase in urinary output. b. discomfort over the lumbar area. c. lethargy. d. rising BUN and creatinine.	Answer: d Rationale: Rising BUN and creatinine levels reflect declining function of the transplanted kidney. A decrease in urinary output and discomfort over the abdominal/groin area would be seen. Lethargy may be seen but is nonspecific. Analysis Assessment Physiological Integrity: Reduction of Risk Potential
11.10 The nurse is preparing a community teaching program aimed at prevention of human immunodeficiency virus (HIV) transmission. The nurse is aware that populations at high risk for becoming infected with HIV are: a. white females from 16 to 26 years of age. b. older Asian and African American males. c. young Puerto Rican females. d. young African American and Hispanic males.	Answer: d Rationale: African American and Hispanic males make up 56% of HIV cases; 78% of women with HIV are African American or Hispanic. Application Planning Health Promotion: Prevention and/or Early Detection of Health Problems

CHAPTER 12

12.1 An 86-year-old client asks the nurse why cancer affects mostly the elderly. An accurate response would be: a. "The elderly have more oncogenes." b. "It may take 10 to 20 years after damage to the DNA for the cancer to appear." c. "The cells of the elderly are more fragile and more susceptible to cancer." d. "The elderly have a longer time to be affected by all carcinogens."	Answer: b Rationale: Since the time between damage to the DNA and manifestation of a tumor may take 10 to 20 years, many cancers tend to occur in older adults. Application Implementation Physiological Integrity: Physiological Adaptation

 © 2007 Pearson Education, Inc.

12.2 An elderly client told the nurse she had been smoking for 70 years and did not have lung cancer. The nurse explained that other factors need to be taken into account, such as: a. genetic predisposition. b. history of alcohol abuse. c. type of cigarettes smoked. d. type of diet.	Answer: a Rationale: Noncontrollable risk factors such as heredity can play a role in cancer development. Application Implementation Physiological Integrity: Physiological Adaptation
12.3 An eighth-grade class is taking a field trip to the beach to explore sea life. The school nurse suggests that the students: a. stay out of the water. b. wear long-sleeved shirts and long pants to protect them from the sun. c. go on the field trip in the evening to avoid exposure to the sun. d. use SPF 15 lotion on their exposed skin to prevent sunburn.	Answer: d Rationale: SPF 15 lotion provides protection against the sun's most damaging ultraviolet radiation and would be the most practical of the suggestions. Application Implementation Health Promotion: Prevention and/or Early Detection of Health Problems
12.4 A 78-year-old client has been diagnosed with prostate cancer. The nurse should educate the client about the prevention or treatment of: a. constipation. b. urinary retention. c. recurrent headaches. d. urinary incontinence.	Answer: b Rationale: Prostatic tumors often obstruct the bladder neck or urethra, causing urinary retention. Application Implementation Physiological Integrity: Basic Care and Comfort
12.5 The client tells the nurse, "The doctor says my breast tumor was at B stage. What does that mean?" The nurse explains the staging describes: a. "The size of the tumor and extent of the cancer." b. "The rate of growth of the cancer cells." c. "Where the tumor tissue first originated." d. "The type of cancer cells."	Answer: a Rationale: Staging of tumors provides the relative size of the tumor and extent of disease. Grading estimates the rate of growth. Classifications identify the tissue or cell origin and type of cancer cell. Application Implementation Physiological Integrity: Physiological Adaptation
12.6 A client suffers from claustrophobia, the fear of being in enclosed places. The nurse knows that the client may have difficulty with the following test: a. CT scan b. ultrasonography c. x-ray imaging d. MRI	Answer: d Rationale: An MRI involves being placed inside a diagnostic imaging machine, similar to being encased in a small tube. Analysis Assessment Physiological Integrity: Reduction of Risk Potential
12.7 The nurse is caring for a hospitalized cancer client with a radiation implant. The nurse plans to take the following precautions: a. Wear a lead apron when administering care. b. Organize care to limit exposure. c. Avoid touching the patient. d. Encourage family involvement with client care.	Answer: b Rationale: It is not necessary to wear a lead apron, but exposure should be limited as much as possible. Family members and visitors should stay 6 feet away from client. Analysis Planning Safe, Effective Care Environment: Safety and Infection Control

© 2007 Pearson Education, Inc.

12.8 Which of the following statements indicates a need for further teaching by the nurse for a client with radiation implants? a. "I need to take good care of the skin around the radiation implant." b. "I may have nausea and vomiting." c. "I will spend some time with my grandson and my daughter who is expecting again." d. "I might feel unusually fatigued."	Answer: c Rationale: Clients with radiation implants should avoid close physical contact with others. The skin around an implant is prone to irritation and breakdown. Fatigue and nausea may occur. Analysis Planning Safe, Effective Care Environment: Safety and Infection Control
12.9 A client with breast cancer who is receiving chemotherapy tells the nurse she does not care what happens to her anymore, since she cannot work or care for her family. The nurse can assist by: a. finding a helper for her. b. referring her to counseling services. c. allowing her to express her feelings, fears, and concerns. d. telling her that she has the right to feel depressed.	Answer: c Rationale: Allowing the client to express her feelings will help diminish anxiety and may help to lay groundwork for new coping behaviors. Application Implementation Psychosocial Integrity: Coping and Adaptation
12.10 A client is being prepared for a bone marrow transplant. The nurse knows to prepare for which of the following administration routes? a. incision and instillation b. intravenous c. intrathecal d. intramuscular	Answer: b Rationale: The client is given an intravenous infusion of cells obtained from a donor or the client himself. Application Implementation Physiological Integrity: Physiological Adaptation

Chapter 13

13.1 A client who has experienced a severe blood loss becomes hypotensive and loses consciousness. The nurse suspects the client is experiencing: a. cardiogenic shock. b. neurogenic shock. c. anaphylactic shock. d. hypovolemic shock.	Answer: d Rationale: Hypovolemic shock is caused by a decrease in intravascular volume secondary to hemorrhage, severe dehydration, or internal fluid shifts. Cardiogenic shock occurs when damage to the heart reduces cardiac output and tissue perfusion. Neurogenic shock results from interruption to the sympathetic nervous system. Anaphylactic shock is caused by a severe allergic reaction. Comprehension Assessment Physiological Integrity: Physiological Adaptation
13.2 The nurse is caring for a client who has suffered a severe trauma with pelvic and femur fractures. Because the injuries may lead to shock the nurse plans for which of the following? a. application of femur and pelvic splints b. multiple transfusions c. endotracheal intubation d. pneumatic antishock garment (PASG)	Answer: d Rationale: PASG, or MAST trousers, stabilize the pelvic and femoral fractures and raise the blood pressure, providing for rapid treatment of shock. Splints would not improve shock. Options b and d may be needed if other complications are present. Application Planning Physiological Integrity: Reduction of Risk Potential
13.3 The nurse assesses crackles in the lungs of a client with shock who is receiving IV therapy. The nurse recognizes this finding is indicative of: a. hypostatic pneumonia. b. hypovolemia. c. hypervolemia. d. renal failure.	Answer: c Rationale: Crackles reflect a shift of excess fluid from the vascular space to interstitial spaces in the lung, indicating the client is receiving an excess of IV fluids. Analysis Assessment Physiological Integrity: Physiological Adaptation

© 2007 Pearson Education, Inc.

Question	Answer
13.4 A client is experiencing shock related to blood loss. When preparing the client for transfusion, it is the nurse's primary responsibility to: a. monitor the client's vital signs. b. determine blood loss. c. correctly identify the client and the blood. d. warm the blood.	Answer: c Rationale: Before a client can receive blood, blood typing and cross-matching must be done to determine donor and recipient ABO types and Rh group. Verification of correct patient with the matched blood is mandatory. Vital signs will be monitored throughout the transfusion. Blood may be warmed under certain conditions. Application Assessment Physiological Integrity: Reduction of Risk Potential
13.5 When caring for a client in cardiogenic shock, the nurse plans to administer which of the following drugs to raise the blood pressure? a. aminophylline b. dopamine c. lanoxin d. furosemide	Answer: b Rationale: Dopamine is a vasopressor drug that produces vasoconstriction and raises the blood pressure. Aminophylline is a bronchodilator. Lanoxin is a cardiac glycoside and strengthens cardiac contractility and slows conduction. Furosemide is a diuretic that promotes flud loss. Application Implementation Physiological Integrity: Pharmacological and Parenteral Therapies
13.6 A 37-year-old client is admitted in shock secondary to blood loss following an auto accident. The nurse places the client in the following position: a. modified Trendelenburg b. Sim's position c. Fowler's d. supine	Answer: a Rationale: By lowering the head and elevating the lower extremities,this position can best increase venous return to the heart. The other positions would not promote venous return. Application Implementation Physiological Integrity: Reduction of Risk Potential
13.7 The nurse is monitoring vital signs on a client receiving a blood transfusion. If a transfusion febrile reaction occurs, the client experiences chills and fever usually within: a. 3 hours. b. 2 hours. c. 60 minutes. d. 15 minutes.	Answer: d Rationale: In a febrile transfusion reaction, the client's antibodies react to the donor's white blood cells, causing fever and chills usually within 15 minutes. Application Assessment Physiological Integrity: Physiological Adaptation
13.8 When performing triage in an emergency department, the nurse would assign the highest priority to which of the following clients? a. one with injuries to the face and neck b. one with multiple fractures of the extremities c. one with abdominal pain d. one with a laceration of the forearm	Answer: a Rationale: Injuries to the face and neck may interfere with airway patency and adequate ventilation. Application Assessment Physiological Integrity: Reduction of Risk Potential
13.9 A 19-year-old client was admitted to the emergency department after a bicycle accident complaining of low back pain. Hematuria was present. For accurate monitoring of output, the nurse should: a. insert a Foley catheter. b. measure all voided urine. c. weigh the sheets and reweigh periodically. d. keep the client on the bedpan.	Answer: a Rationale: An indwelling urinary catheter provides the most accurate method to monitor urine output. Hourly measurements as well as observation of urine color and character can be easily checked. Application Implementation Physiological Integrity: Reduction of Risk Potential

13.10 The family is notified of a client's grave prognosis and the nurse informs the family that the client filled out an organ donor card. It is important for the nurse to: a. tell the family about how the organs will be removed. b. tell the family about the person who will be receiving the organs. c. encourage the family to ask questions and express their feelings. d. provide the family with a brochure on organ donation.	Answer: c Rationale: Organ donation is a difficult decision and this option affords the family the opportunity to have questions answered. The other options do not provide the family an opportunity to express concerns. Application Implementation Psychosocial Integrity: Coping and Adaptation

CHAPTER 14

14.1 A female member of the "I Can Cope" group thanked the nurse, saying that she probably would not be coming to the meetings since she had to get her finances in order and planned to return to school. The nurse understands the client is in which of the following stages, of grief? a. denial b. anger c. depression d. acceptance	Answer: d Rationale: In the acceptance stage the individual comes to terms with loss and resumes activities and displays a positive attitude. Denial is characterized by shock and disbelief. Anger is manifested by resistance and "acting out." During depression the person may withdraw or freely talk about the loss. Analysis Assessment Psychosocial Integrity: Coping and Adaptation
14.2 A client has just lost his girlfriend in an automobile accident. When the nurse asks the client about what happened, the client responds with a firm, "I don't want to talk about it." An appropriate response by the nurse would be: a. to sit quietly with the client. b. "You need to talk about the accident." c. "Not sharing your loss can make you ill." d. "You'll feel better if you talk about the accident."	Answer: a Rationale: Sitting with the client conveys acceptance to the client and lets him know the nurse is available to him. The other options do not show respect for the client's view. Application Implementation Psychosocial Integrity: Coping and Adaptation
14.3 A 17-year-old client whose boyfriend was killed in a car accident says that God punished her by taking her boyfriend because they had been living together and were not married. What kind of response by the nurse would be most helpful? a. "Tell me about your boyfriend." b. "You're right, you should have gotten married." c. "God does not punish people in that manner." d. "What is your religion?"	Answer: a Rationale: This response encourages the client to reflect on the loved one who has been lost and conveys genuine interest. Application Implementation Psychosocial Integrity: Coping and Adaptation
14.4 A client undergoing outpatient chemotherapy for cancer treatment expresses concern about being kept alive on life support. The nurse suggests that the client contact a lawyer to: a. prepare for assisted suicide. b. discuss disposal of her assets.	Answer: d Rationale: Advance directives and living wills are legal documents that can allow clients to express their wishes regarding life-sustaining treatments. Application Implementation Psychosocial Integrity: Coping and Adaptation

© 2007 Pearson Education, Inc.

c. meet with her family to decide what would be best for her. d. prepare advance directives and a living will.	
14.5 An elderly client signs a do-not-resuscitate statement in a living will then, during lunch, chokes on food and loses consciousness. The nurse has a responsibility to: a. perform the Heimlich maneuver and call a code. b. call the doctor to get an order for resuscitation. c. call a code and perform the Heimlich maneuver. d. do nothing, since the client signed a DNR order.	Answer: c Rationale: DNR orders are intended for near-death situations. Since the choking event was accidental, the nurse has a responsibility to treat the client, attempt to remove the obstruction, and preserve life. Application Implementation Safe, Effective Care Environment: Coordinated Care
14.6 In developing an end-of-life plan of care for the client, the nurse identifies which of the following hygiene goals as appropriate? a. Involve the client in 30% of her bath daily. b. Involve family in hygiene care daily to maintain clean, dry skin. c. Maintain clean skin by providing daily whirlpool baths. d. Provide hourly sponge baths for end-of-life comfort.	Answer: b Rationale: Involving the family gives them the opportunity to say good-bye and prepares them for the grieving process. The other options aren't realistic; hourly sponge baths and whirlpool would not be necessary. Analysis Planning Physiological Integrity: Basic Care and Comfort
14.7 The nurse can best provide sensory stimulation for a dying client who is unconscious by: a. having the television tuned to favorite programs. b. leaving the radio on at all times. c. encouraging the family to talk with the client. d. leaving her door open at all times.	Answer: c Rationale: It is believed that hearing is the last sense a dying person loses. Although TV and radio provide sensory stimulation, voices familiar to the client provide emotional and sensory stimuli. Application Implementation Physiological Integrity: Basic Care and Comfort
14.8 A dying client began having periods of absence of breathing alternating with noisy, rattling respirations. The nurse documents that the client is experiencing: a. apnea. b. dyspnea. c. Cheyne-Stokes respirations. d. orthopnea.	Answer: c Rationale: Cheyne-Stokes are characterized by alternating noisy respirations with absence of respirations. Apnea is an absence of respirations. Dyspnea involves labored breathing, and orthopnea is difficulty breathing when lying flat. Comprehension Assessment Physiological Integrity: Physiological Adaptation
14.9 A client who had a DNR order died during the night with no family members present. The nurse's first responsibility is to: a. document the time of death. b. call the physician. c. call the family. d. call the mortuary.	Answer: a Rationale: The nurse initially notes the exact time of death, followed then by options b, c, and d. Application Implementation Safe, Effective Care Environment: Coordinated Care

14.10 The daughters of a deceased client asked the nurse if they could wash their mother's body and dress her. The nurse's response might be: a. "Yes, but please hurry because the mortuary is coming to pick up the body." b. "I'm sorry, but that is my job." c. "Let me know how I can help you, I really liked your mother." d. "I will get you a basin, towels, and a fresh gown."	Answer: d Rationale: Allowing the family to assist with postmortem care provides them the opportunity to begin grieving and yet still play a role in caring for their loved one. Application Implementation Psychosocial Integrity: Coping and Adaptation

CHAPTER 15

15.1 A client is being evaluated for a disorder of the parathyroid glands. The nurse anticipates blood work will be ordered to check: a. calcium levels. b. fasting blood sugar. c. urinary 17-ketosteroids. d. TSH (thyroid stimulating hormone).	Answer: a Rationale: Calcium and phosphorous levels reflect parathyroid function. Fasting blood sugar reflects circulating blood glucose level. Urinary 17-ketosteroids reflect adrenal cortex function, and TSH reflects thyroid function. Comprehension Assessment Physiological Integrity: Reduction of Risk Potential
15.2 The physician orders a urinary 17-ketosteroid test on a client with a suspected adrenal disorder. The nurse is responsible to: a. send the first voided urine specimen of the day to the laboratory. b. keep a 24-hour urine collection on ice. c. obtain a catheterized sterile urine specimen. d. instruct client to avoid drinking any caffeine products.	Answer: b Rationale: Urine for 17-ketosteroids must be collected for 24 hours and kept on ice. It is not a sterile collection and dietary restrictions are not necessary. Application Implementation Physiological Integrity: Reduction of Risk Potential
15.3 A client has an elevated level of urinary microalbumin. The nurse understands this could be an indication of: a. Addison's disease. b. pancreatitis. c. diabetic nephropathy. d. thyroid cancer.	Answer: c Rationale: The presence of microalbumin is an early indication of damage to the nephron, often precipitated by diabetes. It is not related to the conditions listed in the other options. Application Evaluation Physiological Integrity: Reduction of Risk Potential
15.4 A client is scheduled for an MRI (magnetic resonance imaging) of the head. Prior to the procedure the nurse will need to determine if the client: a. is allergic to iodine. b. has had anything to eat in the past 8 hours. c. has a history of seizures. d. has any metallic implants.	Answer: d Rationale: Metallic implants interfere with the magnetic mechanism in the machine and would contraindicate the client having the MRI. Allergy to iodine is of concern when contrast dyes are use. Fasting is not required. Application Assessment Physiological Integrity: Reduction of Risk Potential
15.5 A client scheduled to have a 2-hour glucose tolerance test asks the nurse what is involved in the test. The nurse explains: a. "You will have blood drawn two hours after eating a large meal." b. "You will drink a glucose solution and not eat anything for two hours."	Answer: b Rationale: Client is given 75 grams of a glucose solution and nothing else is eaten for 2 hours; then blood is drawn. Application Implementation Physiological Integrity: Reduction of Risk Potential

© 2007 Pearson Education, Inc.

c. "After your breakfast meal, blood will be drawn every thirty minutes for two hours." d. "Blood is drawn two hours after eating a high carbohydrate meal."	
15.6 A client seen in the clinic is scheduled to have a radioactive iodine (RAI) uptake test. In preparation for the test, it is important for the nurse to instruct the client to: a. avoid drinking dairy products 24 hours prior to the test. b. hold any thyroid medications for 2 weeks prior to the test. c. eat a high fat meal the morning of the test. d. bring a fresh voided urine specimen the day of the test.	Answer: b Rationale: Thyroid drugs interfere with accurate uptake measurements and must be held 2 weeks prior to exam. Dietary restrictions are not necessary; client should be NPO for 8 hours prior to the exam. Application Implementation Physiological Integrity: Reduction of Risk Potential
15.7 A client with type 1 diabetes mellitus has a glycosylated hemoglobin level of 8%. The nurse recognizes that this indicates the client: a. has not been taking his insulin. b. is well controlled in his diet and insulin. c. needs adjustment in diet and/or medication. d. has a low hemoglobin level.	Answer: c Rationale: A normal level is 2.2% to 4.8%. Elevated levels indicate the diabetes is poorly controlled, warranting an adjustment in diet, exercise, and/or medication, or combination of all. Application Evaluation Physiological Integrity: Reduction of Risk Potential
15.8 When reading a client's history, the nurse notes the client has exopthalmos, secondary to hyperthyroidism. An assessment finding the nurse expects to see is: a. ecchymotic areas on the trunk. b. forward protrusion of the eyeballs. c. purple striae over the abdomen. d. a bronze discoloration of the skin.	Answer: b Rationale: Exopthalmos is the forward protrusion of the eyeball, producing a bug-eyed or startled appearance. Comprehension Assessment Physiological Integrity: Physiological Adaptation
15.9 The nurse can anticipate a client suspected of having Cushing's disease to have blood levels checked for: a. calcium. b. phosphorus. c. cortisol. d. glycosylated hemoglobin.	Answer: c Rationale: Cortisol levels are increased in Cushing's disease. Calcium and phosphorus reflect parathyroid function. Glycosylated hemoglobin measures blood sugar control of diabetics. Application Assessment Physiological Integrity: Reduction of Risk Potential
15.10 An active elderly client complains of feeling tired all the time and is frequently constipated. The nurse recognizes that these symptoms: a. are most likely due to normal changes of aging. b. may be indicative of an endocrine imbalance. c. are probably a sign of cancer. d. are frequently signs of dementia.	Answer: b Rationale: Although these can be normal signs of aging and may occur with cancer, they may be related to an endocrine dysfunction and often overlooked or misdiagnosed. They are not signs of dementia. Analysis Assessment Physiological Integrity: Physiological Adaptation

CHAPTER 16

16.1 When caring for a client with an aldosterone deficiency, the nurse should monitor the client for signs of? a. hyperkalemia b. metabolic acidosis c. hypernatremia d. hypertension	Answer: a Rationale: An aldosterone deficit results in increased excretion of sodium and increased reabsorption of potassium. Low sodium and hypotension would be seen. Application Assessment Physiological Integrity: Physiological Adaptation
16.2 In teaching a client with hypoparathyroidism about the disorder, which statement by the nurse best explains how the parathyroid hormone controls calcium levels in the blood? a. "Parathyroid hormone blocks phosphorous excretion by the kidneys, which then decreases the blood calcium level." b. "When blood calcium levels fall, parathyroid hormones stimulate bone resorption and increase calcium in the blood." c. "Parathyroid hormones promote magnesium excretion by the kidneys, which raises blood calcium levels." d. "Parathyroid hormones stimulate cells of the gastrointestinal tract to absorb dietary calcium, raising the blood level."	Answer: d Rationale: Parathyroid hormone is excreted by the parathyroid glands and regulates serum calcium and phosphorous levels; in response to low serum calcium, it stimulates resorption of calcium from the bones. It also stimulates calcium reabsorption from the kidneys and intestines, but does not regulate magnesium levels. Application Implementation Physiological Integrity: Physiological Adaptation
16.3 A client scheduled for a thyroid scan asks the nurse about the test and what will happen after taking the radioactive iodine. Which is the best response by the nurse? a. Several blood samples will be drawn to determine the amount of iodine in the bloodstream. b. The client will be isolated from others for several days. c. The scanner will deliver a radioactive beam to her thyroid to reduce its size. d. A scanner will be passed back and forth across her throat and she will feel no discomfort.	Answer: d Rationale: Option d is an accurate description of a thyroid scan. Blood is not drawn and isolation is not necessary. The radioactive isotope is given via an intravenous injection. Application Implementation Health Promotion: Prevention and/or Early Detection of Health Problems
16.4 An important nursing intervention for the nurse to provide when caring for a client with Addison's disease is: a. regular feedings throughout the day. b. insulin continuously by intravenous drip. c. stimulating recreational activities. d. a vigorous exercise regime.	Answer: a Rationale: Management of Addison's disease focuses on maintenance of fluid and electrolytes and adequate nutrition. Corticosteroid, not insulin, needs to be replaced. Stress and excessive exercise should be avoided. Application Implementation Physiological Integrity: Basic Care and Comfort
16.5 A client asks the nurse about the abnormal growth changes related to acromegaly. The best response by the nurse would be: a. "These changes lead to severe disability and death if untreated."	Answer: d Rationale: The increased growth of bone and connective tissue occurs gradually and is not reversible. Treatment of the hypersecretion may stop growth, but will not reverse growth that has occurred. The changes may cause discomfort. Application Implementation Physiological Integrity: Physiological Adaptation

© 2007 Pearson Education, Inc.

Question	Answer
b. "These changes are minimal and will cause little discomfort." c. "These changes will gradually diminish with proper treatment." d. "These changes are irreversible."	
16.6 A client with Cushing's syndrome was taught by the nurse about safety precautions to use at home. Which of the following comments indicates the client understands the instructions? a. "I will be careful not to hurt myself, since I could break a bone easily." b. "I should avoid direct sunlight to prevent my skin from developing dark patches." c. "I should get up slowly from bed or my chair because I might faint." d. "I should learn some relaxation exercise so that I do not become suicidal."	Answer: a Rationale: Cushing's disease can lead to osteoporosis, making the client vulnerable to fractures. Hypertension, not hypotension, is usually a problem. Mood swings are experienced, but client rarely is suicidal. Analysis Evaluation Physiological Integrity: Reduction of Risk Potential
16.7 A client is scheduled for transsphenoidal microsurgery for removal of a pituitary adenoma. The nurse includes which of the following preoperative instructions? a. Turn, cough, and deep breathe every 2 hours. b. The client must remain supine in bed, with sandbags alongside her head to prevent movement. c. The client may not use a toothbrush for several days after surgery to prevent injury to the surgical site. d. The client will have to take replacement growth hormone for the rest of her life.	Answer: c Rationale: Tooth brushing could disrupt the incision, which is in the roof of the mouth. Coughing increases intracranial pressure.A semi-Fowler's to Fowler's position facilitates breathing. Lifelong replacement of pituitary hormones is necessary. Application Intervention Physiological Integrity: Reduction of Risk Potential
16.8 Following a hypophysectomy for a pituitary tumor, the client is monitored for the presence of diabetes insipidus. Which finding by the nurse indicates this condition? a. hyponatremia b. large amount of dilute urine c. rise in blood pressure d. fluid retention and dependent edema	Answer: b Rationale: Diabetes insipidus results in polyuria, polydipsia, and dehydration secondary to a decreased antidiuretic hormone secretion. Hypernatremia, hypotension, and dehydration also occur. Analysis Assessment Physiological Integrity: Reduction of Risk Potential
16.9 The nurse explains that symptoms the client with hypothyroidism might experience could include: a. intolerance to cold and dry skin and menstrual dysfunction. b. weight loss, oily skin, and periorbital edema. c. intolerance to heat and lethargy and headache. d. tachycardia, hypertension, and rapid respirations.	Answer: a Rationale: Reduced thyroid hormone production results in a decrease in metabolic rate and heat production, causing cold intolerance, dry skin, weight gain, fatigue, and hypotension. Weight loss, oily skin, heat intolerance, tachycardia, and hypertension are symptoms of hyperthyroidism. Application Implementation Physiological Integrity: Physiological Adaptation

16.10 Following a thyroidectomy, the client complains to the nurse that she is having leg spasms and cramps. These symptoms may indicate:
a. postanesthesia reaction.
b. damage to the cervical nerves.
c. damage to the parathyroid glands during surgery.
d. potassium depletion.

Answer: c
Rationale: During a thyroidectomy, the parathyroid glands (which lie under the thyroid gland and regulate calcium balance) can be accidentally damaged or removed. The resulting low serum calcium could lead to tetany, reflected by the leg spasm and cramps. Anesthesia or cervical nerve damage would not cause the spasms. Hypokalemia may manifest as leg cramps, but option b is more related to the surgery.
Analysis
Assessment
Safety: Management of Care

CHAPTER 17

17.1 The client asks the nurse to explain how type 1 diabetes differs from type 2. The nurse explains that with type 2 diabetes:
a. the client depends entirely on an outside source of insulin.
b. there is decreased insulin production by the pancreas or cell resistance to the insulin produced.
c. there are insulin antibodies that destroy the beta cells in the pancreas.
d. the liver destroys the C-peptide chain of proinsulin produced by the pancreas.

Answer: b
Rationale: Type 2 diabetes is characterized by a lack of pancreatic insulin production and/or insulin resistance at the cellular level. Options a and c pertain to type 1.The liver does not destroy the insulin; it is an autoimmune reaction.
Application
Implementation
Physiological Integrity: Physiological Adaptation

17.2 A client was diagnosed as having type 2 diabetes and was treated with diet and exercise. When assisting the client with diet planning, the nurse's instructions include:
a. no substitutes can be made if using the food exchange plan.
b. the greatest number of calories should be from the protein group.
c. the meal plan can be disregarded if "dietetic" foods are used.
d. a consistent number of calories are needed each day.

Answer: d
Rationale: A consistent number of calories are needed daily based on client's ideal weight, activity level, and age. Substitutions can be done within exchange lists. The largest percentage of calories should come from carbohydrates. Dietetic foods have calories and cannot be substituted for a meal plan.
Application
Implementation
Physiolgical Integrity: Reduction of Risk Potential

17.3 A type 1 diabetic was admitted to the emergency room with an elevated temperature and urinary tract infection. The findings were 3+ acetone in the urine and blood glucose of 654 mg/dL. The nurse recognizes the client is probably experiencing:
a. hyperinsulinism.
b. diabetic ketoacidosis.
c. a Somogyi reaction.
d. nonketotic hyperosmolar syndrome.

Answer: b
Rationale: Diabetic ketoacidosis is characterized by hyperglycemia and ketosis. Hyperinsulinism involves insulin resistance by the cells. A Somogyi reaction involves a morning rise in blood sugar, precipitated by a nighttime hypoglycemic event. Option d is characterized by hyperglycemia, diuresis, and dehydration, but not ketosis.
Analysis
Assessment
Physiological Integrity: Physiological Adaptation

17.4 A client hospitalized with diabetic ketoacidosis calls the nurse and reports feeling hungry, shaky, and anxious. Which action by the nurse is most appropriate?
a. Check the client's blood pressure and pulse.
b. Call the lab to draw blood for a glucose level.

Answer: d
Rationale: An alert client with hypoglycemia should be given an immediate treatment of 15 grams of a rapid-acting sugar. A finger-stick blood sugar can be done at the bedside to check blood sugar, followed by vital signs. Glucagon is given intravenously.
Application
Implementation
Physiological Integrity: Reduction of Risk Potential

© 2007 Pearson Education, Inc.

c. Administer 10 mg glucagon intramuscularly. d. Give 6 ounces of orange juice to drink.	
17.5 The client who is self-injecting insulin was advised by the nurse to rotate injection sites because: a. it reduces the danger of nerve damage and decreases absorption. b. insulin can reach all parts of the body and be used more efficiently. c. it reduces the chance of infection and increases absorption. d. it reduces irritation to the tissues and increases absorption.	Answer: d Rationale: If the same injection sites are used repeatedly, lipodystrophy and lipoatrophy of the tissue can result, which will alter insulin absorption. Site selection affects rate of absorption; insulin will reach all body parts eventually. Nerve damage and infection are not related to rotation. Application Implementation Physiological Integrity: Reduction of Risk Potential
17.6 A diabetic client asks the nurse why it is so important to exercise several times a week. Which of the following is the best response by the nurse? a. "Exercise helps to increase blood sugar levels, so the body needs less food." b. "Exercise helps reduce high ketone levels, so the body stays healthier." c. "Exercise brings down high sugar levels, so the body needs less food." d. "Exercise increases the use of insulin in the body, so it requires less insulin."	Answer: d Rationale: Exercise reduces blood glucose levels by increasing glucose utilization by the muscles and thereby reducing the need for insulin. Comprehension Implementation Physiological Integrity: Reduction of Risk Potential
17.7 The father told the nurse that his 11-year-old child with type 1 diabetes has frequent nightmares and wakes up in the middle of the night. Which of the following is probably the cause of the nightmares? a. The child is experiencing anxiety related to the diabetes. b. The child's nightmares have nothing to do with the diabetes. c. The child may be experiencing Somogyi phenomenon, which often occurs at night. d. The child may be experiencing dawn phenomenon with blood sugar elevations.	Answer: c Rationale: The Somogyi phenomenon involves nighttime episodes of hypoglycemia, which cause tremors, restlessness, and night sweats, followed by a morning rise in blood sugar. They are a likely cause of the nightmares, rather than anxiety. Dawn phenomenon is a rise in blood sugar between 5 and 8 A.M. Analysis Assessment Physiological Integrity: Reduction of Risk Potential
17.8 A client with type 1 diabetes who has the flu calls the nurse asking what to do. The best advice by the nurse would be: a. "Measure your blood sugar and urinary ketones every two to four hours while you are sick." b. "You should not take any insulin until you are well again." c. "You should increase your insulin dose for five days, then return to the prescribed dose." d. "You should be hospitalized whenever you have the flu in case it affects your diabetes."	Answer: a Rationale: Illness increases blood glucose levels and they need to monitored closely. Insulin should be taken as usual. Hospitalization may not be necessary. Application Implementation Physiological Integrity: Reduction of Risk Potential

© 2007 Pearson Education, Inc.

Question	Answer
17.9 The nurse instructs a client with type 2 diabetes on foot care. In addition to keeping the feet clean and dry, the nurse may also offer the following advice: a. "Wear nylon socks to keep your feet warm." b. "Walk on bare feet to promote circulation." c. "File your toenails straight across. Avoid using scissors." d. "Wear open-toe shoes to avoid pressure around toenails."	Answer: c Rationale: Cutting nails straight across avoids ingrown nails. Cotton or wool socks allow perspiration to dry. Diabetics should never go barefoot and feet should be covered completely with well-fitting, comfortable shoes. Application Implementation Physiological Integrity: Reduction of Risk Potential
17.10 The physician orders 10 units regular and 40 units NPH insulin subcutaneously. The nurse prepares the injection by: a. injecting 40 units air into the NPH, 10 units air into the regular, aspirate 10 units of regular, then aspirate 40 units NPH. b. injecting air into the regular, air into the NPH, aspirating the NPH, then aspirating the regular. c. injecting air into the regular, aspirating 10 units regular, injecting air into the NPH, then aspirating 40 units NPH. d. aspirating 10 units regular, then aspirating 40 units NPH.	Answer: a Rationale: Option a describes the correct technique when mixing regular and NPH Insulins. The clear insulin is drawn up first to avoid accidentally contaminating the vial with NPH insulin. Application Implementation Physiological Integrity: Pharmacological and Parenteral Therapies

CHAPTER 18

Question	Answer
18.1 A client scheduled to have a urea breath test asks the nurse what the purpose of the test is. The nurse explains: a. "It detects the presence of bacteria that contribute to formation of peptic ulcer disease." b. "It measures the acidity of your esophagus and gastric fluids." c. "It identifies the pressure of the esophageal sphincter." d. "It is done to determine the amount of hydrochloric acid secreted by your stomach."	Answer: a Rationale: Urea breath testing is done to detect infection with *Helicobacter pylori*. Option b describes pH testing; c describes esophageal manometry; and d describes gastric analysis. Comprehension Implementation Physiological Integrity: Reduction of Risk Potential
18.2 A client is scheduled to have esophageal manometry testing. Prior to the test nursing responsibilities will include: a. medicating client with an antihistamine. b. keeping client NPO for 12 hours prior to the test. c. restricting intake to clear liquids for 4 hours prior to the test. d. ensure client has not smoked cigarettes in the past 24 hours.	Answer: d Rationale: Antacids, cholinergic and anticholinergic drugs, alcohol, and tobacco are to be avoided for 24 hours prior to the test because they may increase or decrease esophageal sphincter pressures, and interfere with test results. Fluid restrictions are not required. Application Implementation Physiological Integrity: Reduction of Risk Potential

© 2007 Pearson Education, Inc.

18.3 The nurse is caring for a client being treated for pancreatitis. Which of the following laboratory studies would best indicate the treatment is being effective: a. normal liver function tests. b. elevated amylase level. c. normal lipase level. d. decreased bilirubin level.	Answer: b Rationale: Lipase and amylase levels are increased with pancreatitis. A normal level would indicate inflammation has subsided. Liver function tests and bilirubin reflect liver and gall bladder function predominantly. Application Evaluation Physiological Integrity: Reduction of Risk Potential
18.4 A client's medical record indicates he has presence of the *H. pylori* antibody. The nurse understands the client: a. will be at increased risk for diarrhea. b. has a current or past infection with *H. pylori*. c. will not need to be medicated for gastric reflux. d. has had a recent viral infection.	Answer: b Rationale: Presence of *H. pylori* indicates a past or present infection with the bacteria. It places the client at increased risk for peptic ulcer disease and GERD may be a coexisting condition. Application Assessment Physiological Integrity: Reduction of Risk Potential
18.5 The nurse is caring for an elder client with periodontal disease and recognizes this can be a cause of: a. excessive dryness in the mouth. b. tooth loss. c. excessive craving of salty foods. d. furrows in the tongue.	Answer: b Rationale: Periodontal tissue affects supporting structures of the teeth; diseased tissue contributes to tooth loss. Decreased saliva production contributes to dryness and a decreased taste sensation, which leads to excess salt use. Furrows are usually a sign of dehydration. Application Assessment Physiological Integrity: Physiological Adaptation
18.6 A client is admitted with malnutrition. The nurse can expect laboratory studies to show: a. elevated bilirubin levels. b. elevated blood sugar. c. decreased albumin levels. d. decreased alkaline phosphate level.	Answer: c Rationale: Albumin levels reflect protein stores available in the body. Bilirubin reflects liver and biliary tract function. Blood sugar is related to diabetes and impaired insulin metabolism. Alkaline phosphate levels reflect numerous conditions including bone and liver. Application Assessment Physiological Integrity: Reduction of Risk Potential
18.7 The nurse is assigned to care for a client with cirrhosis of the liver. The nurse recognizes the client's impaired liver function will affect: a. metabolism of drugs. b. formation of hydrochloric acid. c. production of digestive enzymes. d. formation of red blood cells.	Answer: a Rationale: The liver is responsible for detoxification and metabolism of drugs. The stomach produces hydrochloric acid, and the pancreas produces digestive enzymes. Normal kidney and bone marrow function are needed for red blood cell production. Application Assessment Physiological Integrity: Physiological Adaptation
18.8 A client having complaints of right upper quadrant pain is scheduled for an ultrasound of the gallbladder. The nurse explains the test will help to identify: a. presence of gallstones. b. presence of an abdominal aneurysm. c. ability of the gallbladder to store and excrete bile. d. blockages in the common bile duct and sphincter of Oddi.	Answer: a Rationale: An ultrasound of the gallbladder can detect gallstones and help evaluate gallbladder emptying. An abdominal ultrasound would detect an abdominal aneurysm. A cholecystogram is done to check gallbladder functions of storage and excretion. An ERCP is done to explore the common bile duct and pancreatic sphincters. Application Implementation Physiological Integrity: Reduction of Risk Potential

Question	Answer
18.9 An ERCP (endoscopic retrograde cholangiopancreatomy) indicates a client has an obstruction at the sphincter of Oddi. Which of the following client symptoms does the nurse correlate to this finding? a. frequent episodes of hiccoughing b. abdominal distention c. complaints of indigestion after eating d. complaints of heartburn after eating	Answer: c Rationale: Pancreatic digestive enzymes are unable to enter the duodenum and assist with digestion. Hiccoughs are believed to be secondary to irritation of the phrenic nerve in the diaphragm. Abdominal distention can be related to many abdominal conditions. Heartburn is secondary to gastric reflux. Analysis Assessment Physiological Integrity: Physiological Adaptation
18.10 The nurse is instructing a client in preparation for a colonoscopy. The nurse explains that the client: a. will need to be NPO for 8 to 12 hours prior to the exam. b. should eat a low-residue meal the evening before the exam. c. is permitted to drink clear liquids up until the time of the exam. d. will be given a soap-suds water enema shortly before the exam.	Answer: a Rationale: Fasting is required prior to the exam. Only clear liquids are allowed for 24 hours prior to the exam. An oral bowel cleansing preparation is done the evening before the exam and a tap water enema may be given 3 to 4 hours prior to the exam; soap-suds enemas are too irritating to the bowel. Application Implementation Physiological Integrity: Reduction of Risk Potential

CHAPTER 19

Question	Answer
19.1 A client following a vegetarian diet asks a nurse what he can do to get more protein with a meal that consists of a corn tortilla and refried beans. The nurse should suggest complementary protein such as: a. lettuce and tomato salad. b. cooked spinach. c. cheese. d. raisin and oatmeal granola bar.	Answer: c Rationale: The milk, cheese, and yogurt group provides complementary proteins to meat, eggs, beans, and nuts. Options a and b are vegetables, which complement the fruit group. Oatmeal is part of the cereal, pasta, and grains group. Application Implementation Health Promotion: Prevention and/or Early Detection of Health Problems
19.2 A client visits an urgent care center and tells the nurse he has had nausea and vomiting for 3 days and thinks he has the flu. The nurse should assess the client for symptoms of: a. adequate carbohydrate intake. b. chronic fatigue. c. vitamin C deficiency. d. dehydration.	Answer: d Rationale: The loss of fluid and electrolytes though vomiting puts the client at risk for dehydration. The other options are also of concern, but not of highest priority. Analysis Assessment Physiological Integrity: Reduction of Risk Potential
19.3 During assessment of the oral cavity, the nurse notes the presence of swollen gums. The nurse teaches the client about proper oral hygiene in order to assist the client in meeting which of the following outcomes? a. Reduce risk factors for periodontal disease. b. Experience a decrease in dental caries. c. Maintain balanced nutritional intake. d. Maintain healthy oral mucous membranes.	Answer: a Rationale: Swollen gums are a risk factor for periodontal disease. Proper oral hygiene will also contribute to the other outcomes, but the assessment finding is more supportive for periodontal disease. Analysis Assessment Physiological Integrity: Reduction of Risk Potential

© 2007 Pearson Education, Inc.

Question	Answer
19.4 The physician ordered Nystatin oral suspension for a client with candidiasis. Which of the following instructions on the use of Nystatin should the nurse give to the client? a. Dilute the medication with water. b. Drink the medication through a straw. c. Swish the medication throughout the mouth and spit out the excess. d. Swish the medication throughout the mouth and swallow.	Answer: d Rationale: Nystatin is intended to be taken undiluted and swished in the mouth to provide a local, rather than systemic effect. Application Implementation Physiological Integrity: Pharmacological and Parenteral Therapies
19.5 When the nurse inspects a client's oral cavity, which of the following findings would indicate the need to evaluate the client for oral cancer? a. gingivitis b. white, curdlike patches on the mucous membranes c. velvety red patch on inner cheek d. presence of dental caries	Answer: c Rationale: Erythroplakia are slightly raised irregular red patches indicative of oral cancer. Gingivitis and dental caries are related to dental hygiene and gum irritation. White curdlike changes are seen with oral fungal infections. Analysis Assessment Health Promotion: Prevention and/or Early Detection of Health Problems
19.6 A client has an esophagogastroduodenoscopy (EGD) performed for evaluation of dysphagia. Which action by the nurse is most important in postprocedure care? a. Position the client on the left side. b. Provide mouth care with saline rinses and gargles. c. Assess for nausea and vomiting. d. Keep the client NPO until her gag reflex returns.	Answer: d Rationale: A lidocaine solution that anesthetizes the throat is instilled when the EGD is performed, putting the client at risk of aspiration if given anything oral before the gag reflex returns. Analysis Implementation Physiological Integrity: Reduction of Risk Potential
19.7 A client admitted to the emergency department with coffee-grounds emesis and melena develops sudden, severe upper abdominal pain and calls for the nurse. The client is doubled over in pain and is diaphoretic. The nurse suspects a perforated ulcer. The nurse should assess for which other signs or symptoms? a. fever and respiratory depression b. rigid, boardlike abdomen c. bowel sounds increased in frequency and pitch d. diarrhea	Answer: b Rationale: This would be indicative of peritonitis and would support suspicion of a perforated ulcer. An increased respiratory rate would be more likely. Option c would be indicative of a bowel obstruction. Diarrhea would not be suspected. Analysis Assessment Physiological Integrity: Reduction of Risk Potential
19.8 A client undergoes a gastroduodenostomy (Billroth I) for treatment of a perforated ulcer. Postoperatively the nurse cannot detect bowel sounds and there is 200 mL of bright red blood in the nasogastric (NG) drainage container. What is the most appropriate nursing action? a. Assess the client's pain level. b. Irrigate the NG tube. c. Apply an abdominal binder. d. Notify the physician.	Answer: d Rationale: The findings indicate a rupture or bleed of the suture line, necessitating immediate intervention. Assessment of pain level would be a subsequent intervention after notifying the physician. Irrigating the NG and applying a binder could cause further damage. Analysis Implementation Physiological Integrity: Basic Care and Comfort

Question	Answer
19.9 A client is recovering from a gastrojejunostomy (Billroth II) for treatment of duodenal ulcer. About 20 minutes after lunch, the client develops dizziness, weakness, palpitations, and the urge to defecate. To avoid recurrence of these symptoms, which measures does the nurse teach the client? a. Increase fluid intake with meals and lie down 30 minutes after meals. b. Eat a high-carbohydrate, low-fat diet in six small feedings a day. c. Decrease fluid intake with meals and lie down after meals. d. Drink fruit juice after each meal.	Answer: a Rationale: The symptoms indicate dumping syndrome, which is minimimized by limiting carbohydrate intake, eating small meals, drinking liquids separate from solid foods, and assuming a recumbent or semirecumbent position after meals. Analysis Assessment Physiological Integrity: Physiological Adaptation
19.10 The nurse is teaching a client with a history of upper gastrointestinal bleeding to check his stool for occult blood. Which information provided by the nurse is most accurate? a. If a client is vomiting blood, stools will not be black and tarry. b. Stools that are black and tarry occur with prolonged bleeding from the stomach or small intestine. c. Acute bleeding in the upper gastrointestinal tract will result in bright red blood in the stool. d. Blood is never obvious in the stool and must be detected by guaiac testing.	Answer: b Rationale: As the bleeding from the upper GI passes through the intestines, chemical reactions cause it to become black and tarry. Bright red rectal bleeding is indicative of lower GI bleeding. Application Implementation Health Promotion: Prevention and/or Early Detection of Health Problems

CHAPTER 20

Question	Answer
20.1 The client with diarrhea asks the nurse what he can eat, since every time he eats he has more watery stools. The nurse provides the following information: a. "It would be best to give your bowel a rest and not eat anything for 24 hours." b. "Try the 'BRAT' diet: bouillon soup, rice, applesauce, and tea." c. "Soft-boiled eggs and toast for several days should help." d. "You need to talk to the dietician about that."	Answer: a Rationale: Food should be withheld during the first 24 hours of acute diarrhea in order to rest the bowel. Following bowel rest, the BRAT diet is often recommended. A dietician would not be needed. Application Implementation Physiological Integrity: Reduction of Risk Potential
20.2 The physician has suggested that the client try Pepto-Bismol to relieve the diarrhea. The nurse might provide the following information: a. "The Pepto-Bismol will turn your stools yellow." b. "Do not take the Pepto-Bismol for longer than 48 hours." c. "Take the Pepto-Bismol once per day." d. "Take the Pepto-Bismol before meals and at bedtime."	Answer: b Rationale: Any antidiarrheal should not be taken for more than 48 hours. If diarrhea persists, the physician should be notified. Pepto-Bismol may cause tongue and stools to darken. It is best taken at onset of diarrhea and after each loose stool. Application Implementation Physiological Integrity: Reduction of Risk Potential

© 2007 Pearson Education, Inc.

Question	Answer
20.3 The nurse identifies the following priority nursing diagnosis for an elderly client experiencing diarrhea: a. Risk for Fluid Volume Excess related to diarrhea b. Potential for Impaired Skin Integrity related to diarrhea c. Risk for Imbalanced Nutrition less than Body Requirements related to diarrhea d. Risk for Dehydration related to diarrhea	Answer: d Rationale: The elderly become dehydrated quickly from loss of fluids and electrolytes, possibly leading to hypovolemic shock and metabolic acidosis. A fluid volume deficit, not excess would occur. Options b and c are also a concern, but not of highest priority. Analysis Planning Safe, Effective Care Environment: Coordinated Care
20.4 An elderly client complains to the nurse that he experiences constipation. The nurse should suggest that he consume extra: a. milk products. b. eggs. c. carrots. d. tomatoes.	Answer: c Rationale: Of the foods listed, carrots would provide the most fiber, adding bulk to the stool and reducing constipation. Application Implementation Physiological Integrity: Reduction of Risk Potential
20.5 A 57-year-old client was admitted to the emergency room with severe abdominal pain, anorexia, chills, skin pallor, a weak and thready pulse of 118, a blood pressure of 70/40, rebound tenderness, and rigidity of the abdomen. The nurse's initial action is focused on: a. treatment for shock. b. diagnostic testing with barium studies and endoscopy. c. administration of antibiotic. d. preparation for an exploratory laparoscopy.	Answer: a Rationale: The assessment findings suggest a perforated appendix with peritonitis. Stabilization of the shock will be necessary before surgery is performed. Barium studies would be contraindicated. Antibiotics would be administered after shock is treated. Application Implementation Physiological Integrity: Reduction of Risk Potential
20.6 A client had a resection of the small bowel due to obstruction. Two days postoperatively she complains of gas and abdominal distention. The nurse plans care for the client based on the knowledge that postoperative gas pain occurs as a result of: a. hypermotility of the bowel. b. impaired peristalsis. c. nasogastric suctioning. d. inflammation of the bowel at the site of the anastomosis.	Answer: b Rationale: The effect of anesthesia and manipulation of the bowel decrease peristalsis, causing gas and distention postoperatively. Bowel motility will be decreased. The NG tube does not cause the gas, but is needed until bowel motility resumes. Inflammation at the anastomosis site causes pain. Analysis Planning Physiological Integrity: Physiological Adaptation
20.8 A client is hospitalized for acute exacerbation of ulcerative colitis. The client reports 12 to 16 bloody stools per day with cramping abdominal pain. The nurse explains that the order by the physician to promote bowel rest is for the client to: a. have a nasogastric tube inserted. b. receive total parenteral nutrition (TPN) for 2 weeks. c. receive intravenous corticosteroids. d. have nothing by mouth (NPO) for several days.	Answer: b Rationale: During an acute exacerbation, TPN is given to provide nutritional support while the bowel is rested. An NG tube is not necessary. Intermittent doses of corticosteroids may be given. Being NPO for several days without another form of nutritional support is not recommended. Application Implementation Physiological Integrity: Reduction of Risk Potential

20.9 A client had a sigmoid colostomy with abdominal-perineal resection incisions. The perineal resection is partially closed and has two drains attached to Jackson-Pratt suction devices. During the early postoperative period, which goal should be given the highest nursing priority? a. providing a clear liquid diet b. promoting perineal drainage and healing c. teaching colostomy irrigation d. encouraging acceptance of the colostomy	Answer: b Rationale: Care of the wound drains and incisions is a priority to prevent complications and ensure proper wound healing. Fluids would be introduced gradually when bowel sounds have returned. Care of the colostomy will be given attention later in the postoperative recovery period. Analysis Planning Safe, Effective Care Environment: Coordinated Care
20.10 A male client had a herniorrhaphy for an incarcerated inguinal hernia. Postoperatively, the nurse identifies pain as the primary problem associated with edema of the scrotum. Which nursing intervention is appropriate for this problem? a. Elevate the scrotum on a small pillow. b. Apply moist heat to the abdomen. c. Provide warm sitz baths several times a day. d. Administer narcotics for pain.	Answer: a Rationale: Elevation of the scrotum will help to relieve edema, which is causing the pain. Moist heat and sitz baths will not relieve edema and may even increase edema. Non-narcotic pain management may be sufficient. Application Intervention Physiological Integrity: Basic Care and Comfort

CHAPTER 21

21.1 A 45-year-old client has been on oral contraceptives for 24 years. The nurse discusses the possible risk of developing: a. cholelithiasis. b. kidney stones. c. hepatitis. d. cholecystitis.	Answer: a Rationale: Use of oral contraceptives is a risk factor for development of gallstones, or cholelithiais. Application Implementation Health Promotion: Prevention and/or Early Detection of Health Problems
21.2 The nurse is caring for a client post-cholecystectomy with common duct exploration who has a t-tube. The nurse will be responsible for keeping the t-tube: a. clamped. b. patent. c. attached to continuous suction. d. covered with dressings.	Answer: b Rationale: Since the t-tube keeps the common bile duct open and promotes bile flow until edema has subsided, it needs to be kept patent. It is only clamped as ordered by the physician. It drains by gravity, not suction. Only the insertion site is covered with a dressing. Application Implementation Physiological Integrity: Reduction of Risk Potential
21.3 When caring for a client with cholecystitis, the nurse knows to place the client in which of the following positions? a. supine b. Trendelenburg c. lithotomy d. Fowler's	Answer: d Rationale: Fowler's position decreases pressure on the inflamed gallbladder and may decrease pain. Application Implementation Physiological Integrity: Basic Care and Comfort
21.4 The nurse assists the client with chronic cholecystitis to plan meals that are: a. high in calories. b. hot and high in carbohydrates. c. cold, small in quantity, and low in fats. d. cold, large in quantity, and infrequent.	Answer: c Rationale: A diet low in fat, cold, and eaten in small amounts is better tolerated and reduces stimulus for gallbladder contractions. Application Implementation Health Promotion: Prevention and/or Early Detection of Health Problems

© 2007 Pearson Education, Inc.

21.5 The physician orders a nasogastric tube (NGT) for the client with pancreatitis. The nurse explains that the purpose of the tube is:

a. relief from nausea and vomiting.
b. reduction of pancreatic secretions.
c. control of fluid and electrolyte balance.
d. removal of irritants.

Answer: b
Rationale: Keeping the client NPO and inserting an NG tube decrease enzyme production by the pancreas, allowing the organ to rest. It may relieve nausea, but that is not the main purpose of the tube. Fluid and electrolyte balance are established by intravenous fluid therapy.
Application
Implementation
Physiological Integrity: Reduction of Risk Potential

21.6 A client is admitted with pain in the right upper quadrant, jaundice, and nausea, and is diagnosed with hepatitis C. The nurse recognizes the client is in which phase of hepatitis?

a. preicteric or prodromal
b. icteric
c. posticteric
d. terminal

Answer: b
Rationale: The icteric phase is characterized by jaundice, pruritis, and clay-colored stools.
Comprehension
Assessment
Physiological Integrity: Reduction of Risk Potential

21.7 The client's ascites is severe and is causing difficulty breathing and shortness of breath. The nurse prepares the client for a paracentesis to remove excess fluid by instructing the client to:

a. lie on the right side.
b. lie on the left side.
c. empty the bladder.
d. drink nothing by mouth 12 hours prior to the procedure.

Answer: c
Rationale: The client should void immediately prior to the procedure to avoid accidental bladder puncture. The client is usually positioned in a sitting position and does not have to be NPO.
Application
Implementation
Physiological Integrity: Reduction of Risk Potential

21.8 The client with cirrhosis is given lactulose (Cephulac), which causes diarrhea. The client asks the nurse why it is necessary to take this medication. The nurse explains that the medication will:

a. prevent gastrointestinal bleeding.
b. reduce serum ammonia levels.
c. promote excess fluid loss.
d. prevent constipation.

Answer: b
Rationale: Lactulose inhibits ammonia absorption from the bowel and is also an osmotic laxative, thereby promoting excretion of ammonia.
Application
Implementation
Physiological Integrity: Pharmacological and Parenteral Therapies

---

21.9 The nurse assisted the physician with a needle biopsy of the liver. Following the procedure, which action should the nurse take?

a. Have the client lie on the right side with the bed flat.
b. Check the client's coagulation time.
c. Elevate the head of the bed.
d. Instruct the patient to avoid deep breathing to prevent liver pressure.

Answer: a
Rationale: The client is positioned on the right side, which allows client's own body weight to provide downward pressure against the liver and upward pressure from the mattress; this reduces chances of internal bleeding. Coagulation time is checked prior to the procedure. Deep breathing, but not coughing, is advised.
Application
Implementation
Physiological Integrity: Reduction of Risk Potential

21.10 An LPN had a needle-stick injury and had not been immunized for hepatitis B. The infection control nurse advises the LPN to get which of the following treatments?

a. evaluation of liver function tests in 10 days
b. hepatitis B vaccine and hepatitis B immune globulin(HBIG)
c. hepatitis B vaccine
d. hepatitis B immune globulin(HBIG)

Answer: b
Rationale: Following a needle-stick injury, both hepatitis B vaccine and HBIG are recommended as postexposure prophylaxis.
Application
Implementation
Health Promotion: Prevention and/or Early Detection of Health Problems

© 2007 Pearson Education, Inc.

CHAPTER 22

22.1 The nurse is assessing an elderly client who is 2 days postop abdominal surgery. The nurse recognizes alterations in the respiratory system of the elderly put the client at risk for: a. rib fractures. b. upper respiratory infections. c. increased vital capacity. d. pulmonary embolus.	Answer: b Rationale: Decreased mobility of the rib cage, weaker respiratory muscles, and loss of elasticity increase the risk for respiratory infections secondary to inability to clear secretions. Rib fractures could occur with trauma. Vital capacity is decreased. A pulmonary embolus would be related to alterations in the cardiovascular system. Assessment Application Physiological Integrity: Reduction of Risk Potential
22.2 A client has blood drawn for an arterial blood gas. When applying pressure to the puncture site it is important for the nurse to: a. hold the pressure for at least 60 seconds. b. hold pressure for 2 minutes or longer. c. keep the extremity elevated above the heart. d. have a tourniquet available in case bleeding does not stop.	Answer: b Rationale: Since arteries are under high pressure, they may bleed if pressure is not held for 2 to 5 minutes. It is not necessary to keep the extremity elevated or have a tourniquet available. Application Implementation Physiological Integrity: Reduction of Risk Potential
22.3 A client scheduled to have blood drawn for a serum alpha$_1$-antitrypsin level asks the nurse if any special preparation is necessary. Since the client has a history of hyperlipidemia the nurse explains: a. "A low-fat diet should be eaten for twenty-four hours prior to the test." b. "No special preparation is needed." c. "A fasting specimen will be necessary." d. "Any lipid-lowering medications should be held the day of the test."	Answer: c Rationale: Clients with elevated cholesterol or triglyceride levels need to have a fasting specimen drawn. No dietary restrictions are necessary and medications do not need to be held. Comprehension Implementation Physiological Integrity: Reduction of Risk Potential
22.4 A client scheduled for a pulmonary function test asks what is involved in the test. The nurse explains: a. "You will be asked to breathe in breathe in a specific manner and measurements are taken." b. "You will have blood drawn from an artery in your wrist." c. "A sensor is placed on your fingertip or earlobe and your oxygen levels will be measured." d. "An x-ray of your lungs is taken after a dye is injected into your vein."	Answer: a Rationale: Pulmonary function tests measure lung volumes as the client performs specific inhalation and exhalation instructions. Option b describes an arterial blood gas. Option c is pulse oximetry, and option d describes a CT of the lung. Application Implementation Physiological Integrity: Reduction of Risk Potential
22.5 A client has been given instructions on collection of a sputum specimen for analysis of mycobacterium tuberculosis. Which statement by the client indicates he understands the directions? a. "I will need to take a sedative before the secretions are suctioned." b. "They will need to collect three specimens." c. "It is best to collect a specimen after drinking warm liquids." d. "I will need to drink a radioactive dye before coughing up secretions."	Answer: b Rationale: The specimens are obtained in the early morning, upon arising. A dye is not given. Secretions may need to be suctioned if client is unable to expectorate them. Assessment Application Physiological Integrity: Reduction of Risk Potential

© 2007 Pearson Education, Inc.

Question	Answer
22.6 The nurse caring for a client who has sustained a head trauma closely monitors respirations because: a. the client will be lethargic and forget to breathe. b. the trauma may cause the client to be disoriented. c. breathing is controlled by the respiratory center in the brain. d. the client will be unable to cough and clear secretions.	Answer: c Rationale: The brain injury may have impacted chemoreceptors in the respiratory center of the brain, which controls breathing. Options b and d may be true but do not explain why respirations are monitored. Breathing is a function of the autonomic nervous system; absence would indicate a neurologic impairment. Application Implementation Physiological Integrity: Reduction of Risk Potential
22.7 When assessing the respiratory status of a client, the nurse auscultates the lungs by: a. listening for air exchange in the bronchus and anterior lobes. b. checking breath sounds in the anterior and posterior thorax. c. listening to breath sounds in the anterior and posterior lung bases. d. checking for adventitious sounds while having client cough.	Answer: b Rationale: Option b describes the correct method; all areas of the anterior and posterior lobes are checked for type of and presence of breath sounds. Application Implementation Physiological Integrity: Reduction of Risk Potential
22.8 The nurse obtains a pulse oximetry reading of 95% on a client 2 days postoperative. Which of the following actions should be taken by the nurse? a. Encourage client to do more coughing and deep breathing. b. Increase level of oxygen delivery by 1 L/min. c. Document the findings. d. Recheck the pulse oximetry after ambulating client.	Answer: c Rationale: A SA O_2 of 95% or higher indicates adequate lung ventilation and gas exchange. No further action is necessary. Application Implementation Physiological Integrity: Reduction of Risk Potential
22.9 The nurse observes the serum alpha$_1$-antitrypsin level of a client is 40 mg/dL and recognizes this reading could be influenced by which of the following client conditions? a. osteoporosis b. migraine headaches c. gastroesophageal reflux disease d. cellulitis of a lower extremity	Answer: d Rationale: Inflammatory conditions and exercise can increase the blood level of alpha$_1$-antitrypsin. Analysis Assessment Physiological Integrity: Physiological Adaptation
22.10 The nurse uses palpation of the chest in order to assess the client for: a. retractions and bulging. b. use of accessory muscles. c. tactile fremitus. d. pleural rub.	Answer: c Rationale: Tactile fremitus is palpated by noting presence of subcutaneous emphysema, felt as air pockets under the skin. Options a and b are observed. Option d is heard on auscultation. Application Assessment Physiological Integrity: Reduction of Risk Potential

CHAPTER 23

Question	Answer
23.1 When assessing a client with streptococcal pharyngitis, the nurse can expect the client to complain of pain and: a. headache. b. nausea and vomiting. c. palpitations d. dysphagia.	Answer: d Rationale: Streptococcal pharyngitis is an inflammatory condition caused by bacteria, which produces inflammation, pain, and fever; the inflammation often leads to dysphagia, or painful swallowing. Analysis Assessment Physiological Integrity: Physiological Adaptation

© 2007 Pearson Education, Inc.

23.2 The client with chronic rhinitis asks the nurse why he cannot use his nasal spray as often as he needs. The nurse's best response is: a. "Continuous use of nasal spray causes nosebleeds." b. "Continuous use causes rebound congestion, which increases frequency of use." c. "Prolonged use of nasal spray dries the nasal mucosa." d. "Too much medication is absorbed through the mucosa and has a systemic effect on the circulation."	Answer: b Rationale: Rebound congestion can occur when decongestant nasal sprays are used for more than 3 to 5 days. Increased congestion results in excessive and more frequent use of the nasal spray. Application Implementation Physiological Integrity: Pharmacological and Parenteral Therapies
23.3 The nurse is preparing a client for discharge who has had endoscopic sinus surgery for obstruction. The nurse instructs the client: a. "Sleep on your back or in a semireclining position only." b. "Irrigate your sinuses with warm saline solution." c. "Avoid blowing your nose and strenuous exercising for a week." d. "Sneeze with your mouth closed."	Answer: c Rationale: These restrictions will reduce the chance of disrupting the surgical site and maintain patency of the sinuses. Sleep position is not restricted. A humidifier or saline spray is recommended. The mouth should be open when sneezing. Application Implementation Physiological Integrity: Reduction of Risk Potential
23.4 The nurse is caring for a patient who develops epistaxis. Which of the following nursing interventions is advisable? a. Have the client tilt his head back and hold pressure to the nose by pinching the nares toward the septum. b. Apply heat to the client's nose. c. Have the client tilt the head forward and apply pressure by pinching the nares toward the septum. d. Have the client lie supine and place ice packs to the forehead.	Answer: c Rationale: Leaning forward drains blood into the nasopharynx and reduces the chance of swallowing blood. Applying pressure at the nares reduces bleeding. Ice packs to the nose and forehead cause vasoconstriction, helping to reduce bleeding. A sitting, not supine, position decreases blood flow to the head. Application Implementation Physiological Integrity: Reduction of Risk Potential
23.5 The nurse provides discharge teaching to a client with laryngitis. Which of the following statements by the client indicates an understanding of the instruction? a. "I should massage my throat to stimulate the vocal cords." b. "I can speak as much as I want as long as it is not painful." c. "I should rest my voice by not speaking." d. "I can whisper but not speak in a regular voice."	Answer: c Rationale: Speaking aggravates and prolongs the inflammation of laryngitis. Massaging would not help. Whispering strains the vocal cords. Analysis Evaluation Physiological Integrity: Reduction of Risk Potential
23.6 A postoperative laryngectomy and radical neck dissection client has a nursing diagnosis of Impaired Verbal Communication. Which of the following interventions should be included in the care plan? a. Provide uninterrupted time for the client to attempt communication with the nurse and health care team.	Answer: d Rationale: This provides client with an easy and immediate means of communication. The client will be unable to speak until alternate methods of speech are established. Application Intervention Physiological Integrity: Physiological Adaptation

 © 2007 Pearson Education, Inc.

Question	Answer
b. Instruct the client to speak softly when talking. c. Teach the client to read lips. d. Provide the client with a pen and paper for writing.	
23.7 When caring for clients who have had a tonsillectomy, the nurse should monitor closely for which of the following complications: a. throat pain and headache b. temperature elevation of 100.6°F c. nausea and vomiting d. hemorrhage	Answer: d Rationale: All of the problems listed are possible following a tonsillectomy, but hemorrhage constitutes an emergency. Analysis Assessment Physiological Integrity: Reduction of Risk Potential
23.8 The nurse monitors a client with suspected nasal bone fractures for cerebrospinal fluid leakage by: a. checking nasal or ear drainage for glucose. b. checking the nasal drainage for blood. c. determining the amount of postnasal drainage. d. gently palpating nose for presence of crepitus.	Answer: a Rationale: Cerebrospinal fluid tests positive for glucose. Postnasal drainage cannot be measured. Crepitus is the grating sound from the bone fracture. Analysis Assessment Physiological Integrity: Reduction of Risk Potential
23.9 A cyanotic client with an unknown diagnosis is admitted to the emergency department. In relation to oxygen, the first nursing action would be to: a. not administer oxygen unless ordered by the physician. b. administer oxygen at a flow of 6 L/min and check O_2 sats. c. wait until the client's STAT lab work is completed. d. administer oxygen at a flow of 2 L/min.	Answer: d Rationale: Oxygenation is a priority for the cyanotic client; oxygen delivered at 2 L/min is a safe amount to give until labs are obtained. Application Implementation Physiological Integrity: Physiological Adaptation
23.10 A postoperative client with a tracheostomy requires tracheal suctioning. The first intervention in completing this procedure would be to: a. change the tracheostomy dressing. b. deflate the tracheal cuff. c. perform oral or nasal suctioning. d. provide humidity with a trach mask.	Answer: c Rationale: This reduces the chance of secretions entering the trachea when the cuff is deflated. Humidity is applied in between suctioning. Dressing is applied after suctioning is done. Application Implementation Physiological Integrity: Reduction of Risk Potential

CHAPTER 24

Question	Answer
24.1 A client with tuberculosis has been on drug therapy for several months, but his sputum is still positive for tuberculosis bacilli. It would be most important for the nurse to ask which of the following questions? a. "When did you last take your medications?" b. "Have you had any reaction to your medications?" c. "Are you feeling better now that you are taking medicine?" d. "Have you taken all of your medicines as prescribed?"	Answer: d Rationale: This would best help to determine if client has stopped taking the medication all together or has been skipping doses, since three to four medications need to be taken for 6 to 12 months to effectively treat tuberculosis. Application Assessment Physiological Integrity: Reduction of Risk Potential

24.2 The nurse is caring for a client admitted with pneumonia. Which of the following assessment findings would provide the most accurate information about the type of pneumonia the client has? a. productive cough with large amounts of rust-colored sputum b. client's complaint of chest pain c. client's complaint of shortness of breath d. temperature of 38.3°C (101°F)	Answer: a Rationale: The various types of pneumonia differ in onset, character of cough, presence of fever, and pain. The specific finding of rust-colored sputum is indicative of pneumococcal pneumonia. Shortness of breath and low-grade fever are seen with various other types of pneumonia. Analysis Assessment Physiological Integrity: Physiological Adaptation
24.3 A client informs the nurse he is having pleuritic pain. Before documenting this complaint, the nurse should verify if the pain: a. increases with expiration. b. is constant along the costal borders. c. increases with deep breathing. d. subsides when client coughs.	Answer: c Rationale: Pleuritic pain is sharp and stabbing, aggravated by deep breathing, coughing, and movement. Analysis Assessment Physiological Integrity: Physiological Adaptation
24.4 The nurse assesses a client suspected of having chronic bronchitis. It would be most important for the nurse to question the client about which of the following? a. pain location b. medication history c. occupation history d. characteristics of the cough	Answer: d Rationale: Chronic bronchitis is manifested by persistent, productive cough. Pain is not always present. Medications do not usually induce or cause bronchitis. Occupations may be a risk factor, although the primary cause is smoking. Analysis Assessment Health Promotion: Prevention and/or Early Detection of Health Problems
24.5 The nurse instructs the client with chronic obstructive pulmonary disease (COPD) to practice pursed-lip breathing and explains that this breathing technique is done: a. to prolong exhalation to help remove carbon dioxide from the lungs. b. to prolong inhalation to help bring more oxygen to the lungs. c. to use the abdominal muscles to breathe, giving the diaphragm a rest. d. to break up mucus that has accumulated in the airway.	Answer: a Rationale: The alveoli become less elastic and tend to collapse with expiration, causing air to be trapped in the lungs. Expiration, not inspiration is prolonged. Use of abdominal muscles improves diaphragmatic movement. It does not help to break up mucus. Application Implementation Physiological Integrity: Reduction of Risk Potential
24.6 A client has just been diagnosed with a pulmonary embolism. The nurse anticipates the physician will order which of the following medication therapies? a. antibiotic therapy b. bronchodilator and nebulizer treatments c. heparin therapy d. nitroglycerin therapy	Answer: c Rationale: Anticoagulation therapy is initiated to prevent further clotting and embolization. Application Implementation Physiological Integrity: Reduction of Risk Potential
24.7 The nurse auscultates crackles at the bases of the lungs of a client with adult respiratory distress syndrome (ARDS). The nurse knows that these adventitious lung sounds are due to: a. mucus in the airways. b. constriction of the airways. c. hyperinflated alveoli. d. fluid in the alveoli.	Answer: d Rationale: Massive inflammation damages the alveolar capillary membranes, allowing plasma and blood cells to leak into the alveoli. Application Assessment Physiological Integrity: Physiological Adaptation

 © 2007 Pearson Education, Inc.

24.8 A client is brought in with a gunshot wound to the chest. The nurse assesses for tension pneumothorax. What signs and symptoms of tension pneumothorax can the nurse expect to find? a. deviated trachea b. high blood pressure c. wheezes in all lung fields d. audible sucking sounds on inspiration	Answer: a Rationale: As air enters the pleural space, it is unable to escape and accumulates, causing collapse of the lung on the affected side and shifting of the heart, trachea, and esophagus to the unaffected side. Analysis Assessment Physiological Integrity: Physiological Adaptation
24.9 The nurse assesses the client's chest tube drainage system. Which of the following findings should be reported to the physician? a. serosanguinous drainage in the collection chamber b. bubbling in the water seal chamber when the client coughs c. bubbling in the suction control chamber d. fluid in the water seal chamber that rises and falls with respirations	Answer: b Rationale: This indicates a leak in the closed drainage system. Serosanguinous drainage is normal. Options c and d are normal or expected findings. Application Assessment Physiological Integrity: Reduction of Risk Potential
24.10 The nurse caring for a client admitted with a diagnosis of suspected lung cancer might expect to find which of the following on assessment? a. hemoptysis b. night sweats c. dysphagia d. cyanosis	Answer: a Rationale: Coughing up blood is a common sign of lung cancer. Night sweats are seen with tuberculosis. Dysphagia is common with disorders of the throat. Cyanosis is a sign of impaired gas exchange, secondary to many respiratory and cardiac conditions. Comprehension Assessment Physiological Integrity: Physiological Adaptation

Chapter 25

25.1 A client with a history of deep venous thrombosis (DVT) is seen in the clinic. Since the client is planning a long airplane flight, the nurse instructs the client to: a. restrict intake of fluids during the flight. b. perform isometric exercises of the lower extremities every 2 hours. c. do deep-breathing exercises every hour while awake. d. keep the lower extremities elevated as much as possible during the flight	Answer: b Rationale: Contraction of the skeletal muscles will help to open valves in the veins and propel blood back to the heart, thereby preventing stasis of blood. Fluids should be encouraged. Deep breathing will not help to promote venous return of blood. Keeping the legs elevated will help some, but does not provide the pumping action that isometric exercise would. Application Implementation Physiological Integrity: Reduction of Risk Potential
25.2 The nurse is performing a cardiovascular assessment on an elderly client. Which of the following findings should be reported to the charge nurse? a. presence of bruising on upper extremities b. sparse hair growth on lower extremities c. weak, thready, irregular pulse d. thin, pale facial hair	Answer: c Rationale: It is not unusual for the elderly to have irregular beats, but the pulse should not be weak and thready. The other findings are normal for an elderly client. Application Assessment Physiological Integrity: Physiological Adaptation

Question	Answer
25.3 A client being seen in the office is scheduled to have an ankle-brachial index test. When the client asks what the purpose of the test is, the nurse explains that it: a. measures the pressure of varicose veins. b. will determine if atherosclerosis is present. c. measures cardiac ejection fraction. d. predicts the likelihood of developing hypertension.	Answer: b Rationale: The ankle-brachial index test provides information of circulation to the lower extremities and helps to identify changes caused by atherosclerosis. It does not provide information about venous pressure, ejection fraction, or hypertension. Comprehension Implementation Physiological Integrity: Reduction of Risk Potential
25.4 A client with chest pain is seen in the emergency department and is scheduled for blood work to check his heart damage. The nurse anticipates which of the following laboratory studies will be ordered? a. creantine kinase (CK) b. cardiac muscle troponin c. B-naturetic peptide (BNP) d. atrial nuturetic factor (ANF)	Answer: b Rationale: Cardiac muscle troponin is a sensitive indicator of heart muscle damage. CK is more general, found in both cardiac and skeletal muscle. ANF and BNP are more indicative of heart failure. Comprehension Planning Physiological Integrity: Reduction of Risk Potential
25.5 The nurse instructs the client scheduled to have blood drawn for a C-reactive protein level to do which of the following prior to the test? a. Fast for 8 hours prior to the test. b. No special fasting or preparation is required. c. Restrict intake of caffeine containing products 24 hours prior to the test. d. Hold any cardiac medication for 24 hours prior to the test.	Answer: b Rationale: No special preparation is necessary. Application Implementation Physiological Integrity: Reduction of Risk Potential
25.6 A client has returned to the nursing unit following a transesophageal echocardiogram (TEE). Nursing responsibilities include: a. keeping client sedated for the remainder of the shift. b. removing chest electrodes and checking for skin irritation. c. checking for return of a gag reflex. d. encouraging client to drink 8 ounces of water every hour.	Answer: c Rationale: Since the client is sedated during the procedure, presence of a gag reflex must be determined prior to resuming fluid or food intake. Further sedation is not necessary. A transducer is mounted endoscopically in the esophagus; electrodes are not applied. Application Implementation Physiological Integrity: Reduction of Risk Potential
25.7 A client being seen in the outpatient clinic has had a radionuclear scan of the heart. Upon discharge the client should be instructed to: a. increase fluid intake to 2000 mL in 24 hours. b. avoid close physical contact with others for 24 hours. c. return in 24 hours for follow up x-rays. d. dispose of urine in specially provided containers.	Answer: a Rationale: Fluids are encouraged in order to promote excretion of the radioactive dye from the kidneys and body, thereby reducing contrast-induced renal failure. The amount of radioactive substance is very small and special exposure precautions are not needed. Follow-up x-rays are not done. Application Implementation Physiological Integrity: Reduction of Risk Potential

© 2007 Pearson Education, Inc.

Question	Answer
25.8 A client is being sent home with a 24-hour Holter monitor device. The nurse instructs the client to: a. change the chest electrodes every 4 hours. b. record any unusual symptoms you may experience. c. remove the Holter monitor when sleeping. d. avoid drinking any alcoholic beverages.	Answer: b Rationale: Activity and unusual symptoms should be recorded in order to provide a record to correlate with the ECG tracings. Electrodes are only changed if needed. The monitor is kept on the entire 24 hours. Food and beverage restrictions are not indicated. Application Implementation Physiological Integrity: Reduction of Risk Potential
25.9 A client tells the nurse his recent blood work indicated his high density lipids (HDLs) were 40 mg/dL and asks if this is a "good level"? The nurse should respond: a. "You should ask your primary care provider to explain the results." b. "That is a good level. You must be eating healthy." c. "It is desirable to have a level above 60 mg/dL." d. "HDLs should be lower than your cholesterol level."	Answer: c Rationale: This provides the most accurate statement. HDL levels are generally lower than the total cholesterol level, but option d does not provide the best answer. Deferring to the primary care provider does not answer the client's question, although client should be encouraged to discuss the results of the entire lipid profile. Analysis Implementation Physiological Integrity: Reduction of Risk Potential
25.10 Before an electron beam computed tomography (EBCT) study is done, the nurse needs to determine if the client: a. is pregnant. b. has an allergy to iodine or shellfish. c. has any metal implants. d. is taking any antihypertensive medications.	Answer: a Rationale: This test, which is done to detect calcium deposits in the coronary arteries, can be harmful to a fetus and is contraindicated if pregnant. Application Assessment Physiological Integrity: Reduction of Risk Potential

CHAPTER 26

Question	Answer
26.1 A client admitted with chest pain is being evaluated for a myocardial infarction (MI). Which of the following comments made by the client would best indicate the pain is angina rather than an MI? a. "The pain went away when I took a nap." b. "I took nitroglycerin but the pain was not relieved." c. "I was very short of breath and sweating with the pain." d. "The pain started when I was watching television."	Answer: a Rationale: Anginal pain is usually relieved by rest and/or nitroglycerin. A MI is usually not relieved by nitroglycerin and often is accompanied by shortness of breath and diaphoresis. Unstable angina may occur at rest, but option a is the best indicator. Analysis Assessment Physiological Integrity: Physiological Adaptation
26.2 The nurse is checking the laboratory results on a client suspected of having a myocardial infarction (MI). Which of the following would provide the most specific information for this diagnosis? a. low density lipids (LDLs) b. CK-MB c. AST and ALT d. C-reactive protein	Answer: b Rationale: Creatinine kinase-MB is the most specific for diagnosis of a MI; CK levels rise rapidly following the event and the MB fraction is specific to the heart muscle. LDLs identify a risk factor for coronary artery disease (CAD). AST and ALT are more specific to the liver. C-reactive protein indicates inflammation and is another screening test for CAD risk. Application Assessment Physiological Integrity: Reduction of Risk Potential

26.3 The nurse is teaching a client with angina about taking nitroglycerin (NTG) tablets. The nurse instructs the client to: a. take the tablet with a large glass of water. b. place a tablet under the tongue as soon as chest pain starts. c. call 911 if pain is not relieved after taking one pill. d. discard any tablets if produce a tingling sensation.	Answer: b Rationale: NTG should be taken as soon as pain begins and is placed sublingually. If no relief is obtained after taking three tablets, then emergency help is sought. A tingling sensation is normal. Application Implementation Physiological Integrity: Pharmacological and Parenteral Therapies
26.4 A female client with coronary heart disease asks the nurse, "How will I know if I am having a heart attack if the symptoms are different for women?" The nurse informs the client that women's symptoms may differ in the following way: a. "Women usually do not become short of breath." b. "The pain is not always precipitated by activity." c. "The pain is often experienced as nausea and heartburn." d. "Fatigue and weakness in the lower extremities often occurs just before the chest pain."	Answer: c Rationale: Chest pain in females is often atypical; it may be silent, experienced as epigastric pain and nausea. It can occur when resting. Shortness of breath is common as well as fatigue and weakness of the shoulders and upper arms. Analysis Implementation Physiological Integrity: Reduction of Risk Potential
26.5 When caring for a client who has just experienced an acute myocardial infarction (MI), the nurse places highest priority on which of the following nursing diagnoses: a. Acute Pain b. Ineffective Coping: Denial c. Anxiety d. Ineffective Breathing Pattern	Answer: a Rationale: Reduction of cardiac workload is essential to protect cardiac muscle cells from further damage; relief of pain will also help to reduce anxiety and improve breathing. Denial may initially help to ease anxiety as well and is a normal coping skill in the early stage. Application Planning Physiological Integrity: Reduction of Risk Potential
26.6 A client with coronary artery disease (CAD) is having frequent premature ventricular contractions (PVCs) and dysrhythmias. It is most important for the nurse to: a. administer prn antianxiety medications. b. maintain client on complete bed rest. c. document the ECG rhythm hourly. d. maintain patency of the intravenous line.	Answer: d Rationale: Many drugs used to treat dysrhythmias must be given intravenously; an existing line must be available in an emergency. The other options may be indicated, but bed rest is not always necessary. Application Implementation Physiological Integrity: Reduction of Risk Potential
26.7 Blood work done to identify risk factors for coronary heart disease reveals a client has elevated cholesterol and low density lipid (LDL) levels. The nurse should make the following suggestions for changes in dietary habits: a. Switch from whole milk to skim milk. b. Eliminate all red meat from the diet. c. Eliminate all simple sugars from the diet. d. Avoid eating eggs or any foods prepared with eggs.	Answer: a Rationale: This offers a realistic option and reduces saturated fat, which contributes to cholesterol and lipid production. Total abstinence from meat is not necessary; the total intake of cholesterol should be less than 25% to 30% of total daily calories. Simple sugars contribute to elevation of triglyceride levels. It is recommended to restrict eggs to two per week. Application Implementation Physiological Integrity: Reduction of Risk Potential

© 2007 Pearson Education, Inc.

Question	Answer
26.8 A client is started on "statin" therapy for reduction of high cholesterol. When the client ask why he needs to have blood work done routinely to monitor his liver functions, the nurse explains: a. "The drugs have been known to cause hepatitis in some people." b. "All drugs are metabolized in the liver and it is just a safe practice." c. "The drugs inhibit cholesterol synthesis in the liver and may produce harmful effects." d. "It helps to monitor the response of the drug."	Answer: c Rationale: Because they affect a chemical pathway in the liver, damage can occur to liver cells, which is reflected by abnormal liver function tests. Application Implementation Physiological Integrity: Reduction of Risk Potential
26.9 The nurse is teaching a community class on cardiopulmonary resuscitation (CPR) and discusses sudden cardiac death. The nurse informs the group that: a. CPR must be initiated within 8 to 10 minutes of a cardiac arrest. b. automatic electrical defribillators (AED) should only be used in health care settings. c. the risk of sudden cardiac death is greatest 6 to 18 months after having an MI. d. only people with coronary heart disease are at risk of having a cardiac arrest.	Answer: c Rationale: This is a correct statement. CPR should be initiated within 2 to 4 minutes. AEDs are available in public places and can be used by non–health care people. Anyone could have a cardiac arrest. Application Implementation Physiological Integrity: Reduction of Risk Potential
26.10 A client with a complete heart block receives a permanent pacemaker. Which of the following discharge instructions should be given by the nurse? a. "Do not fly on commercial airplanes as long as you have the pacemaker." b. "You will be taught to take your pulse, and should check it daily when you get home." c. "Do not use a microwave to cook your food even if you stand 10 feet from the oven." d. "Do not use your right arm for six weeks to avoid injury to the pacemaker incision."	Answer: b Rationale: It is important to monitor the pulse and report a pulse rate greater or lesser than five beats of the preset pulse. Airplane flights are not restricted. Microwaves may be used as long as proper distance is maintained. Restriction of movement is only for 24 hours. Application Implementation Physiological Integrity: Reduction of Risk Potential

CHAPTER 27

Question	Answer
27.1 A 78-year-old client is admitted with a diagnosis of left-sided congestive heart failure. When assessing the client, what signs and symptoms can the nurse expect to find? a. peripheral dependent edema and bradycardia b. signs of fluid volume deficit, hypokalemia, and hypernatremia c. dyspnea, orthopnea, and cough d. enlarged liver, venous congestion, and distended neck veins	Answer: c Rationale: Manifestations of left-sided heart failure are the result of pulmonary congestion and decreased cardiac output. Impaired left ventricular emptying causes a backup of fluids in the pulmonary vascular system. Peripheral edema, liver congestion, and distended neck veins are seen with right-sided failure. Signs of fluid volume excess, not deficit, would be seen. Application Assessment Physiological Integrity: Physiological Adaptation

Question	Answer
27.2 The nurse is teaching a client recently started on digitalis preparation the signs and symptoms of toxicity. The client is instructed to notify the physician if he experiences: a. vision disturbances, abdominal cramps, and pulse above 80. b. anorexia, nausea, malaise, and blurred vision. c. anorexia, anxiety, and pulse rate below 70. d. loss of night vision, anxiety, and leg cramps.	Answer: b Rationale: Signs and symptoms of digoxin toxicity include palpitations, abdominal pain, anorexia, nausea, weakness, irregular heart rate and/or slow heart rate, and blurred, colored, or double vision. Analysis Assessment Physiological Integrity: Pharmacological and Parenteral Therapies
27.3 In caring for a client with rheumatic heart disease, the nurse knows that priority interventions will be to: a. administer cardiotonic and diuretic medications. b. promote bed rest and administer scheduled antibiotics. c. schedule regular exercise periods and administer narcotics as ordered. d. administer oxygen and tranquilizers as ordered.	Answer: b Rationale: Activity is restricted to decrease stress on the heart, and antibiotics are needed to eliminate the streptococcal infection. Cardiotonics and oxygen are not part of the treatment generally. Anti-inflammatory drugs are given to treat the inflammation and pain. Application Implementation Physiological Integrity: Reduction of Risk Potential
27.4 A client is diagnosed with mitral insufficiency, and the nurse detects a murmur with a musical quality over the apex of the heart. The nurse recognizes this is caused by: a. regurgitation of blood from the left ventricle into the left atrium. b. enlargement of the right ventricle due to increased pressure in the right atrium. c. regurgitation of blood from the right ventricle into the right atrium. d. regurgitation of blood from the aorta into the left ventricle.	Answer: a Rationale: Mitral insufficiency involves the mitral valve, located between the left atrium and left ventricle. Comprehension Assessment Physiological Integrity: Physiological Adaptation
27.5 A client with a history of rheumatic heart disease is being evaluated for mitral stenosis. To identify symptoms that support the diagnosis of mitral stenosis, the nurse should ask which of the following questions? a. "How often do you get short of breath?" b. "Do you have to urinate often during the night?" c. "Have you had a lot of headaches recently?" d. "Do you experience numbness or tingling in your extremities?"	Answer: a Rationale: Dyspnea on exertion is often an early sign of mitral stenosis. The other options would be indicative of mitral stenosis. Application Implementation Physiological Integrity: Physiological Adaptation

 © 2007 Pearson Education, Inc.

Question	Answer
27.6 The nurse is providing discharge teaching to a client with cardiomyopathy. The nurse instructs the client that he must: a. maintain a daily intake of vegetables high in vitamin K. b. avoid strenuous activity and allow time for rest periods. c. take Vitamin B_{12} supplements daily. d. keep the lower extremities elevated whenever sitting.	Answer: b Rationale: Strenuous physical activity may precipitate dysrhythmias and/or sudden cardiac death. Dietary and sodium restriction may help to reduce symptoms, but vitamin K and B_{12} are not recommended. Keeping extremities elevated helps to reduce dependent edema, but is not the highest priority to teach. Application Implementation Physiological Integrity: Reduction of Risk Potential
27.7 A client has been treated with a cardiac glycoside and diuretics for congestive heart failure (CHF). The nurse determines the treatment has been successful when the client experiences: a. weight loss. b. an increase in energy level. c. clear lung sounds. d. improved level of consciousness.	Answer: c Rationale: Successful treatment of CHF is indicated by absence of the symptoms of pulmonary congestion. Weight loss, increased energy, and improved mental state may occur without improvement of the CHF. Analysis Assessment Physiological Integrity: Pharmacological and Parenteral Therapies
27.8 The nurse is preparing a client for discharge who has had an artificial valve placement and will be taking an oral anticoagulant. The nurse instructs the client to: a. "Use only electric toothbrushes." b. "Avoid taking acetaminophen (Tylenol) while on the medication." c. "Take your pulse every day at the same time." d. "Wear a Medic-Alert bracelet indicating your medication."	Answer: d Rationale: The bracelet informs others that client is on an anticoagulant and alerts them to potential risks of bleeding. Soft toothbrushes may be used. ASA and NSAIDS should be avoided. The pulse does not have to be checked. Application Implementation Physiological Integrity: Reduction of Risk Potential
27.9 When obtaining a nursing history on a client with myocarditis, the nurse should question the client about: a. prior use of beta blockers for treatment of hypertension. b. a recent viral infection. c. a recent streptococcal infection. d. a history of coronary heart disease (CAD).	Answer: b Rationale: Myocarditis frequently occurs following a viral, bacterial, or protozoal infection. Beta blockers and CAD are not precipitating factors. Streptococcal infections usually lead to rheumatic heart disease. Application Implementation Physiological Integrity: Physiological Adaptation
27.10 A client with rheumatic heart disease is concerned she will need to take antibiotics for the rest of her life. The nurse explains that antibiotic prophylaxis: a. will be required whenever she has dental care. b. is not necessary in adults, only children. c. needs to be taken if the client travels abroad. d. is only needed if client is malnourished or underweight.	Answer: a Rationale: Antibiotic prophylaxis is needed with any dental work or invasive procedure to prevent bacterial endocarditis, irregardless of nutritional state. Antibiotics may be recommended for travel, depending on countries to be visited. Application Implementation Physiological Integrity: Reduction of Risk Potential

CHAPTER 28

Question	Answer
28.1 During early treatment, the client with hypertension experienced postural hypotension. The nurse can minimize symptoms of this problem by instructing the client to: a. rise slowly when changing from sitting or lying positions. b. limit Na in the diet. c. increase fluid intake. d. lie down for 1 hour after taking antihypertensive medications.	Answer: a Rationale: Changing positions slowly allows for adjustment of vascular smooth muscle and ensures safety. Limiting sodium may help to reduce the blood pressure and maintain it at appropriate levels. Increasing fluids may be contraindicated. Postural hypotension can occur at any time, not just an hour after taking the med. Application Implementation Physiological Integrity: Reduction of Risk Potential
28.2 The nurse instructs clients with hypertension to drink beverages with caffeine (coffee, tea, cola drinks) in moderation because caffeine causes: a. accumulation of plaque in blood vessels. b. hardening of the arteries. c. constriction of blood vessels. d. dilation of blood vessels.	Answer: c Rationale: Caffeine causes vasoconstriction, causing an increase in peripheral vascular resistance, which will increase the workload of the heart and increase blood pressure. Comprehension Implementation Physiological Integrity: Reduction of Risk Potential
28.3 The nursing assessment determines that a client has hypertension risk factors. The most significant risk factor(s) include: a. maternal grandmother died of complications related to malignant hypertension. b. client smokes two packs of cigarettes per day and is obese. c. client only exercises three times per weeks and is 15 pounds overweight. d. client is a manager at Microsoft.	Answer: b Rationale: Smoking and obesity present two risk factors, both of which will increase workload of heart. The other options identify only one risk factor each: genetics, decreased activity, and stress. Analysis Assessment Health Promotion: Prevention and/or Early Detection of Health Problems
28.4 In management of a newly diagnosed, low-risk client with hypertension, the nurse understands that the initial treatment generally consists of: a. aggressive treatment with diuretics, beta blockers, and 1,000-calorie diet. b. restriction of fluid and sodium intake. c. dietary management; exercise regimen; and stress reduction. d. lifestyle modification and a diuretic medication.	Answer: c Rationale: Lifestyle modification of diet, exercise, and stress managment for up to 1 year is initially recommended. When that is unsuccessful, medications are added. Analysis Planning Physiological Integrity: Reduction of Risk Potential
28.5 A client with PVD tells the nurse that even short walks cause leg pain and muscle cramps. The nurse recommends to the client: a. "Stop and rest when your legs start to hurt." b. "Wear elastic hose to prevent the leg pain." c. "Take pain medication before you go walking." d. "You might try using an exercise bicycle instead of walking."	Answer: a Rationale: The pain is secondary to a reduction in blood flow and is relieved by rest. Elastic hose promote venous return; leg pain is caused by arterial ischemia. Pain medications will not provide oxygen and blood supply to the muscles, which is needed. An exercise bike may also precipitate the pain. Application Implementation Physiological Integrity: Basic Care and Comfort

 © 2007 Pearson Education, Inc.

28.6 The nurse prepares to discharge a client with deep venous thrombophlebitis. Which information does the nurse include in the teaching plan? a. Bed rest should be maintained to prevent pulmonary emboli. b. Sitting instead of standing relieves pressure on the veins. c. Thromboembolism device (TED) hose should be worn to prevent venous stasis. d. Venous circulation is improved by decreasing activity.	Answer: c Rationale: TED hose promotes venous return to the heart by gently compressing the extremities. Bed rest would not be necessary after discharge and contraindicated, because activity is needed to promote venous circulation. Sitting would promote venous stasis also. Analysis Planning Physiological Integrity: Reduction of Risk Potential
28.7 When performing a circulatory system assessment, the nurse suspects the client has a total arterial occlusion based on the following findings: a. Extremity suddenly became white, cold, and painful. b. Client complained of absence of sensation or ability to move the extremity. c. Client complained of pain and numbness in the extremity. d. Extremity became deep red and cool to touch.	Answer: b Rationale: The sudden onset of symptoms with coldness, pallor, and pain suggest an arterial thrombus or emboli. The other options describe signs and symptoms of impaired blood flow or neurovascular function. Application Implementation Physiological Integrity: Physiological Adaptation
28.8 When caring for a client with Raynaud's disease, the nurse provides the following instructions: a. Restrict your fluid intake to <1,500 mL of liquids daily. b. Wear gloves and warm socks during cold weather. c. Engage in high activity and stressful situations to promote circulation. d. Drink red wine because it is a vasodilator and would be helpful.	Answer: b Rationale: Symptoms of Raynaud's occur after exposure to cold; the extremities should be kept warm and protected from injury. Fluids should be encouraged, not restricted. Excessive exercise could precipitate an event of vasospasm. Alcohol will not help to relieve the vasospasms. Application Implementation Physiological Integrity: Reduction of Risk Potential
28.9 A client with surgical repair with synthetic graft of an abdominal aortic aneurysm develops bruising of the scrotum and penis. The nurse's findings may indicate: a. altered renal perfusion. b. expected postoperative signs and symptoms. c. disruption of the graft anastomosis. d. accumulation of fluid in the perineum.	Answer: c Rationale: Bruising of the scrotum, perineum, or penis is indicative of a graft leakage and must be reported immediately. Analysis Assessment Physiological Integrity: Physiological Adaptation
28.10 A client being discharged following treatment for a deep venous thrombosis (DVT), will be taking warfarin (Coumadin) at home. The nurse instructs the client to: a. "Avoid drinking any alcohol while taking this med." b. "Include a lot of dark green leafy vegetables in your diet." c. "If you miss a dose of the drug, wait until the next day to take the next dose." d. "Use over-the-counter anti-inflammatory drugs for pain or a headache."	Answer: a Rationale: Alcohol, ASA, and NSAIDs interact with Coumadin and can prolong bleeding times. Green leafy vegetables are high in vitamin K and will also prolong bleeding times with Coumadin. If a dose is missed, the pill should be taken as soon as possible. Application Implementation Physiological Integrity: Pharmacologic and Parenteral Therapies

Chapter 29

Question	Answer
29.1 It is reported a client has leukocytosis. When checking the laboratory results, the nurse will expect to find: a. white blood cell count is less than 5,000/mm^3. b. white blood cell count is greater than 10,000/mm^3. c. eosinophil count is less than 5%. d. neutrophil count is greater than 50%.	Answer: b Rationale: Leukocytosis reflects an elevated WBC; normal is 5,000 to 10,000 mm^3. A normal eosinophil count is 1% to 3%. A normal neutrophil count is 60% to 70%. Comprehension Assessment Physiological Integrity: Reduction of Risk Potential
29.2 When checking laboratory values, the nurse notes the client's platelet count is 100,000 mm^3. The nurse should include which of the following actions in the clients' plan of care? a. Encourage client to increase ambulation to prevent a deep venous thrombosis. b. Instruct client to increase intake of vitamin C to assist in blood coagulation. c. Hold pressure over injection sites to ensure clotting has occurred. d. Use strict sterile technique with wound care in order to prevent infection.	Answer: c Rationale: A platelet count of 100,000 is less than the norm of 150,000 to 450,000, putting client at risk of bleeding secondary to decreased clotting ability. Vitamin K, not C, is needed for clot formation. A reduced WBC increases risk of infection. Analysis Implementation Physiological Integrity: Reduction of Risk Potential
29.3 While bathing the client, the nurse observes large purple-colored rashes on the client's chest. The nurse documents that the client has: a. petechiae. b. eythema. c. purpura. d. papules.	Answer: c Rationale: Purpura are purple rashes caused by blood leaking under the skin. Petechiae are pinpoint red discolorations. Erythema is a redness of the skin and papules are raised red lesions. Comprehension Assessment Physiological Integrity: Physiological Adaptation
29.4 The physician has informed the parents that the results of a hemoglobin electrophoresis perfomed on their child indicate the presence of hemoglobin S. When the parent asks what this means, the nurse explains: a. "It is indicative of sickle cell disease or trait." b. "It verifies the presence of hemolytic anemia." c. Hemoglobin S is found in people with pernicious anemia." d. "Hemoglobin S is a type of immature red blood cell."	Answer: a Rationale: Hemoglobin S is an abnormal form of the hemoglobin molecule found in people with sickle cell trait or disease. Coombs' test is done to diagnose hemolytic anemia. Schilling's test is done to detect pernicious anemia. Application Implementation Physiological Integrity: Reduction of Risk Potential
29.5 The nurse checks the results of a client's Schilling's test and notes the excretion of vitamin B_{12} is less than 10% in 24 hours. The nurse should plan to: a. instruct client to increase intake of foods high in iron. b. explain the need and rationale for supplemental vitamin B_{12}.	Answer: b Rationale: The expected excretion rate of vitamin B_{12} is greater than 10%; less than 10% indicates pernicious anemia, which would indicate a need for vitamin B_{12} supplementation. Iron replacement would be indicated for iron deficiency anemias. Platelet deficiencies warrant close monitoring for bleeding and decreased hemoglobin levels affect oxygenation. Analysis Planning Physiological Integrity: Reduction of Risk Potential

© 2007 Pearson Education, Inc.

c. observe client for signs of bleeding tendencies. d. measure client's oxygen saturation levels.	
29.6 The nurse checks the coagulation studies on a client who is not receiving any type of anticoagulant therapy. Which of the following findings should be reported to the physician? a. INR is 2.5. b. APPT is 25 seconds. c. Platelet count is 250,000 mm^3. d. Prothrombin time is 20 seconds.	Answer: d Rationale: A prothrombin time of 20 seconds is prolonged; normal is 10 to 13 seconds. A normal INR is 2.0 to 3.0. Platelets are 150,000 to 450,000 mm^3 and APTT is 25 to 35 seconds. Application Assessment Physiological Integrity: Reduction of Risk Potential
29.7 A nurse is bathing a client who had a bone marrow aspiration from the right iliac crest 5 days ago. Which of the following findings would be of concern to the nurse? a. The needle aspiration site is ecchymotic. b. The client complains of moderate pain in the right iliac crest. c. The needle insertion site is scabbed over and without drainage. d. The client is doing isometric leg exercises.	Answer: b Rationale: Continued pain after 3 to 4 days is abnormal and should be reported. Ecchymosis of the site would be normal at 5 days. Isometric exercises would not be contraindicated. Analysis Evaluation Physiological Integrity: Reduction of Risk Potential
29.8 A client in the outpatient clinic is scheduled to have blood drawn for an iron level. Recognizing that certain medications will affect the results, the nurse should determine if the client is taking: a. oral contraceptives. b. acetaminophen. c. antihypertensives. d. antidepressants.	Answer: a Rationale: Drugs most affecting iron levels include antibiotics, estrogen and testosterone, oral contraceptives, alcohol, and aspirin. Application Assessment Physiological Integrity: Pharmacological and Parenteral Therapies
29.9 During the change-of-shift report the nurse learns that an assigned client has a hemoglobin level of 8 g/dL. Based on this information the nurse plans to: a. space activities in order to conserve energy. b. keep the client on strict bed rest to restrict activity. c. encourage ambulation to prevent thrombophlebitis. d. prevent exposure to infectious diseases.	Answer: a Rationale: Hemoglobin is the oxygen-carrying protein in red blood cells; 8 g/dL is well below the normal level of 12 to 15 g/dL and would predispose the client to dyspnea, fatigue, and weakness. Strict bed rest would not be necessary. Platelet abnormalities and inactivity place client at risk for thrombophlebitis. Application Planning Physiological Integrity: Reduction of Risk Potential
29.10 A client being prepared to have a bone marrow transplant expresses concern the procedure will be painful. The nurse explains: a. "A local anesthetic is given and so you won't feel any pain." b. "The procedure is very quick and not very painful." c. "You will be given some analgesic since it can be painful." d. "It should not be any more painful than having an injection."	Answer: c Rationale: The procedure can be painful and analgesics are given to control pain. A local anesthetic is used, but it may not totally prevent pain and pressure felt during the procedure. Application Implementation Physiological Integrity: Reduction of Risk Potential

Chapter 30

Question	Answer
30.1 When caring for the client with a history of pica the nurse assesses the client for signs of chronic iron deficiency anemia. These may include: a. chelosis. b. clubbing of the fingernails. c. petechiae. d. jaundice.	Answer: a Rationale: Chelosis, cracks at the corner of the mouth, are indicative of chronic iron deficiency anemia. Clubbing of the fingers is seen with chronic hypoxemia. Petechiae may be seen with platelet disorders, and jaundice may be seen with aplastic anemia. Application Assessment Physiological Integrity: Reduction of Risk Potential
30.2 The nurse is preparing a client recovering from sickle cell crisis for discharge. To prevent future crises from occurring, the nurse instructs the client to: a. avoid doing any types of exercise. b. keep well hydrated. c. abstain from alcohol use. d. eat a high-protein diet.	Answer: b Rationale: Dehydration can trigger a sickle cell crisis. Excessive exercise and alcohol intake should be avoided, but not totally avoided. Overall good nutrition should be encouraged. Application Implementation Physiological Integrity: Reduction of Risk Potential
30.3 A client with multiple myeloma has been started on filgrastin (Neupogen) for treatment of neutropenia. The nurse identifies the drug is being effective when: a. the client no longer has bone pain. b. the hemoglobin level is within normal limits. c. an increase in the white blood cell count occurs. d. the client is no longer hypotensive.	Answer: c Rationale: Neupogen stimulates the growth and development of WBCs. It does not affect red blood cells or hemoglobin. Bone pain is a side effect of Neupogen. It does not affect the blood pressure. Analysis Assessment Phsyiological Integrity: Pharmacological and Parenteral Therapies
30.4 A client with secondary polycythemia being seen in the clinic informs the nurse he will be taking a long flight overseas in the near future. The nurse reminds the client: a. to be sure to wear support stockings during the flight. b. that he will need supplemental oxygen when at a higher altitude. c. that he should start taking an antibiotic 1 week before leaving. d. to restrict intake of high-protein foods the day of the flight.	Answer: a Rationale: Support stockings would help to prevent blood stasis and possible thrombus when activity will be restricted. Supplemental oxygen and antibiotics are not needed. There is no indication for restriction of protein. Analysis Implementation Physiological Integrity: Reduction of Risk Potential
30.5 When making morning rounds, a client with acute leukemia reports having nosebleeds off and on throughout the night. Which of the following actions should be taken by the nurse? a. Determine if client has pain anywhere. b. Report the findings to the physician. c. Check the client's blood pressure and pulse. d. Apply a water-soluble lubricant to the nares.	Answer: b Rationale: Manifestations of bleeding such as bleeding gums and nosebleeds should be reported promptly, since bleeding can lead to death in acute leukemia. Options a and c should be done after b. Analysis Implementation Physiological Integrity: Reduction of Risk Potential

© 2007 Pearson Education, Inc.

30.6 A client with hemophilia A is being prepared to receive a transfusion of clotting factors and expresses concern about contracting HIV from the transfusion. The best explanation the nurse can provide is: a. "That certainly is always a concern. You can refuse the treatment if you prefer." b. "The blood that is donated is screened so you should not worry." c. "Rigorous screening of donors and treatment of donated blood has significantly reduced the risk." d. "You won't be receiving whole blood so you shouldn't worry about HIV contamination."	Answer: c Rationale: Since 1985 rigorous screening of donors and heat treating of blood products has significantly reduced the risk of HIV transmission. The clotting factors are prepared from fresh frozen plasma, not whole blood. It is best to be honest with the client and acknowledge there is still a risk involved. Application Implementation Physiological Integrity: Reduction of Risk Potential
30.7 The nurse learns a client with sepsis has developed disseminated intravascular coagulation (DIC). The nurse should plan to: a. encourage frequent ambulation in the hallway. b. check peripheral pulses and capillary refill frequently. c. keep client in a low-Fowler's position to promote venous return. d. restrict fluid intake to prevent vascular fluid overload.	Answer: b Rationale: Identification of impaired circulation will alert the nurse to impaired tissue perfusion secondary to microvascular blood clotting. Bed rest should be maintained to decrease oxygen demand. Semi-Fowler's position improves lung expansion and oxygenation. Fluids should not be restricted. Analysis Planning Physiological Integrity: Reduction of Risk Potential
30.8 A client with chronic lymphangitis of the lower extremities asks the nurse how often she should wear elastic stockings. The nurse explains: a. "You should wear them at all times, only taking them off to bathe." b. "It is best to wear them during the waking hours and remove them when sleeping." c. "You should wear them when your legs feel heavy or are painful for you." d. "It is only necessary to wear them if you notice an increase in swelling."	Answer: b Rationale: Management of chronic lymphangitis includes use of intermittent pressure devices or elastic stockings. They should be removed while sleeping since legs will be elevated and this allows for air circulation to the skin. Application Implementation Physiological Integrity: Reduction of Risk Potential
30.9 Infectious mononucleosis is suspected in a client being seen in the clinic. In addition to swollen lymph glands and an increased lymphocyte count, the nurse can expect the client to: a. complain of headaches and malaise. b. have an enlarged liver. c. have petechiae over the anterior chest. d. report having insomnia.	Answer: a Rationale: Common manifestations include headaches, malaise, fatigue, fever, sore throat, and an enlarged spleen. Comprehension Assessment Physiological Integrity: Physiological Adaptation

30.10 When caring for a client with a history of alcoholism the nurse recognizes the client is at increased risk for which of the following conditions?
a. pernicious anemia
b. folic acid deficiency
c. hemolytic anemia
d. Von Willibrand's disease

Answer: b
Rationale: Excess alcohol intake increases folic acid requirements. Pernicious anemia is caused by vitamin B_{12} deficiency. Hemolytic anemia is seen following trauma, immune responses, antibody reactions, and certain drugs and toxic agents. Von Willibrand's disease is a hereditary bleeding disorder.
Application
Assessment
Physiological Integrity: Reduction of Risk Potential

Chapter 31

31.1 The nurse is preparing a client for a renal scan. It will be necessary for the nurse to:
a. determine if the client has allergies to iodine.
b. instruct the client to drink two to three glasses of water.
c. keep client NPO for 8 hours prior to the procedure.
d. medicate client with a mild tranquilizer.

Answer: b
Rationale: Fluids are necessary to promote flushing of the radioactive substance used. It is not necessary to keep client NPO or to give a tranquilizer. It is not an iodine-based dye.
Application
Implementation
Physiological Integrity: Reduction of Risk Potential

31.2 The nurse is preparing to do a portable ultrasonic bladder scan to check for residual urine in a client who voids very frequently. The nurse should plan to do the scan:
a. just before the client is ready to void.
b. immediately upon awakening in the am.
c. within 15 minutes of voiding.
d. immediately after the client has voided.

Answer: c
Rationale: Measurements for residual urine need to be done within 15 minutes of voiding to provide accurate information.
Comprehension
Planning
Physiological Integrity: Reduction of Risk Potential

31.3 Following a cystoscopy of the bladder the nurse provides the following teaching:
a. "Taking a sitz bath may help to ease discomfort."
b. "Contact your physician if you experience burning with urination."
c. "It is not unusual to have chills and a fever for a few days."
d. "Avoid taking any laxatives or straining with defecation."

Answer: a
Rationale: Sitz baths and analgesics may help to relieve local urethral discomfort. Burning on urination for 1 to 2 days is normal. Chills and fever are indicative of an infection. Laxatives may be taken to prevent straining.
Application
Implementation
Physiological Integrity: Reduction of Risk Potential

31.4 When reviewing results of a client's urinalysis, the nurse notes the specific gravity is 1.050. The nurse is aware this level is:
a. within normal limits.
b. could be indicative of diabetes.
c. could be a sign of dehydration.
d. the result of a contaminated specimen.

Answer: c
Rationale: This is an elevated level, indicating concentrated urine, which could be secondary to dehydration. The presence of glucose and ketones is indicative of diabetes.
Analysis
Evaluation
Physiological Integrity: Reduction of Risk Potential

31.5 A client became hypotensive following a surgical procedure. When assessing the urinary system the nurse should expect to find:
a. presence of blood in the urine.

Answer: b
Rationale: A drop in blood volume or blood pressure will cause a decrease in glomerular filtration rate and urine output.
Application

© 2007 Pearson Education, Inc.

b. a decrease in urine output. c. episodes of frequent urination. d. painful urination.	Assessment Physiological Integrity: Physiological Adaptation
31.6 The nurse is instructing a female client on the proper method for a midstream clean-catch urine specimen. The nurse stresses the importance of: a. cleansing the meatus in a circular motion with an antiseptic towelette. b. wiping the meatus with an antiseptic towelette from front to back. c. using an iodine solution to cleanse the outer labia. d. using antibacterial foam to cleanse the labia and meatus.	Answer: b Rationale: Females cleanse the meatus from front to back to avoid spreading any rectal contamination. Application Implementation Physiological Integrity: Reduction of Risk Potential
31.7 A client scheduled to have a uroflometry asks the nurse why the test is being done. The nurse explains that the test: a. is used to evaluate urinary retention and incontinence. b. can identify types of bladder infections. c. will determine the presence of bladder tumors. d. can evaluate need for urethral surgery.	Answer: a Rationale: Cystometry, or uroflometry, evaluates the motor and sensory function of the bladder, which can contribute to urinary incontinence. It can provide information about bladder structure and function, but is not used to determine infections, tumors, or urethral conditions. Application Assessment Physiological Integrity: Reduction of Risk Potential
31.8 The nurse recognizes the client with reduced renal function should also be assessed for: a. a decrease in red blood cell production. b. an increase in white blood cell production. c. a low blood pressure. d. signs of dehydration.	Answer: a Rationale: Decreased kidney function reduces erythropoietin production, which is needed to stimulate red blood production. WBC production is not affected. Blood pressure is usually elevated due to fluid retention, not dehydration. Analysis Assessment Physiological Integrity: Reduction of Risk Potential
31.9 Following an intravenous pyelogram (IVP) nursing responsibilities will include: a. informing client a warm flushed feeling may occur at the IV site. b. checking injection site for redness and warmth. c. keeping client NPO for 4 hours. d. explaining urine may be pink tinged for 24 hours.	Answer: b Rationale: The injection site should be assessed for signs of phlebitis or dye reaction because dye may be irritating to the vein. The flushed feeling occurs during the procedure when the dye is injected. Fluids are encouraged, not restricted. Urine should be clear. Application Implementation Physiological Integrity: Reduction of Risk Potential
31.10 A client is voiding 50 to 100 mL of urine every few hours and reports urgency with voiding. The nurse reports this as an abnormal finding based on the understanding that: a. the urge to void occurs at 300 to 500 mL in the bladder. b. it is abnormal to urinate every few hours. c. it is normal to void at least 600 to 700 mL with each bladder emptying. d. urgency is always a sign of a bladder infection.	Answer: a Rationale: Voiding is usually stimulated when bladder contains 300 to 500 mL. Frequency and urgency of voiding are influenced by many factors and the cause should be determined. Analysis Evaluation Physiological Integrity: Reduction of Risk Potential

Chapter 32

Question	Answer
32.1 A young female client presents with UTI. Which of the following questions by the nurse will provide information that might help to prevent future UTI infections? a. "How long have you been married?" b. "Do you urinate after having sexual intercourse?" c. "Are you pregnant?" d. "What kind of bath soap do you use?"	Answer: b Rationale: Personal hygiene following intercourse is important: Voiding is encouraged to wash away bacteria that could ascend the urethra. The other questions do not address risk factors for preventing UTIs. Analysis Assessment Physiological Integrity: Reduction of Risk Potential
32.2 A client informs the nurse that he frequently experiences stress incontinence. The nurse plans the following interventions: a. Have a bedside commode readily available to the client. b. Provide client with absorbent pads or panty liners. c. Toilet client every 2 hours. d. Catheterize client every shift for residual urine.	Answer: b Rationale: Stress incontinence involves loss of small amounts of urine when intra-abdominal pressure increases, as with sneezing or coughing. The pads help to keep undergarments dry. Option a would help with urge incontinence. Option c helps with functional incontinence, and option d would be done for overflow incontinence. Analysis Planning Physiological Integrity: Basic Care and Comfort
32.3 An adult client is admitted with acute glomerulonephritis with symptoms of fatigue, anorexia, and blood pressure of 140/94. The nurse identifies the initial goal of treatment as follows: a. to reduce the hypertension b. providing a 5,000-calorie daily diet c. energy conservation and bed rest during the acute phase d. urinary output of at least 3,000 mL daily	Answer: c Rationale: Preservation of renal function is a primary goal; bed rest lowers metabolic demands on the body and conserves energy reserves. If present, hypertension should be controlled. Protein may be restricted in the dict and intake and output are closely monitored. Analysis Planning Physiolgical Integrity: Reduction of Risk Potential
32.4 The nurse obtains a urine specimen from the client with glomerulonephritis and expects to find the urine is: a. clear and very dilute. b. dark brown. c. cloudy with some hematuria. d. clear amber with a foul odor.	Answer: c Rationale: Damage to the capillary membrane allows blood cells and protein to escape. Comprehension Assessment Physiological Integrity: Physiological Adaptation
32.5 The nurse is caring for a client who has had a cystectomy for bladder cancer. Postoperative nursing interventions should include: a. limit fluid intake to less than 1,000 mL in 24 hours to promote healing. b. secure catheters and stents with tape; keep drainage bags lower than the kidneys. c. label all catheters and stents; keep drainage bags at kidney level. d. reduce activity levels and keep client on strict bed rest.	Answer: b Rationale: Securing catheters and stents prevents kinking or occlusion; gravity flow is maintained by keeping the drainage bag below the level of the kidneys. Fluids and activity are not restricted. Application Implementation Physiological Integrity: Reduction of Risk Potential

© 2007 Pearson Education, Inc.

32.6 The nurse is checking lab values on a client who has just had a hemodialysis treatment. Which of the following would indicate to the nurse that the client's renal dialysis was effective? a. an increase in hemoglobin level b. a decrease in white cell count c. a decrease in potassium level d. an increase in serum creatinine	Answer: d Analysis Assessment Physiological Integrity: Physiological Adaptation
32.7 The nurse monitors a client receiving peritoneal dialysis for signs of peritonitis. Which of the following assessment findings should be reported to the physician? a. Skin is pale and dry. b. Abdomen is tender to palpation. c. Dialysate return is cloudy and yellow. d. Temperature is 36.8°C.	Answer: c Rationale: Cloudy dialysate fluid is indicative of peritonitis; the fluid should be clear and pale yellow. The abdomen may be tender due to distention from the fluid; severe pain would be a concern. Application Assessment Physiological Integrity: Physiological Adaptation
32.8 Following an intravenous pyelogram (IVP) the nurse encourages fluid intake, recognizing this is necessary to prevent which of the following renal complications? a. glomerulonephritis b. acute renal failure c. chronic renal failure d. polycystic kidney disease	Answer: b Rationale: The contrast media used in the IVP can precipitate prerenal failure; increasing fluids promotes excretion of the dye. Application Implementation Physiological Integrity: Reduction of Risk Potential
32.9 When caring for a client with chronic renal failure (CRF) the nurse should plan to administer which of the following medications? a. antidiarrheals b. folic acid supplements c. opioid analgesics d. antiarrhythmic agents	Answer: b Rationale: Folic acid is given to stimulate red blood cell production since clients with CRF are often anemic. Clients tend to be constipated, not have diarrhea. Opioid analgesics and antiarrhythmics are not routinely needed. Analysis Planning Physiological Integrity: Pharmacological and Parenteral Therapies
32.10 The nurse is giving discharge instructions to a client treated for renal calculi. The nurse explains that the stones can be prevented in many cases by: a. engaging in frequent aerobic exercise. b. restricting protein and acid foods in the diet. c. taking urinary antiseptic agents to prevent urinary tract infections. d. drinking 8 to 10 glasses of water daily.	Answer: d Rationale: High fluid intake keeps urine dilute and prevents stasis of urine. Stone analysis must be done for specific dietary restrictions to be appropriate. Application Implementation Physiological Integrity: Reduction of Risk Potential

CHAPTER 33

33.1 When a client calls to schedule a mammogram, the nurse informs the client the following preparation is necessary: a. Avoid having sexual intercourse for 24 hours prior to the exam. b. Wear a loose-fitting top and bra that opens in the front. c. Jewelry worn above the waist may need to be removed. d. Do not use any aluminum-containing deodorants.	Answer: c Rationale: Jewelry may interfere with adequate reading of the exam. Sexual abstinence is not necessary. The client is given a hospital gown, so clothing will be removed. It is recommended to avoid all deodorants and powders, not just those containing aluminum. Application Implementation Health Promotion and Maintenance: Prevention and Early Detection of Disease

Question	Answer
33.2 Following an abdominal laparascopic procedure to examine the pelvic cavity, a client is concerned because she is passing gas through her vagina. The nurse should offer which of the following responses: a. "This is normal following the procedure you had done." b. "I'll give you some perineal pads in case fluid is also expelled." c. "As long as you don't have severe pain or bleeding, it should be okay." d. "That is quite unusual. I'll let your physician know."	Answer: a Rationale: The peritoneal cavity is filled with gas during the procedure and is normally expelled through the vagina. Options b and c would not be incorrect, but do not offer the best response. Application Implementation Physiological Integrity: Physiological Adaptation
33.3 Following a report of abnormal findings on a Pap exam, a client is scheduled to have a colposcopy. Nursing responsibilities prior to the exam include: a. obtain an informed consent. b. place client in a left lateral Sims' position. c. premedicate client with a non-narcotic analgesic. d. give client a tap water enema.	Answer: a Rationale: Colposcopy is an invasive procedure requiring an informed consent. The client is placed in a lithotomy position. Premedicating and enemas are not necessary; the client might need non-narcotic analgesia following the procedure. Application Implementation Physiological Integrity: Reduction of Risk Potential
33.4 Estradiol levels are drawn on a 55-year-old female who stopped menstruating 2 years ago. The nurse anticipates the levels will be: a. between 0 and 30 pg/mL. b. less than 100 pg/mL. c. between 200 and 400 pg/mL. d. greater than 400 pg/mL.	Answer: a Rationale: Normal postmenopausal levels are 0 to 30 pg/mL. Comprehension Assessment Physiological Integrity: Physiological Adaptation
33.5 An 18-year-old client is scheduling her first Pap smear exam. The nurse should provide the following instructions: a. Abstain from having sexual relations for 1 week prior to the exam. b. Schedule the exam for when your next menstrual cycle will just be starting. c. Restrict alcohol intake 24 hours prior to the exam. d. Avoid use of any vaginal medications 24 hours prior to the exam.	Answer: d Rationale: Sexual intercourse, douching, and vaginal medications should be avoided 24 hours prior to the exam, because they may interfere with tissue samples. The exam should be done when not menstruating. No food or drink restrictions are necessary. Application Implementation Physiological Integrity: Reduction of Risk Potential
33.6 A 58-year-old female asks the nurse how often she should have a mammogram. The nurse states she should have one done: a. every year. b. every other year until age 75, then yearly. c. every 5 years if her current one is negative. d. only if she feels a lump or has a strong family history of breast cancer.	Answer: a Rationale: The American Cancer Society recommends mammograms every other year between ages 40 and 50, and then yearly after age 50. Comprehension Implementation Health Promotion and Maintenance: Prevention and Early Detection of Disease

© 2007 Pearson Education, Inc.

33.7 A client who had an abnormal mammogram is scheduled to have a breast ultrasonogram and asks the nurse how this test differs from the mammogram. The nurse explains that the ultrasonogram: a. can locate possible metastatic cancer. b. is used to confirm breast cancer. c. can distinguish between solid and cystic masses. d. will confirm the findings of the mammogram.	Answer: c Rationale: Ultrasongraphy uses sound waves to obtain a cross-sectional view of breast tissue and can distinguish between solid and cystic masses. A CT scan would be done to detect metastasis. A needle biopsy is done to confirm diagnosis of type of masses. Application Implementation Physiological Integrity: Reduction of Risk Potential
33.8 When performing a physical assessment of the male reproductive system, it is important for the nurse to determine: a. when the client last had sexual intercourse. b. if client has any difficulty with urination. c. when the client last had a bowel movement. d. if the client has more than one sexual partner.	Answer: b Rationale: Since the urinary and reproductive systems are closely linked, a problem in the reproductive system may produce urinary tract symptoms. Options a and c would not be pertinent to the exam. History of sexual partners is determined when assessing risk factors. Analysis Assessment Health Promotion and Maintenance: Prevention and Early Detection of Disease
33.9 A nurse is participating in a community education program. The nurse explains that premenopausal women should perform breast self-examination (BSE): a. shortly after the menstrual period. b. just before the menstrual period. c. during the menstrual period. d. during ovulation.	Answer: a Rationale: Premenstrual women should perform the exam after the menstrual period since hormonal changes increase breast tenderness and lumpiness just before menses. Application Implementation Health Promotion: Prevention and/or Early Detection of Health Problems
33.10 The nurse instructing a woman on breast self-examination (BSE) informs her that most breast lumps or masses are found in the: a. upper inner quadrant of the breast. b. lower inner quadrant of the breast. c. upper outer quadrant of the breast. d. lower outer quadrant of the breast.	Answer: c Rationale: This is the area of highest frequency. Comprehension Implementation Health Promotion: Prevention and/or Early Detection of Health Problems

CHAPTER 34

34.1 The client being started on the medication finasteride (Proscar) asks the nurse how the medication will help to treat his enlarged prostate. The nurse provides the following explanation: a. "Proscar decreases the inflammation of the prostate gland." b. "Proscar decreases the production of urine." c. "Proscar promotes contraction of the bladder to help expel the urine more easily." d. "Proscar reduces the production of a hormone that normally stimulates prostate growth."	Answer: d Rationale: Proscar inhibits the conversion of testosterone to dihidrotestosterone, which stimulates growth of the prostate. Application Implementation Physiological Integrity: Pharmacological and Parenteral Therapies

Question	Answer
34.2 In caring for the client who has had a transurethral resection of the prostate (TURP), the nurse assesses the client frequently for which of the following complications? a. bright red blood and large clots in the urine b. large amounts of dilute, light pink urine c. increased hemoglobin and hematocrit d. hypertension and bradycardia	Answer: a Rationale: Frank red blood, large clots, decreased urinary output, a decrease in hemoglobin and hematocrit, tachycardia, and hypotension could indicate hemorrhage. Analysis Assessment Physiological Integrity: Reduction of Risk Potential
34.3 When caring for a client who has had a prostatectomy, discharge teaching by the nurse should include: a. Kegel exercises and bladder training for incontinence. b. restriction of fluids to reduce incontinence. c. provision of a list of absorbent products for urinary incontinence. d. use of a condom catheter for incontinence.	Answer: a Rationale: Because stress incontinence often occurs following a prostatectomy, Kegel exercises can improve urine retention. A referral to a physical therapist or continence specialist may be indicated. Fluids should not be restricted; a condom catheter may be indicated for total incontinence. Application Implementation Physiological Integrity: Reduction of Risk Potential
34.4 A client with cryptorchidism is being seen at the infertility clinic. The nurse gives high priorty to including which of the following instructions? a. teaching testicular self-exam (TSE) due to risk for testicular cancer b. advising the client to seek the assistance of a sex counselor c. avoiding the use of scrotal support devices d. avoiding strenuous activity	Answer: a Rationale: Testicular cancer risk is increased with cryptorchidism. It may cause problems with fertility, which should be addressed by a fertility specialist. Scrotal supports are not needed. Activity is not restricted. Application Implementation Health Promotion: Prevention and/or Early Detection of Health Problems
34.5 The client with epididymitis gets a prescription for antibiotics and the nurse provides the following discharge instructions: a. "You may resume sexual activity after forty-eight hours." b. "Take warm sitz baths three to four times a day." c. "Take the antibiotics until the swelling subsides." d. "Use ice packs on your scrotum and wear scrotal support."	Answer: d Rationale: Ice packs and scrotal supports are recommended to relieve pain. Client should be counseled regarding sexually transmitted diseases. Warm sitz baths would increase pain. The complete course of antibiotics should be taken. Application Implementation Physiological Integrity: Reduction of Risk Potential
34.6 A 38-year-old male client tells the nurse that he is afraid that he is sterile. Which of the following responses by the client helps the nurse determine that the client is sterile and not infertile? a. "I was treated for a sexually transmitted disease a few years ago." b. "I only have one orgasm while having intercourse." c. "I have had unprotected sex for the past ten years with my wife who has a child from a previous marriage." d. "I have had unprotected sex with my wife for eight months and she has not conceived."	Answer: c Rationale: Since client has not conceived a child in 10 years and knowing the wife is not infertile supports sterility. Infertility is an inability to conceive during a one-year period of unprotected intercourse; if caused by testicular or systemic disorders it may be reversible. Some STDs can cause infertility, but further information would be necessary. Analysis Assessment Physiological Integrity: Physiological Adaptation

 © 2007 Pearson Education, Inc.

34.7 The nurse is conducting a community education program on testicular cancer. The nurse informs the clients that early signs and symptoms of testicular cancer include: a. difficulty maintaining an erection. b. a painless, hard nodule on a testicle. c. severe pain in the groin. d. enlargement of the scrotum.	Answer: b Rationale: Enlargement of one testicle, hard lumps, or an irregular shape are signs of testicular cancer. Comprehension Assessment Health Promotion: Prevention and/or Early Detection of Health Problems
34.8 The nurse provides the following instructions for a client with phimosis: a. "Retract the foreskin behind the glans for an hour at least three times a day." b. "You will need to contact your physician to schedule a circumcision." c. "Keep your penis clean and dry and contact the doctor if you develop pain and redness." d. "Do not take tub baths, because they may increase the possibility of infection."	Answer: c Rationale: Retraction of the foreskin could cause it to become trapped and impair blood flow to the glans. Circumcision may be needed. Tub baths can be taken. Application Implementation Health Promotion: Prevention and/or Early Detection of Health Problems
34.9 The nurse is evaluating the effectiveness of teaching on a client with erectile dysfunction. Which of the following comments made by the client should be addressed by the nurse? a. "I'm not embarrassed to tell you I'm unable to have an erection." b. "I don't want to upset my wife so I'll share my concerns with you." c. "I know I need to take the sildenafil, Viagra, about an hour before having sex." d. "I know there are surgical options if I can't tolerate the pills."	Answer: b Rationale: Clients should express a willingness to share concerns with their partners, since the problem affects both parties and fosters communication. Willingness to discuss with health care worker is positive. Option c is a correct statement and an implantable prosthesis is a surgical option. Analysis Evaluation Health Promotion: Prevention and Early Detection of Disease
34.10 A nurse is preparing to give a presentation at a community screening program on prostate cancer. The nurse plans to include the following information: a. Annual digital rectal exams, DRE, are recommended after age 65. b. African Americans are considered at highest risk for this cancer. c. Prostate cancer has a low incidence of metastasis to other organs. d. A diet high in dairy products is a risk factor.	Answer: b Rationale: African American males have a high incidence of prostate cancer. DREs are recommended at age 50. Metastasis is common. A diet high in animal fat is a risk factor. Application Planning Health Promotion: Prevention and Early Detection of Disease

CHAPTER 35

35.1 The nurse instructs the lactating mother with mastitis about preventing future episodes by: a. feeding the infant from only one breast during each feeding. b. alternating breasts every 2 minutes during each feeding. c. not breastfeeding the infant at night. d. thoroughly emptying both breasts to prevent engorgement.	Answer: d Rationale: Thorough emptying of breasts keeps milk from lying in the ducts and providing a medium for growth of organisms, which are usually spread from the infant's nose and throat. Application Implementation Physiological Integrity: Reduction of Risk Potential

© 2007 Pearson Education, Inc.

35.2 The young woman asks the nurse about breast augmentation surgery. An appropriate response by the nurse would be: a. "It is a very common surgery and the technique has been perfected." b. "It has been proven that women who have breast augmentation are at greater risk for breast cancer." c. "There is no evidence of implants causing cancer, but the implants do make detection of cancer more difficult." d. "You might want to think about it, because the scar tissue distorts the breasts."	Answer: c Rationale: This provides honest and accurate information to the client. Scar tissue may cause excessive firmness and distortion of the breast. Application Implementation Health Promotion: Prevention and Early Detection of Health Problems
35.3 A female client who has had a recurrence of breast cancer is prescribed tamoxifen (Nolvadex) therapy. What would the nurse include in the instructions for taking this medication? a. Take before meals with orange juice. b. Medication will cause chills; dress warmly. c. Stop smoking while taking this medication. d. Maintain a 1,500-calorie diet; medication causes weight loss.	Answer: c Rationale: Smoking can increase the risk of thromboembolic events, which are sometimes increased with tamoxifen. The medication may cause weight gain and fluid retention. It is not necessary to take it with orange juice and it does not cause chills. Application Implementation Physiological Integrity: Pharmacological and Parenteral Therapies
35.4 The newly diagnosed client with breast cancer asks the nurse if they diagnosed the cancer too late, since the surgeon recommended surgery and radiation therapy. The appropriate response by the nurse is: a. "Surgery and radiation are recommended in the later stages of breast cancer." b. "Surgery and radiation are recommended in cancer that has not metastasized." c. "Chemotherapy is only used in the first stage." d. "You need to discuss that with your doctor."	Answer: b Rationale: Radiation is typically used following surgery to destroy any remaining cancer cells that could reoccur or mestastasize. Application Implementation Health Promotion: Prevention and/or Early Detection of Health Problems
35.5 A client with premenstrual syndrome (PMS) has been on diet therapy, diuretics, and medications such as danazol (Danocrine) and fluoxetine (Prozac) and still finds no relief from the symptoms. The nurse recognizes the client may benefit from: a. belonging to a PMS support group. b. oophorectomy to relieve the hormonal imbalance. c. a vigorous, daily exercise regimen. d. alternative therapies such as acupuncture and relaxation exercises.	Answer: d Rationale: Since diet and medication have not been helpful, alternative therapies provide options that have been helpful to other women with PMS. An oophorectomy would not be indicated. Exercise should be balanced with rest. Analysis Planning Physiological Integrity: Basic Care and Comfort

 © 2007 Pearson Education, Inc.

Question	Answer
35.6 A client with ongoing metrorrhagia asks the nurse what she should do about the problem. Which of the following responses by the nurse is most appropriate? a. "If it a small amount of bleeding you shouldn't worry." b. "Wearing a tampon and a perineal pad will help with absorption of the drainage." c. "It may help to cut back on your physical exercise." d. "When was the last time you had a pelvic examination?"	Answer: d Rationale: Metorrhagia may be a sign of cervical or uterine cancer and should be evaluated promptly. Application Implementation Physiological Integrity: Reduction of Risk Potential
35.7 When caring for the client with uterine prolapse nursing interventions should include: a. recommending laxatives to prevent constipation. b. have the client lie in knee-chest position for an hour, twice daily. c. have the client lie in a high-Fowler's position when experiencing low back pain. d. teach the client Kegel exercises.	Answer: d Rationale: Kegel exercises help to strengthen pelvic floor muscles, helping to minimize urinary leakage and descent of the bladder and rectum into the vagina. Although prolapse may cause constipation, option d provides a specific intervention that can be done to help the prolapse and prevent other complications. Application Implementation Physiological Integrity: Reduction of Risk Potential
35.8 The client diagnosed with endometriosis asks the nurse to explain what it is. The nurse provides the following explanation: a. "It is inflammation of the inside of your uterus." b. "It is a condition in which the tissue found inside the uterus grows outside the uterus." c. "It is an infection of the tissue that connects your intestines." d. "It is inflammation of the outside lining of your uterus."	Answer: b Rationale: Endometrial tissue is found outside the uterus, often on the ovary or other pelvic organs and tissues. Comprehension Implementation Physiological Integrity: Physiological Adaptation
35.9 When assisting in a community education program the nurse knows that early cancer of the uterus or cervix causes no symptoms and focuses interventions on: a. promoting screening and early detection with Papanicolaou (Pap) smear. b. providing sex education programs for high school students. c. distribution of pamphlets describing risk factors for cervical cancer. d. promoting annual physical examinations for all females.	Answer: a Rationale: The Pap smear is used to screen for cervical cancer, and when it is performed, manual palpation of the uterus is also done to assess for uterine abnormalities. Application Implementation Health Promotion: Prevention and/or Early Detection of Health Problems

35.10 When caring for a client with pelvic inflammatory disease (PID), nursing interventions will include: a. having the client take sitz baths b.i.d. b. keeping the client on bed rest in a semi-Fowler's position. c. instructing client to use tampons. d. ambulating client frequently.	Answer: b Rationale: PID can have severe life-threatening complications. This position promotes drainage and localizes infection to the pelvic cavity. Tampons would interfere with flow of drainage. Antibiotics and rest are also part of the treatment. Application Implementation Physiological Integrity: Reduction of Risk Potential

CHAPTER 36

36.1 A client whose child was diagnosed with a sexually transmitted disease (STD) shouted at the nurse, saying it was impossible for children to have STDs. The nurse's response is based on her knowledge that: a. sexually transmitted diseases can only be spread through sexual contact. b. organisms can be contacted from public bathrooms. c. laboratory samples are sometimes contaminated. d. children can be infected at birth or through sexual abuse.	Answer: d Rationale: STDs can be passed onto infants and children though the birth canal, incest, or sexual abuse. Application Implementation Health Promotion: Prevention and/or Early Detection of Health Problems
36.2 The nurse working in a Planned Parenthood program recognizes chlamydial infections are often asymptomatic, so the nurse focuses on: a. care of the persons who have symptoms and can be diagnosed and treated. b. talking to high school students about the disease. c. talking to parents of teenagers about the disease. d. identification and screening of women at high risk for chlamydia.	Answer: d Rationale: Since the infection is asymptomatic, incidence is much higher than reported. It is the leading cause of pelvic inflammatory disease and screening should be aimed at clients with risk factors. Application Implementation Health Promotion: Prevention and/or Early Detection of Health Problems
36.3 The nurse knows that a young woman needs further instructions about genital herpes when she says: a. "There is no cure for genital herpes." b. "You can't get genital herpes with oral-genital sex." c. "You won't know for three to seven days after intercourse if you have genital herpes." d. "You'll know you have it because you get painful blisters in the genital area."	Answer: b Rationale: Genital herpes is spread by vaginal, anal, or oral-genital contact. The other statements are correct. Analysis Evaluation Physiological Integrity: Reduction of Risk Potential
36.4 When obtaining a client's history, the nurse suspects that the client is manifesting the prodromal symptoms of genital herpes when the client describes: a. nausea and vomiting. b. suprapubic pain radiating toward the small of the back.	Answer: d Rationale: Prodromal symptoms, or warning signs, include burning, itching or throbbing at sites where lesions occur, usually the labia, vagina, or cervix in women. Pain may radiate to legs, buttocks, and groin. Dysuria is seen with recurrent infections.

© 2007 Pearson Education, Inc.

c. dysuria and difficulty starting and stopping the stream of urine. d. burning, throbbing pain in the genital area.	Analysis Assessment Physiological Integrity: Physiological Adaptation
36.5 The nurse gives the client with genital herpes who has painful, open ulcerations the following suggestions: a. Clean the lesions with a solution of cold water, soap, and dilute alcohol three times a day. b. Drink at least three or four glasses of cranberry juice daily. c. Keep moist dressings on the lesions at all times. d. Keep the lesions dry using a hair dryer at a cool setting.	Answer: d Rationale: Keeping lesions clean and dry promotes healing and reduces risk of a secondary infection. Lesions should be cleaned with warm water, soap, and hydrogen peroxide. Fluids that increase acidity of the urine should be avoided. Application Implementation Physiological Integrity: Basic Care and Comfort
36.6 The nurse examines the genital area of a young man with lesions on the penis. The nurse suspects genital warts caused by the human papillomavirus (HPV), because the lesions appear: a. like blisters in clusters. b. singularly as pustules. c. like strawberries. d. like cauliflower growths.	Answer: d Rationale: Genital warts have a cauliflower growth-like appearance. Option a describes genital herpes. Warts do not look like pustules or strawberries. Comprehension Assessment Physiological Integrity: Physiological Adaptation
36.7 When assessing the male client with complaints of dysuria, the nurse suspects gonorrhea based on which of the following additional symptoms? a. milky urethral discharge b. bloody urethral discharge c. blister-like lesions on the penis d. cauliflower-like lesions on the penis	Answer: a Rationale: In addition to dysuria, a serous, milky, or purulent urethral discharge occurs. Option c describes genital herpes; option d describes HPV lesions. Comprehension Assessment Physiological Integrity: Physiological Adaptation
36.8 A male client being treated for gonorrhea asks the nurse if he will experience any complications from the infection. The nurse informs him: a. "As long as you complete your course of antibiotics you should not have a problem." b. "It can lead to inflammation of the prostate and other glans." c. "If you are concerned about sterility, it only occurs in females." d. "There are no complications but you will need to use a condom when having sexual relations.	Answer: b Rationale: Gonorrhea, especially when untreated, can cause acute, painful inflammation of the prostate, epididymis, and periurethral glands and can lead to sterility. Application Implementation Physiological Integrity: Physiological Adaptation
36.9 A male client informs the nurse his partner is infected with chlamydia and he is concerned he may be infected as well. The nurse questions him to determine if he has any of the following manifestations: a. urinary retention b. blisters on the penis c. painful intercourse d. urethral discharge	Answer: d Rationale: Manifestation of chlamydia in males include dysuria, urethral discharge, and testicular pain. Application Implementation Physiological Integrity: Reduction of Risk Potential

36.10 A client being seen in the clinic is diagnosed with primary syphilis. The nurse prepares to administer: a. intravenous cefotetan. b. a loading dose of oral tetracycline. c. an intramuscular injection of Penicillin G. d. a urethral suppository of clindamycin.	Answer: c Rationale: The treatment of primary syphilis is a single IM dose of penicillin G. Comprehension Planning Physiological Integrity: Pharmacological and Parenteral Therapies

CHAPTER 37

37.1 A client's CT scan indicates the presence of an abnormal mass near the hypothalamus. The nurse understands this could affect the client's: a. speech. b. problem-solving skills. c. fluid balance. d. ability to follow simple directions.	Answer: c Rationale: The hypothalamus regulates temperature, fluid balance, thirst, appetite, emotions, and the sleep–wake cycle. The other options are controlled by tissues in the left hemisphere of the brain. Application Assessment Physiological Integrity: Physiological Adaptation
37.2 The nurse checks the laboratory report on a client who recently had a spinal tap. The presence of which of the following cerebral spinal fluid (CSF) contents should be of concern to the nurse? a. many red blood cells b. few white blood cells c. high glucose content d. high water content	Answer: a Rationale: CSF should not contain red blood cells. A high glucose and water content are normal as are a few white blood cells. Comprehension Assessment Physiological Integrity: Reduction of Risk Potential
37.3 A client scheduled for an electromyography (EMG) study asks the nurse what the purpose of the test is. The nurse explains that it: a. measures brain electrical activity. b. will identify velocity of blood flow in a vessel. c. records electrical activity of muscles. d. stimulates contraction of muscle fibers.	Answer: a Rationale: During an EMG needles are inserted into muscles and recordings are made of the electrical activity. Option a describes an EEG. Option b describes a carotid duplex study. Comprehension Implementation Physiological Integrity: Reduction of Risk Potential
37.4 When caring for a client who has experienced a massive trauma, the nurse recognizes that the response of the autonomic nervous system to stress correlates with the following assessment finding: a. increased peristalsis b. decreased pulse c. dilated pupils d. urinary urgency	Answer: c Rationale: Stress stimulates the sympathetic branch of the autonomic nervous system, causing increased pulse and BP and pupil and bronchial dilatation.The parasympathetic branch regulates digestion and elimination and would increase GI motility and bladder emptying. Application Assessment Physiological Integrity: Physiological Adaptation
37.5 The nurse notes that a client was treated for labyrinthitis on previous admission. To determine if the problem has resolved, the nurse asks the client: a. "Have you noticed any drainage from your ears?" b. "Are you still having earaches?" c. "Do you ever have ringing in your ears?" d. "Are you having difficulty with your balance?"	Answer: d Rationale: The inner ear, or labyrinth, contains receptors that respond to gravity and head position, helping to maintain balance. Drainage and earaches would relate to an ear infection and/or ruptured ear drum. Ringing in the ears can be a sign of ASA toxicity. Application Evaluation Physiological Integrity: Reduction of Risk Potential

© 2007 Pearson Education, Inc.

Question	Answer
37.6 The nurse recognizes that a client with a tumor in the temporal lobe may exhibit which of the following symptoms? a. receptive aphasia b. global aphasia c. personality changes d. mood swings	Answer: a Rationale: Wernicke's area, which is responsible for understanding the written and spoken word, is located in the temporal lobe. Global aphasia involves damage to both Broca and Wernicke's areas. Options c and d are functions controlled by the frontal lobe. Application Assessment Physiological Integrity: Physiological Adaptation
37.7 The nurse is explaining the preparation needed for a positive emission tomography (PET) scan. The client is told he will: a. need to drink several glasses of contrast media. b. have an intravenous line inserted just before the test. c. be given a mild sedative 1 hour before the test. d. only be allowed to drink water the morning of the test.	Answer: b Rationale: A radioisotope is given via an intravenous line at the time of the test. Contrast media and sedatives are not given. Food and fluids are held for 4 hours prior to the test. Application Implementation Physiological Integrity: Reduction of Risk Potential
37.8 A client has sustained damage to the ventral root of the lower thoracic spinal cord. When the client's wife asks if her husband will be paralyzed, the nurse explains: a. "Your husband will not have any sensation from the neck down." b. "His kind of damage will cause flaccid paralysis in the lower extremities." c. "He will have flaccid paralysis from the neck down." d. "He will be able to move his extremities, but he won't be able to feel anything."	Answer: b Rationale: Damage to the ventral root of the spinal cord results in flaccid paralysis. Since injury is at the thoracic level, the lower extremities only will be involved. Application Implementation Physiological Integrity: Physiological Adaptation
37.9 During a neurologic examination of the older client the nurse would expect to see which of the following age-related findings? a. a decreased sense of touch and temperature b. an increase in deep tendon reflexes c. a depressed mood d. disorientation to person and place	Answer: a Rationale: Brain atrophy in the elderly reduces perception to touch, movement, sensation, and temperature. Reflexes would be decreased. A depressed mood and confusion would signal an underlying disease. Application Assessment Physiological Integrity: Physiological Adaptation
37.10 The nurse is checking results of a neurologic assessment on a client. Abnormal results to testing of the abducens nerve indicate the client may have difficulty with: a. chewing food properly. b. taste sensation. c. adequate tear production d. peripheral vision.	Answer: d Rationale: The abducens, or seventh cranial nerve, controls lateral movement of the eyeball. The trigeminal nerve controls chewing. The facial nerve controls taste and tear production. Application Assessment Physiological Integrity: Reduction of Risk Potential

CHAPTER 38

38.1 The nurse is planning to assist with a lumbar puncture. The most vital nursing action prior to the procedure is: a. starting an IV and connecting a heart monitor. b. contacting the lab for a blood type and cross-match. c. emphasizing the importance of not moving during the procedure. d. obtaining a lumbar puncture kit.	Answer: c Rationale: Clients need to be prepared for the position that must be maintained throughout the procedure to ensure safety. Options a and b would not be necessary. Application Planning Physiological Integrity: Reduction of Risk Potential
38.2 The client with a head injury has multiple nursing needs. To promote venous drainage and alleviate pressure, the nurse should: a. encourage the client to cough. b. elevate the head of the bed 30 degrees. c. use oxygen at 2 L/min. d. monitor the temperature every 15 minutes.	Answer: b Rationale: Elevation of 30 degrees promotes venous drainage. Coughing would increase ICP. Oxygen is given at a rate to maintain saturation of 94% or better. Temperature should be monitored every 2 hours. Application Implementation Physiological Integrity: Reduction of Risk Potential
38.3 A client begins to have a seizure during your assessment. Which of the following interventions should be initiated first? a. Turn the client onto his side. b. Monitor seizure and give appropriate medication. c. Place protective pads on the bed. d. Protect the client from injuring himself.	Answer: a Rationale: Turning the client allows secretions, which could pool at the back of the mouth, to drain from the mouth. The other measures could than be initiated. Application Implementation Physiological Integrity: Reduction of Risk Potential
38.4 The nurse instructs the client with a minor head injury to return to the emergency room if which of the following occur? a. increased appetite and fluid consumption b. slight headache that continues for 24 hours c. slight nausea for several hours after injury d. becomes drowsy or confused	Answer: d Rationale: A change in level of consciousness and orientation is a sign of increased intracranial pressure. An increased appetite would not be of concern. Slight headache or nausea may be experienced after a head injury. Application Implementation Physiological Integrity: Reduction of Risk Potential
38.5 The family of a client diagnosed with encephalitis asks the nurse how the disease is treated. The nurse explains that treatment will include: a. strict isolation to prevent spread. b. use of broad-spectrum antibiotics. c. use of antiviral medications. d. a combination of antibiotics and diuretics.	Answer: c Rationale: Antiviral medications are used since it is almost always caused by a virus. Isolation is not necessary as it is not transmitted person to person. Application Implementation Physiological Integrity: Reduction of Risk Potential
38.6 A client informs the nurse he has suddenly developed a headache. The nurse's first priority of care in treating a client with a headache is to: a. give pain medication. b. identify the underlying cause.	Answer: b Rationale: Identifying the underlying cause helps to determine the type of treatment that will be most beneficial and could identify any critical risk factors. Application Assessment Physiological Integrity: Reduction of Risk Potential

© 2007 Pearson Education, Inc.

c. monitor vital signs. d. obtain laboratory values, including drug screens.	
38.7 When caring for a client with left-sided hemianopsia, the nurse should: a. place the food tray on the client's left side. b. check the left side of the mouth for food pocketing. c. place client's personal belongings on the client's right side. d. keep client positioned on the back or left side only.	Answer: a Rationale: Hemianopsia involves loss of one-half of the vision field. The client will only see the food on the left side of the tray if it is placed directly in front. Options b and d are not related to the visual fields. Application Implementation Physiological Integrity: Physiological Adaptation
38.8 Family members are upset and frightened over a client's use of profane language and verbal abusive behavior. The nurse explains that the behavior is related to the location of the client's brain tumor in the: a. frontal lobe. b. parietal lobe. c. occipital lobe. d. temporal lobe.	Answer: a Rationale: Frontal lobe tumors often cause loss of emotional control, confusion, and personality changes. Comprehension Implementation Physiological Integrity: Physiological Adaptation
38.9 When caring for a client who has had a subarachnoid hemorrhage, the nurse focuses nursing interventions on preventing: a. rebleeding. b. seizures. c. aphasia. d. meningitis.	Answer: a Rationale: The major complications following a subarachnoid hemorrhage are rebleeding and vasospasm. Medications are given to prevent seizures. Aphasia and meningitis would not be related to a subarachnoid hemorrhage. Application Implementation Physiological Integrity: Reduction of Risk Potential
38.10 The nurse is caring for a client with a subdural hematoma. To reduce intracranial pressure (ICP), the nurse anticipates giving the following medications: a. loop diuretics and beta blockers b. osmotic diuretics and corticosteroids c. histamine 2 antagonists and antibiotics d. calcium channel blockers and anticonvulsants	Answer: b Rationale: Loop and osmotic diuretics will draw water from the edematous brain tissue. Corticosteroids reduce edema through their anti-inflammatory action. Application Planning Physiological Integrity: Pharmacological and Parenteral Therapies

CHAPTER 39

39.1 When planning to discharge a client with multiple sclerosis (MS), the nurse should teach the client to: a. perform tasks in the morning. b. increase exercises in the afternoon. c. take showers or tub baths in hot water. d. decrease medication as symptoms improve.	Answer: a Rationale: Fatigue is usually worse in the afternoon. Hot water may produce vasodilatation contributing to postural hypotension and increased risk of falls. Medication should be taken on a maintenance basis to decrease incidence of exacerbations. Application Planning Physiological Integrity: Reduction of Risk Potential

39.2 When doing a physical assessment of a client, the nurse should expect to find which symptom related to a diagnosis of Parkinson's disease? a. bradykinesia b. dry skin c. polyuria d. elevated blood pressure	Answer: a Rationale: The three cardinal symptoms of Parkinson's are tremors, rigidity and bradykinesia (slowed voluntary movements and speech). Comprehension Assessment Physiological Integrity: Physiological Adaptation
39.3 A client is admitted with the following symptoms: visual changes, muscular weakness, and numbness and tingling in the extremities. Based on theses findings, the nurse should suspect the client of having which of the following diseases? a. myasthenia gravis b. amyotrophic lateral sclerosis c. multiple sclerosis d. guillain-Barré syndrome	Answer: c Rationale: All of these symptoms are seen with multiple sclerosis. Signs of myasthenia gravis include speech, chewing, and motor impairments. AMLS involves muscle fasiculations and muscle wasting. Guillain-Barré symptoms begin in the lower extremities and move upward. Analysis Assessment Physiological Integrity: Physiological Adaptation
39.4 When caring for a client with herniated disk disease, the nurse's priority of focus is to: a. take precautions to prevent further injury. b. teach the client log-rolling techniques. c. assess the degree to which the disease affects daily activities. d. decrease intervertebral disk pressure.	Answer: a Rationale: Further trauma or herniation of the disk can reduce mobility and sensation, leading to further injury. Treatment focuses on medication and bed rest. Options b, c, and d will all be part of the nursing care. Comprehension Planning Safe, Effective Care Environment: Coordinated Care
39.5 When a client has trigeminal neuralgia, the client should be carefully assessed for: a. signs and symptoms of acute cholinergic crisis. b. symptoms of acute respiratory distress. c. changes in the level of consciousness. d. trigger zones that cause pain when stimulated.	Answer: d Rationale: Clients with trigeminal neuralgia experience severe pain and burning sensations when specific sites near the nose and cheek are stimulated. Identifying exactly where these areas are for a specific client enables the nurse to avoid triggering the sites. Option a refers to MS. Options b and c are not pertinent to trigeminal neuralgia. Comprehension Assessment Physiologic Integrity: Basic Care & Comfort
39.6 A client diagnosed with Parkinson's disease is prescribed to take levodopa. The nurse should instruct the client about possible side effects which include: a. orthostatic hypotension and confusion. b. acute hypertension and glycosuria. c. diarrhea. d. bradycardia.	Answer: a Rationale: The client is instructed to change positions slowly to avoid postural hypotension and to be aware the drug may cause confusion at times. It does not cause diarrhea or bradycardia. Comprehension Implementation Physiological Integrity: Pharmacological and Parenteral Therapies
39.7 When teaching the client and family about the disease myasthenia gravis, the nurse should include which of the following? a. strategies to improve memory b. signs and symptoms of fluid volume excess c. methods to increase fluid intake d. signs and symptoms of cholinergic crisis	Answer: d Rationale: Cholinergic crisis is caused by overmedication with cholinergic medications. Symptoms will include excessive sweating, bradycardia, severe muscle weakness, cramps, and salivations. Application Implementation Physiological Integrity: Reduction of Risk Potential

© 2007 Pearson Education, Inc.

39.8 The family of a client with Alzheimer's disease expresses concern that their mother is becoming worse. The nurse identifies the following manifestations as indicating the client is advancing to stage 2 of Alzheimer's disease: a. short-term memory loss b. has difficulty using objects c. has difficulty learning new information d. forgets the location and names of objects	Answer: b Rationale: Difficulty using objects correctly, reading, writing, and speech are seen in stage 2. Options a, c, and d are all seen in stage 1. Analysis Assessment Physiological Integrity: Physiological Adaptation
39.9 When planning the care for a client who has a spinal cord injury, the nurse should give priority to which of these treatment measures first? a. monitoring the client's blood pressure b. listening for bowel sounds c. testing for motor strength d. palpating the client's bladder for fullness	Answer: a Rationale: An exaggerated sympathetic response leads to autonomic dysreflexia, which can lead to a hypertensive crisis. A full bladder or distended bowel can trigger the response. Analysis Planning Physiological Integrity: Reduction of Risk Potential
39.10 After administering diazepam (Valium) PO to a client who has a spinal cord injury the nurse should expect to observe which of these client responses? a. improved swallowing ability b. a decrease in salivation and sweating c. decrease in muscle spasm and pain d. improved motor coordination	Answer: c Rationale: Diazepam is given to control the muscle spasms and pain associated with musculoskeletal injuries. It would not affect saliva and sweating. It is not given to improve swallowing or coordination. Application Evaluation Physiological Integrity: Pharmacological and Parenteral Therapies

CHAPTER 40

40.1 During the eye assessment, the nurse takes a history of the client's use of eye medications, recognizing many of them can affect which of the following body systems? a. cardiovascular and respiratory b. endocrine and digestive c. gastrointestinal and endocrine d. urinary and reproductive	Answer: a Rationale: Systemic absorption of various eyedrop medications can have adverse effects. The sympathomimetic drugs, i.e., Alphagan and Epitrate, can increase blood pressure and cause irregular pulse rates or chest pain. The beta blockers, i.e., Betoptic and Timolol, can exacerbate COPD, asthma and heart failure. Analysis Assessment Health Promotion: Prevention and Early Detection of Health Problems
40.2 A client working in a laboratory accidentally splashed chemicals in both eyes. The occupational health nurse should instruct this client to: a. wash the eyes with antibacterial solution. b. flush both eyes with water using an eyedropper and see the family doctor if pain persists. c. wipe both eyes with a sterile cotton ball saturated with normal saline and proceed to the emergency room. d. flush both eyes with large amounts of water immediately, then report to a physician as soon as possible.	Answer: d Rationale: Chemical burns require flushing with copious amounts of fluid in an effort to remove as much chemical as possible. An antibiotic would not be needed to flush the eye. An eyedropper or cotton balls would not provide sufficient flushing pressure. Application Implementation Physiological Integrity: Reduction of Risk Potential

Question	Answer
40.3 Clients with chronic, open-angle glaucoma should be instructed by the nurse to: **a.** use over-the-counter medications for eye pain. **b.** use mild boric acid solution to irrigate the eyes periodically. **c.** sleep with the head of the bed elevated to reduce eye pressure. **d.** avoid over-the-counter cold or allergy medications.	Answer: d Rationale: Over-the-counter preparations have sympathomimetic action, causing pupil dilation, which blocks the trabecular meshwork and flow of aqueous humor, leading to increased intraocular pressure. Chronic glaucoma is painless. Irrigations are not necessary. Sleep position won't affect the eye pressure associated with glaucoma. Application Implementation Physiological Integrity: Reduction of Risk Potential
40.4 A client in seen in the emergency department and is diagnosed as having acute glaucoma. What symptoms could the nurse expect to find in the client's history related to the glaucoma? **a.** acute eye pain **b.** loss of peripheral vision **c.** diplopia **d.** no symptoms of pain or pressure	Answer: a Rationale: Acute glaucoma causes severe eye pain, blurred vision, nausea, vomiting, and halos. Comprehension Assessment Physiological Integrity: Physiological Adaptation
40.5 The client who has just had cataract extraction surgery suddenly complains of sharp pain in the eye. The nurse responds by: **a.** administering pain medication. **b.** notifying the physician. **c.** placing an ice pack over the eye. **d.** removing the dressing to examine the eye.	Answer: b Rationale: The pain could be secondary to a surgical complication and must be assessed by the physician. Application Implementation Physiological Integrity: Reduction of Risk Potential
40.6 A client is suspected of having a detached retina. The nurse assesses the client for which of the following findings that would support the diagnosis? **a.** total loss of vision **b.** strabismus and eye pain **c.** burning and eye dryness **d.** flashes of light and floaters	Answer: d Rationale: Common manifestations of a detached retina include a sense of curtain or veil across vision, flashes of light, and floaters. Comprehension Assessment Physiological Integrity: Physiological Adaptation
40.7 The nurse should instruct clients with conjunctivitis to: **a.** use over-the-counter eyedrops to reducc the redness in the eyes. **b.** wash around the eyes with mild soap and water. **c.** keep the hands away from the eyes and not rub the eyes. **d.** use an eye patch until the redness disappears.	Answer: c Rationale: The bacteria or fungal organisms causing conjunctivitis are frequently spread by hand contact. Rubbing the eye causes further irritation. Corticosteroid and topical antiseptics are used to treat the infection and inflammation. An eye patch is not necessary. Application Implementation Physiological Integrity: Reduction of Risk Potential
40.8 The nurse cautions the client who just had a stapedectomy with prosthesis not to blow the nose hard because: **a.** it may cause bleeding in the middle ear. **b.** it may cause vertigo. **c.** it may rupture the tympanic membrane. **d.** it may dislodge the prosthesis.	Answer: d Rationale: Blowing the nose can increase pressure within the middle ear and dislodge or disrupt the prosthesis. Application Implementation Physiological Integrity: Reduction of Risk Potential

© 2007 Pearson Education, Inc.

40.9 A client with Ménière's disease is hospitalized for severe vertigo. The nurse plans the following nursing interventions to assist in management of the vertigo and nausea: a. administration of stool softeners b. bed rest in a quiet, darkened room c. encouraging frequent ambulation in the hall d. offering frequent warm beverages containing caffeine	Answer: b Rationale: Minimal movement and minimal sensory stimuli provide comfort and help to reduce nausea. Antiemetics are administered. Activity should be reduced or limited. Caffeine may precipitate an attack. Application Planning Physiological Integrity: Reduction of Risk Potential
40.10 A client phones into the physician's office and reports an insect has flown into his ear and asks the nurse what he should do. The nurse instructs him to: a. irrigate the ear with water to flush out the insect. b. instill mineral oil into the ear canal and try to gently remove insect with tweezers. c. attempt to remove the insect with a cotton-tipped applicator that has been dipped in hydrogen peroxide. d. apply Vaseline to smother and kill the insect.	Answer: b Rationale: Mineral oil helps to immobilize the insect, making removal easier. Water may cause the insect to swell, making removal more difficult. Cotton-tipped applicators may push the insect further into the ear canal. Vaseline would be difficult to insert; mineral oil is a better option. Application Implementation Physiological Integrity: Reduction of Risk Potential

CHAPTER 41

41.1 Following an arthrocentesis of the right knee in the physician's office, the nurse gives the following instructions to the client: a. Apply warm moist heat as needed for pain relief. b. Remove the pressure dressing when you get home. c. Limit use of the joint for 2 to 3 days. d. Begin range-of-motion exercises to the knee in 24 hours.	Answer: c Rationale: The affected joint is rested for 2 to 3 days to allow for healing and reduce swelling. Heat would increase swelling; cold packs should be applied. The pressure dressing should be removed after 8 to 24 hours. ROM exercises would be started in about a week. Application Implementation Physiological Integrity: Reduction of Risk Potential
41.2 A client scheduled for a magnetic resonance imaging (MRI) of the shoulder expresses concern over radiation exposure. The nurse provides the following information: a. "Most of your body will be covered with a lead apron." b. "Drinking a lot of water after the procedure helps to flush it out of the body." c. "The amount of radiation is no more than when you have a dental x-ray. d. "You will not be exposed to any radiation."	Answer: d Rationale: A super magnet and radio-frequency signals are used in an MRI; radiation is not used. Comprehension Implementation Physiological Integrity: Reduction of Risk Potential

41.3 The nurse determines a client has understood instructions given following a lung scan when the client states: a. "I won't play with the grandchildren for at least forty-eight hours." b. "I need to drink a lot of fluids." c. "I'll avoid close contact with my family for one week." d. "I won't eat foods with any artificial colors or dyes."	Answer: b Rationale: Increased fluid intake is necessary to promote excretion of the radioactive material and prevent renal complications. Radioactive precautions are not necessary as the amount is minimal. Comprehension Evaluation Physiological Integrity: Reduction of Risk Potential
41.4 The nurse is preparing a client scheduled for an arthroscopy of the elbow. When the client asks if there will be any restrictions after the procedure, the nurse explains: a. "There are no restrictions, unless you have a lot of pain." b. "You will need to keep the elbow elevated for one to two days." c. "The elbow will be kept in a sling for two weeks." d. "You will need to limit range of motion in the joint until the sutures are removed."	Answer: b Rationale: Elevation of the involved extremity is necessary for 24 to 48 hours to prevent swelling. Range-of-motion exercises and physical therapy may be indicated. Sutures are usually not necessary. Application Implementation Physiological Integrity: Reduction of Risk Potential
41.5 When assessing the musculoskeletal system of an elderly client, it would be important for the nurse to report which of the following findings? a. Crepitus is heard when bending the knee. b. Client complains of numbness in the hands. c. Client is unable to fully extend arms about the head. d. Client complains of stiffness and mild pain in the knee joints.	Answer: b Rationale: Numbness could indicate a neurologic or musculoskeletal disorder, because these systems are closely related. It would not be considered a normal age-related finding. Crepitus is a grating noise heard due to loss of cartilage over ends of bones and can occur with age and osteoarthritis. Full range of motion and flexibility are decreased with age. Osteoarthritis causes pain and stiffness in the joints. Analysis Assessment Physiological Integrity: Physiological Adaptation
41.6 Following a motor vehicle accident, a client with injuries to the face is tested for muscle strength. The nurse determines there is adequate strength of the eyes and eyelids when the client is able to: a. blink rapidly. b. keep eyelids closed for 30 seconds. c. follow the nurse's finger movements with eyes. d. close eyes tightly.	Answer: d Rationale: Ability to shut eyes tightly indicates intact use of both eye and eyelid muscles. Blinking and closing eyelids indicates muscle movement but does not measure strength. Following fingers with the eyes measures eye muscles, but not the eyelids. Application Evaluation Physiological Integrity: Physiological Adaptation
41.7 The nurse determines a client's treatment for hypoparathyroidism has been effective for correction of electrolyte imbalances when laboratory values indicate the: a. calcium level has increased from 8.2 mg/dL to 8.9 mg/dL. b. calcium level has decreased from 8.6 mg/dL to 8.0 mg/dL. c. phosphate levels are 3.0 mg/dL. d. alkaline phosphate is within normal limits.	Answer: a Rationale: Low calcium levels are seen with hypoparathyroidism; an increase to a normal level would indicate treatment is effective for correction of the low serum calcium. The phosphate level is normal and alkaline phosphatase levels would not be evaluated. Analysis Evaluation Physiological Adaptation: Reduction of Risk Potential

© 2007 Pearson Education, Inc.

Question	Answer
41.8 When checking laboratory values on a client recovering from a fracture of the left femur, the nurse would expect to find which of the following changes? a. an increase in alkaline phosphatase b. an increase in uric acid c. a decrease in erythrocyte sedimentation rate (ESR) d. a positive antinuclear antibody (ANA)	Answer: a Rationale: Alkaline phosphatase levels increase during bone healing and with bone tumors. Elevated uric acid levels are seen in gout. ESR is a nonspecific marker of inflammation; it may be elevated secondary to the trauma, but would not be specific to bone. ANA is found in autoimmune disorders. Application Assessment Physiological Integrity: Physiological Adaptation
41.9 The nurse is assisting a client who is having a Thomas test performed. When the client's left knee is brought to the chest, the nurse recognizes a hip flexion contracture is present when: a. the right leg externally rotates. b. the right leg rises off the bed. c. the client complains of sharp pain radiating down the left leg. d. the client complains of pain in the lumbar spine.	Answer: b Rationale: When the left leg is brought to the chest, the right leg should be kept straight. When the leg rises off the bed, a hip flexion contracture is indicated. Pain may be present, but would not support diagnosis of the contracture. Comprehension Assessment Physiological Integrity: Physiological Adaptation
41.10 When assessing a client's lateral flexion of the cervical spine, the nurse asks the client to: a. look at the ceiling. b. touch the chin to the chest. c. turn the head and look to the left. d. touch the ear to the shoulder.	Answer: d Rationale: Bending the neck laterally tests flexion of the cervical spine. Looking at the ceiling tests extension. Touching chin to chest tests flexion. Turning head to the side tests rotation. Application Assessment Physiological Integrity: Physiological Integrity

CHAPTER 42

Question	Answer
42.1 Four hours after a total knee replacement, a 78-year-old client is found to have a heart rate of 110 bpm. The nurse should assess the client for: a. cardiac arrhythmia. b. pain. c. hypothermia. d. elevated blood pressure.	Answer: b Rationale: Tachycardia is often a sympathetic nervous system response to pain, which commonly occurs following this type of surgery. Detection of cardiac arrhythmias requires telemetry monitoring. If pain is not found, then client should be monitored for temperature and blood pressure changes. Analysis Assessment Physiological Integrity: Reduction of risk potential
42.2 The nurse performs frequent neurovascular assessments for clients with musculoskeletal trauma in order to prevent: a. CVA. b. compartment syndrome. c. DVT. d. fat embolus.	Answer: b Rationale: Compartment syndrome results in nerve damage and impaired tissue perfusion if not identified and treated promptly. A CVA is not a typical complication of musculoskeletal trauma. Frequent circulatory and respiratory assessments are done to detect DVT and fat emboli. Application Implementation Physiological Integrity: Reduction of Risk Potential
42.3 Following an above-the-knee amputation, the client continues to complain of pain in the amputated leg. The nurse determines that the client is experiencing which of the following types of pain: a. psychosomatic. b. referred. c. myofascial. d. phantom limb.	Answer: d Rationale: Trauma to the nerves serving the amputated body parts often produce sensations of pain, burning, and/or numbness, which is called phantom pain. Application Assessment Physiological Integrity: Physiological Adaptation

42.4 When caring for a client with multiple fractures requiring prolonged bed rest, the nurse knows a priority nursing diagnosis will be: **a.** Risk for Injury related to orthostatic hypotension. **b.** Hypovolemia related to multiple traumatic injuries. **c.** Potential for Impaired Tissue Perfusion related to immobility. **d.** Risk for Social Isolation related to prolonged bed rest.	Answer: c Rationale: Immobility can contribute to development of DVTs, PEs, edema, and compartment syndrome, all of which could result in impaired tissue perfusion. Options a and d are not as high a priority. Hypovolemia is not caused by immobility. Application Analysis/Diagnosis Physiological Integrity: Reduction of Risk Potential
42.5 A client on prolonged bed rest asks why ROM exercises are necessary. The nurse explains that prolonged bed rest can result in: **a.** decreased body mechanics. **b.** increased skeletal pain. **c.** increased muscle spasms. **d.** decreased muscle tone.	Answer: d Rationale: Adequate muscle tone is required to promote venous return, reducing risk of DVT and edema. Application Implementation Physiological Integrity: Reduction in Risk Potential
42.6 A client with a hip fracture is experiencing muscle spasms. The nurse anticipates that the following type of traction may be utilized preoperatively to reduce the spasms: **a.** skeletal traction **b.** manual traction **c.** Buck's traction **d.** balanced suspension traction	Answer: c Rationale: Buck's traction applies a pulling force to the leg and maintains traction; the pulling force helps to reduce spasms. Skeletal traction involves use of pins for realignment. Manual traction is used to reduce a fracture. Balanced suspension uses more than one force and allows for easier turning. Application Planning Physiological Integrity: Reduction of Risk Potential
42.7 A client with an above-the-knee amputation asks the nurse why he has a prosthesis so soon after surgery. The nurse explains that the advantage of immediate prosthesis fitting postamputation is: **a.** client's ability to ambulate sooner. **b.** less frequent dressing changes. **c.** better fit of the prosthesis. **d.** decreased chance of phantom limb sensation or pain.	Answer: a Rationale: This allows limited weight bearing within 24 to 48 hours of surgery. It does not alter the need to do dressing changes or reduce phantom limb pain. Additional adjustments to the prosthesis will be made once healing of the stump has occurred. Comprehension Planning Physiological Integrity: Physiological Adaptation
42.8 To maintain proper alignment of a client's Buck's traction, the nurse performs the following interventions: **a.** Ensure the weights hang freely over the end of the bed. **b.** Lift the weights when assisting client to move up in bed. **c.** Keep the leg in traction externally rotated. **d.** Instruct the client to do ankle rotation exercises.	Answer: a Rationale: The weights should be hanging freely without touching the floor or bed. Lifting the weights breaks the traction. The client should be moved up in bed allowing weights to freely move with client. The leg should be kept in straight alignment. Ankle exercises could cause the leg to go out of alignment. Application Implementation Physiological Integrity: Reduction of Risk Potential
42.9 The nurse is instructing a family member on how to properly position her mother following a total hip replacement. The nurse explains the client's hip should always be kept: **a.** straight with the knee flexed and no pillows.	Answer: b Rationale: This position keeps the joint from being displaced out of the socket. An adducted or totally straight position may cause the new joint to become dislocated. The leg can be kept straight and fixed if an abductor pillow is used. Application Implementation Physiological Integrity: Reduction of Risk Potential

 © 2007 Pearson Education, Inc.

b. in an abducted position. c. in an adducted position. d. totally straight without any pillow between legs.	
42.10 The nurse is caring for a client with a fracture of the right humerus. Which of the following assessment findings could be an early sign of fat emboli? a. abdominal cramping b. confusion c. numbness in the right hand d. headache	Answer: b Rationale: Irritation and confusion are signs of hypoxia, caused by fat emboli that have traveled to the lungs, causing inflammation to lung tissue. The other symptoms would not be indicative of fat emboli. Analysis Assessment Physiological Integrity: Reduction of Risk Potential

CHAPTER 43

43.1 When caring for a client with an arthroplasy, the nurse needs to monitor the client for which major complication? a. mobility postsurgery b. monitoring postoperative pain c. infection postsurgery, because it impairs healing d. cardiac arrhythmias	Answer: c Rationale: Infection is a major complication, leading to impaired healing and the possible need for removal of prosthesis. The other options identify components that need to be monitored, but are not of highest priority. Application Implementation Physiological Integrity: Reduction of Risk Potential
43.2 When caring for a client with systemic lupus erythematosus the nurse should provide teaching that addresses: a. the need to adhere to a high-protein diet. b. the need for daily aerobic exercises. c. skin care and limiting of sun exposure. d. the use of birth control to prevent pregnancy.	Answer: c Rationale: Sun exposure can worsen both skin and systemic manifestations of SLE. Excessive drying of skin and sun exposure should be avoided. A special diet is not indicated; supplements may be needed. Exercise and rest must be balanced. Pregnancy is not contraindicated, but client will need close medical supervision during the pregnancy. Application Implementation Physiological Integrity: Reduction of Risk Potential
43.3 A client seen in the clinic expresses concern she may have Lyme disease. The nurse explains that some common symptoms in the early stage include: a. severe swelling at tick bite mark within 24 hours. b. erythema, headache, fever, and chills. c. slight temperature and nausea. d. progressive confusion and disorientation.	Answer: b Rationale: Erythema migrans, a flat or slightly raised red lesion, is the initial manifestation seen at the site of the tick bite. Client may also experience headache, fever, muscle aches, and fatigue. Comprehension Assessment Physiological Integrity: Physiological Adaptation
43.4 A client with rheumatoid arthritis (RA) says to the nurse: "I thought I had osteoarthritis. How is this different?" The nurse explains it differs from osteoarthritis in that rheumatoid arthritis: a. has an abrupt onset of red, swollen joints. b. is slower to progress than osteoarthritis. c. affects only one joint at a time. d. does not cause fever or malaise.	Answer: a Rationale: RA has an abrupt or insidious onset, whereas osteoarthritis can be more gradual and insidious. RA progresses more rapidly and affects multiple joints, causing fever, weight loss, fatigue, and anemia. Application Assessment Physiological Integrity: Physiological Adaptation

Question	Answer
43.5 The nurse is instructing a client who has been started on colchicine for the treatment of gout. The following information should be included: a. Limit fluid intake with the medicine. b. Take with food. c. Report any GI distress and fatigue. d. Have serum uric acid levels checked.	Answer: c Rationale: Colchicine can cause serious GI, kidney, liver, and heart disease. Fluids should be encouraged. It should be taken on an empty stomach for best absorption. It does not lower serum uric acid levels. Application Implementation Physiological Integrity: Pharmacological and Parenteral Therapies
43.6 When collecting a client's drug history, the nurse recognizes that both bone and muscle function may be most impaired if the client reports taking: a. corticosteroids. b. oral hypoglycemic agents. c. aspirin. d. potassium sparing diuretics.	Answer: a Rationale: Corticosteroids cause protein catabolism with skeletal muscle wasting and contribute to osteoporosis, secondary to increased osteoclast activity. Analysis Assessment Physiological Integrity: Pharmacological and Parenteral Therapies
43.7 The nurse is assisting at an athletic team function at her child's school. The nurse understands the use of cold, compression, and elevation will be indicated if a student has which of the following injuries? a. muscle spasm b. dislocation of the elbow c. a repetitive-use strain of the wrist d. an ankle sprain.	Answer: d Rationale: Rest, ice, compression, and elevation (RICE) help to reduce the edema associated with sprains and strains. Muscle spasms should be treated with ice. Repetitive strain injuries require rest and limitation of movement. A dislocation needs immobilization. Application Assessment Physiological Integrity: Reduction of Risk Potential
43.8 The nurse is preparing a client with osteomyelitis of the left tibia for discharge. The nurse stresses the importance of the following information: a. "You will need to continue to take antibiotics for another four to eight weeks." b. "You can start to do light weight bearing on the leg in one week." c. "Be sure to do active range-of-motion exercises to the left leg daily." d. "You can apply heat to the leg if you are having a lot of pain and discomfort."	Answer: a Rationale: Prolonged antibiotic therapy will be necessary for adequate eradication of the organism, usually staphylococcus. Weight bearing should be avoided to prevent fracture. Range-of-motion exercises and heat increase circulation and encourage spread of the organism. Application Implementation Physiological Integrity: Reduction of Risk Potential
43.9 The nurse is speaking with the mother of a child with muscular dystrophy at a local health fair. The nurse emphasizes the importance of: a. preventing respiratory infections. b. avoiding pneumococcal vaccines. c. using braces as little as possible. d. keeping child isolated from other children.	Answer: a Rationale: Because the muscles of respiration may be affected, they are at risk of upper respiratory infections. Pneumococcal vaccines are recommended. The use of braces promotes independence and mobility. Socialization is encouraged. Application Implementation Physiological Integrity: Reduction of Risk Potential
43.10 A nurse who is caring for a client with Paget's disease plans the following nursing interventions: a. Keep client on bed rest. b. Do all client care activities at one time. c. Encourage client to stay out of bed most of the day. d. Teach client how to apply a back brace.	Answer: d Rationale: Since the client with Paget's disease is at risk for pathological fractures and spinal deformities, back braces are used for support. Activity and rest should be balanced, allowing client time to rest between activities. Application Planning Physiological Integrity: Reduction of Risk Potential

© 2007 Pearson Education, Inc.

Chapter 44

44.1 When assessing a client of African American descent for jaundice, the nurse should check the: a. palms of the hands. b. abdomen. c. sclera. d. mucous membranes of the mouth.	Answer: c Rationale: Jaundice can be seen in the sclera of dark-skinned individuals. Comprehension Assessment Physiological Integrity: Physiological Adaptation
44.2 A client is admitted with third-degree burns of the upper arms and chest. When assessing the client, the nurse will expect the skin to be: a. reddened and covered with blisters. b. white with patches of blackened skin. c. bluish-purple with blisters. d. diffusely bright red and swollen.	Answer: b Rationale: Third-degree burns produce charring of the skin, appearing as white with black necrotic patches. Option a describes second-degree burns. Option d describes first-degree burns. Comprehension Assessment Physiological Integrity: Physiological Adaptation
44.3 A client recently started on steroids has been reading about the medication and asks the nurse: "The book says I could have hirsutism as a side effect. How will I know if this happens?" The nurse explains: a. "You will notice a pinpoint red rash on your chest." b. "Your hair will start to comc out in clumps." c. "You will notice excess facial and body hair." d. "Your breasts will become enlarged and swollen."	Answer: c Rationale: Hirsutism is a growth of fine downy body hair, usually seen on the face and chest. Option a decribes a rash. Option b describes the start of alopecia. Option d describes gynecomastia. Application Implementation Physiological Integrity: Pharmacological and Parenteral Therapies
44.4 While bathing an elderly client, the nurse observes the presence of various age-related skin changes. Which of the following skin changes should be of concern to the nurse? a. senile lentigines b. seborrheic keratosis c. actinic keratosis d. skin tags	Answer: c Rationale: Actinic keratoses are reddish raised plaques that can become malignant and should be checked frequently. Senile lentigines (liver spots), seborrheic keratosis (dark raised lesions), and skin tags (excess flaps of skin) are normal with aging and benign. Analysis Assessment Physiological Integrity: Physiological Adaptation
44.5 When performing an assessment of the integumentary system on a client, the nurse should: a. check for skin turgor on the forearm. b. palpate for edema over the knee. c. check color, quantity, and distribution of hair. d. inspect inside of the mouth for skin tags.	Answer: c Rationale: Overall assessment of the hair is part of the integumentary system. Turgor should be checked on the forehead or collarbone. Edema is palpated best over the ankle. Skin tags are found on the external surface of skin. Application Assessment Physiological Integrity: Reduction of Risk Potential
44.6 The nurse observes that a client has a deep, irregularly shaped area of skin loss extending into the dermis on the lower extremity. The nurse documents that the client has: a. an ulcer. b. a fissure. c. a wheal. d. a macule.	Answer: a Rationale: The description defines the characteristics of an ulcer. Fissures are linear cracks with sharp edges. A wheal is elevated and fluid filled, with an irregular border. A macule is a flat, nonpalpable change in skin color. Application Assessment Physiological Integrity: Physiological Adaptation

© 2007 Pearson Education, Inc.

44.7 Which of the following assessment findings on an African American client should be reported to the primary nurse? **a.** red splinter hemorrhages on the nails **b.** keloid formation over an appendectomy scar **c.** pigmented bands on the fingernails **d.** a pustule on the right hand	Answer: d Rationale: A pustule is a pus-filled vesicle and could be indicative of an infection. The nail abnormalities are normal in 90% of African Americans. Keloids develop more easily in this race as well and are benign. Analysis Assessment Physiological Integrity: Physiological Adaptation
44.8 The nurse is assisting in the collection of fluid from a client's blister. The nurse explains the specimen will be sent for a Tzanck test, which is done to: **a.** identify herpes infections. **b.** diagnose fungal infections. **c.** diagnose scabies. **d.** identify bacterial infections.	Answer: a Rationale: The Tzanck test identifies herpes infection. Identification of fungal infections and scabies requires a skin scraping. Bacterial infections are identified through culture and sensitivity testing. Comprehension Implementation Physiological Integrity: Reduction of Risk Potential
44.9 A client has a patch test done to determine degree of allergic reaction to suspected allergens. After the patches are applied the nurse instructs the client to: **a.** return in 48 hours to have the patches removed. **b.** leave patches on until they fall off on their own. **c.** return in 1 week to have skin reactions assessed. **d.** avoid contact with anyone else for 48 hours.	Answer: a Rationale: Patches are removed and sites assessed for reaction in 48 hours. No contact restrictions are necessary. Application Implementation Physiological Integrity: Reduction of Risk Potential
44.10 A client seen in the clinic is being evaluated for a scabies infection. To confirm the diagnosis, the nurse informs the client he will need to have which of the following tests performed? **a.** Tzank test **b.** patch test **c.** skin scraping **d.** Wood's light examination	Answer: c Rationale: Tissue samples are scraped from the lesion and examined for the presence of the mite. The Tzanck test identifies herpes infections. Patch tests are done to diagnose allergies. The Wood's light exam distinguishes hyperpigmented from hypopigmented lesions. Application Implementation Physiological Integrity: Physiological Adaptation

CHAPTER 45

45.1 The nurse has instructed an adult client with diabetes about proper foot care. The nurse determines that the client understood the instructions when the nurse observes the client: **a.** cutting the toenails at the corners. **b.** trimming toenails with scissors. **c.** using a file to trim the toenails. **d.** wearing open toe sandals.	Answer: c Rationale: Filing nails is the safest way to prevent skin trauma. Toenails should be cut straight across to avoid ingrown nails. Proper cutters or having nail care done by a podiatrist is safest for a diabetic. Closed toe shoes are safest to protect feet and toes from trauma. Comprehension Evaluation Physiological Integrity: Reduction of Risk Potential
45.2 After turning a bedridden client from her side to her back, the nurse observes that the area over the trochanter is red and does not blanch with finger pressure. The nurse should document this observation as: **a.** a stage I pressure ulcer. **b.** ischemia. **c.** eschar. **d.** hyperemia.	Answer: a Rationale: Nonblanchable erythema with intact skin is characteristic of a stage 1 pressure ulcer. Ischemia indicates lack of blood flow, and erythema is not present. Eschar indicates dead necrotic tissue. Hyperemia is redness from increased blood flow to a site which resolves when pressure is removed. Application Implementation Safe, Effective Care Environment: Coordinated Care

© 2007 Pearson Education, Inc.

45.3 While inspecting a pressure ulcer of a 90-year-old client, the nurse observes new tissue growth around the area, which is pinkish-red in color. The nurse documents the presence of: a. epithelialization. b. granulation. c. eschar. d. slough.	Answer: b Rationale: The pinkish-red tissue is new tissue growth in the wound bed, called granulation tissue. Epithelialization is a process of new cell growth. Eschar appears as black or brown, dried and hardened necrotic tissue. Slough is the semiliquid white and yellow tissue seen in a wound bed. Analysis Assessment Physiological Integrity: Physiological Adaptation
45.4 The nurse is preparing to cleanse a pressure ulcer over the sacrum of a client. The nurse chooses which of the following solutions? a. povidone–iodine (Betadine) b. normal saline solution c. hydrogen peroxide d. Dakin's solution	Answer: b Rationale: Normal saline is an isotonic solution equal to the tonicity of body fluids and used for cleansing wounds. Diluted hydrogen peroxide and betadine may be used for cleansing of infected wounds, but need to be followed with saline cleansing to remove any irritating chemicals harmful to the tissue. Dakin's solution is used when specifically ordered to change the pH of the wound environment. Application Implementation Physiological Integrity: Pharmacological and Parenteral Therapies
45.5 A dark-skinned client was admitted in respiratory distress. When planning to assess for cyanosis the nurse recognizes that: a. cyanosis in clients with dark skin will need to be checked. b. it is not possible to assess color changes in clients with dark skin. c. cyanosis can be seen on the lips and mucous membranes of clients with dark skin. d. cyanosis will blanch with direct pressure to the soles of the feet in dark-skinned clients.	Answer: c Rationale: A bluish discoloration of the mucous membranes indicates cyanosis in clients with dark skin. Application Assessment Physiological Integrity: Physiological Adaptation
45.6 When taking a history on a client who has had a severe flare-up of psoriasis, the nurse should determine which of the following factors? a. age at onset of his psoriasis b. allergy history c. recent changes in work or home environment d. where the symptoms first appeared	Answer: c Rationale: The exact cause of psoriasis is unknown, but many factors appear to make the condition worse, including stress, sunlight, seasonal changes, and various medications. Determining contributing factors to the flare-up will help the client to prevent future exposures. The other factors do not have an impact on the current flare-up. Analysis Assessment Health Promotion: Prevention and/or Early Detection of Health Problems
45.7 A female client with acne vulgaris is given a prescription for Retin-A. The client should be instructed to: a. avoid chocolate, cola drinks, and peanuts. b. take larger doses if acne gets worse before menstrual periods. c. do not take if pregnant and limit exposure to sunlight. d. increase intake of vitamin A and calcium.	Answer: c Rationale: Retin-A is not safe for the developing fetus and causes increased sensitivity to the sun. Vitamin A is a fat-soluble vitamin and may be toxic if excessive doses are taken. Vitamin A supplements and alcohol should be avoided; there are no restrictions on caffeine-containing products or peanuts. Application Implementation Physiological Integrity: Pharmacological and Parenteral Therapies

© 2007 Pearson Education, Inc.

Question	Answer
45.8 A client has crusty vesicopustular lesions over her face diagnosed as furuncles. When teaching the client to how prevent reoccurrences, the nurse identifies a common contributing factor: a. excessively dry skin b. impaired immune response c. inadequate personal hygiene d. deficiency in vitamin A in the diet	Answer: c Rationale: The causative agent is frequently *Staphylococcus aureas,* a bacteria easily spread through skin contact. Other causes are skin trauma and excessive skin oiliness or perspiration. Application Planning Health Promotion: Prevention and/or Early Detection of Health Problems
45.9 A nurse is planning to teach about early recognition of malignant melanoma at a local health fair. A poster using which of the following acronyms would be appropriate? a. Know your ABCDs. b. Watch the SUN. c. Eat RICE. d. Don't be a BRAT.	Answer: a Rationale: The acronym represents A for asymmetry, border irregularity, C for color variations, and D for greater than 6 cm in diameter. These are the markers indicative of malignant melanoma. RICE is used for treatment of sprains and strains: rest, elevation, compression, and elevation. The BRAT diet is advised for diarrhea and gastroenteritis: broth, rice, applesauce, and tea. Application Planning Health Promotion: Prevention and/or Early Detection of Health Problems
45.10 A client has been treated for pediculosis capitis and is concerned about spreading the infestation. The nurse explains that it can be spread: a. through sexual activity. b. by sharing personal hygiene items. c. through your clothing and bed linens. d. by sharing drinks and eating utensils.	Answer: b Rationale: Pediculosis capitis is transmitted through contact with the infected person or by sharing items used on the head, such as combs and brushes. Pediculosis pubis is spread through sexual activity and bed linens. Comprehension Implementation Physiological Integrity: Reduction of Risk Potential

CHAPTER 46

Question	Answer
46.1 The nurse plans interventions knowing the client with first-degree burns over a large part of her body surface may experience symptoms such as: a. dehydration and thirst. b. headache, chills, nausea, and vomiting. c. pain and temporary memory loss. d. chest pain and dyspnea.	Answer: b Rationale: These are the symptoms experienced with first-degree burns. Dehydration and thirst occur more with more severe burns when fluid is lost or sequestered in interstitial spaces. Pain can occur, but not memory loss. Chest pain and dyspnea would not typically be seen. Comprehension Assessment Physiological Integrity: Physiological Adaptation
46.2 A client with first- and second-degree burns of the cheek was very concerned about permanent damage. The nurse might focus the client teaching on: a. prevention of infection to reduce scarring. b. use of vitamin E to prevent scarring. c. scrubbing the burned area daily to promote new skin growth. d. use of plastic surgery to relieve scarring.	Answer: a Rationale: Infection of the burn injury can cause further damage and scarring. Vitamin E is used keep skin softer and more supple, but not to prevent scarring. The skin is too fragile for scrubbing. Plastic surgery may be an option after primary healing has occurred. Application Implementation Physiological Integrity: Reduction of Risk Potential
46.3 The client told the nurse that he was thankful that the burns were not bad since they did not hurt much. The best response by the nurse would be: a. "Yes, you are fortunate not have a lot of pain" b. "I'm afraid you are mistaken. These are severe burns."	Answer: c Rationale: Deep partial-thickness burns are less painful than superficial burns due to damage to the pain and nerve receptors. Options a and c are not incorrect statements, but do not provide the best response. Application Implementation Physiological Integrity: Physiological Adaptation

© 2007 Pearson Education, Inc.

c. "Your burns are pretty deep and have destroyed some of the pain receptors." d. "I'm glad you have such a positive attitude; it's going to be helpful during your recovery."	
46.4 A burn client experiences excessive fluid in the interstitial spaces causing edema. Because the fluid accumulation impairs peripheral circulation, the nurse assesses the client for which of the following complications? a. increase in cardiac output b. tissue necrosis c. increased diuresis d. impaired mobility	Answer: b Rationale: The impaired circulation caused by the edema leads to a decrease in blood flow to tissues, which can in turn cause tissue death. Fluid trapped in the interstitial spaces is pulled from the vascular volume, resulting in a decrease in cardiac output and diuresis. Analysis Assessment Physiological Integrity: Reduction of Risk Potential
46.5 The nurse notices that the burn client develops a dysrhythmia. The nurse recognizes that the probable cause of this complication is: a. increased cardiac output. b. decrease in sodium levels related to diuresis. c. loss of potassium ion related to cell injury. d. increase of intracellular magnesium ions.	Answer: c Rationale: Potassium is an intracellular ion and is lost when cells are destroyed, as with a burn. Potassium is required for proper cardiac contractility; low levels put client at risk for dysrhythmias. Analysis Assessment Physiological Integrity: Reduction of Risk Potential
46.6 The nurse admits a severely burned client who is unconscious, dyspneic, and cyanotic. The blood test shows decreased levels of oxyhemoglobin, which occur secondary to: a. carbon monoxide poisoning. b. smoke inhalation. c. cardiac arrest. d. pulmonary collapse.	Answer: a Rationale: Smoke inhalation can result in inhalation of carbon monoxide, an asphyxiant that displaces oxygen and binds with hemoglobin. This causes hypoxemia in the client. Comprehension Assessment Physiological Integrity: Physiological Adaptation
46.7 A 42-year-old client was admitted with second- and third-degree burns over 45% of the body. The nurse identifies the initial goal in treatment for these burns as: a. preventing scarring and infection. b. preventing dehydration and infection. c. combating shock and preventing infection. d. preventing hemorrhage and shock.	Answer: c Rationale: Loss of fluids puts the client with major burns at great risk for shock; loss of tissue integrity puts the client at risk for infection. These are higher priorities initially than scarring. Dehydration occurs in the diuretic stage of burns. Application Implementation Physiological Integrity: Reduction of Risk Potential
46.8 Before applying mafenide acetate (Sulfamylon) to a client's burns, the nurse should plan to: a. premedicate client with pain medication. b. check client for allergies to codeine. c. wear protective clothing to avoid staining. d. have client wear a facial mask.	Answer: a Rationale: Application of this drug is painful and often causes burning. Client should be checked for sulfa allergies. Silver nitrate solutions cause staining. A mask is not necessary. Application Implementation Physiological Integrity: Pharmacological and Parenteral therapies

Question	Answer
46.9 During the acute stage of burns, nursing interventions should focus on: **a.** assessment of shock. **b.** treatment of respiratory distress. **c.** application of topical antimicrobial agents. **d.** prevention of contractures.	Answer: c Rationale: During the acute phase, interventions focus on treatment of the burns, nutritional support, skin grafting, wound debridement, and pain control. Shock and respiratory distress are addressed in the emergent or initial burn phase. Contractures are addressed in the rehabilitative stage. Application Implementation Physiological Integrity: Reduction of Risk Potential
46.10 The nurse is observing a client with major burn injuries for signs of Curling's ulcer, a common complication. The nurse should assess the client for: **a.** purulent drainage from wound sites. **b.** frequent headaches. **c.** hypertension. **d.** black, tarry stools.	Answer: d Rationale: Black, tarry stools would be indicative of GI bleeding from the ulcer. The other options would not be indicative of an ulcer. Analysis Implementation Physiological Integrity: Reduction of Risk Potential

CHAPTER 47

Question	Answer
47.1 The nurse observes that a client shows no emotional expression and speaks in a monotone. The nurse documents the client as having: **a.** a flat affect. **b.** a labile affect. **c.** a catatonic reaction. **d.** a broad affect.	Answer: a Rationale: A flat affect is conveyed by an absence of facial expression and emotions. Labile affect is expressed by rapidly changing emotional expressions. A catatonic reaction involves slow or absence of responses and expressions. A broad affect involves a full range of emotions. Comprehension Assessment Psychosocial Integrity: Psychosocial Adaptation
47.2 Family members are upset when their mother, who is being treated for diverticulitis, begins to yell at the nurse and refuses to eat. They apologize and say "We don't understand her behavior. She is always such a sweet person." The nurse's response is based on the knowledge that: **a.** physical health may be altered by the client's emotional state of health. **b.** the stress of illness may alter the client's normal emotional reactions. **c.** the client most likely is expressing emotions that have been suppressed for years. **d.** physical illness will often cause psychotic symptoms.	Answer: b Rationale: Clients often exhibit emotional responses and coping mechanisms different from their normal pattern when experiencing a stressful event, pain, and/or hospitalization. Option a can occur also, but this doesn't explain the behavior in this scenario. Psychotic symptoms may occur on occasion, but are not often seen. Analysis Implementation Psychosocial Integrity: Coping and Adaptation
47.3 To best determine how a client copes with stressors, the nurse should ask which of the following questions? **a.** "What do you do when you are confronted with a major change in your life?" **b.** "Do you turn to drugs or alcohol to help you cope with stressful events?" **c.** "Have you had many crises in your life?" **d.** "Have you ever been seriously depressed or suicidal?"	Answer: a Rationale: This question solicits information the nurse can use to best help the client draw upon when the client needs to deal with stress. The other options ask about specific coping strategies and previous crises and would not provide as much useful information. Application Assessment Psychosocial Integrity: Coping and Adaptation

© 2007 Pearson Education, Inc.

47.4 When collecting information for a psychosocial assessment, the nurse should question which of the following clients about their history of alcohol and drug use? a. clients who have a history of substance abuse b. clients admitted with elevated drug or alcohol levels c. all clients d. clients who display unhealthy coping skills	Answer: c Rationale: All clients should be asked. Even though the questions may not always be answered honestly, it provides an opportunity to help clients who do have questions about alcohol and drug use or would like to share more information with the nurse. Application Assessment Psychosocial Integrity: Coping and Adaptation
47.5 The nurse is performing a psychosocial assessment and asks the client to interpret a proverb, such as "slow and steady wins the race." The nurse uses the client's response to evaluate the client's: a. ability to think abstractly. b. ability to problem solve. c. memory recall. d. judgment skills.	Answer: a Rationale: Proverbs are frequently used to assess a client's ability to think abstractly vs. concretely and provides some insight into the presence of disorganized thinking. Problem solving and judgment require examples where the client explains what should be done in a certain situation. Memory recall involves recall of a list of words, objects, etc. Application Evaluation Psychosocial Integrity: Psychosocial Adaptation
47.6 When assessing a client's ability to cope with major stressors, the nurse recognizes that the most important influence on this ability is the: a. specific nature of the stressor b. person's problem-solving abilities. c. person's perception of the stressor. d. availability of resources.	Answer: c Rationale: An individual's perception must first be determined, since what one person perceives to be a stressor may not be the same for everyone. Once the perception is established, the other options can be applied in assisting the client to deal with a stressor. Application Assessment Psychosocial Integrity: Coping and Adaptation
47.7 As part of a psychosocial assessment, the nurse determines a client's ability to make judgments. To do this, the nurse might ask the client: a. "Can you explain what 'The early bird gets the worm' means?" b. "What would you do if the fire alarm went off just now?" c. "Can you repeat these five words back to me: lecture, ketchup, pickle, broom, and door?" d. "How do you feel about persons of a different cultural background than yourself?"	Answer: b Rationale: This question requires the client to provide information that involves problem solving and decision making. Option a tests abstract thinking. Option c tests memory recall. Option d assesses attitude and self-concept. Application Implementation Psychosocial Integrity: Psychosocial Adaptation
47.8 The nurse understands that neurotransmitters have a direct relationship to many mental health disorders and explains to a family member that the client's depression may be related to a deficiency of: a. serotonin. b. epinephrine. c. acetylcholine. d. histamine.	Answer: a Rationale: Serotonin, norepinephrine, and dopamine are often decreased in depression. Comprehension Implementation Psychosocial Integrity: Psychosocial Adaptation

47.9 When performing a client's mental status examination, the nurse will obtain information about the client's: a. culture and family. b. employment history. c. ability to perform bathing and hygiene needs. d. insurance.	Answer: a Rationale: Assessment of mental status includes cognitive function, feelings, coping skills, relationships, family, and support systems. Employment and insurance are part of the socioeconomic assessment. Ability to perform ADLs is part of a physical exam. Comprehension Assessment Psychosocial Integrity: Coping and Adaptation
47.10 The nurse is participating in a mental health information session at a local health fair. In an effort to reduce the stigma of mental health illness, the nurse promotes the following philosophy: a. Mental illness can often be treated in the same way as a physical illness. b. People with a mental illness can't help or control their behavior. c. Most mental illnesses have a genetic link. d. The public should view mental illness as a disability.	Answer: a Rationale: Many members of the public view mental illness as untreatable. With proper medication and therapy, many people can control their behavior just as a diabetic controls his blood sugar. There can be a genetic link, but not always. Stereotypes such as a disability should be avoided. Application Implementation Psychosocial Integrity: Coping and Adaptation

CHAPTER 48

48.1 The sibling of a client with schizophrenia states to the nurse: "I understand there is a genetic link to this disorder. Can you tell me anything more about that?" The nurse should respond: a. "Recent research indicates schizophrenia is linked mainly to an excess in brain neurotransmitters, not genetics." b. "As long as you are not identical twins, the occurrence in siblings is just a coincidence." c. "Siblings of people with schizophrenia have a much higher incidence of the having the disease as well." d. "You should have gene testing if you are concerned you will develop the disease."	Answer: c Rationale: The causes of schizophrenia are multifactorial, including imbalances of neurotransmitters, genetic components, structural brain changes, and environmental factors. Siblings having a ninefold increased risk of having the disease. Genetic testing may help identify susceptibility for the disease, but this option does not provide the best answer to the client's question. Application Implementation Psychosocial Integrity: Psychosocial Adaptation
48.2 The nurse is discussing the employment history of a client with schizophrenia. Due to cognitive impairment associated with the disease, the nurse understands that the client may have difficulty: a. remembering what kind of work he did 10 years ago. b. explaining what things he likes to do. c. describing the repetitive tasks involved in the job. d. understanding why he was terminated by an employer.	Answer: d Rationale: Difficulty with abstract thinking and having insight into his illness are affected so he may not be able to understand why he has lost a job. Short-term memory, not long term, is usually affected. Such clients usually have intact concrete thinking and can tell you what they like to do and describe repetitive type skills. Application Assessment Psychosocial Integrity: Psychosocial Adaptation

© 2007 Pearson Education, Inc.

Question	Answer
48.3 A client in the mental health unit is being evaluated for schizophrenia. In addition to having hallucinations, the nurse identifies which of the following observations that would support the diagnosis? a. The client has frequent outbursts of yelling and shouting. b. The client has had symptoms for over 30 days. c. The client is convinced he is Elvis Presley. d. The client refuses to eat and come out of his room.	Answer: c Rationale: Delusions are a symptom characteristic of schizophrenia. Outburst of anger and refusal to come out of his room could be associated with many other mental health illnesses or a coping mechanism. Symptoms must be present for more than 6 months to support the diagnosis. Application Assessment Psychosocial Integrity: Psychosocial Adaptation
48.4 During a conversation with a client with schizophrenia, the nurse realizes that the client's disorganized thinking is frequently manifested by looseness of association when the client states: a. "I hate all these speaking engagements required of me as the President of Hungary." b. "I had a good lunch. I love ice cream. My aunt visited yesterday." c. "Newspaper, ghetto, cat, rat, silly girl." d. "I wish they would clean the spiders off the wall."	Answer: b Rationale: Looseness of association, or derailment, involves a pattern of speech in which ideas move from one track to another, often loosely connected. Option a describes delusional thinking. Option c is an example of a word salad. Option d may be a hallucination, or real. Application Assessment Psychosocial Integrity: Psychosocial Adaptation
48.5 A client with schizophrenia has developed tardive dyskinesia secondary to a psychotropic medication. When a family member ask the nurse if anything can be done to stop the symptoms, the nurse explains: a. "The physician will probably order an anticholinergic medication to reduce the symptoms." b. "If the antipsychotic medication is stopped, these symptoms are reversible." c. "If the lowest effective dose of the medication is given, the symptoms may decrease." d. "Another atypical antipsychotic medication will be given that doesn't have these side effects."	Answer: c Rationale: If the lowest effective dose is given, the symptoms can sometimes be prevented. Giving anticholinergics does not help tardive dyskinesia. It is often irreversible. Changing to another psychotropic medication may stop the progression of the tardive dyskinesia. Application Implementation Psychosocial Integrity: Psychosocial Adaptation
48.6 The physician asks the nurse if the client with schizophrenia is experiencing any negative symptoms. The nurse says that the client frequently: a. has visual hallucinations of seeing polar bears in the room b. is still delusional and believes she is Marilyn Monroe. c. answers questions in one- and two-word phrases with little expression. d. dresses in brightly colored, mismatched outfits.	Answer: c Rationale: A reduction in speech with brief responses and without emotion describes alogia, a negative symptom that involves a deficit or decrease in normal function. Positive symptoms involve an excess of normal function, as occurs with hallucinations, disorganized thinking, and flamboyant behavior. Analysis Assessment Psychosocial Integrity: Psychosocial Adaptation

Question	Answer
48.7 The nurse recognizes that the client with schizophrenia often stops taking her medication secondary to side effects. To prevent this from occurring, the nurse should plan to teach the client which of the following? a. Avoid prolonged exposure to sunlight and wear sunscreen. b. Take an over-the-counter analgesic as needed for headaches. c. Dress lightly to keep from getting too warm. d. Eat a high-calorie, high-protein diet to avoid weight loss.	Answer: a Rationale: Some clients experience photosensitivity, becoming severly sunburned with just minimal sun exposure. Headaches and being too warm are not typical side effects. Weight gain, not loss, is common. Application Implementation Physiological Integrity: Pharmacological Parenteral Therapies
48.8 Which of the following actions by a nurse would be most effective when dealing with a client with schizophrenia who is shouting and verbally aggressive? a. Take the client's arms and gently but firmly guide him to a safe place. b. Approach the client with hands at her side and talk calmly to the client. c. Encourage the client to come into the dayroom and watch television. d. Ignore client's behavior unless it escalates or client threatens another person.	Answer: b Rationale: A nonthreatening, calm, and controlled approach can be contagious to the client. Touching the client might make him defensive and become violent. A quiet environment is best until the client has calmed down. Early intervention is necessary with psychotic clients to prevent escalation of behavior. Application Implementation Psychosocial Integrity: Psychosocial Adaptation
48.9 A client with schizophrenia who frequently has auditory hallucinations has been taught strategies to deal with them. The nurse documents that the client demonstrates use of the interacting strategy when observing the client: a. talking to the voice and pretending to use a mobile phone. b. playing the piano and singing loudly. c. reading out loud while reading the newspaper. d. sitting quietly and listening to what the voices have to say.	Answer: a Rationale: Talking to the voices or telling them to stop is way of interacting with them, allowing the client to acknowledge they are not real. Playing the piano is an activity strategy. Reading out loud is a form of distraction strategy. Actively listening to the voices is not a strategy. Application Evaluation Psychosocial Integrity: Psychosocial Adaptation
48.10 The brother of a client with schizophrenia says to the nurse: "I would like to help my brother, but he just doesn't seem to understand he has a serious psychological problem. He tells me he is fine and just gets a little weird occasionally." The nurse explains: a. "Many people with schizophrenia use denial as a coping mechanism." b. "This is why it is so difficult to treat since lack of insight is a large part of the disease." c. "Because of the stigma attached to mental illness most people with schizophrenia won't tell others they have the disease." d. "They need to take their medications when having psychotic episodes."	Answer: b Rationale: Lack of insight is one of the cognitive defects present and keeps clients from seeking and maintaining treatment, because they do not see themselves as being sick. Denial is not the problem, but rather a lack of self-understanding. Because of the lack of insight they are often not aware of the stigma attached to the illness. Since they do not see themselves as ill they frequently stop medications, especially when stable; medications need to be take even when not having psychotic episodes. Analysis Implementation Psychosocial Integrity: Psychosocial Adaptation

© 2007 Pearson Education, Inc.

Chapter 49

49.1 A friend shares with a nurse that her mother has been in a very depressed mood lately and is concerned she should see a psychiatrist. To best determine if the client might be experiencing a major depressive disorder, the nurse should ask the friend: a. "Does your mother cry a lot or is just quiet and sad most of the time?" b. "Has she been depressed for more than a solid week?" c. "Has her depressed mood caused significant interruption of daily routines?" d. "How often does she attend social events outside of the home?"	Answer: c Rationale: Diagnostic criteria for a major depressive disorder include a client must have five different depression-related symptoms lasting for more than 2 weeks and the symptoms must cause significant impairment to everyday functions. Application Assessment Psychosocial Integrity: Psychosocial Adaptation
49.2 A client being seen in the mental health clinic is being started on tricyclic antidepressants for treatment of depression. Which of the following conditions in the client's history should be brought to the attention of the primary care provider? a. The client has a history of previous suicide attempts. b. The client lives alone. c. The client was unresponsive to treatment with selective serotonin reuptake inhibitors (SSRIs). d. The client smokes cigarettes.	Answer: a Rationale: Tricyclics can be fatal if an overdose is taken; clients sometimes take the medications to commit suicide. Living alone and smoking would not be significant. Tricyclics are sometimes effective for people unresponsive to other antidepressants. Analysis Implementation Psychosocial Integrity: Psychosocial Adaptation
49.3 The nurse instructs a client being started on a SSRI for possible side effects. The nurse explains that the most frequent side effects include: a. headaches, nausea, and insomnia. b. postural hypotension and diarrhea. c. cardiac arrhythmias and postural hypotension. d. urinary retention, dry mouth, and drowsiness.	Answer: a Rationale: The most frequent side effects are headache, anxiety, nausea, diarrhea, and insomnia. The other options include side effects associated with tricyclic antidepressants. Comprehension Implementation Physiological Integrity: Pharmacological and Parenteral Therapies
49.4 A client being treated for depression with a selective serotonin reuptake inhibitor (SSRI) becomes agitated, diaphoretic, and complains of muscle spasms and tremors. The client's sister confides to the nurse her sister has been taking St. John's wort daily for the last 6 months. Which of the following actions should be taken by the nurse? a. Withhold any scheduled doses of the SSRI and notify the physician. b. Ask the client to give the St. John's wort tablets to the staff. c. Have the laboratory draw blood work for a serotonin level. d. Discuss the dangers of taking over-the-counter herbal preparations with the client.	Answer: a Rationale: The symptoms are suggestive of serotonin syndrome as a result of excess serotonin activity from the St. John's wort and SSRI. It can be fatal and needs to be reported immediately. The other options do not address the critical nature of the situation. Analysis Implementation Physiological Integrity: Pharmacological and Parenteral Therapies

49.5 A client is seen in the emergency department complaining of sudden onset of a throbbing headache. The client is taking a monoamine oxidase inhibitor (MAOI) and admits to having eaten a lot of aged cheese recently. The nurse should assess the client for which other symptoms? a. diaphoresis b. hypotension c. abdominal cramping d. stiff neck	Answer: d Rationale: The combination of tyramine-containing foods (aged cheese) and MAOIs can cause a hypertensive crisis, manifested by a throbbing headache, heart palpitations, hypertension, and a stiff neck. Analysis Assessment Physiological Integrity: Pharmacological and Parenteral Therapies
49.6 Which of the following symptoms would a nurse most expect to identify when assessing a client with bipolar disorder who is in the manic phase? a. pressured speech b. hallucinations c. napping throughout the day d. thoughts of inferiority	Answer: a Rationale: During the manic phase, clients are very talkative and express pressure to keep talking. Hallucinations are seen more in people with psychoses and schizophrenia. Mania is characterized by a decreased need to sleep and an inflated self-esteem and grandiosity. Application Assessment Psychosocial Integrity: Psychosocial Adaptation
49.7 The nurse is caring for a client with bipolar disorder who is experiencing a manic episode. To assist the client in reducing the hyperactive behavior, the nurse should plan to do which of the following? a. Allow the client to set her own limits on behavior. b. Provide a calm, quiet area for client to sit or walk around in. c. Engage the client in a quiet game of cards or puzzle solving. d. Encourage the client to get involved in a game of volleyball.	Answer: b Rationale: Providing a calm, quiet environment reduces excessive stimuli and helps the client to be less hyperactive. People in a manic state are unable to safely set their own limits. Cards and puzzles require concentration, which is difficult for the manic person to do and may actually increase agitation. Playing volleyball would probably cause more stimulation. Application Planning Psychosocial Integrity: Psychosocial Adaptation
49.8 A client confides in the nurse that he is going to kill himself. Which of the following questions should the nurse ask the client? a. "Have you ever attempted suicide before?" b. "What has happened to make you feel this way?" c. "How will you kill yourself?" d. "Do you think this will solve your problems?"	Answer: c Rationale: Since the client has expressed suicidal ideation, it is necessary to determine if the client has organized his thoughts enough to have an actual plan. The other options would not provide this information. Application Implementation Psychosocial Integrity: Psychosocial Adaptation
49.9 The nurse has determined that a client with a bipolar disorder has a nursing diagnosis of hopelessness. Which of the following therapeutic communication skills should the nurse use? a. Encourage the client to engage in a social activity. b. Arrange for the client to go on a group outing to the mall. c. Ask the client how she has overcome obstacles in the past. d. Sit quietly with the client and hold her hand.	Answer: c Rationale: Encouraging clients to identify some coping strategies and strengths help them to see they have survived difficulties in the past. Options a and b are interventions, not communication skills. Sitting with the client can be therapeutic, but doesn't offer specific, in dealing with the hopelessness.

© 2007 Pearson Education, Inc.

49.10 A client who was experiencing symptoms of early lithium toxicity has had the dosage of medication reduced. The nurse determines the dosage reduction was effective when the client demonstrates: a. a coarse hand tremor. b. a return of normal speech. c. a decrease in urine output. d. a decrease in blood pressure.	Answer: b Rationale: Slurred speech is seen with early lithium toxicity. A coarse hand tremor is a sign of early lithium toxicity. Decreased urine output and hypotension are seen in severe lithium toxicity. Analysis Evaluation Physiological Integrity: Pharmacological and Parenteral Therapies

CHAPTER 50

50.1 A client scheduled for an operation later in the day tells the nurse she is anxious and wants the surgery to be over. The nurse correlates the following physical findings to the client's moderate degree of anxiety: a. blood pressure and pulse are elevated from baseline b. pacing in the hall c. crying uncontrollably d. difficulty arousing	Answer: a Rationale: The sympathetic nervous system reacts in response to the anxiety, as manifested by the increase in BP and pulse. Crying and pacing would be seen with severe anxiety. Anxiety produces a state of alertness; client would not be sleeping. Application Assessment Psychosocial Integrity: Psychosocial Adaptation
50.2 The nurse initially employs which of the following nursing interventions to reduce anxiety in a client demonstrating severe anxiety? a. Encourage client to identify the source of the anxiety. b. Ask the client to verbalize his feelings. c. Instruct client to do deep-breathing exercises. d. Allow client to be alone in a quiet environment.	Answer: c Rationale: During an acute attack of anxiety the client should be stabilized. Deep breathing and relaxation are done initially to interrupt the autonomic anxiety response. The client should not be left alone during an acute episode of anxiety, but monitored for indications of self-harm. After client is stabilized, verbalization of feelings and discussion of the source of anxiety would be appropriate. Application Implementation Psychosocial Integrity: Psychosocial Adaptation
50.3 A client just recently diagnosed with having panic disorder asks the nurse if there is any way to predict when an attack will occur. The nurse explains: a. "If you are stressed in any way you are more likely to have an attack." b. "Unfortunately attacks can occur at anytime without warning." c. "People usually experience attacks in surroundings where a previous attack occurred." d. "Many people will have an aura, such as flashes of light or a strange smell, just before the attack occurs."	Answer: b Rationale: Panic attacks occur without warning in people with panic disorder. They are not necessarily triggered by stress but can be. Many people fear returning to a location where an attack was experienced, but attacks occur anywhere. Auras are experienced before seizures.

50.4 A client on the mental health unit has agoraphobia and refuses to go to the dayroom for a scheduled unit activity. The nurse can best reduce the client's anxiety by doing which of the following? a. Offer to accompany the client and stay with her. b. Premedicate the client with a benzodiazepine. c. Reinforce that the client knows everyone else on the unit. d. Require the client to go and only stay for 10 minutes.	Answer: a Rationale: Accompanying the client offers assurance someone will be present to help if a severe anxiety or panic attack occurs. The other options do not help the client as much to deal with the fear. Medications should not be used when adaptive practices can be used to solve the problem. Application Implementation Psychosocial Integrity: Psychosocial Adaptation
50.5 A client with obsessive compulsive disorder (OCD) occupies much of the day with rituals involved with washing hands and frequently misses breakfast because of the behavior. The nurse should: a. make the client stop washing and go to breakfast with the other clients. b. wake the client an hour early, allowing time to complete the ritual. c. allow the client to miss breakfast since the ritual is more important than a missed meal. d. bring the meal to the client's room and allow as much time as needed for washing.	Answer: b Rationale: The compulsive action helps to reduce the stress. Waking the client early allows time to complete the activity while setting limits and expectations. The other options do not set limits and allow for reduction of stress. Application Implementation Psychosocial Integrity: Psychosocial Adaptation
50.6 A friend confides he goes around his house three to four times to check that all lights are turned off before leaving for work in the morning. He asks the nurse "Do you think I have an obsessive compulsive disorder (OCD)?" To help identify criteria defining the disorder, the nurse should ask: a. "Do you do this on the weekends as well?" b. "How much time do you spend doing this activity?" c. "How long have you been doing this?" d. "Have you ever considered purchasing an automatic timing device to turn out the lights at a designated time?"	Answer: b Rationale: Compulsive behavior doesn't become OCD until it is distressful, consumes more than one hour a day, or interferes with an individual's daily life. Options a and c do not address specific criteria that define OCD. Option d does not relate to the obsessive behavior. Application Implementation Psychosocial Integrity: Psychosocial Adaptation
50.7 The nurse notes that a client has a diagnosis of post-traumatic stress syndrome (PTSD). When developing a plan of care, the nurse anticipates the client may have the following nursing diagnosis: a. Disturbed Body Image related to trauma of imprisonment b. Anxiety related to flashbacks of torture c. Self-Care Deficit related to refusal to bathe self d. Acute Pain related to nerve damage secondary to torture	Answer: b Rationale: Flashbacks cause extreme distress and anxiety in individuals with PTSD. The other options are possible, but they do not relate to the psychosocial aspects associated with PTSD. Analysis Planning Psychosocial Integrity: Psychosocial Adaptation

 © 2007 Pearson Education, Inc.

50.8 The nurse is preparing to draw blood from a client who states, "Oh, I hate needles. I hope I don't faint this time." The nurse should take the following action: a. Be sure to have aromatic spirits available. b. Ensure client is in a recumbent position. c. Have another nurse present. d. Keep client distracted while drawing the blood.	Answer: b Rationale: A phobia of blood or needles frequently results in a vasovagal response, which can lead to loss of consciousness. The recumbent position offers the best safety option. Application Implementation Physiological Integrity: Reduction of Risk Potential
50.9 A client given a benzodiazepine for general anxiety disorder has a paradoxical reaction to the medication. When planning to administer the next scheduled dose of the benzodiazepine the nurse should: a. hold the drug and inform the physician of the client's reaction. b. observe client closely since the reaction may occur a second time. c. notify physician and request a lower dose of the benzodiazepine. d. explain to the client the reactions will decrease as the body adjusts to the medication.	Answer: a Rationale: A drug should be discontinued when a paradoxical reaction occurs. Altering the dose or repeated use of the drug will not lessen the chance of another reaction. Analysis Planning Physiological Integrity: Pharmacological and Parenteral Therapies
50.10 A client is being started on busprione (Buspar), a nonbenzodizepine antidepressant agent. The client should be given the following information about use of the drug: a. It may cause extreme drowsiness initially. b. It may lead to dependence. c. It may take up to 6 weeks to see full effects. d. It may cause euphoria in some people.	Answer: c Rationale: It may take 7 to 10 days to begin to see effects and up to 6 weeks to see full effects. Drowsiness, dependence, and euphoria are not seen with this medication. Application Implementation Physiological Integrity: Pharmacological and Parenteral Therapies

CHAPTER 51

51.1 A client admitted with Paranoid Personality Disorder insists the food is contaminated with pesticides. Which of the following communication techniques should the nurse plan to use to encourage the client to eat? a. Encourage identification of foods preferred by the client. b. Identify reasons why the client should eat. c. Ask client open-ended questions and sit with client. d. Describe how the food is prepared at the institution.	Answer: c Rationale: Open-ended questions encourage communication with the client. Options a and b encourage client to talk about the food, but do not encourage client to express feelings and anxieties. Explaining how food is prepared does not involve the client. Application Implementation Psychosocial Integrity: Coping and Adaptation.

Question	Answer
51.2 The nurse is working with a group of clients with personality disorders who are attending a cognitive behavioral therapy session. The nurse recognizes that the clients who are most responsive to this type of therapy have the following personality trait: a. eccentric b. dramatic c. agreeableness d. inflexible	Answer: c Rationale: Personality traits of agreeableness and conscientiousness tend to make people more responsive to therapy. Eccentric, dramatic, and inflexible behaviors are exhibited by people with personality disorders. Application Assessment Psychosocial Integrity: Coping and Adaptation
51.3 The nurse is developing a plan of care for a client with an Avoidant Personality Disorder. The nurse decides an appropriate goal would be for the client to: a. improve social skills. b. make a decision about their care. c. be free from self-harm. d. refrain from harming others.	Answer: a Rationale: People with this disorder display social shyness, fear rejection, and view themselves as socially inept. Making decisions applies to Dependent Personality Disorders. Remaining free of self-harm is appropriate for Borderline Personality Disorder. Not hurting others is a goal for people with Antisocial Personality Disorder. Analysis Planning Psychosocial Integrity: Psychosocial Adaptation
51.4 A client with a personality disorder has a nursing diagnosis of Disturbed Thought Processes. The nurse should implement which of the following skills when interacting with the client? a. Approach client in a friendly, jovial manner. b. Reassure client she is in a safe place. c. Allow visitors to stay longer than designated visiting hours. d. Ignore suspicions and fears verbalized by the client.	Answer: b Rationale: Reassurance of a safe environment may help allay client's underlying fear and insecurity. Clients should be approached in a matter-of-fact, professional manner; excessive friendliness may be interpreted as a weakness or deceit. Strict adherence to rules conveys assurance of safety. Suspicions and fears shouldn't be ignored, but also not overemphasized. Application Implementation Psychosocial Integrity: Psychosocial Adaptation
51.5 A client with a Histrionic Personality Disorder is admitted to the mental health unit. The nurse expects the client will display which of the following behaviors? a. detachment from staff and other clients b. hostile and suspicious of others c. impulsive and frequently aggressive with others d. being the center of attention	Answer: d Rationale: People with this disorder display attention-seeking behavior and often create a scene to bring attention to themselves. Detachment is seen with schizoid disorders. Hostility and suspiciousness are seen with paranoid disorders. Impulsivity and aggression are seen with antisocial disorders. Application Assessment Psychosocial Integrity: Psychosocial Adaptation
51.6 When developing a plan of care for the client with Paranoid Personality Disorder, the nurse recognizes that a hallmark of the disorder is the client's: a. preoccupation with delusions of persecution. b. difficulty with interpersonal relationships. c. violation of the rights of others. d. impulsive behavior.	Answer: b Rationale: People with this disorder are so vigilant to the imagined malicious intentions of others that they can't develop satisfying relationships. At times they may express feelings of persecution or feel they are being plotted against. Impulsive behavior and violation of others' rights are characteristics of Antisocial Personality Disorder. Analysis Planning Psychosocial Integrity: Psychosocial Adaptation
51.7 The nurse is doing group therapy with a group of clients on a mental health unit. The nurse determines that a client with Schizotypal Personality	Answer: c Rationale: Inappropriate affect occurs when an emotional response is not culturally appropriate to the situation. The other options describe inappropriate behaviors.

© 2007 Pearson Education, Inc.

Disorder is displaying an inappropriate affect when the client: a. sits off to the side and refuses to participate. b. sings loudly while the other clients are trying to talk. c. cries when another client tells a silly joke. d. rocks back and forth in the chair throughout the meeting.	Application Assessment Psychosocial Integrity: Coping and Adaptation
51.8 When caring for a client with a Dependent Personality Disorder, the nurse plans nursing interventions based on the knowledge that the client: a. has an unrealistic fear of abandonment. b. will frequently display attention-seeking behaviors. c. has an inflated sense of self-importance. d. often engages in self-harm activities.	Answer: a Rationale: People with this disorder are preoccupied with a fear of being forced to care for themselves and fear abandonment. Option a is seen with a histrionic personality. Option b is seen with narcisstic personalities. Option c is seen in borderline personalities. Analysis Planning Psychosocial Integrity: Psychosocial Adaptation
51.9 A client with an obsessive compulsive personality tells the nurse, "I become so anxious and stressed and then I start my compulsive ritual. I wish I could stop it." To help the client reduce the anxiety, the nurse offers the following suggestions: a. "Make a list of things that provoke anxiety for you." b. "Hold an ice cube in each hand for ten minutes when you are tempted to do a ritual." c. "Set a rigid timetable of your daily schedule." d. "Keep distracted by playing the television and radio loudly."	Answer: a Rationale: Early recognition of situations associated with anxiety can help the client take action to avoid them or to use adaptive behaviors. Holding an ice cube is a technique suggested for clients who are tempted to harm themselves. Rigidity only supports the compulsive behavior. Reduction of environmental stimuli helps to reduce anxiety. Application Implementation Psychosocial Integrity: Coping and Adaptation
51.10 When working with a client with personality disorders the nurse recognizes that the behavior displayed by the client must have the following characteristics: a. It can occur at anytime during adulthood. b. It is frequently characterized by psychotic behaviors. c. The behavior is very different from what is expected of the client's culture. d. Daily functioning is rarely affected by the disorders.	Answer: c Rationale: Some behaviors, such as dependency, may be normal within a culture; behaviors seen with personality disorders deviate markedly from one's cultural norms. It begins in adolescence or young adulthood. It is characterized by inflexible and inappropriate behaviors and occasionally psychotic behavior. The disorders impair day-to-day functioning. Analysis Assessment Psychosocial Integrity: Psychosocial Adaptation

CHAPTER 52

Question	Answer
52.1 The nurse working with clients who have a history of substance abuse understands that a major reason they are not readily identified or do not seek help from health professionals is: a. denial that they have a problem. b. fear that they will be subject to legal charges. c. fear of health interventions against their will. d. fear that family members will reject them.	Answer: a Rationale: Denial is a common coping mechanism used by people with substance abuse. The fears may also contribute to their avoidance, but they are not the main reason. Comprehension Assessment Psychosocial Integrity: Psychosocial Adaptation
52.2 In obtaining a teenage client's history, which of the following would the nurse consider an early indicator of substance abuse? a. six absences from school in 1 year b. drinking beer with friends after a football game c. an increasing tolerance for alcohol d. a desire to stop drinking	Answer: c Rationale: An increased tolerance indicates a maladaptive pattern and can progress to substance dependency. Absences from school can be attributed to many things. Drinking with friends is not a positive sign, but is typical teenage behavior and would not be the best indicator of an abuse problem. A desire to stop is positive. Comprehension Assessment Psychosocial Integrity: Psychosocial Adaptation
52.3 A client admitted with a long history of alcohol abuse is at risk to go through withdrawal and suffer delirium tremens (DTs). The nurse knows to assess the client for: a. lethargy and fine tremors. b. fever, diaphoresis, and hyperactivity. c. grand mal seizures. d. confusion, delusions, and hallucinations.	Answer: d Rationale: When the substance is withdrawn, the central nervous system is stimulated; withdrawal associated with long-term alcohol use is also associated with cognitive symptoms. Application Assessment Physiological Integrity: Physiological Adaptation
52.4 The nurse recognizes that the following assessment finding in the alcoholic client indicates a gastrointestinal complication: a. nausea and vomiting b. loss of appetite c. dental caries d. tarry, black stools	Answer: d Rationale: Excessive intake of alcohol can lead to gastritis and GI bleeding; the latter will be manifested by tarry, black stools. The other options are GI symptoms and side effects of excessive drinking. Analysis Assessment Physiological Integrity: Physiological Adaptation
52.5 An alcoholic client is admitted with Wernicke's syndrome (alcoholic encephalopathy). The nurse prepares to administer: a. vitamin C. b. vitamin B_1. c. vitamin E. d. vitamin A.	Answer: b Rationale: Wernicke's syndrome occurs as a result of a severe vitamin B_1 (thiamine) deficiency secondary to lack of adequate nutritional intake. Application Implementation Physiological Integrity: Pharmacological and Parenteral Therapies
52.6 In obtaining a history from a male client who abuses codeine, the nurse might expect the client to describe which of the following symptoms? a. "I eat at least three meals a day." b. "I can't sleep more than a few hours a day." c. "I have a persistent cough." d. "I can no longer maintain an erection."	Answer: d Rationale: Use of opioids, such as codeine, in high doses often causes a decrease in libido and impotence. Codeine acts as a cough suppressant. Options a and b might be seen with amphetamine abuse. Application Assessment Health Promotion: Prevention and/or Early Detection of Health Problems

© 2007 Pearson Education, Inc.

Question	Answer
52.7 In planning the care of a postoperative client who uses caffeine and nicotine in large quantities, the nurse may want to observe for signs and symptoms of: a. cardiac arrhythmias. b. depression. c. physical and psychological withdrawal. d. lower pain threshold.	Answer: c Rationale: These substances cause both physical (headaches, nervousness, and anxiety) and psychological (cravings) withdrawal symptoms. Tapering the use of the substance helps to reduce the symptoms. Analysis Planning Physiological Integrity: Reduction of Risk Potential
52.8 The nurse understands that the ultimate goals of substance dependence treatment are abstinence from the drug and: a. having a close relationship with a counselor. b. development of coping mechanisms to replace the use of drugs as solutions to problems. c. involvement of the entire family in drug rehabilitation. d. belonging to a support group and maintaining a close affiliation with the members.	Answer: b Rationale: Clients must learn how to cope with situations that prompt inappropriate use of the substance. The other options can also play a large role in helping the client to recover. Comprehension Planning Psychosocial Integrity: Psychosocial Adaptation
52.9 A client who has a history of amphetamine abuse comes to the clinic and informs the nurse she has stopped taking all drugs. To ensure the client's safety, the nurse informs her withdrawal from amphetamines can cause: a. lethargy and depression. b. life-threatening respiratory depression. c. an extreme increase in appetite. d. nausea and vomiting.	Answer: a Rationale: Withdrawal commonly causes clients to feel lethargic and experience depression. Withdrawal is uncomfortable but not life threatening. The other symptoms are not associated with stimulant withdrawal. Application Implementation Physiological Integrity: Reduction of Risk Potential
52.10 The nurse is providing an educational seminar at a high school on the abuse of anabolic steroids. The nurse explains that some dangerous complications can include: a. increased risk of prostate cancer. b. hypotension. c. severe acne. d. a deepened voice.	Answer: a Rationale: Increased risks of prostate and liver cancer are potential dangerous complications. Acne and a deep voice are side effects, but not dangerous. Hypertension, not hypotension, is a major side effect. Comprehension Implementation Physiological Integrity: Reduction of Risk Potential